CURRENT

Rheumatology

CURRENT
Rheumatology
Diagnosis &
Treatment

second edition

John B. Imboden, MD
Professor of Medicine
University of California, San Francisco
Chief, Division of Rheumatology
San Francisco General Hospital

David B. Hellmann, MD, MACP
Vice Dean & Chairman
Department of Medicine
Johns Hopkins Bayview Medical Center
Aliki Perroti Professor of Medicine
Johns Hopkins University School of Medicine
Baltimore, Maryland

John H. Stone, MD, MPH
Deputy Editor for Rheumatology
UpToDate, Inc.
Waltham, Massachusetts

Lange Medical Books/McGraw-Hill
Medical Publishing Division

New York   Chicago   San Francisco   Lisbon   London   Madrid
Mexico City   Milan   New Delhi   San Juan   Seoul   Singapore   Sydney   Toronto

Current Rheumatology Diagnosis & Treatment, Second Edition

1 2 3 4 5 6 7 8 9 0 DOC/DOC 0 9 8 7 6

ISBN-13: 9780071460408
ISBN-10: 0-07-146040-3

Notice

This book was set in Adobe Garamond by Techbooks.
The editors were James F. Shanahan, Maya Barahona, & Heather Cooper.
The production supervisor was Sherri Souffrance.
The index was prepared by Robert Swanson.
RR Donnelley was the printer and binder.

This book is printed on acid-free paper.

INTERNATIONAL EDITION ISBN-13: 0-071104542 ISBN-10: 9780071104548

In this, as in all of our endeavors, we are grateful for the love and support of our wives and children: Dolores Shoback and Tom and Elizabeth Imboden; Linda, Matthew, and Jessica Hellmann; and Martha, Sarah, and William Stone.

Contents

8. Approach to the Painful Shoulder 80
Robin V. West, MD, & Mark W. Rodosky, MD

9. Approach to the Patient with Neck Pain 93
David Borenstein, MD

10. Approach to the Patient with Low Back Pain 100
Rajiv K. Dixit, MD

11. The Patient with Hip Pain 111
Ilksen Gurkan, MD, & Simon Mears, MD, PhD

12. Approach to the Patient with Knee Pain 123
Carl A. Johnson, MD

Contributors

Jeffrey S. Alderman, MD
Assistant Professor of Medicine, Department of
    Medicine, University of Oklahoma College of
    Medicine, Tulsa
jeffrey-alderman@ouhsc.edu
*Pseudogout: Calcium Pyrophosphate Dihydrate Crystal
Deposition Disease*

Sharon E. Banks, DO
Assistant Professor of Medicine, Division of
    Rheumatology, Penn State Milton S. Hershey
    Medical Center, Hershey, Pennsylvania
sbanks@psu.edu
*Rheumatic Manifestations of Acute & Chronic Viral
Arthritis*

Ralf Baron, MD
Professor, Vice-Director, Neurology Clinic,
    Christian-Albrechts-University, Kiel, Germany
r.baron@neurologie.uni-kiel.de
*Complex Regional Pain Syndromes: Reflex Sympathetic
Dystrophy & Causalgia*

Linda K. Bockenstedt, MD
Harold W. Jockers Associate Professor, Section of
    Rheumatology, Yale University School of
    Medicine, New Haven, Connecticut
linda.bockenstedt@yale.edu
Lyme Disease

Phyllis N. Bonaminio, MD
Rheumatology Fellow, Northwestern University/
    The Feinberg School of Medicine,
    Chicago, Illinois
pnbonaminio@aol.com
Pregnancy & Rheumatic Diseases

David Borenstein, MD
Clinical Professor of Medicine, the
George Washington University Medical Center,
    Washington, DC
dborenstein715@aol.com
Approach to the Patient with Neck Pain

Calvin R. Brown, Jr., MD
Associate Professor of Medicine and Orthopaedic
    Surgery, Rush Medical College, Chicago, Illinois
cbrown@rush.edu
Common Injuries from Running

Victor R. Cotton, MD, JD
Adjunct Professor of Law, Widener University
    School of Law, Hummelstown, Pennsylvania
cottonmdjd@aol.com
Legal Issues

Jeff Critchfield, MD
Assistant Clinical Professor of Medicine, University of
    California, San Francisco; Vice-Chief of Medicine,
    San Francisco General Hospital
jeff@itsa.ucsf.edu
*Evaluation of Rheumatic Complaints in Patients
with HIV*

David I. Daikh, MD, PhD
Assistant Professor of Medicine, University of
    California, San Francisco and Veterans Affairs
    Medical Center, San Francisco, California
daikh@itsa.ucsf.edu
*Practical Guide to the Use of Assistive Devices, Physical
Therapy, & Occupational Therapy*

E. Gene Deune, MD
Assistant Professor, Division of Plastic Surgery, and
    Co-Director, Section of Hand Surgery, The Johns
    Hopkins University School of Medicine, Baltimore,
    Maryland
egdeune@jhmi.edu
The Patient with Hand, Wrist, or Elbow Pain

Rajiv K. Dixit, MD
Associate Clinical Professor of Medicine, University of
    California, San Francisco; Director, Northern
    California Arthritis Center, Walnut Creek,
    California
ncarthritiscenter@hotmail.com
Approach to the Patient with Low Back Pain

Fiona A. Donald, MD, FRCP(C)
Attending Physician, Department of Medicine,
    Division of Rheumatology, University of California,
    San Francisco
fdonald@itsa.ucsf.edu
Rheumatic Manifestations of Malignancy;
Medications: Intravenous Immune Globulin (IVIG)

Kenneth H. Fye, MD
Clinical Professor of Medicine, Division of
    Rheumatology, University of California,
    San Francisco
kenfye@itsa.ucsf.edu
Aspiration & Joint Injection; Sjögren Syndrome

Monica Gandhi, MD, MPH
Assistant Professor, Division of Infectious Diseases,
    Department of Medicine, University of California,
    San Francisco
mgandhi@itsa.ucsf.edu
Septic Arthritis & Disseminated Gonococcal Infection

Allan C. Gelber, MD, MPH, PhD
Associate Professor of Medicine, Division of
    Rheumatology, The Johns Hopkins University
    School of Medicine, Baltimore, Maryland
agelber@jhmi.edu
Osteoarthritis

Jennifer D. Gorman, MD, MPH
Assistant Adjunct Professor of Medicine, Division of
    Rheumatology, University of California,
    San Francisco
gormanj@itsa.ucsf.edu
Spondyloarthropathies

Jonathan Graf, MD
Assistant Adjunct Professor of Medicine,
    Department of Medicine, University of California,
    San Francisco; Division of Rheumatology,
    San Francisco General Hospital
grafj@itsa.ucsf.edu
Endocrine & Metabolic Disorders; Medications:
Anti-Tumor Necrosis Factor Agents: Etanercept (Enbrel),
Infliximab (Remicade), and Adalimumab (Humira)

Ilksen Gurkan, MD
Fellow, Department of Orthopedic Surgery, The Johns
    Hopkins University/Johns Hopkins Bayview
    Medical Center, Baltimore, Maryland
ilksen@doctor.com
The Patient with Hip Pain

David B. Hellmann, MD
Mary Betty Stevens Professor of Medicine and
    Chairman, Department of Medicine, Johns Hopkins
    Bayview Medical Center, The Johns Hopkins
    University School of Medicine, Baltimore, Maryland
hellmann@jhmi.edu
Introduction to Vasculitis: Classification & Clinical Clues;
Giant Cell Arteritis & Polymyalgia Rheumatica; Takayasu
Arteritis; Behçet Disease; Vasculitis of the Central Nervous
System; Medications: Allopurinol; Medications: Colchicine

Laura K. Hummers, MD
Instructor of Medicine, Division of Rheumatology,
    The Johns Hopkins University School of Medicine,
    Baltimore, Maryland
lhummers@jhmi.edu
Scleroderma

John B. Imboden, MD
Professor of Medicine, University of California,
    San Francisco; Chief, Division of Rheumatology,
    San Francisco General Hospital
imboden@itsa.ucsf.edu
Laboratory Diagnosis; The Approach to the Patient with
Arthritis; Mycobacterial & Fungal Infections of Bone &
Joints; Medications: Nonsteroidal Anti-Inflammatory
Drugs; Medications: Systemic Glucocorticoid Therapy:
Prednisone, Prednisolone, & Methylprednisolone;
Medications: Methotrexate (MTX); Medications:
Leflunomide (Arava); Medications: Sulfasalazine (SSA);
Medications: Antimalarial Drugs: Hydroxychloroquine
(Plaquenil) & Chloroquine

Richard Jacobs, MD, PhD
Clinical Professor of Medicine and Clinical Pharmacy,
    University of California, San Francisco
jacobsd@medicine.ucsf.edu
Septic Arthritis & Disseminated Gonococcal Infection

William M. Jenkin, DPM
Professor and Chair, Department of Podiatric Surgery,
    California School of Podiatric Medicine at Samuel
    Merritt College, Oakland, California
bjenkin@samuelmerritt.edu
Approach to the Patient with Ankle & Foot Pain

Carl A. Johnson, MD
Associate Professor of Orthopaedic Surgery,
The Johns Hopkins University School of Medicine,
Baltimore, Maryland
cjohnsoa@jhmi.edu
Approach to the Patient with Knee Pain

Sharon L. Kolasinski, MD
Chief of Clinical Service and Assistant Professor of
Medicine, Division of Rheumatology,
University of Pennsylvania School of Medicine,
Philadelphia
sharonk@mail.med.upenn.edu
Complementary & Alternative Therapies

Jon D. Levine, MD, PhD
Professor of Medicine, University of California,
San Francisco
levine@itsa.ucsf.edu
*Complex Regional Pain Syndromes: Reflex Sympathetic
Dystrophy & Causalgia*

Steven A. Lietman, MD
Department of Orthopaedic Surgery, The Cleveland
Clinic Foundation, Cleveland, Ohio
lietmans@ccf.org
The Approach to the Patient with a Painful Prosthetic Joint

David R. Moller, MD
Associate Professor, Division of Pulmonary and
Critical Care Medicine, Department of Medicine,
The Johns Hopkins University School of Medicine,
Baltimore, Maryland
dmoller@jhmi.edu
Sarcoidosis

Daniel Most, MD
Chief Resident, Division of Plastic Surgery,
The Johns Hopkins University
School of Medicine, Baltimore, Maryland
danmost@yahoo.com
The Patient with Hand, Wrist, or Elbow Pain

Paul S. Mueller, MD, MPH
Assistant Professor of Medicine, Mayo Clinic College of
Medicine and Consultant, Division of General
Internal Medicine, Mayo Clinic, Rochester,
Minnesota
mueller.pauls@mayo.edu
Amyloidosis

Stanley J. Naides, MD
Thomas B. Hallowell Professor of Medicine;
Professor of Microbiology & Immunology, and
Pharmacology; Chief, Division of Rheumatology,
Department of Medicine, Penn State Milton
S. Hershey Medical Center, Hershey, Pennsylvania
snaides@psu.edu
*Rheumatic Manifestations of Acute & Chronic Viral
Arthritis*

Meg Newman, MD
Associate Professor of Clinical Medicine, University of
California, San Francisco; Director, HIV Clinical
Scholars Program and AIDS Eduction Program,
University of California, San Francisco Positive
Health Program at San Francisco General Hospital
mnewman@php.ucsf.edu
Evaluation of Rheumatic Complaints in Patients with HIV

James R. O'Dell
Professor and Vice-Chairman, Section of
Rheumatology, Department of Internal Medicine,
University of Nebraska Medical Center, Omaha
jrodell@unmc.edu
Rheumatoid Arthritis

Irina Petrache, MD
Assistant Professor of Medicine, Division of
Pulmonary and Critical Care Medicine,
Department of Medicine, The Johns Hopkins
University School of Medicine, Baltimore,
Maryland
ipetra@jhmi.edu
Sarcoidosis

Michelle Petri, MD, MPH
Professor of Medicine, Division of Rheumatology,
Department of Medicine, The Johns Hopkins
University School of Medicine, Baltimore, Maryland
mpetri@jhmi.edu
*Systemic Lupus Erythematosus; Antiphospholipid Antibody
Syndrome*

Rosalind Ramsey-Goldman, MD, DrPH
Professor of Medicine, Northwestern University,
The Feinberg School of Medicine,
Chicago, Illinois
rgramsey@northwestern.edu
Pregnancy & Rheumatic Diseases

Mark W. Rodosky, MD
Chief, Division of Shoulder and Elbow Surgery,
    University of Pittsburgh Center for Sports
    Medicine; Assistant Team Physician, Pittsburgh
    Penguins, Pittsburgh, Pennsylvania
rodoskymw@msx.upmc.edu
Approach to the Painful shoulder

Kenneth E. Sack, MD
Professor of Clinical Medicine, Department of
    Rheumatology, University of California,
    San Francisco
kensac@medicine.ucsf.edu
Physical Examination of the Musculoskeletal System

Sherri Sanders, MD
Assistant Professor, Department of Internal Medicine
    University of Oklahoma College of Medicine, Tulsa
sherri-sanders@ouhsc.edu
Gout

Peggy Schlesinger, MD
Clinical Associate Professor, University of
    Washington School of Medicine
p.schlesinger@earthlink.net
*Approach to the Adolescent with Arthritis; Adult Still
Disease*

Philip Seo, MD
Post-Doctoral Fellow, The Johns Hopkins University
    School of Medicine, Baltimore, Maryland
seo@jhmi.edu
*Miscellaneous Forms of Vasculitis; Medications:
Azathioprine (AZA; Imuran); Medications:
Mycophenolate Mofetil (MMF; CellCept)*

Dolores Shoback, MD
Professor of Medicine, University of California,
    San Francisco; Staff Physician, San Francisco
    Veterans Affairs Medical Center
dolores@itsa.ucsf.edu
*Endocrine & Metabolic Disorders; Osteoporosis &
Glucocorticoid-Induced Osteoporosis; Medications:
Bisphosphonates: Etidronate (Didronel), Pamidronate
(Aredia), Alendronate (Fosamax), Risedronate (Actonel),
Zoledronic acid (Zometa)*

John H. Stone, MD, MPH
Associate Professor of Medicine, Division of
    Rheumatology, The Johns Hopkins University
    School of Medicine; Director, The Johns Hopkins
    University Vasculitis Center, Baltimore, Maryland
jstone@mail.jhmi.edu
*Relapsing Polychondritis; Wegener Granulomatosis;
Microscopic Polyangiitis; Churg-Strauss Syndrome;
Polyarteritis Nodosa; Mixed Cryoglobulinemia;
Hypersensitivity Vasculitis; Henoch-Schönlein Purpura;
Buerger Disease; Miscellaneous Forms of Vasculitis;
Medications: Cyclophosphamide(CYC; Cytoxan);
Medications: Chlorambucil (CHL; Leukeran);
Medications: Azathioprine (AZA; Imuran); Medications:
Mycophenolate Mofetil (MMF; CellCept)*

Sangeeta Dileep Sule, MD
Instructor in Rheumatology and Pediatrics,
    The Johns Hopkins University School of Medicine,
    Baltimore, Maryland
ssule@jhmi.edu
Raynaud Phenomenon

James F. Wenz, MD[†]
Chairman, Department of Orthopaedic Surgery,
    The Johns Hopkins University/Johns Hopkins
    Bayview Medical Center, Baltimore, Maryland
The Patient with Hip Pain

Robin V. West, MD
Assistant Professor, University of Pittsburgh,
    UPMC Sports Medicine; Head Team Physician,
    The University of Pittsburgh Mens Basketball Team;
    Assistant Team Physician, The Pittsburgh Steelers,
    Pennsylvania
westrv@msx.upmc.edu
Approach to the Painful shoulder

Fredrick M. Wigley, MD
Professor of Medicine, Johns Hopkins University
    School of Medicine; Associate Director,
    Division of Rheumatology, and Director,
    The Johns Hopkins Scleroderma Center,
    Baltimore, Maryland
fwig@jhmi.edu
Raynaud Phenomenon; Scleroderma

[†]Deceased

John B. Winfield, MD
Herman & Louise Smith Distinguished Professor of
Medicine, and Attending Physician, University of
North Carolina School of Medicine, Chapel Hill
john_winfield@med.unc.edu
The Patient with Diffuse Pain

Robert L. Wortmann, MD
Professor of Medicine and Chair, Department of
Internal Medicine, University of Oklahoma
College of Medicine, Tulsa
robert-wortmann@ouhsc.edu
Polymyositis & Dermatomyositis; Gout; Pseudogout:
Calcium Pyrophosphate Dihydrate Crystal Deposition
Disease

Carol M. Ziminski, MD
Associate Professor of Medicine, Division of
Rheumatology, The Johns Hopkins University School
of Medicine; Deputy Director, Johns Hopkins
Rheumatology at Good Samaritan Hospital,
Baltimore, Maryland
ziminski@jhmi.edu
Osteonecrosis

Preface

Current Rheumatology Diagnosis and Treatment is the only rheumatology textbook written with the practicing clinician foremost in mind. The book is a practical guide to the diagnosis and management of the complete range of rheumatological problems encountered in clinical medicine, from common musculoskeletal complaints to complex, multi-organ system inflammatory diseases.

Distinguishing Features

- Thoroughly-illustrated and detailed "How To" chapter on the aspiration and injection of joints.
- Practical chapters devoted to the evaluation of common musculoskeletal symptoms.
- Concise, authoritative reviews of major rheumatic diseases.
- Consistent format that facilitates access to clinical information.
- Thorough guide to medications used in the treatment of rheumatic disease, including the latest biologic therapies.
- Unique chapters on clinical topics of special interest, including:

    Common rheumatologic problems encountered by the hospitalist: Pearls & Myths

    Pregnancy and rheumatic disease

    The red eye

    Immune-mediated sensorineural hearing loss

    Common running injuries

    Rheumatic complaints in the patient with HIV

    Complementary and alternative therapies

    Minimizing lawsuits and others legal entanglements

- Guidance in minimizing lawsuits and other legal entanglements.

Intended Audience

- Primary care physicians will appreciate the books problem-oriented approach to musculoskeletal symptoms and its emphasis on the clinical features, laboratory findings, differential diagnosis, and treatment of specific rheumatic diseases.
- Rheumatologists will find the book to be a quick, reliable, and up-to-date reference.
- For other specialists the book will serve as a primary textbook in rheumatology.
- Fellows, house officers, and medical students will appreciate this engaging introduction to clinical rheumatology.
- Physician assistants and nurse practitioners will find the book sufficiently comprehensive to guide their care of patients with rheumatic disease.
- The book will prove to be invaluable for those studying for board certification or recertification in rheumatology.

Acknowledgments

Dr. Imboden wishes to acknowledge the ongoing support of the Rosalind Russell Medical Research Center for Arthritis.

Dr. Stone wished to acknowledge his support as Hugh and Renna Cosner Scholar in the Center for Innovative Medicine at the Johns Hopkins Bayview Medical Center.

December 2006

SECTION I

Approach to the Patient with Rheumatic Disease

Physical Examination of the Musculoskeletal System

Kenneth E. Sack, MD

The physical examination begins when the physician meets the patient. The physician can assess posture, gait, skin texture, and gross muscle strength by shaking hands, accompanying the patient into the office, and watching him or her move. A comprehensive assessment of the musculoskeletal system includes inspection and palpation of joints and soft tissues as well as evaluation of joint range of motion and neuromuscular function.

INSPECTION

Joint swelling, color, and alignment, as well as skin rashes and muscle wasting, are usually obvious in a glance. Comparing similar joints and muscle groups on opposite sides of the body helps detect subtle abnormalities.

Swelling

The hallmark of inflammation is swelling, which, when present in a joint, indicates that **arthralgia** has become **arthritis.** An increase in synovial fluid causes generalized joint swelling unless fluid accumulates in a contiguous synovial pouch (eg, suprapatellar space) or bursa (eg, gastrocnemius-semimembranous popliteal bursa [Baker cyst]). Inflammation of a tendon sheath may cause soft, localized para-articular swelling. Soft tissue edema tends to be more diffuse.

Well-defined swelling over a bony prominence such as the olecranon process or patella may represent an inflamed subcutaneous bursa, a rheumatoid nodule, a gouty tophus, or rarely, a xanthoma or an amyloid deposit. Bony enlargements (osteophytes) adjacent to joints are typical of osteoarthritis and occur as a result of cartilage damage. Occasionally, such overgrowths are a product of chronic inflammation. Osteophytes may be palpable and visible at the distal interphalangeal and proximal interphalangeal (PIP) joints, where they are called Heberden and Bouchard nodes, respectively.

Color Changes

Acute inflammation of a joint may impart an erythematous hue to the overlying skin, reflecting vasodilation of cutaneous vessels. In some cases of crystal-induced disease, such as gout, the joint and surrounding areas have an intense red-violet color mimicking that seen in infectious cellulitis and septic arthritis.

Deformity

Inflamed joints tend to assume positions that maximize intrasynovial volume, thereby minimizing intrasynovial pressure and reducing pain. In chronic arthritis, when such positions are held for prolonged periods, flexion deformities may ensue. Chronic arthritis can also lead to destruction of supporting structures with consequent malalignment of adjacent bones.

Muscle Wasting

Atrophy of muscles may result from lack of use, neurologic disease, inflammation of an adjacent joint, or myositis associated with an underlying disease. Thus, atrophy of the intrinsic muscles of the hand commonly accompanies inflammation of the fingers or wrists and is visible as depressions between the extensor tendons on the dorsum of the hand. Similarly, synovitis of the knee typically causes atrophy of the quadriceps muscles, resulting in a concavity just above the knee, particularly on the medial aspect.

PALPATION

A "hands on" examination is vital to the detection of inflammation and structural damage in a joint.

Tenderness

Joint tenderness is the most sensitive but the least specific indicator of inflammation. During examination, apply similar pressure to all joint groups and surrounding structures. (Some experts suggest exerting pressure sufficient to blanch the examiner's fingernail bed.) When indicated, test normal structures to determine the patient's baseline pain threshold. Remember that the joint capsule and periosteum are pain-sensitive structures, but the articular cartilage and meniscus are not.

Swelling

A tense synovial effusion has the consistency of a hollow rubber ball, whereas synovial hypertrophy feels more doughy. Inflammation of a tendon sheath results in soft, para-articular swelling in the distribution of the tendon, and the associated subcutaneous edema tends to be more diffuse. Osteophytes produce the bony swelling typical of Heberden and Bouchard nodes. Simultaneous swelling of different joint components can confuse even the most experienced examiner.

Temperature

An increase in the surface temperature of the joint usually indicates underlying inflammation. By using the dorsum of the hand to palpate the same joint on each side of the body, temperature changes as small as 0.5°C can be detected. Note that surface temperatures of superficial joints such as the knee are normally *lower* than those of the surrounding tissue (unless there is extra subcutaneous fat overlying the joint). Thus, an equalization of temperatures often indicates joint inflammation.

Crepitus

Joint motion may produce a crackling sound or a crunching sensation on palpation. This phenomenon, called crepitus, occurs when the surfaces of degenerated cartilage rub together or when bone rubs against bone after extensive loss of cartilage. Inflammation of tendon sheaths also can cause crepitus. In normal joints, crepitus usually reflects motion of tendon over bone.

RANGE OF MOTION

A number of mechanisms can reduce joint motion (Table 1–1). Excessive joint motion may result from destruction of supporting structures or subchondral bone or from joint dislocation. Active range of motion (by the patient) allows rapid assessment of joint mobility, while passive range of motion (by the examiner) permits a more complete evaluation of joint function.

Normal range of joint motion varies according to age and gender. Flexibility tends to diminish with age, and women are typically more flexible than men.

NEUROLOGIC TESTING

A complete musculoskeletal evaluation includes a neurologic examination with specific attention to the sensorimotor components. Inflammatory myopathies typically cause weakness or wasting of proximal muscles. Immune-mediated diseases tend to affect the central or peripheral nervous systems. Degenerative processes affecting the spine or extremities may lead to impingement on nerve roots or various portions of peripheral nerves.

THE PHYSICAL EXAMINATION

Having a consistent routine facilitates thoroughness without sacrificing speed, but the nature of the patient's problem will dictate emphasis on any given aspect of the examination. Evaluating the back and the neuromuscular system of the lower extremity is a reasonable starting point.

Back & Neuromuscular System of the Lower Extremity

Begin with the patient seated in a chair. Ask him or her to stand without using the arms. This gives you a good idea of the patient's proximal lower extremity strength.

Table 1–1. Factors That Reduce Joint Motion

Damage to articular cartilage or bone
Large synovial effusions
Loose bodies within the joint cavity
Joint subluxation
Fibrous or bony ankylosis
Contracture of the capsule or contiguous tendons
Irritation of pain-sensitive structure in and about the joint

If the patient has trouble rising, ask whether it is because of pain or weakness. If a psychogenic reason is suspected, ask the patient to sit down slowly without using the arms. Because the same muscles that facilitate rising allow sitting, the person with true weakness will fall into the chair early in the process. Now have the patient take one or two steps on the heels and then on the toes. This indicates strength in the distal muscles and gives some idea of coordination.

With the patient standing comfortably, evaluate the configuration of the spine and lower extremities from the front and back. This is the best way to look for structural abnormalities in the back (eg, scoliosis or kyphosis), legs (eg, genu valgum or varum), and feet (eg, pes planus). Prominence of one shoulder or scapula suggests **scoliosis.** If this asymmetry vanishes when the patient bends forward, the vertebral column is probably normal, and the scoliosis is "functional" (ie, caused by such processes as hip disease, leg-length discrepancy, or nerve root irritation). Structural scoliosis results from abnormalities of the vertebral column and rib cage consequent to disorders of bone, nerve, or muscle. It may also have no obvious cause (idiopathic). Associated skin lesions, such as café-au-lait spots, patches of hair, dimpling, or lipomata, may be clues to an underlying causative abnormality. The direction of spinal convexity defines the scoliosis—compensated (the first thoracic vertebra is centered over the sacrum) or uncompensated (the first thoracic vertebra is to the right or left of the sacrum). To quantitate the degree of list, drop a plumb line from the first thoracic vertebra and measure the distance from this line to the midgluteal crease.

Check whether the iliac crests are level. Asymmetry may reflect real or apparent leg-length discrepancy. The relationship of the hip to the pelvis affects functional leg length. Thus, an adducted hip raises the pelvis and makes the leg appear shorter. Conversely, an abducted hip lowers the pelvis and "lengthens" the leg. Fixed obliquity of the pelvis also causes relative changes in leg length. Measuring the distance from the anterior superior iliac spine to the ipsilateral medial malleolus detects real differences in leg length. (This measurement can also be performed later when the patient is lying supine.)

Note the mobility of the thoracolumbar spine by asking the patient to bend forward as far as possible with the knees straight; also determine the amount of lumbar extension and lateral bending. Limited motion or pain consequent to these maneuvers may indicate disease of spinal articulations or supporting structures, as well as irritation of a muscle or nerve root. To quantify the amount of lumbar mobility, use the **modified Schober maneuver** (Figure 1–1). Mark a spot in the midline 5 cm below the level of the buttock dimples. Using a tape measure, place a mark 15 cm directly above the first mark and ask the patient to bend forward as far as possible. The distance between the two marks should increase at least 5 cm. Periodic measurements are useful in monitoring patients with inflammatory back disease,

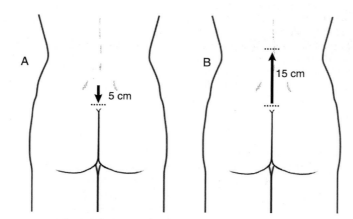

Figure 1–1. Modified Schober test of flexion of the lumbar spine. With the patient standing upright, the examiner makes a mark on the skin 5 cm below an imaginary line drawn between the buttock dimples that overlie the posterior superior iliac spines (**A**). A second mark is made 15 cm above the first (**B**). The distance between the two marks is then measured while the patient bends over and attempts to touch his or her toes while keeping the knees fully extended. The distance between the marks increases to at least 20 cm if there is normal flexion of the lumbar spine. In the original Schober test, the first mark is placed between the buttock dimples and a second mark is made 10 cm above that; the distance between these marks should increase to at least 15 cm when the patient bends over.

such as ankylosing spondylitis. Test thoracolumbar function by having the patient rotate the upper torso from side to side. Determine chest expansion by holding the tape measure at approximately nipple level and measuring the difference between full expiration and inspiration. Chest expansion, which is normally at least 5 cm, diminishes with costovertebral disease, a frequent early component of ankylosing spondylitis.

Press firmly over the spinous processes and interspinous ligaments for areas of tenderness or bony defects. Full palpation of the coccyx requires a rectal examination. Although it is possible to palpate the lower portion of the sacroiliac (SI) joint between the posterior inferior iliac spine and the sciatic notch, tenderness in this area may represent irritation of a tendon, bursa, or the sciatic nerve. Therefore indirect maneuvers (performed later in the examination) are necessary to elicit pain in the SI joint. When indicated, palpate the ischial tuberosities or the posterior portions of the greater trochanters for bursal tenderness.

Analysis of the patient's gait can localize a neurologic or musculoskeletal disorder in the lower extremities. Have the patient walk several steps in a straight line and then return. The normal gait is narrow-based (2–4 inches between the feet) with a shift in the pelvis of no more than 1–2 inches in the vertical or horizontal direction. Table 1–2 outlines the causes of several common gait abnormalities.

Upper Extremities

A. HANDS

With the patient seated at the end of the examination table, examine the hands. Look closely at the fingernails for clubbing, discoloration, dilated periungual capillaries, and pitting or other dystrophic changes. Palpate the distal interphalangeal, PIP, and metacarpophalangeal (MCP) joints for swelling, tenderness, and warmth (Figures 1–2 and 1–3). Have the patient make a full fist for gross evaluation of hand function. Test separately any abnormal joints, and palpate the flexor tendons for nodules or crepitance.

Inability to flex the fingers may result not only from a damaged joint, but also from abnormalities in tendons or supporting structures. When active flexion is diminished but passive flexion remains, consider adhesions between the flexor profundus and sublimis digitorum tendons. Also, when flexion of a PIP joint is difficult, attempt to flex the joint while at the same time flexing the MCP joint. If PIP flexion *increases* during this maneuver, suspect tightening of the intrinsic muscles (lumbricaleis and interossei). If flexion of the MCPs *decreases* flexion of the PIPs, tightness of the extrinsic extensor tendons may be the culprit. Examine the palm for skin lesions, soft tissue nodules, and muscle atrophy.

Table 1–2. Common Gait Abnormalities and Their Causes

Gait	Description	Cause
Antalgic	Rapid shift from painful extremity (short stance phase)	Pain in foot, knee, or hip
Abductor (gluteus medius)	Shift of thorax over involved hip	Weakened gluteus maximus unable to fully extend hip
Extensor (gluteus maximus)	Excessive shift of thorax posteriorly	Weakened gluteus maximus unable to fully extend hip
Quadriceps weakness	Shift of trunk anteriorly (sometimes with patient pushing knee manually into extension)	Weakened quadriceps unable to extend knees
Excessive lateral foot contact	Diminished pronation of foot during stance phase	Weakened peroneus or painful medial foot
Excessive medial foot contact	Diminished supination of foot during stance phase	Weakness of invertors or tight peroneus
Hip hiking	Vertical lifting of hip during swing phase	Increased leg length, hamstring weakness, or fused knee
Steppage	Excessive flexion of knee to enable foot to clear ground (may be a accompanied by foot slap)	Weakened dorsiflexors
Insufficient push-off	Entire foot leaves ground at once	Weakness of gastrocnemius or painful foot

B. WRISTS

Palpate the dorsum of the wrist (Figure 1–4). Thickened tissue occupying the normal depression just distal to the radial styloid may indicate early synovitis. Swelling, tenderness, or increased mobility of the ulnar styloid is typical of rheumatoid arthritis. Flex and extend the wrist to determine range of motion. These maneuvers also may bring into prominence a ganglion cyst on the dorsal or volar aspects of the wrist.

Pain and tenderness along the radial aspect of the wrist are characteristic of tenosynovitis of the abductor pollicis longus and extensor pollicis brevis, both of which conjoin to form the volar aspect of the anatomic snuffbox. To distinguish this process from degenerative disease of the first carpometacarpal joint, have the patient make a fist

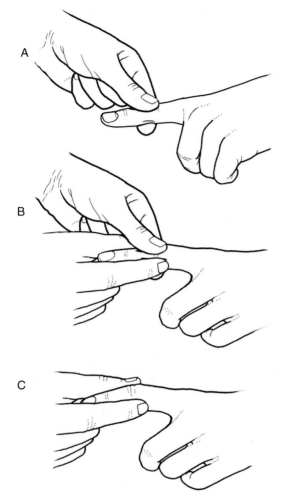

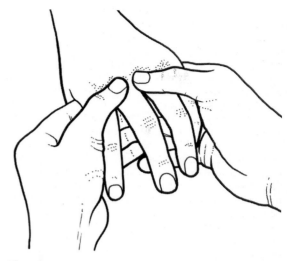

Figure 1–3. Examination of the metacarpophalangeal joints. With the metacarpophalangeal joints partially flexed to approximately 60 degrees, the joint lines should be easily palpable just below the heads of the metacarpals.

Figure 1–2. Method for detecting subtle synovitis of the proximal interphalangeal joints. The examiner firmly compresses the proximal interphalangeal joint with the thumb and forefinger of one hand (**A**) and then palpates the lateral aspects of the joint with the thumb and forefinger of the other hand (**B**). Palpation of the lateral aspect of the joint is repeated without compression (**C**). When synovitis is present, there is a sensation of bogginess overlying the lateral surface of the joint that is more pronounced when the joint is compressed.

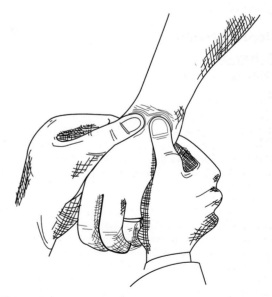

Figure 1–4. Palpation of the dorsum of the wrist. Using both thumbs and firm pressure, the examiner begins palpating just distal to the wrist and then slides proximally into the joint space. The thumbs will easily drop into the depression of a normal joint space, but will encounter bogginess or thickened tissue if there is wrist synovitis.

with the thumb tucked inside the fingers. Then, deviate the wrist in the ulnar direction (**Finkelstein maneuver**) (Figure 1–5). A sharp pain along the distal radial border confirms tenosynovitis.

To test for carpal tunnel syndrome, hold the wrist in slight extension and tap the volar aspect at the distal end

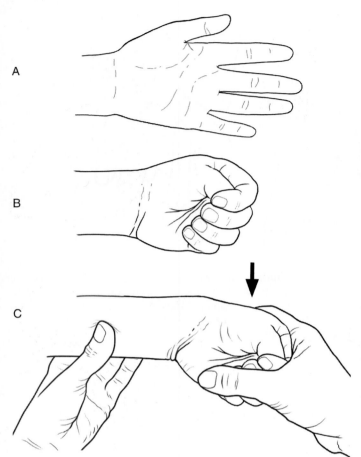

A

B

C

Figure 1–5. Finkelstein maneuver. After the patient makes a fist with the thumb inside the fingers (**A, B**), the examiner forces the wrist in an ulnar direction (**C**). This maneuver elicits pain along the distal radial aspect of the wrist when there is tenosynovitis of the abductor pollicis longus. (From Hoppenfeld S. *Physical Examination of the Spine and Extremities.* Appleton-Century-Crofts, 1976, Figure 49. With permission.)

of the palmaris longus tendon. A tingling feeling either up the arm or in any of the first three digits indicates irritation of the median nerve (a positive **Tinel sign**). If this test is negative or equivocal, hold the wrist in full flexion for at least 1 minute (**Phalen test**) to elicit similar symptoms.

C. Elbows

Palpate along the proximal ulna and over the olecranon process for nodules. Olecranon bursitis manifests as a swelling—often golf-ball-like—directly over the olecranon process. Synovial thickening or joint effusions are easily palpable in the grooves between the olecranon process and the lateral and medial epicondyles. Tenderness along the medial epicondyle usually indicates injury to the tendinous origins of the flexors of the wrist (**medial epicondylitis**). Confirm this by attempting to reproduce the pain on resisted flexion of the wrist. Conversely, tenderness along the lateral epicondyle usually reflects in-

flammation at the tendinous origins of the extensors of the wrist (**lateral epicondylitis**); resisted extension of the wrist usually elicits pain. Assess maximum flexion and extension of the elbow; test pronation and supination with the elbow held at 90 degrees of flexion and close to the waist to prevent shoulder motion.

D. Shoulders

Test active shoulder abduction by having the patient touch his or her outstretched palms over the head. Similarly, test internal rotation and adduction by having the patient reach behind the back to touch the opposite scapula, and test external rotation and abduction by having the patient reach behind the head for the opposite scapula (Figure 1–6). Pursue abnormalities noted on active motion by performing passive tests of glenohumeral motion (Figure 1–7). Pain on these maneuvers may arise from an inflamed bursa or an injured rotator cuff tendon. To evaluate glenohumeral motion, have the patient relax his or her arm at the side with the elbow held at

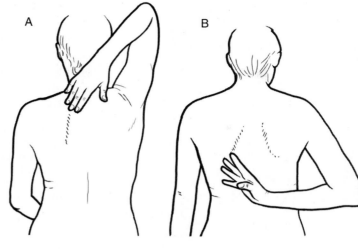

Figure 1–6. Examination of the shoulder: active range of motion. To test external rotation and abduction of the shoulder, ask the patient to reach behind the back and touch the top of the opposite scapula (**A**). To examine internal rotation and adduction ask the patient to reach behind the back and touch the inferior aspect of the shoulder (**B**).

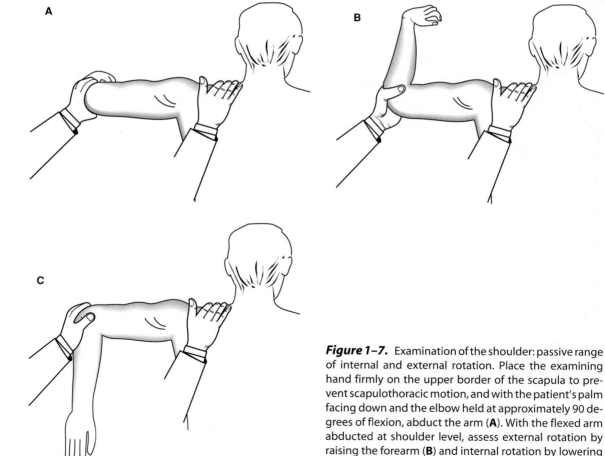

Figure 1–7. Examination of the shoulder: passive range of internal and external rotation. Place the examining hand firmly on the upper border of the scapula to prevent scapulothoracic motion, and with the patient's palm facing down and the elbow held at approximately 90 degrees of flexion, abduct the arm (**A**). With the flexed arm abducted at shoulder level, assess external rotation by raising the forearm (**B**) and internal rotation by lowering the forearm (**C**).

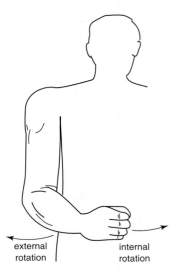

Figure 1–8. Internal and external rotation of the gleno-humeral joint.

90 degrees of flexion; the forearm should externally and internally rotate about 90 degrees (Figure 1–8).

Palpate for tender areas, particularly under the lateral acromion (near the subacromial bursa and the insertion of the supraspinatus tendon), and over the acromioclavicular joint, the anterior capsule overlying the humeral head, and the long head of the biceps tendon lying in the bicipital groove. Search for tender areas that may serve as trigger points for pain that is difficult to localize. Such areas include the medial border of the scapula and the upper trapezius as well as the ligaments joining the transverse processes of the lower cervical vertebrae.

E. Sternum

Palpate along the sternal border at the sternoclavicular and costosternal junctions, as well as over the sternomanubrial junction.

F. Temporomandibular Joints

Place index fingers in front of the patient's ears below the zygomatic arch (or insert the tips of the fifth fingers in the ear canals) and have the patient open and close his or her mouth. Assess for asymmetric or painful motion, tenderness, or crepitus. Inability to fully open the jaw (about three fingerbreadths or 5 cm between the teeth) may reflect tightening of the skin (as in scleroderma), dysfunction of muscles of mastication, or an abnormality of the temporomandibular joint.

G. Neck

Palpate the cervical spinous processes and paraspinal muscles for tenderness and assess range of motion in all directions. Approximately 50% of cervical flexion and extension occurs at the atlanto-occipital joint; 50% involves the remaining lower vertebrae. Normal flexion brings the chin to within a fingerbreadth of the chest. Normal extension permits an imaginary vertical line to be drawn between the outer canthus of the eye, the ear lobe, and the shoulder (Figure 1–9). The atlantoaxial articulation and the lower cervical vertebrae contribute equally to cervical rotation, normally about 75 degrees. Lateral bending, normally about 45 degrees, involves all of the cervical vertebrae.

H. Hips

With the patient supine and the leg extended, check abduction and adduction of the hip. Test flexion by bringing the patient's fully flexed knee as close as possible to the

A

B

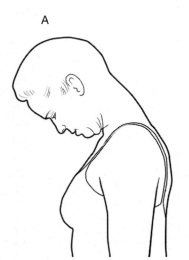

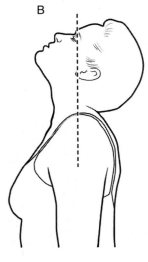

Figure 1–9. Flexion and extension of the cervical spine. Normal flexion brings the chin to within a fingerbreadth of the chest (**A**). With normal extension of the neck, an imaginary line should connect the eye, ear lobe, and shoulder (**B**).

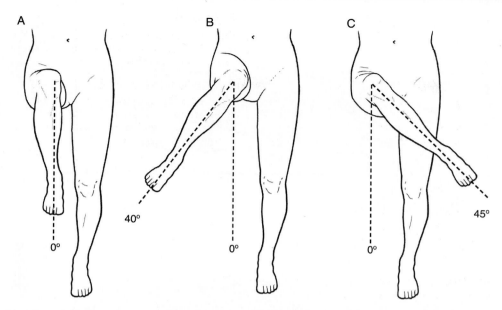

Figure 1–10. Internal and external rotation of the hip. The patient is positioned supine with the both the hip and knee flexed to 90 degrees (**A**). To test internal rotation, the examiner swings the foot outward with one hand while keeping the knee positioned over the hip with the other hand (**B**). Normal external rotation is approximately 40 degrees. To test external rotation, the examiner swings the foot inward while keeping the knee positioned over the hip (**C**). Normal external rotation is 45 degrees. (From Polley HF, Hunder GS. *Rheumatologic Interviewing and Physical Examination of the Joints.* 2nd ed. WB Saunders, 1978, Figure 12–8. With permission.)

abdomen. To assess rotation, position the leg vertically with the knee directly over the hip and flexed to about 90 degrees. Swing the foot from right to left; normal rotation is approximately 45 degrees (Figure 1–10). It is important to compare both hips; remember that women tend to be more flexible than men and that flexibility tends to diminish with age. To bring out a subtle flexion contracture of the hip, have the patient grasp his or her opposite knee and bring it to the chest. This flattens the lumbar lordosis, and the thigh on the affected side will rise from the table. Palpate for tender areas, particularly over the anterior hip and along the posterior aspect of the greater trochanter. Tenderness in this latter region may arise from the trochanteric bursa or from nearby tendons. To elicit pain in the SI joint, press down on the supine patient's iliac crests, or fully abduct and externally rotate the flexed hip. These maneuvers will cause pain in the buttock on the affected side.

I. KNEES

Examine the knee for swelling, being careful not to mistake infrapatellar fat for hypertrophied synovium. Look for an effusion by alternately squeezing the suprapatellar and infrapatellar aspects of the knee with each hand. To demonstrate a small effusion, rub several times along the medial patellofemoral junction in a cephalad direction to "milk" the fluid into the lateral side. Then gently press the superolateral aspect of the knee and watch for fluid to bulge out on the medial aspect. Check the popliteal fossa for swelling of the gastrocnemius-semimembranous bursa (Baker cyst).

Look for atrophy of the medial aspect of the distal quadriceps muscle, an early indicator of inflammation or pain in the knee. Test flexion and extension while placing a hand on the patella to detect crepitus. With the knee flexed, check for tenderness medially and laterally over the femoral condyles and tibial plateaus and tubercle and along the joint articulations, collateral ligaments, and infrapatellar tendon. Tenderness 2–3 cm inferior to the medial tibial plateau may indicate inflammation in the anserine bursa.

With the knee extended and relaxed, move the patella from side to side while applying firm pressure downward toward the table; pain or crepitus indicates patellofemoral disease. However, a more sensitive indicator of such disease is the **patellar inhibition test,** performed by pressing downward on the upper patellar border while at the same time pushing the patella toward the feet. Even with

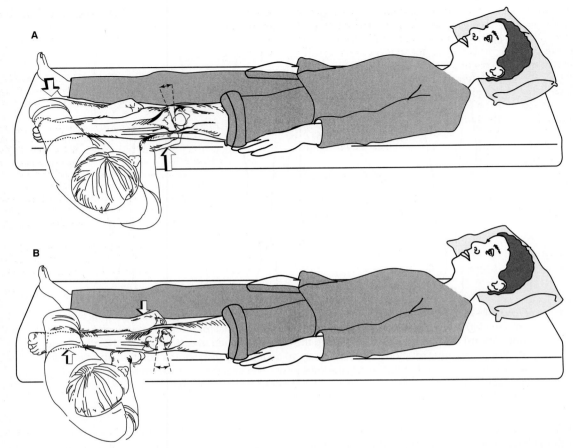

Figure 1–11. Tests for stability of the medial and lateral collateral ligaments of the knee. With the patient supine on the examining table and the knee slightly flexed to loosen the posterior joint capsule, stabilize the lateral femoral condyle while applying valgus force to the lower leg (**A**). Excessive motion or a palpable gap along the medial joint line indicates laxity of the medial collateral ligament. Repeat this maneuver in the opposite direction to test the lateral collateral ligament (**B**). (From Hoppenfeld S. *Physical Examination of the Spine and Extremities.* Appleton-Century-Crofts, 1976. Figures 44 and 45. With permission.)

mild patellofemoral arthritis, pain will occur when the patient contracts his or her quadriceps muscle (elicited by asking the patient to lift the leg while keeping the knee extended) and the patella moves under the examiner's fingers.

For suspected recurrent patellar subluxation, push the relaxed patella laterally and note whether the patient actively resists or appears anxious (positive "anxiety sign").

Check for laxity of the medial and lateral collateral ligaments by first having the patient flex the knee slightly to loosen the posterior joint capsule (Figure 1–11). Then press the lateral femoral condyle while applying valgus force to the lower leg. Excessive motion or a palpable

gap along the medial joint line indicates laxity of the medial collateral ligament. Repeat this maneuver in the opposite direction to test the lateral collateral ligament. Finally, with the knee in slight flexion, check for laxity of the anterior cruciate ligament by pulling the upper tibia in the anterior direction; push backward to test the posterior cruciate ligament. Excessive motion in either direction is a positive **drawer sign.**

J. FEET AND ANKLES

Evaluate these areas first with the patient standing (ie, during the initial part of the examination). From behind the patient, check for excessive pronation (outward turning) of the foot by noting the amount of lateral slope of the heel. Note also any loss of the normal longitudinal arch. With the patient supine, palpate the areas around the malleoli for tenderness, synovial thickening, or effusion. Check the calcaneal insertion of the Achilles tendon for nodules or tenderness. Also, look for tenderness at the insertion of the plantar aponeurosis into the medial plantar surface of the calcaneus. Dorsiflex and plantarflex the ankle. Pain or limitation of motion indicates disease in the tibiotalar joint. To test the subtalar joint, bring the foot into the neutral position to stabilize the talus; then invert and evert the ankle.

Palpate the midfoot for tarsal tenderness. Squeeze the forefoot at the level of the metatarsal heads. If this causes pain, press each metatarsal head from above and below to elicit tenderness. Metatarsophalangeal swelling is sometimes manifested by widening of the space between adjacent toes. For a suspected Morton neuroma, press between the metatarsal heads from the plantar surface with a blunt object, such as a pencil eraser. Such lesions occur most commonly between the third and fourth metatarsals.

REFERENCES

Hoppenfeld S. *Physical Examination of the Spine and Extremities.* Appleton-Century-Crofts, 1976. (A superbly illustrated treatise on physical examination of the musculoskeletal system. Contains countless "pearls.")

McCarty D. Differential diagnosis of arthritis: analysis of signs and symptoms. In: Koopman W, ed. *Arthritis and Allied Conditions.* 15th ed. Lippincott Williams & Wilkins, 2005:37–49. (An easy-to-read description of important symptoms and physical findings in rheumatic diseases by a master rheumatologist. Includes illustrations of normal joint range of motion.)

Polley H, Hunder G. *Rheumatologic Interviewing and Physical Examination of the Joints.* 2nd ed. WB Saunders, 1978. (A timeless, well-illustrated textbook describing the musculoskeletal examination.)

Sack K, Miller C. Examining adults and children for rheumatic disease. *J Musculoskel Med.* 1986;3(5):19–30; 3(6):14–20. (A step-by-step approach to the musculoskeletal examination.)

Joint Aspiration & Injection

2

Kenneth H. Fye, MD, & Kirsten Morehead, MD

 ESSENTIAL FEATURES

- *Joint aspiration and synovial fluid analysis are essential to the diagnoses of microcrystalline and infectious forms of arthritis.*
- *Glucocorticoid injections are often the swiftest means of providing relief to patients with inflamed joints.*
- *Aspiration should be performed with the joint positioned to maximize intra-articular pressure, allowing easier withdrawal of synovial fluid.*
- *The four major components of synovial fluid analysis are assessment of fluid clarity and color, cell count, crystals, and culture.*
- *Culture is more sensitive than Gram stain for identifying an infection. Thus, sending fluid for culture takes priority over Gram stain when a limited quantity of synovial fluid is available.*

Joint aspiration and synovial fluid analysis are essential tools in the diagnosis of arthritic conditions. Local injection of therapeutic agents into articular or periarticular structures can lead to rapid decreases in pain and inflammation without many of the side effects associated with systemic medications. The removal of inflammatory cells and destructive enzymes from an inflamed joint may decrease the likelihood of permanent articular damage. As with any diagnostic or therapeutic procedure, success depends on the expertise of the clinician.

Diagnostic Indications for Aspiration

Aspiration and synovial fluid analysis are most crucial in the initial evaluation of an acute monarticular arthritis because of the importance of ruling out septic arthritis. A septic joint signals the presence of a life-threatening illness. Without immediate and aggressive antibiotic therapy, a bacterial infection can lead rapidly to joint destruction and long-term disability. Analysis of synovial fluid from a septic joint usually reveals white blood cell (WBC)

counts of 100,000/mL or higher, with greater than 95% polymorphonuclear leukocytes. Gram stain, culture, and sensitivity studies are essential to the selection of appropriate antibiotic therapy.

A. DIFFERENTIAL DIAGNOSIS

The major differential diagnoses in patients with monarticular arthritis are the crystal-induced arthropathies, particularly gout. In gout, examination of synovial fluid with a polarized light microscope will reveal uric acid crystals in 80–90% of patients; gout can also—albeit rarely—result in WBC counts of up to $100,000/\mu L$. Even when crystals are identified, it is important to obtain culture and sensitivity studies, because superinfections can occur in patients with gouty arthropathy. Severe trauma can lead to an acute monarthritis as a result of bleeding into a joint. In such cases, arthrocentesis will reveal a hemarthrosis.

Even degenerative arthritis can sometimes appear clinically as a monarticular process. Although the monarthritis in these cases is not usually inflammatory, arthrocentesis may be necessary to exclude indolent infections. Arthrocentesis plays a significant diagnostic role in other, less common causes of monarticular disease, including malignancy (either primary in the joint or as a result of metastasis), pigmented villonodular synovitis, and clotting disorders with recurrent hemarthrosis.

Synovial fluid analysis is often the only way to make the distinction between a noninflammatory polyarticular disease such as osteoarthritis, and inflammatory polyarticular conditions, such as rheumatoid or psoriatic arthritis. In addition, some crystal-induced arthritides, such as calcium pyrophosphate dihydrate deposition disease (CPPD) or oxalosis, may present as polyarticular disease.

B. CLASSES OF SYNOVIAL FLUID

The four classes of synovial fluid are described in Table 2–1. The classes are differentiated by characteristics that define inflammation.

Class I (noninflammatory) fluid is transparent with a color ranging from clear to yellow, has a high viscosity, and a normal string test. The WBC count is $2000/\mu L$ (normal synovial fluid has $<200/\mu L$), and $<25\%$ are

Table 2–1. Classes of Synovial Fluid

	Class I (Noninflammatory)	Class II (Inflammatory)	Class III (Septic)	Class IV (Hemorrhagic)
Color	Clear/yellow	Yellow/white	Yellow/white	Red
Clarity	Transparent	Translucent/opaque	Opaque	Opaque
Viscosity	High	Variable	Low	NA
Mucin clot	Firm	Variable	Friable	NA
White blood cell count	<2000/μL	2000–75,000/μL[a]	>100,000/μL	NA
Differential	<25% PMNs	>50% PMNs	>90% PMNs	NA
Culture	Negative	Negative	Positive	Variable

[a]In rare instances the count may be as high as 100,000/μL.
NA, not applicable; PMNs, polymorphonuclear leukocytes.
Reprinted from *The Primer on the Rheumatic Diseases,* 12th ed., with permission of the Arthritis Foundation.

polymorphonuclear leukocytes. Gram stain and culture and sensitivity studies are all negative. Class I synovial fluid is typical of osteoarthritis.

Class II (inflammatory) synovial fluid ranges from translucent to opaque and is yellow or white. The WBC count generally ranges from 2000 to 75,000/μL although in rare instances counts may range up to 100,000/μL. More than 50% are polymorphonuclear leukocytes. Gram stain and culture and sensitivity studies are negative. Class II synovial fluid is characteristic of all of the autoimmune arthropathies, such as rheumatoid arthritis and systemic lupus erythematosus; the spondyloarthropathies; the crystal-induced arthropathies; postinfectious arthropathies; indolent infections; and a variety of noninfectious arthropathies that are not easily categorized (Table 2–2.)

Class III (septic) synovial fluid is opaque and yellow (sometimes white) with a low viscosity. WBC counts are generally >100,000/μL, although counts as low 50,000/μL are not uncommon. Gram stain, culture, and sensitivity studies may all be positive. Class III synovial fluid is typical of bacterial joint infections.

Table 2–2. Diagnosis by Synovial Fluid Class

Class I	Class II	Class III	Class IV
Osteoarthritis	RA	Bacterial arthritis	Trauma
Traumatic	SLE		Pigmented villonodular synovitis
Osteonecrosis	Poly/dermatomyositis		Tuberculosis
Charcot arthropathy	Scleroderma		Tumor
	Systemic necrotizing vasculitides		Coagulopathy
	Polychondritis		Charcot arthropathy
	Gout		
	CPPD		
	Hydroxyapatite deposition disease		
	Juvenile RA		
	Ankylosing spondylitis		
	Psoriatic arthritis		
	Reactive arthritis		
	Chronic inflammatory bowel disease		
	Hypogammaglobulinemia		
	Sarcoidosis		
	Rheumatic fever		
	Indolent/low virulence infections (Viral, mycobacterial, fungal, Whipple disease, Lyme arthritis)		

RA, rheumatoid arthritis; SLE, systemic lupus erythematosus; CPPD, calcium pyrophosphate dihydrate deposition disease.
Reprinted from *The Primer on the Rheumatic Diseases,* 12th ed., with permission of the Arthritis Foundation.

Class IV (hemorrhagic) fluid is red and opaque. Culture is negative except in patients with tuberculosis. Class IV synovial fluid is typical of trauma, tuberculosis, pigmented villonodular synovitis, neoplasia, coagulopathies, and Charcot arthropathy.

Therapeutic Indications for Aspiration or Injection

The response to joint injection can have diagnostic implications. For example, in patients with equivocal low back or hip pain, injection of lidocaine into the hip or epidural space will enable the clinician to determine the source of the pain. If injection of the hip alleviates the pain, the hip is probably the source of the problem. If an epidural injection alleviates the symptoms, the pain is probably the result of back disease.

A. ASPIRATION

The removal of synovial fluid from an acutely inflamed joint may provide significant benefit. This is particularly true in infected joints, from which removal of synovial fluid will decrease intra-articular synovial pressure, the number of activated inflammatory cells, and the concentration of destructive enzymes and cytokines that can damage articular and periarticular structures. Septic joints may need to be aspirated daily to prevent reaccumulation of inflammatory synovial fluid. Removing blood from a hemarthrosis may also be beneficial. A significant collection of blood may increase intra-articular pressure, thereby stretching periarticular supporting structures and resulting in subsequent joint laxity. Intra-articular blood can also lead to the development of adhesions, eventually resulting in decreased range of motion.

B. INJECTION

A number of locally injected pharmacologic agents have been used in the treatment of rheumatic disorders. Local glucocorticoids in conjunction with lidocaine are valuable in the treatment of the arthritic conditions. Joints, tenosynovium, bursae, soft tissue tender points (such as the medial and lateral epicondyles in tennis or golfer elbow or the lateral thigh in meralgia paresthetica), and even the epidural space can be injected with a reasonable expectation of benefit. Although most target tissues can be injected without radiographic help, it is always wise to inject the hip or the epidural space under computed tomographic guidance to ensure that the medication is delivered to the proper tissue space. In refractory septic arthritis that does not respond to systemic antibiotics and serial aspirations, surgical drainage and washing with local antibiotics are indicated. The injection of any of a variety of hyaluronic acid preparations into a joint, although expensive, has been shown to be of short-term benefit in the treatment of osteoarthritis.

Technique

A. EQUIPMENT

The specific procedure and size of the joint will determine the size of the syringe needed for aspiration. Syringes 3 mL and smaller are usually adequate for injecting lidocaine and glucocorticoids into a peripheral target. Three- to 10-mL syringes are preferred for aspiration of small joints, and 10- to 20-mL syringes are best for intermediate joints, such as the elbow or ankle (Figures 2–1 and 2–5). For larger joints, such as the knee (Figure 2–4) or glenohumeral joint (Figure 2–2), or when copious amounts of synovial fluid must be aspirated, a 60-mL syringe may be more appropriate. When using a large syringe, it is important to break the vacuum in the syringe before introducing it into the joint. Aspiration should be performed slowly to avoid generating significant negative pressure that can draw synovial tissue into the opening of the needle and actually prevent adequate withdrawal of fluid. To aspirate ≥100 mL from an arthritic joint, several large syringes or a stopcock on the end of a syringe may be used. If using several syringes, a Kelly clamp can stabilize the needle (which can be left in place) while the syringes are changed.

The size of the needle also depends on the procedure. Needles as small as 25 or 30 gauge are most appropriate for injecting lidocaine into articular or periarticular structures before aspiration or for injecting glucocorticoids into small joints. A 25-gauge needle also can be used to aspirate synovial fluid or periarticular interstitial fluid from small, acutely inflamed joints, such as the first metatarsophalangeal joint in podagra. A 1.5-inch, 22-gauge needle is useful for injecting large joints, such as the knee, or deep structures, such as the supraspinatus tendon (see Figure 2–2A) and trochanteric bursa (Figure 2–7). These 22-gauge needles also can be used to aspirate small joints, but 19- or 20-gauge needles are indicated for the aspiration of large joints, joints with large amounts of synovial fluid, or joints or cysts with inspissated synovial fluid.

Gloves are important in protecting the clinician from the patient's body fluids. With proper antiseptic technique, the likelihood of an infection after an aspiration or injection is so low that sterile gloves are not generally necessary. Usually the clinician simply marks the injection target with a ballpoint pen, applies appropriate antisepsis, and then proceeds using nonsterile gloves. Sterile gloves are indicated only if the anatomy is equivocal and the clinician must reexamine the procedure site after prepping the area with povidone-iodine. Joint infection after aspiration or injection is extremely rare, but the possibility of complications must always be minimized.

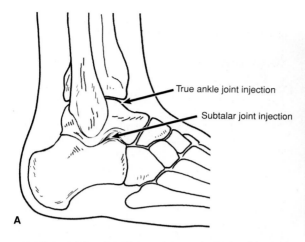

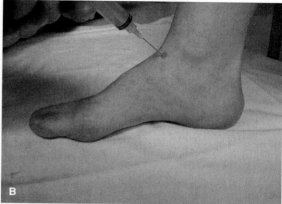

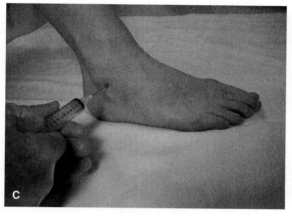

Figure 2–1. A: Lateral view of the ankle. **B:** Injection of the true ankle joint, just medial to the extensor hallucis longus. **C:** Injection of the sub-talar joint, just inferior and anterior to the tip of the lateral malleolus.

Povidone-iodine should be applied to the arthrocentesis site and allowed to dry. An alcohol swab then should be used to wipe off the excess to prevent skin irritation in those patients sensitive to iodine or iodine derivatives. It is also appropriate to use an alcohol swab for hemostasis after the procedure.

B. MEDICATIONS

Many clinicians use ethyl chloride to numb the skin before the procedure. However, this technique is somewhat cumbersome and of equivocal benefit. The value of ethyl chloride is its cooling effect on cutaneous pain fibers. A similar effect may be achieved with the use of refrigerated needles, which in plastic surgery has been reported to be less painful for the injection of local anesthesia.

Lidocaine (1–2%, without epinephrine) is a safe and effective local anesthetic, and 5–10 mg should be injected into the capsule and periarticular supporting structures before aspiration is attempted. Aspiration without ben-

efit of anesthesia can be quite painful. Because serial aspirations may be necessary in the treatment of arthritic conditions, the clinician should attempt to make the first aspiration as painless as possible. A similar amount of lidocaine should be drawn up with the glucocorticoids to be injected. This will provide anesthesia as the glucocorticoids are being injected into the target tissue. Single-dose vials of lidocaine, although more costly, are less likely to be contaminated.

Local injections are an efficient way to administer high concentrations of glucocorticoids directly into target tissues, maximizing the desired anti-inflammatory effects of the medication and minimizing the many unpleasant side effects associated with systemic glucocorticoids. Glucocorticoids can be injected with reasonable expectation of clinical benefit into joints, synovial cysts, peritendinous structures, bursal sacs, ligamentous attachments, tender points, and periarticular tissues. Patients should be aware that injection of local glucocorticoids, although

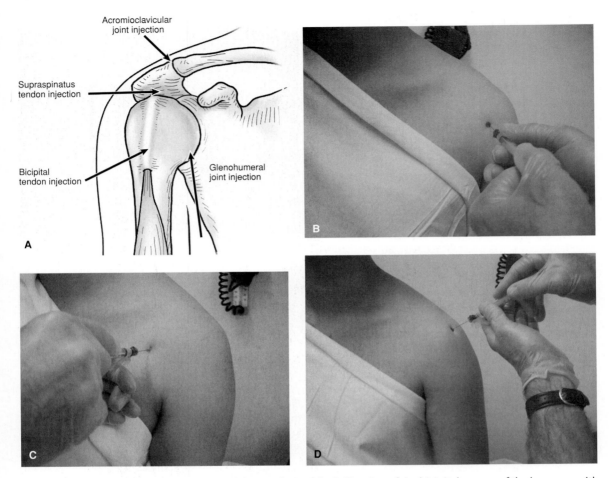

Figure 2–2. **A:** Anterior view of the shoulder. **B:** Technique for infiltration of the bicipital groove of the humerus with a glucocorticoid preparation (treatment for biceps tendinitis). **C:** Injection of the glenohumeral joint from the anterior position. **D:** Injection of the shoulder just inferior to the acromion (the preferred approach to shoulder injection).

frequently helpful, is not always curative. The long-term efficacy of the procedure depends in large part on the nature of the underlying problem.

Several preparations of glucocorticoids are available. Dexamethasone can be obtained in a crystalloid solution, dissolved in lidocaine. It is short acting and less likely to lead to atrophy, even when injected into soft tissues. Both dexamethasone and triamcinolone diacetate are available as colloidal suspensions. These suspensions remain in target tissues longer and may be more effective in the treatment of chronic inflammatory processes. However, they are more likely to lead to atrophy or cutaneous pigment changes when injected into superficial structures, such as the lateral epicondyle in the treatment of lateral epicondylitis. Some very stable (and therefore

extremely long-acting) agents, such as triamcinolone hexacetonide, should be used only for the injection of large joints or deep structures, because of the possibility of atrophy of superficial tissues. Repeat glucocorticoid injections should be administered judiciously. Too many injections sometimes lead to laxity of the periarticular supporting structures, soft tissue atrophy, or bone dissolution. No solid data provide guidance on which to base definitive recommendations. However, a single joint or soft tissue target probably should not be injected more than 3 times a year.

Several preparations of injectable hyaluronic acid are available. Evidence suggests that a series of 3 injections of hyaluronic acid into an affected joint (particularly the knee) in a patient with degenerative arthritis can give

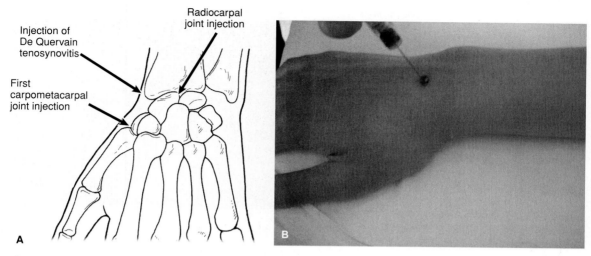

Figure 2–3. A: Dorsum of the left wrist. **B:** Injection of the radiocarpal joint.

short-term relief of pain equal to the response observed in patients receiving glucocorticoid injections into the joint. However, 6 months after injection, no significant difference in pain or function was noted among groups of patients receiving hyaluronic acid, glucocorticoids, or placebo. Although no difference has been reported in the long-term clinical benefits of hyaluronic acid and glucocorticoid injections, the cost difference is significant. The prohibitive expense of a series of hyaluronic acid injections makes glucocorticoid injection the preferable therapeutic modality.

C. Approach

The optimal approaches to the ankle, shoulder, wrist, knee, elbow, and metacarpophalangeal joints are shown in Figures 2–1 through 2–6. The optimal approach to the trochanteric bursa is shown in Figure 2–7.

Aspiration of a joint should be performed with the joint positioned to maximize intra-articular pressure, allowing easier withdrawal of synovial fluid. Intra-articular pressure is usually highest at maximum extension or flexion. For example, in the knee, the intra-articular pressure is highest when the knee is in full extension (see Figure 2–4B). Conversely, joint injection (without aspiration) is performed most easily with the joint semiflexed to minimize intra-articular pressure (see Figure 2–4C). The simplest approach for a knee injection is to seat the patient on an examining table, with the leg dangling down and the knee flexed at a 90-degree angle. This flexed position minimizes intra-articular pressure. Gravity pulls the lower leg down, thus opening the joint and facilitating introduction of the needle. The best position for aspira-

tion alone or with injection depends on the anatomy of the specific target joint.

The best approach for aspiration or injection of soft tissues also depends on the anatomy of the target. Aspiration or injection of the olecranon or prepatellar bursae is performed most effectively with the elbow or knee in full flexion, thereby maximizing intrabursal pressure. Positioning is less important when injecting ligaments or tendinous attachments, such as the lateral epicondyle in tennis elbow (see Figure 2–5), because the target is a tissue plane or area of swelling, nodularity, tenderness, or pain, rather than a distinct structure. When treating tendinitis, the target tissue is the tendon sheath, not the tendon itself.

Care must be taken *not* to inject against resistance, because an unusual degree of resistance may indicate that the tip of the needle is in the tendon. Injection directly into an inflamed tendon may increase the likelihood of tendon rupture.

D. Difficulty in Obtaining Adequate Samples

On occasion, initial efforts at aspiration may fail to produce an adequate sample of synovial fluid. This may occur because the needle is not in the joint space, and simple repositioning of the needle may result in a successful aspiration. If the needle is properly positioned but the synovial fluid is too viscous to be withdrawn easily, a larger gauge needle must be used.

Sometimes chronic inflammatory arthritis results in the formation of loculations that make adequate joint drainage difficult. In such cases arthroscopic surgery should be considered.

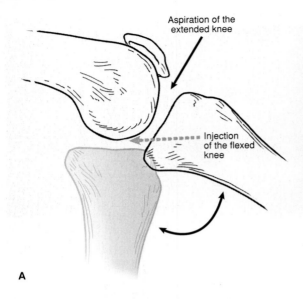

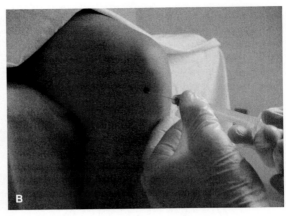

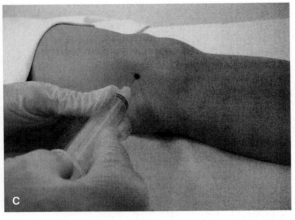

Figure 2–4. A: Lateral view of the knee. **B:** Optimal positioning of the knee for joint injection. **C:** Optimal positioning of the knee for joint aspiration.

In some attempts at aspiration, synovial fluid flows easily at first and then stops. This may be the result of too much negative pressure and can be resolved either by slowing the rate of fluid withdrawal or using a smaller syringe.

Synovial fluid debris can easily clog the needle. The needle can be cleared by reinjecting a small amount of synovial fluid from the syringe; aspiration is then resumed.

When enough synovial fluid has been removed to significantly lower intra-articular pressure, aspiration becomes increasingly difficult. In aspiration from the knee, an assistant can apply external pressure to the joint,

thereby increasing intra-articular pressure and facilitating the aspiration.

Synovial Fluid Analysis

A. CLARITY AND COLOR

Examination of the synovial fluid begins with a visual determination of clarity and color. Although various crystals (such as monosodium urate, calcium pyrophosphate dihydrate, and hydroxyapatite), lipids, and even cellular debris may affect clarity, the major determinant of synovial fluid clarity and color is the cell count. Noninflammatory

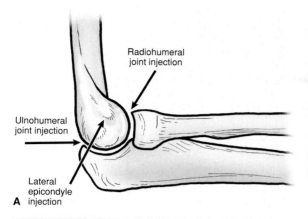

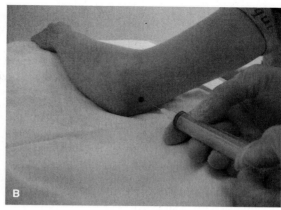

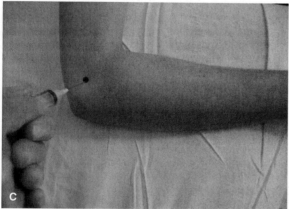

Figure 2–5. **A:** Lateral view of the elbow flexed to 90 degrees. **B:** Injection of the ulnohumeral joint, into the olecranon fossa. **C:** Injection of the lateral epicondyle, just proximal to the radial head.

fluid, such as that associated with osteoarthritis, has a low cell count and is clear. Synovial fluid from moderately inflammatory forms of arthritis, such as systemic lupus erythematosus or mild rheumatoid arthritis, has higher cell counts and is translucent and yellow. Fluid from intensely inflammatory processes, such as septic joints or crystal-induced arthropathies, has very high cell counts and is opaque and white to yellow. Bleeding into a joint leads to a hemarthrosis with characteristic opaque, red synovial fluid (see Table 2–1).

The physical characteristics of synovial fluid depend largely on the integrity of the hyaluronan and lubricin produced by synoviocytes. The WBCs in inflammatory arthritis release activated enzymes that digest the hyaluronan, decreasing the high viscosity typical of normal synovial fluid. A single drop of normal synovial fluid expressed from a needle will form a "tail" or "string" that will stretch to 10 cm long before surface tension is broken. Increasing degrees of inflammation lead to higher cell counts, greater concentrations of activated enzymes in the synovial fluid, lower concentrations of intact hyaluro-

nan, and shorter strings. Inflammatory synovial fluid may have a string test of only 5 cm or shorter.

B. Cell Count

The WBC count and differential are among the most valuable pieces of information derived from synovial fluid. Normal synovial fluid has <200 cells/μL, most of which are mononuclear. In contrast, synovial fluid from patients with noninflammatory arthritis may contain up to 2000 cells/μL, almost half of which may be polymorphonuclear leukocytes. Cell counts in mildly inflammatory synovial fluid, such as that from a patient with systemic lupus erythematosus or mild reactive arthritis, generally range from 2000–30,000 cells/μL.

Cell counts may be as high as 50,000 cells/μL in rheumatoid arthritis or a destructive seronegative arthropathy such as psoriatic arthritis. In crystal-induced arthropathies, cell counts of 30,000–50,000 cells/μL are typical, but $\geq$100,000 cells/μL are sometimes observed. Early or partially treated bacterial or chronic infections, such as those caused by mycobacteria or fungi, may

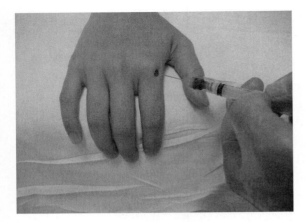

Figure 2–6. Injection of the metacarpophalangeal joint.

have cell counts as low as 50,000 cells/μL. Patients with chronic inflammatory arthritides, such as rheumatoid or psoriatic arthritis or the crystal-induced arthropathies, are more susceptible to bacterial superinfection. A Gram stain and culture and sensitivity studies should be performed on synovial fluid from any patient in whom infection is suspected, even when accompanied by a history of known nonseptic chronic inflammatory arthritis.

C. CRYSTALS

Crystal analysis is best performed on a fresh wet preparation with a clean slide and cover slip. Synovial fluid analysis for crystals is performed under polarized light. The strength of birefringence and shape of the crystals are helpful in distinguishing among the different forms of microcrystalline disease.

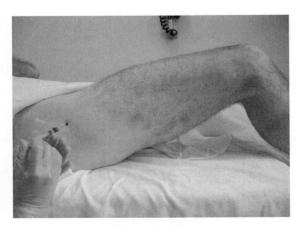

Figure 2–7. Injection of the trochanteric bursa.

- Monosodium urate crystals are needle-shaped and negatively birefringent (ie, the crystal is yellow when the long axis of the crystal is parallel to the slow axis of vibration of the red compensator used with polarized lenses to identify crystals under the microscope). Because of their strong birefringence, monosodium urate crystals are easily seen with a polarized light microscope.
- Calcium pyrophosphate dihydrate crystals are rhomboid-shaped and positively birefringent (ie, the crystal is blue when the long axis of the crystal is parallel to the slow axis of vibration of the red compensator used with polarized lenses to identify crystals under the microscope). Because they are weakly bifringent, calcium pyrophosphate dihydrate crystals are dim and difficult to detect even with a polarized light microscope.
- Calcium oxalate crystals can be seen in patients with primary oxalosis or in renal failure. These crystals are rod or tetrahedron shaped and positively birefringent.
- Cholesterol crystals are rectangular and tend to have notched corners. Lipids form spherules with birefringence in the shape of a Maltese cross. Because the arms of the cross that parallel the slow axis of vibration of the red compensator are blue, these spherules are positively birefringent.
- Hydroxyapatite crystals are not birefringent and form amorphous clumps that stain red with alizarin red S.
- Glucocorticoids from previous joint injections, talc from gloves, and even debris can form birefringent crystals and lead to mistaken diagnoses of microcrystalline disease.

The presence of intracellular crystals in synovial fluid inflammatory cells is diagnostic of a crystal-induced arthropathy. However, this diagnosis does not rule out infection, so it is always wise to culture the fluid from an acute monarticular arthritis even when crystals are identified. In addition, a patient may have more than one crystal-induced arthropathy. Fifteen percent of patients with gout also have CPPD. Appropriate short- and long-term therapies depend on proper diagnosis. A superinfected gouty joint will require aggressive antibiosis as well as anti-inflammatory therapy. A patient with gout and CPPD may require long-term anti-inflammatory therapy and a hypouricemic agent.

When aspirating a small joint, such as the first metatarsophalangeal joint, it is important to remember that monosodium urate crystals can be identified in interstitial fluid. Even when synovial fluid cannot be drawn into the syringe, negative pressure maintained as the needle is withdrawn will allow enough interstitial fluid for crystal analysis to be pulled into the needle. The needle is then removed, the syringe is filled with air, the needle is replaced, and the air is used to express the contents of the needle onto a slide. The small amount of material obtained is often enough to allow detection of monosodium urate crystals.

D. CULTURE

Any inflammatory monarticular arthritis must be considered infectious until proven otherwise. The best way to rule out infection is Gram stain and culture and sensitivity studies of synovial fluid. Microbiologic analysis usually is performed on fluid collected in a sterile tube. However, if the aspiration is difficult, material in the needle may be expressed onto a swab and sent for culture and sensitivity studies. It is important to remember that many significant pathogens are difficult to culture. For example, two-thirds of patients with gonococcal arthritis have negative cultures, even when the specimen is cultured directly onto chocolate agar. Tuberculosis and other mycobacterial infections, fungal infections, and anaerobic infections are difficult to detect from synovial fluid analysis, and diagnosis may depend on synovial biopsy. Because septic arthritis can be so quickly destructive it is wise to initiate antibiotic therapy based on the clinical picture, WBC count, differential, and Gram stain, and if necessary, make subsequent appropriate adjustments in therapy based on culture and sensitivity study results.

Synovial Biopsy

Sometimes an arthritic condition cannot be diagnosed by synovial fluid analysis. Diagnoses of indolent infections or noninfectious forms of granulomatous arthritis (such as sarcoidosis) usually require synovial biopsy. Although synovial fluid cytologic studies can sometimes reveal the presence of malignant cells, neoplastic arthritic conditions are usually diagnosed by histologic analysis of synovial biopsy material. Finally, a host of infiltrative, metabolic, or presumably infectious disorders, such as amyloidosis, ochronosis, hemochromatosis, Wilson disease, and Whipple disease, that can affect the joints are difficult to detect by synovial fluid analysis but are easily recognized by synovial biopsy.

REFERENCES

American College of Rheumatology Ad Hoc Committee on Clinical Guidelines. Guidelines for the initial evaluation of the adult patient with acute musculoskeletal symptoms. *Arthritis Rheum.* 1996;39:1. [PMID: 8546717]

Gatter RA, Schumacher HR Jr. *A Practical Handbook of Joint Fluid Analysis.* 2nd ed. Lea & Febiger, 1991.

Shmerling RH. Synovial fluid analysis: a critical reappraisal. *Rheum Dis Clin North Am.* 1994;20:503. [PMID: 8016423]

Laboratory Diagnosis

John B. Imboden, MD

3

■ AUTOANTIBODIES

METHODS FOR DETECTING AUTOANTIBODIES

A variety of basic assays are used to detect autoantibodies. More than one type of assay may be available for any given autoantibody, and the particular test used may vary from institution to institution. In general, there has been a trend away from labor-intensive tests, such as agglutination assays and countercurrent immunoelectrophoresis, and toward assays amenable to automation, such as nephelometry and enzyme-linked immunosorbent assay (ELISA).

Indirect immunofluorescence assays identify autoantibodies reactive with antigens in particular tissues or subcellular compartments (eg, nuclear antigens). Fixed tissue samples or cells are overlayed with patient sera and then washed. The presence of autoantibodies that have bound to the tissue sample is then revealed by staining with a fluorescein-labeled antiserum to human immunoglobulin (Ig).

Agglutination assays identify autoantibodies through the aggregation of particles, such as latex beads, coated with a defined autoantigen.

Immunodiffusion assays detect the formation of immune complexes in a semisolid support, such as an agar gel. Patient sera and antigen, placed in separate wells in the gel, diffuse toward one another and form a line of precipitation when insoluble immune complexes form. Placing the gel in an electrical field (**countercurrent immunoelectrophoresis**) increases the rate of diffusion and facilitates complex formation.

Nephelometry measures the interaction of antibodies and antigens in solution, detecting immune complex formation by monitoring changes in the scattering of an incident light.

ELISA uses an enzymatic readout to detect reactive antibodies. Sera to be tested for an autoantibody is incubated with the relevant autoantigen immobilized on a surface. After extensive washing, a detecting antibody (eg, an antiserum to human immunoglobulin) that has been conjugated to an enzyme is added. In the final step, substrate is added, and the product of the enzymatic reaction is measured. The amount of product reflects the quantity of detecting antibody bound to the autoantibody. There are several modifications of the basic ELISA test, but all take advantage of the remarkable sensitivity imparted by the enzymatic readout.

RHEUMATOID FACTOR

Rheumatoid factor is an autoantibody directed against the Fc region of IgG. The most commonly used methods of detecting rheumatoid factor are latex fixation (using latex beads coated with human IgG) and nephelometry (using human IgG as the target antigen). Both assays primarily detect IgM rheumatoid factors. The results of latex fixation assays are reported as the greatest dilution that retains agglutination activity; in most laboratories, sera with titers of >1:40 are considered abnormal. Rheumatoid factor measured by nephelometry is quantified in international units, with ≥20 IU reported as abnormal in most laboratories. ELISAs for rheumatoid factor are also available but are not in wide use. ELISAs can measure IgG, IgA, and IgM rheumatoid factors.

Associated Conditions

Rheumatoid factor is present in 70–90% of patients with rheumatoid arthritis. Despite its name, rheumatoid factor is not specific for rheumatoid arthritis. Positive tests for rheumatoid factor occur in a wide range of autoimmune disorders, inflammatory diseases, and chronic infections (Table 3–1). Also, the prevalence of positive rheumatoid factor tests increases with age; as many as 25% of persons over the age of 65 may test positive. In the absence of disease, the titer for rheumatoid factor is usually low (≤1:160). High titer for rheumatoid factor (≥1:640) almost always reflects an underlying disease.

Indication

Rheumatoid factor should be ordered when there is clinical suspicion of rheumatoid arthritis.

Table 3–1. Disorders Associated with a Positive Test for Rheumatoid Factor

Autoimmune Disorders
 Rheumatoid arthritis[a]
 Primary Sjögren syndrome[a]
 Mixed connective tissue disease[a]
 Polymyositis/dermatomyositis
 Scleroderma
 ANCA-associated vasculitis[a]
 Polyarteritis nodosa
 Primary biliary cirrhosis[a]
Chronic Infections
 Subacute bacterial endocarditis[a]
 Tuberculosis
 Leprosy
 Syphilis
 Hepatitis C[a] (with or without mixed
  cryoglobulinemia)
 Hepatitis B[a]
 Other viral infections
 Parasitic infections
Miscellaneous conditions
 Sarcoidosis
 Idiopathic pulmonary fibrosis
 Silicosis
 Asbestosis
 Malignancy
 Age ≥65

[a] Prevalence of rheumatoid factor >50% in most series.
ANCA, antineutrophilic cytoplasmic antibodies.

Interpretation of Results

Because of the large number of disorders associated with rheumatoid factor (see Table 3–1), the value of a positive test for rheumatoid factor depends on the pretest probability of the disease. In the proper clinical setting a positive test provides strong support for the diagnosis of rheumatoid arthritis. However, it should be kept in mind that the combination of arthritis and a positive test for rheumatoid factor is not specific for rheumatoid arthritis and can be seen in patients with systemic lupus erythematosus (SLE), mixed connective tissue disease, systemic vasculitis, polymyositis, dermatomyositis, sarcoidosis, subacute bacterial endocarditis, and viral infections, particularly hepatitis C.

A negative test for rheumatoid factor should not be the only reason to rule out the possibility of rheumatoid arthritis. From 10–30% of patients with long-standing disease are seronegative. At the time of presentation, however, the prevalence of a positive rheumatoid factor test is substantially lower (in the range of 50%). Therefore, the sensitivity of the test is lowest when the diagnosis is most likely to be in doubt.

ANTIBODIES TO CYCLIC CITRULLINATED PEPTIDES

Proteins that contain citrulline are the target of an autoantibody response that is highly specific for rheumatoid arthritis. Citrulline, a neutral amino acid, is not genetically encoded. Citrullinated proteins arise through a posttranslational modification in which arginine residues are converted enzymatically to citrulline. Currently autoantibodies to citrullinated proteins are detected using ELISA with synthetic cyclic citrullinated peptides (CCP).

Associated Conditions

The presence of anti-CCP antibodies appears to be quite specific for rheumatoid arthritis. The second-generation ELISA tests for anti-CCP antibodies (anti-CCP2) have a specificity for rheumatoid arthritis as high as 97%. The sensitivities of anti-CCP tests are in the range of 70–80% for established rheumatoid arthritis and 50% for early-onset rheumatoid arthritis. Thus, compared to rheumatoid factor, the currently available anti-CCP ELISA tests have superior specificity and comparable sensitivity for the diagnosis of rheumatoid arthritis. Most patients with rheumatoid arthritis are positive for both anti-CCP antibodies and rheumatoid factor, but some have only one of these autoantibodies, and others have neither.

Indication

Anti-CCP antibodies should be ordered when there is clinical suspicion of rheumatoid arthritis.

Interpretation of Results

The presence of anti-CCP antibodies provides strong support for the diagnosis of rheumatoid arthritis. Moreover, in patients with early-onset, undifferentiated, inflammatory arthritis, the presence of anti-CCP antibodies is a strong predictor of progression to rheumatoid arthritis and for the development of joint erosions.

A negative test for anti-CCP antibodies does not exclude the possibility of rheumatoid arthritis, particularly at the time of initial presentation when approximately 50% of patients lack detectable anti-CCP antibodies.

The specificity of the anti-CCP ELISA test suggests that this test will prove useful when determinations of rheumatoid factor are not. For example, initial studies indicate that anti-CCP antibodies are not associated with chronic hepatitis C infection. In contrast to rheumatoid factor, therefore, testing for anti-CCP antibodies may help to distinguish concomitant rheumatoid arthritis from viral arthritis in patients infected with hepatitis C.

ANTINUCLEAR ANTIBODIES

Antinuclear antibodies (ANA) are autoantibodies directed against histones, double-stranded and single-stranded DNA, ribonucleoprotein (RNP) complexes, and other nuclear components. Current indirect immunofluorescence assays for ANA use HEp-2 cells, a human epithelial cell line, as the source of nuclei and are more sensitive than older tests that used rodent liver and kidney.

Indirect immunofluorescence assays for ANA report the titer of the ANA and the pattern of nuclear staining. In most laboratories, ANA with titers ≥1:40 are considered positive. The staining patterns are diffuse or homogeneous (due to antibodies to histone), rim (an uncommon pattern due to antibodies to nuclear envelope proteins and to double-stranded [ds] DNA), speckled (due to antibodies to Sm, RNP, Ro/SS-A, La/SS-B, and other antigens), nucleolar (see the section on antibodies to nucleolar antigens, below), and centromeric. In general, there is a poor correlation between the pattern of the ANA and the identity of the underlying disease. An exception is the centromeric pattern, which has considerable specificity for limited scleroderma (see the section on anticentromere antibodies, below). Patients often have antibodies to multiple nuclear components, and the staining pattern of certain autoantibodies (eg, antihistone antibodies) can prevent detection of others. The pattern of the ANA should not preclude, or substitute for, the ordering of more specific tests that are otherwise indicated.

Associated Conditions

Positive tests for ANA occur in wide range of conditions, including SLE and other rheumatic diseases, organ-specific autoimmune diseases, lymphoproliferative diseases, and chronic infections (Table 3–2). A number of drugs induce ANA, and less commonly, a lupuslike syndrome (see Table 3–2). Low-titer ANA are relatively common among healthy adults; in one analysis, an ANA titer of ≥1:40 was seen in 32% of healthy adults and ≥1:160 was seen in 5%.

Indications

Testing for ANA by indirect immunofluorescence is a very useful initial laboratory investigation when there is clinical suspicion of SLE, drug-induced lupus, mixed connective tissue disease, or scleroderma. The ANA may provide useful prognostic information for patients with isolated Raynaud phenomenon, identifying those at greater risk for systemic rheumatic disease.

Interpretation of Results

The sensitivity of the immunofluorescent ANA for SLE is very high (>95%). A negative result, therefore, is very

Table 3–2. Conditions Associated with Positive ANA Detected by Indirect Immunofluorescence Assays

Rheumatic Diseases
Systemic lupus erythematosus
Mixed connective tissue disease
Scleroderma
Sjögren syndrome
Rheumatoid arthritis
Polymyositis
Dermatomyositis
Discoid lupus

Organ-Specific Autoimmune Diseases
Autoimmune thyroid disease
Autoimmune hepatitis
Primary biliary cirrhosis
Autoimmune cholangitis

Other
Drug-induced lupus[a]
Asymptomatic drug-induced ANA[a]
Chronic infections
Idiopathic pulmonary fibrosis
Primary pulmonary hypertension
Lymphoproliferative disorders

[a] Drugs that can induce lupus or positive tests for ANA include procainamide, hydralazine, minocycline, antitumor necrosis factor agents, interferon-α, isoniazid, quinidine, methyldopa, chlorpromazine, quinidine, penicillamine, and anticonvulsants.
ANA, antinuclear antibodies.

strong evidence against this diagnosis and usually precludes the need to pursue tests for antibodies to specific nuclear antigens (eg, dsDNA, Sm, or RNP). A positive ANA test is one of the diagnostic criteria for drug-induced lupus and mixed connective tissue disease. The sensitivity of the ANA for scleroderma is >85%.

In general, the probability of an underlying autoimmune disease increases with the titer of the ANA. Nonetheless, because the specificity of the ANA is limited, the value of a positive test depends on the pretest probability of disease. In the proper clinical context, a positive ANA by immunofluorescence provides supportive evidence of disease and should prompt tests for antibodies to specific nuclear antigens (Table 3–3).

Serial determinations of ANA by immunofluorescence are not useful for monitoring disease activity.

ANTIBODIES TO DEFINED NUCLEAR ANTIGENS

Antibodies to Double-Stranded DNA

Antibodies to dsDNA recognize its base pairs, its ribose-phosphate backbone, and the structure of its double

Table 3–3. Selected Antinuclear Antibodies with High Sensitivity or Specificity for Rheumatic Diseases

Condition	High Sensitivity[a]	High Specificity[b]
Systemic lupus erythematosus	ANA[c]	Anti-dsDNA, anti-Sm
Drug-induced lupus	ANA, antihistone[d]	—
Neonatal cutaneous lupus	Maternal anti-Ro/SS-A (90%)	—
Congenital complete heart block	Maternal anti-Ro/SS-A	—
Mixed connective tissue disease	ANA, anti-RNP[e]	—
Primary Sjogren syndrome	Anti-Ro/SS-A (75%)	—
Limited and diffuse scleroderma	ANA (>85%)	Anticentromere, anti-Scl-70, and other antinucleolar antibodies

[a]Sensitivity (probability of a positive test result in a patient with the disease) > 95% except where noted.
[b]Specificity (probability of a negative test result in a patient without the disease) >95%.
[c]ANA: antinuclear antibodies determined by immunofluorescence using HEp-2 cells.
[d]Anti-histone antibodies occur in only a minority of cases of minocycline-induced lupus.
[e]The presence of antibodies to ribonucleoprotein (RNP) is required for diagnosis.

helix. ELISA is the most commonly used method to detect antibodies to dsDNA and has largely supplanted the Farr radioimmunoassay and the crithidia immunofluorescence assay, which measures binding to the dsDNA of the protozoan *Crithidia luciliae.*

A. ASSOCIATED CONDITIONS

Antibodies to dsDNA occur in SLE and are rare in other diseases and in healthy persons. When detected outside the context of SLE, antibodies to dsDNA are almost always of low titer. Antibodies to dsDNA do not occur in most forms of drug-induced lupus but have been observed during treatment with penicillamine, minocycline, and anti–tumor necrosis factor agents.

B. INDICATIONS

Antibodies to dsDNA should be measured when there is clinical suspicion of SLE and the ANA is positive. The yield of testing for anti-dsDNA antibodies is extremely low when ANA are not detected by indirect immunofluorescence on HEp-2 cells. Longitudinal determinations of the levels of antibodies to dsDNA may aid in the analysis of disease activity for patients with known SLE.

C. INTERPRETATION OF RESULTS

The specificity of anti-dsDNA antibodies for SLE is 97% overall and approaches 100% when the antibody titer is high. A positive test, therefore, is a very strong argument for the diagnosis of SLE.

Antibodies to dsDNA occur in 60–80% of patients with SLE. Because titers can fluctuate in and out of the normal range over time, the sensitivity of an isolated test for anti-dsDNA antibodies is probably in the range of 50% for SLE. A negative test, therefore, does not argue strongly against the diagnosis of SLE.

Studies of patient populations indicate that the level of anti-dsDNA antibodies correlates with certain manifestations of SLE activity, such as lupus nephritis, but not others. The strength of this relationship, however, varies from patient to patient. For most patients, a rise in antibody titer often precedes—or occurs concomitantly with—a disease flare. However, there are subsets of patients who manifest disease flares in the absence of anti-dsDNA antibodies, and others whose disease is quiescent despite elevated levels of this autoantibody.

Antibodies to Sm & RNP

Smith (Sm) and RNP were initially identified as extractable nuclear antigens. Antibodies to Sm recognize nuclear proteins that bind to small nuclear RNAs, forming complexes involved in the processing of messenger RNA. Antibodies to RNP recognize a complex of protein and the small nuclear RNA designated U1. ELISA has largely replaced immunodiffusion assays for the measurement of antibodies to Sm and RNP. Antibodies to Sm or to RNP produce a speckled pattern on indirect immunofluorescence assays for ANA.

A. ASSOCIATED CONDITIONS

Antibodies to Sm are specific for SLE. Antibodies to RNP occur in SLE and mixed connective tissue disease. The prevalence of these autoantibodies in other conditions is very low.

B. INDICATIONS

Antibodies to Sm and RNP should be determined when there is clinical suspicion of SLE or mixed connective tissue disease and the ANA are positive by indirect immunofluorescence.

C. INTERPRETATION OF RESULTS

Antibodies to Sm are highly specific for SLE but occur in only 10–40% of patients. The prevalence of anti-Sm antibodies appears to be lower in white patients than in African American and Asian patients.

Antibodies to RNP occur in 30–40% of patients with SLE. The diagnosis of mixed connective tissue disease requires the presence of antibodies to RNP; by definition, therefore, 100% of patients with this disease have anti-RNP antibodies.

Serial determinations of antibodies to Sm and RNP are not useful for monitoring disease activity.

Antibodies to Ro (SS-A) & La (SS-B)

The Ro (also known as Sjögren syndrome A or SS-A) and La (SS-B or Sjögren syndrome B) antigens are distinct RNP particles. ELISA and immunoblot assays are supplanting the older immunodiffusion assays for detection of anti-Ro and anti-La antibodies. Antibodies to Ro and La produce a speckled pattern on immunofluorescence assays for ANA. When rodent tissues were used for this assay, antibodies to Ro often went undetected and were a cause of "ANA-negative" lupus if these were the dominant autoantibody system. The use of HEp-2 cells enhances detection of anti-Ro antibodies and has led to a decline in the prevalence of ANA-negative lupus.

A. Associated Conditions

Antibodies to Ro are uncommon in the normal population and in patients with rheumatic diseases other than Sjögren syndrome and SLE. Antibodies to Ro are present in 75% of patients with primary Sjögren syndrome but only in 10–15% of patients with rheumatoid arthritis and secondary Sjögren syndrome. In SLE, anti-Ro antibodies are present in up to 50% of patients and are associated with photosensitivity, subacute cutaneous lupus, and interstitial lung disease. Transfer of maternal anti-Ro antibodies across the placenta appears to be important in the pathogenesis of neonatal cutaneous lupus and congenital complete heart block (see Table 3–3).

Antibodies to La occur, almost always in association with anti-Ro antibodies, in primary Sjögren syndrome (40–50%), SLE (10–15%), congenital complete heart block (90%), and neonatal cutaneous lupus (70%).

B. Indications

Antibodies to Ro and La should be measured when there is clinical suspicion of primary Sjögren syndrome or SLE. Even when ANA are not detected by indirect immunofluorescence, testing for anti-Ro antibodies is still indicated for patients with suspected subacute cutaneous lupus or with recurrent photosensitive rashes. Mothers of children with neonatal cutaneous lupus and congenital complete heart block should be tested for antibodies to Ro and La; many of these women are asymptomatic. Testing is also indicated for patients with SLE who become pregnant or who are planning to become pregnant.

C. Interpretation of Results

The presence of antibodies to Ro, or to Ro and La, is a strong argument for the diagnosis of Sjögren syndrome in a patient with sicca symptoms. Although not a sensitive test for SLE, a positive test for anti-Ro antibodies can facilitate a diagnosis of subacute cutaneous lupus. Chapter 14 reviews the monitoring of pregnancy in the setting of maternal antibodies to Ro and the evaluation of asymptomatic mothers found to have anti-Ro antibodies.

Anticentromere Antibodies

Antibodies to centromere proteins produce a characteristic pattern of staining in indirect immunofluorescence assays using HEp-2 cells. Anticentromere antibodies can be measured by ELISA, but indirect immunofluorescence is the most commonly used method of detection.

A. Associated Conditions

Anticentromere antibodies occur in limited scleroderma and scleroderma. They are very rare in other rheumatic conditions and in healthy persons.

B. Indications

Anticentromere antibodies should be determined when there is clinical suspicion of scleroderma or its CREST variant (**c**alcinosis, **R**aynaud phenomenon, **e**sophageal dysmotility, **s**clerodactyly, and **t**elangiectasias).

C. Interpretation of Results

Anticentromere antibodies occur in approximately 60% of patients with CREST and in 15% of those with scleroderma. The specificity of this test is remarkable (>98%). Therefore a positive test for anticentromere antibodies is a very strong argument for the presence of CREST or scleroderma. The presence of anticentromere antibodies early in the course of disease predicts limited cutaneous involvement and a decreased likelihood of interstitial lung disease. Anticentromere antibodies and antibodies to Scl-70 rarely coexist. Serial determinations of anticentromere antibodies are not useful for monitoring disease activity.

ANTIBODIES TO NUCLEOLAR ANTIGENS

Antibodies to Scl-70 (Topoisomerase-I)

Antibodies to Scl-70 (or topoisomerase I) produce nucleolar staining on indirect immunofluorescence and are measured by immunodiffusion assays, immunoblotting, and ELISA.

A. Associated Conditions

Antibodies to Scl-70 occur in scleroderma and are rare in patients with other systemic rheumatic diseases and in healthy persons.

B. INDICATIONS

Antibodies to Scl-70 should be measured when there is clinical suspicion of scleroderma.

C. INTERPRETATION OF RESULTS

Immunodiffusion assays identify antibodies to Scl-70 in 20–30% of patients with scleroderma; approximately 40% of patients have antibodies to Scl-70 detectable by immunoblotting or ELISA. The specificity of anti-Scl-70 antibodies approaches 100% for the immunoblotting and immunodiffusion assays. Therefore a positive test by these assays is a very strong argument for the diagnosis of scleroderma. The specificity of ELISA is not certain but it may be lower. The presence of antibodies to Scl-70 has prognostic value in scleroderma and carries an increased likelihood of diffuse skin involvement and of interstitial lung disease. Serial determinations of anti-Scl-70 antibodies are not useful for monitoring the disease.

Antibodies to Other Nucleolar Antigens

Antibodies to nucleolar antigens other than Scl-70 occur in scleroderma. Antibodies with high specificity for scleroderma include anti-RNA polymerase I, anti-RNA polymerase III, anti-U3 small nucleolar RNP (or anti-fibrillarin), and anti-Th small nucleolar RNP. The low sensitivity of these antibodies limits their usefulness in the diagnosis of scleroderma. Antibodies to RNA polymerase II are present in scleroderma, SLE, and overlap syndromes. Antibodies to PM-Scl occur in scleroderma and in an overlap syndrome of myositis and scleroderma.

ANTIBODIES TO HISTONES

Antibodies to histones usually produce a homogeneous staining on indirect immunofluorescence assays for ANA. Antihistone antibodies are almost always present in lupus induced by drugs such as procainamide, hydralazine, and isoniazid (sensitivity >95%). An important exception is minocycline-induced lupus; antihistone antibodies are present in only a minority of patients with this disorder. Antibodies to histones are common in SLE (prevalence 50–70%) and occur at low frequency in a range of rheumatic and nonrheumatic disorders. The clinical usefulness of testing for antibodies to histones is limited. Antihistone antibodies are nonspecific and do not distinguish drug-induced lupus from SLE. Although the absence of antihistone antibodies is strong evidence against most forms of drug-induced lupus, the clinical diagnosis of drug-induced lupus is based on the clinical manifestations, a positive test for ANA by indirect immunofluorescence, and resolution of symptoms following withdrawal of the implicated drug.

MYOSITIS-ASSOCIATED ANTIBODIES (SEE CHAPTER 35)

Anti-Jo-1 & Other Antisynthetase Antibodies

Autoantibodies against amino acyl-tRNA synthetases occur almost exclusively in inflammatory myositis and can cause cytoplasmic staining when sera are analyzed for ANA by indirect immunofluorescence. The most common of these autoantibodies (anti-Jo-1) is directed against histidyl-tRNA synthetase and is present in 20–30% of patients with polymyositis. Patients with antisynthetase antibodies tend to have interstitial lung disease, arthritis, mechanic's hands, and Raynaud phenomenon, as well as myositis.

Antibodies to Signal Recognition Particle

These antibodies recognize a cytoplasmic RNP, occur in 4% of myositis patients, and are associated with acute onset and severe disease.

Anti-Mi-2 Antibodies

These antibodies are directed against helicase activities and produce homogeneous nuclear staining on indirect immunofluorescence assays for ANA. Anti-Mi-2 antibodies have high specificity for dermatomyositis and occur in 15–20% of patients with that disorder.

ANTINEUTROPHILIC CYTOPLASMIC ANTIBODIES

Antineutrophilic cytoplasmic antibodies are reviewed in Chapter 40.

■ MEASUREMENT OF THE ACUTE PHASE RESPONSE

The acute phase response develops in the setting of a wide range of acute and chronic inflammatory conditions: severe bacterial, viral, or fungal infections; rheumatic and other inflammatory diseases; malignancy; and tissue injury or necrosis. These conditions elicit a response in which interleukin-6 and other cytokines trigger the synthesis by the liver of a variety of plasma proteins, including C-reactive protein (CRP) and fibrinogen. The detection and monitoring of this response can be clinically useful and is accomplished by measuring the level of CRP or by determining the erythrocyte sedimentation rate (ESR), which is influenced by the binding of fibrinogen to erythrocytes. As a general rule, CRP is a more sensitive and accurate reflection of the acute phase response than the ESR.

C-REACTIVE PROTEIN

CRP likely has a physiologic role in the innate immune response to infection and may participate in the clearance of necrotic and apoptotic cells. The availability of highly sensitive assays of CRP has allowed accurate determination of baseline CRP levels and has revealed a correlation between baseline CRP and cardiovascular disease. The median baseline level for young adults is 0.8 mg/L, and the 90th percentile is 3.0 mg/L. The baseline levels of CRP increase with age and with body mass index. Laboratories sometimes offer a choice between a routine CRP assay (suitable for the detection and monitoring of inflammatory disease) and a highly sensitive CRP assay for the determination of cardiac risk.

During the acute phase response, levels of CRP rapidly increase up to 1000-fold, reaching a peak at 48 hours. With resolution of the acute phase response, CRP declines with a relatively short half-life of 18 hours. Because there are a large number of disparate conditions that can induce CRP production, an elevated CRP level does not have diagnostic specificity. An elevated CRP level, however, can provide support for the presence of a clinically suspected inflammatory disease, such as polymyalgia rheumatica or giant cell arteritis, when other objective findings are absent. Values >10 mg/L are generally thought to indicate clinically significant inflammation. Monitoring CRP levels can provide useful information on the activity of diseases such as rheumatoid arthritis and giant cell arteritis.

Despite their apparent inflammatory nature, scleroderma, polymyositis, and dermatomyositis often elicit little or no CRP response. CRP levels also tend not to be elevated in SLE unless serositis or synovitis is present.

Elevations of CRP in the absence of clinically significant inflammation can occur in renal failure.

ERYTHROCYTE SEDIMENTATION RATE

The ESR is determined by allowing anticoagulated blood to sediment for 1 hour in a glass tube (200 mm in length for the commonly used Westergren method; 100 mm for the Wintrobe method). Normal ranges for the ESR are 0–10 mm/h and 0–15 mm/h for men and women, respectively, but the upper limit of normal increases with age and with obesity.

Because fibrinogen and certain other acute phase proteins (not including CRP) bind to erythrocytes and increase their sedimentation rate, the ESR is a measure of the acute phase response. The ESR responds slower (over days) to the onset and resolution of an acute phase response than does the level of CRP, and the dynamic range of the ESR is less than that of CRP. More so than CRP, the ESR can be influenced by factors other than the acute phase response.

The ESR is a useful diagnostic test when there is clinical suspicion of polymyalgia rheumatica or giant cell arteritis; it also is commonly used to monitor the activity of these conditions as well as that of rheumatoid arthritis. Due to the wide range of disorders associated with an acute phase response, elevations of the ESR have little diagnostic specificity. Moreover, transient mild to moderate elevations can occur in the absence of other indications of disease. Marked elevations of the ESR (>100 mm/h by the Westergren method), however, are almost always due to a clinically significant condition, usually infection, malignancy, or rheumatic disease.

The ESR is of very limited value in patients with the nephrotic syndrome or end-stage renal disease because virtually all have an elevated ESR (some >100 mm/h), probably due to high levels of fibrinogen. Elevations of the ESR in the absence of clinically significant inflammation also occur in pregnancy, anemia, erythrocyte macrocytosis, and hypercholesterolemia. Conversely, hypofibrinogenemia, polycythemia, microcytosis, sickle cell disease, and congestive heart failure lower the ESR.

■ MEASUREMENTS OF COMPLEMENT

THE COMPLEMENT SYSTEM

Complement is a complex system of at least 30 proteins that play key roles in the innate and adaptive immune responses. Effector functions of complement include opsonization, chemotaxis and activation of leukocytes, lysis of bacteria and cells, promotion of antibody responses, and clearance of immune complexes and apoptotic cells. Three enzymatic complement cascades (the classical pathway, the alternative pathway, and the mannose-binding lectin pathway) lead to the generation of a convertase that cleaves C3, releasing C3a (an anaphylatoxin) and producing C3b, which binds to the target surface. C3b, a potent opsonin, forms a complex that cleaves C5 to C5a (another anaphylatoxin) and C5b, which sequentially binds C6, C7, C8, and C9 to form the membrane attack complex, a channel that can induce osmotic lysis of the target cell.

INDICATIONS FOR MEASUREMENTS OF COMPLEMENT

Complement should be measured when there is clinical suspicion of a disease that is associated with

Table 3–4. Immune Complex Diseases Associated with Hypocomplementemia

---

Systemic lupus erythematosus
Vasculitis
    Hypocomplementemic urticarial vasculitis
    Polyarteritis nodosa (especially hepatitis B-associated)
Glomerulonephritis
    Post-streptococcal
    Membranoproliferative
Cryoglobulinemia (type II and III)
Subacute bacterial endocarditis
Serum sickness

---

hypocomplementemia (Table 3–4) or an inherited or acquired abnormality of the complement system (Table 3–5). Complement levels also can be used to monitor the activity of diseases such as SLE. Some components of the complement system, including C3 and C4, are acute phase proteins, and their synthesis increases during the acute phase response. Because the liver synthesizes many complement components, severe hepatic failure can produce hypocomplementemia.

There are three commonly used measurements of complement in clinical practice: the CH50 and determination of the levels of C3 and C4.

CH50

The CH50 is a functional assay for the classical pathway (components C1 through C9) of complement activation (Figure 3–1). The test measures the complement-dependent lysis of sheep red blood cells, using patient sera as a source of complement and rabbit antibodies to sheep red blood cells. Units are standardized with a known source of complement and may vary from laboratory to laboratory if the standard reagents differ. Immune complex diseases (see Table 3–4) can lead to the

Table 3–5. Clinical Syndromes Associated with Deficiences of Components of the Classical Pathway of Complement Activation

Component	Syndrome
Pathway components	
C1q, C4, C2	Lupus-like syndromes
C3	Recurrent pyogenic infections; immune complex glomerulonephritis
C5, C6, C7, C8	Recurrent neisserial infections
Regulatory proteins	
C1 inhibitor	Angioedema

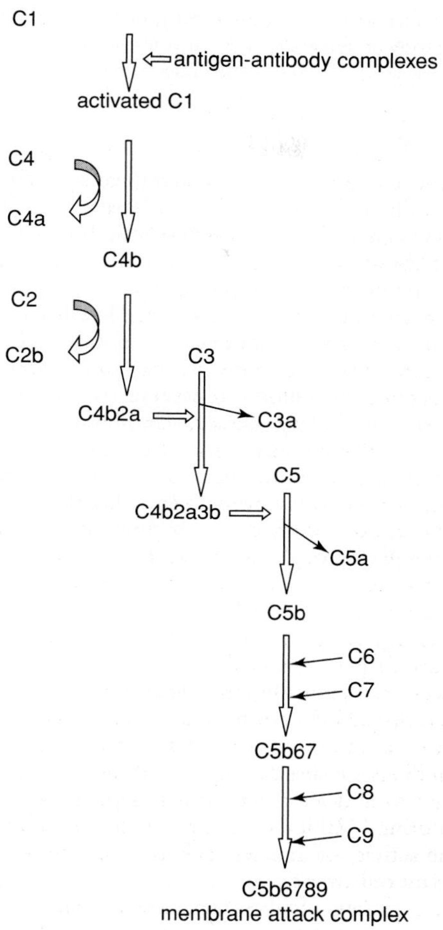

Figure 3–1. Classical pathway of complement activation. Antigen-antibody complexes activate C1 esterase, which acts on C4 and then C2, forming the C3 convertase (C4b2a) that cleaves C3. C4b2a3b acts on C5, releasing C5a and generating C5b, which interacts with C6, C7, C8, and C9 to form the membrane attack complex. (Adapted from Parslow T, Stites D, Terr A, Imboden J, eds. *Medical Immunology.* McGraw-Hill, 2001.)

activation of the classical pathway, the depletion of complement components, and a depressed CH50. In general, a reduction in the CH50 requires at least a 50% reduction of one or more components. Because each component of the classical pathway has an essential role in this assay, the CH50 is an excellent screen for deficiencies of the classical pathway (see Table 3–5). The CH50 is undetectable when there is complete deficiency of any individual component, and a persistently undetectable

CH50 should raise the possibility of such a deficiency. Conversely, a detectable CH50 rules out complete deficiency of components of the classical pathway.

C4 Levels

The concentration of C4 is determined by immunoassay, usually by rate nephelometry. Low levels of C4, or of both C4 and C3, usually reflect activation of the classical pathway by immune complex disease. Deficiency in C1 inhibitor leads to unregulated C1 esterase activity and to depression of C4 levels. Thus C4 is an excellent screen for C1 inhibitor deficiency and should be performed before more specific (and costly) determinations of C1 inhibitor protein levels and enzymatic activity. Two tandem genes on chromosome 6 encode C4. Although null alleles for these genes are relatively common, complete deficiency of C4 is rare, because four genes encode C4 protein. Partial deficiencies (due to the presence of one, two, or three null alleles) can produce persistently low levels of C4 and predispose to SLE.

C3 Levels

The concentration of C3 is determined by immunoassay, usually by rate nephelometry. The classical and alternative pathways converge on C3. Depression of both C4 and C3 indicates activation of the classical pathway. A depressed C3 with normal C4 suggests activation of the alternative pathway. Complete deficiency of C3 is rare and usually manifests in childhood as severe, recurrent infections with pyogenic organisms. C3 nephritic factor, an autoantibody associated with membranoproliferative glomerulonephritis and partial lipodystrophy, stabilizes the alternative pathway C3 convertase, leading to dysregulated cleavage of C3 and low levels of C3.

■ CRYOGLOBULINS

CLASSIFICATION

Cryoglobulins are cold-insoluble immunoglobulins that dissolve on rewarming. The Brouet classification describes three categories.

Type I is a monoclonal immunoglobulin that precipitates in the cold. Type I cryoglobulins are often associated with underlying lymphoproliferative disorders and may cause cold-induced hyperviscosity symptoms if the monoclonal immunoglobulin precipitates at physiologically relevant temperatures.

Type II cryoglobulins are immune complexes composed of a monoclonal immunoglobulin (usually IgMκ) with rheumatoid factor activity and polyclonal IgG. Most cases of type II cryoglobulinemia are associated with chronic hepatitis C infection and manifest clinically as an immune complex–mediated vasculitis with palpable purpura (see Chapter 44). The levels of C4 are usually low. Tests for serum rheumatoid factor are positive unless handling of the sample at lower than 37°C produces a false-negative test.

Type III cryoglobulins are immune complexes composed of polyclonal rheumatoid factor and polyclonal IgG. Type III cryoglobulinemia occurs in hepatitis C, other chronic infections including subacute bacterial endocarditis, and autoimmune diseases such as SLE and rheumatoid arthritis.

MEASUREMENT

Blood to be tested for cryoglobulins is drawn in prewarmed tubes, is allowed to clot at 37°C, and then is centrifuged at 37°C; exposure to temperatures lower than 37°C during these steps can result in a false-negative test due to premature precipitation of the cryoglobulin. The resulting serum is placed at 4°C for 2–7 days (usually 2–3 days) and then is examined for a precipitate. A "cryocrit" provides a crude estimate of the quantity of cryoglobulin. The highest levels are usually seen in type I cryoglobulinemia, but in general the cryocrit correlates poorly with clinical severity. Analysis of resolubilized cryoglobulins by immunofixation electrophoresis permits classification as type I, II, or III.

REFERENCES

Bathon J, Graves J, Jens P, Hamrick, R, Mayes M. The erythrocyte sedimentation rate in end-stage renal failure. *Am J Kidney Dis.* 1987;10:34. [PMID: 3605082]

Kavanaugh AF, Solomon DH, and the American College of Rheumatology Ad Hoc Committee on Immunologic Testing Guidelines. Guidelines for immunologic laboratory testing in the rheumatic diseases: anti-DNA antibody tests. *Arthritis Rheum.* 2002;47:546. [PMID: 12382306]

Nijenhuis S, Zendman AJ, Vossenaar ER, Pruijn GJ, van Venrooij WJ. Autoantibodies to citrullinated proteins in rheumatoid arthritis: clinical performance and biochemical aspects of an RA-specific marker. *Clin Chim Acta.* 2004;350:17–34. [PMID: 15530456]

Pepys MB, Hirschfield GM. C-reactive protein: a critical update. *J Clin Invest.* 2003;111:1805. [PMID: 12813013]

Reveille JD, Solomon DH, and the American College of Rheumatology Ad Hoc Committee of Immunologic Testing Guidelines. Evidence-based guidelines for the use of immunologic tests: anticentromere, Scl-70, and nucleolar antibodies. *Arthritis Rheum.* 2003;49:399. [PMID: 12794797]

Solomon DH, et al, and the American College of Rheumatology Ad Hoc Committee on Immunologic Testing Guidelines.

Evidence-based guidelines for the use of immunologic tests: antinuclear antibody testing. *Arthritis Rheum.* 2002;47:434. [PMID: 12209492]

Sox HC Jr, Liang MH. The erythrocyte sedimentation rate. Guidelines for rational use. *Ann Intern Med.* 1986;104:515. [PMID: 3954279]

Walport MJ. Complement. *N Engl J Med.* 2001;344:1140, 1058. [PMID: 11297706, 11287977]

Wener MH, Hutchinson K, Morishima C, Gretch DR. Absence of antibodies to cyclic citrullinated peptide in sera of patients with hepatitis C virus infection and cryoglobulinemia *Arthritis Rheum.* 2004;50:2305–2308. [PMID: 15248231]

Approach to the Patient with Arthritis

4

John Imboden, MD

TYPES OF ARTHRITIS

When a patient presents with joint symptoms, the first order of business is to ascertain whether or not arthritis is present. The history and examination should determine whether the symptoms are due to an articular process and not to bursitis, tendinitis, or other soft tissue conditions, and whether there are objective findings of arthritis, such as swelling, in the symptomatic joints. Arthralgias in the absence of objective arthritis commonly occur in systemic lupus erythematosus and acute viral illnesses but have less diagnostic significance than true arthritis.

A remarkable variety of diseases can cause arthritis. Accurate characterization of the arthritis and appreciation of the clinical context are the first steps toward the correct diagnosis and allow the clinician to approach the differential diagnosis in a focused, logical fashion (Table 4–1).

Inflammatory versus Noninflammatory Arthritis

The distinction between inflammatory arthritis and non-inflammatory arthritis is critical. The most reliable means for making this distinction is analysis of the white blood cell (WBC) count in the synovial fluid. The synovial fluid WBC count is >2000/mm³ in inflammatory arthritis and is <2000/mm³ in noninflammatory arthritis. Arthrocentesis should be performed whenever feasible because although clinical features and other laboratory investigations also help distinguish inflammatory and noninflammatory arthritis, no single finding is definitive.

Patients with an inflammatory arthritis usually complain of pain and stiffness in involved joints; typically these symptoms are worse in the morning or after periods of inactivity (the so-called "gel phenomenon") and improve with mild to moderate activity. On examination, the larger joints can be warm, and when severely inflamed as in acute gout or septic arthritis, can have erythema of the overlying skin. Laboratory investigations often reveal an elevated erythrocyte sedimentation rate (ESR) and a high C-reactive protein (CRP) level. In contrast, patients with noninflammatory arthritis have pain that worsens with activity and improves with rest. Stiffness is generally mild and usually not a prominent symptom. The ESR and CRP are usually normal.

Constitutional Symptoms

The presence of fever raises the possibility of infection. The majority of patients with septic arthritis or disseminated gonococcal infection are febrile. Fever also can accompany arthritis that is not due to active infection (Table 4–2). Indeed, intermittent high-grade fever >39°C is characteristic of Still disease. Systemic lupus erythematosus (SLE) also can cause fever to >39°C, but fever more often occurs when serositis, rather than polyarthritis, is the major manifestation of SLE. On the other hand, fever >38.3°C is unusual in rheumatoid arthritis, occurring in <1% of patients.

Significant weight loss is common at the initial presentation of reactive arthritis, systemic vasculitis, enteropathic arthritis, and paraneoplastic arthritis, but is unusual in rheumatoid arthritis of recent onset. Constitutional symptoms rarely accompany noninflammatory forms of arthritis.

Extra-Articular Manifestations

Extra-articular manifestations, such as glomerulonephritis, pulmonary abnormalities, ocular inflammation, and peripheral neuropathy may signal that arthritis is a manifestation of a systemic rheumatic disease or vasculitis. The presence of rash can be a very helpful clue to the diagnosis (Table 4–3).

Comorbid Conditions

Certain chronic conditions predispose to the development of particular musculoskeletal problems. For example, patients with long-standing, poorly controlled diabetes mellitus are at greatly increased risk for Charcot arthropathy in the feet and limited joint mobility in the hands. Prior glucocorticoid therapy and alcohol abuse are the leading risk factors for osteonecrosis, which

Table 4–1. Initial Clinical Characterization of Arthritis

- Duration: acute (presenting within hours to days) or chronic (persisting for weeks or longer)
- Number of joints involved: monarticular, oligoarticular (2–4 joints), or polyarticular (5 joints or more)
- If more than one joint is involved: symmetric or asymmetric; additive or migratory
- Accurate delineation of the involved joints
- Inflammatory or noninflammatory
- Constitutional symptoms
- Extra-articular disease
- Comorbid conditions

commonly presents as hip pain (see Chapter 58). Injection drug use carries the risk of septic arthritis, endocarditis, and infection with hepatitis B, hepatitis C, and human immunodeficiency virus, each of which is associated with rheumatic conditions.

ACUTE ARTHRITIS

Except in cases of trauma, arthritis that is acute in onset is usually inflammatory. Septic arthritis and crystal-induced arthritis typically have an acute onset, and patients often present within hours to days after the onset of symptoms. Therefore, these disease processes always

Table 4–2. Fever and Arthritis

- Active infection
  Septic arthritis
  Disseminated gonococcal infection
  Endocarditis
  Acute viral infections
  Mycobacterial
  Fungal
- Not due to active infection
  Systemic lupus erythematosus
  Drug-induced lupus
  Still disease
  Gout
  Pseudogout
  Reactive arthritis (particularly in its early phases)
  Acute rheumatic fever and poststreptococcal arthritis
  Inflammatory bowel disease
  Acute sarcoidosis
  Systemic vasculitis
  Familial Mediterranean fever and other inherited periodic fever syndromes
  Paraneoplastic arthritis

Table 4–3. Rash and Arthritis

- Erythematous maculopapular rash
  Superimposed drug reaction
  Still disease
  Viral syndromes
  Kawasaki disease
  Secondary syphilis
  Chronic meningococcemia
- Urticaria
  Systemic lupus erythematosus (SLE)
  Hypocomplementemic urticarial vasculitis
  Serum sickness
  Acute hepatitis B
  Still disease
  Schnitzler syndrome
- Palpable purpura
  Antineutrophilic cytoplasmic antibody (ANCA)-associated vasculitis
  SLE
  Hypersensitivity vasculitis
  Cryoglobulinemia
  Henoch-Schönlein purpura
  Subacute bacterial endocarditis
- Papulosquamous lesions
  Psoriatic arthritis
  Reactive arthritis
  Discoid lupus
  Subacute cutaneous lupus erythematosus
  Secondary syphilis
- Annular lesions
  Subacute cutaneous lupus erythematosus
  Lyme disease (erythema chronicum migrans)
  Acute rheumatic fever (erythema marginatum)
- Pustular lesions
  Disseminated gonococcal infection
  Pustular psoriasis
  Reactive arthritis (keratoderma blenorrhagicum)
  Behçet disease
  Acne-associated rheumatic syndromes
  Sweet syndrome (also painful papule/nodules)
- Subcutaneous nodular lesions
  Erythema nodosum
    Sarcoidosis
    Inflammatory bowel disease
    Behçet disease
  SLE (lupus profundus)
  Polyarteritis nodosa
  Weber-Christian disease

warrant serious consideration in cases of acute arthritis. Nonetheless, the differential diagnosis of acute arthritis is broad and includes entities such as rheumatoid arthritis and the spondyloarthropathies, that more commonly have a chronic presentation.

ACUTE MONARTHRITIS

 ESSENTIAL FEATURES

- *Septic arthritis is the major diagnostic concern.*
- *Arthrocentesis is the most important diagnostic test.*

Initial Clinical Evaluation

The history and physical examination should determine whether the process is acute (onset over hours to days), involves the joint rather than surrounding tissues or bone, and is truly monarticular. The most common causes of acute monarthritis are infection, crystal-induced arthritis, and trauma (Table 4–4). In cases of suspected trauma it is important to ascertain whether the reported trauma is sufficiently severe to account for the joint findings (patients with new-onset joint effusions often attribute the joint abnormality to incidental bumps, turns, or other minor trauma). The foremost concern in the evaluation of a patient with acute pain and swelling in a single joint not clearly due to trauma is the possibility of a joint space infection.

A. LABORATORY EVALUATION

Arthrocentesis is indicated for all cases of unexplained acute monarthritis. Synovial fluid should be sent for culture (for bacteria, mycobacteria, and fungus), cell count, Gram stain, and examination for crystals by polarized light microscopy. Routine laboratory determinations (eg, complete blood cell count, serum electrolytes and creatinine, and urinalysis) can provide helpful ancillary information. Blood cultures should be obtained if septic arthritis is suspected.

The characteristics of the synovial fluid guide the initial differential diagnosis. Nongonococcal septic arthritis

Table 4–4. Common Causes of Acute Monarthritis

- Bacterial infection of the joint space
  Nongonococcal: especially *Staphylococcus aureus*,
    β-hemolytic streptococci, *Streptococcus
    pneumoniae*, gram-negative organisms
  Gonococcal: often preceded by a migratory
    tenosynovitis or oligoarthritis associated with
    characteristic skin lesions
- Crystal-induced arthritis
  Gout (monosodium urate crystals)
  Pseudogout (calcium pyrophosphate dihydrate crystals)
- Trauma

usually causes synovial fluid WBC counts $> 50,000/\text{mm}^3$ and often generates very high counts ($> 100,000/\text{mm}^3$). The synovial fluid WBC count in gonococcal arthritis is generally lower than in nongonococcal septic arthritis (mean synovial fluid WBC count as low as $34,000/\text{mm}^3$ in some series). Crystal-induced arthritis is also very inflammatory, with synovial fluid WBC counts often $> 50,000/\text{mm}^3$; WBC counts $> 100,000/\text{mm}^3$, however, are uncommon.

Gram staining for bacteria in synovial fluid is relatively insensitive (false-negative rates range from 25–50% for nongonococcal septic arthritis and are substantially higher for gonococcal infections). On the other hand, examination of synovial fluid by polarized light microscopy is a sensitive test for urate crystals. Calcium pyrophosphate dihydrate crystals are somewhat more difficult to visualize due to their weaker birefringence, but their detection should not present difficulties for the experienced observer. Thus the absence of crystals is a strong argument against microcrystalline disease, but a negative Gram stain does not exclude infection. Occasionally infection and microcrystalline disease coexist; therefore the finding of crystals in the synovial fluid does not exclude the possibility of infection.

Properly performed cultures of synovial fluid are a sensitive test for nongonococcal septic arthritis (positive in up to 90% of cases). In contrast, synovial fluid cultures are positive in only 20–50% of cases of gonococcal arthritis, and the diagnosis often depends on culture of *Neisseria gonorrhoeae* from the pharynx, urethra, cervix, or rectum (in aggregate, positive in 80–90%) or in some cases, the response to appropriate antibiotics.

B. IMAGING STUDIES

Radiographs can demonstrate fractures in cases of trauma but usually contribute little to the diagnosis of nontraumatic monarthritis if the process is truly acute. Radiographic evidence of chondrocalcinosis can be seen in cases of pseudogout, and when there have been recurrent attacks of gout, radiographs may reveal erosions characteristic of gout. Occasionally imaging studies can be misleading. For example, radiographs may demonstrate osteoarthritis or other chronic conditions that predispose to the development of septic arthritis but are not the proximal cause of the acute joint inflammation.

Differential Diagnosis

A. INFLAMMATORY MONARTHRITIS

The leading causes of acute inflammatory monarthritis—infection and crystal-induced arthritis—are difficult to differentiate in the absence of synovial fluid analysis and culture. Patients with septic arthritis may be afebrile and may not manifest a peripheral leukocytosis. Conversely, patients with crystal-induced arthritis can have fever and an elevated peripheral blood WBC count. An elevated serum uric acid level does not establish a diagnosis of gout, and patients with gout can have a normal serum uric acid level at the time of an acute attack.

Septic arthritis indicates the presence of a potentially life-threatening infection and requires prompt treatment with appropriate antibiotics. Delay in the treatment of nongonococcal septic arthritis also can cause substantial morbidity due to the rapid destruction of articular cartilage. Therefore, acute inflammatory monarthritis should be considered septic arthritis until there is compelling evidence either against bacterial infection or in favor of an alternative diagnosis.

The differential diagnosis of acute inflammatory monarthritis not due to septic arthritis, gout, or pseudogout is broad. Many of these entities more commonly present as subacute or chronic processes (see below). Diseases that are typically oligoarticular or polyarticular, such as the spondyloarthropathies, rheumatoid arthritis, and adult-onset Still disease, occasionally begin as an inflammatory monarthritis.

B. NONINFLAMMATORY MONARTHRITIS

Noninflammatory synovial fluid can be seen with internal derangements (ie, torn meniscus of the knee). Osteoarthritis of a single joint usually presents with chronic complaints, but on occasion can cause the acute onset of pain. Similarly, neuropathic arthropathy, amyloidosis, and osteonecrosis usually cause chronic noninflammatory arthritis of one or several joints, but occasionally present with acute symptoms.

C. HEMARTHROSIS

Frank blood on arthrocentesis can be indicative of a fracture or other joint trauma. Hemarthrosis also occurs in patients who are on anticoagulant therapy or have a clotting factor deficiency such as hemophilia. Bloody synovial fluid can be seen in pigmented villonodular synovitis, a rare proliferative disorder of the synovium that presents as a chronic monarthritis, typically of the knee, in young adulthood.

ACUTE OLIGOARTHRITIS

 ESSENTIAL FEATURES

- *Disseminated gonococcal infection, nongonococcal septic arthritis, and the spondyloarthropathies are leading causes of acute inflammatory oligoarthritis.*
- *Arthrocentesis and appropriate cultures are important diagnostic tests.*

Table 4–5. Differential Diagnosis of Acute Inflammatory Oligoarthritis

- Infection
    Disseminated gonococcal infection[a]
    Nongonococcal septic arthritis
    Bacterial endocarditis[b]
    Viral[c]
- Postinfection
    Reactive arthritis[b]
    Rheumatic fever (poststreptococcal arthritis)[d]
- Spondyloarthropathy
    Reactive arthritis[b]
    Ankylosing spondylitis[b]
    Psoriatic arthritis[b]
    Inflammatory bowel disease[b]
- Oligoarticular presentation of rheumatoid arthritis, systemic lupus erythematosus,[a] adult-onset Still Disease, relapsing polychondritis,[a] or other polyarthritis
- Gout and pseudogout

[a]Often migratory.
[b]Can be associated with back pain.
[c]Usually causes polyarthritis but occasionally oligoarticular and sometimes noninflammatory.
[d]Migratory in children but usually not in adults.

Initial Clinical Evaluation

Acute oligoarthritis is usually due to an inflammatory process (Table 4–5). Infectious causes of the arthritis need to be ruled out. Disseminated gonococcal infection is the most common cause of acute oligoarthritis in sexually active young people. Nongonococcal septic arthritis is usually monarticular but involves more than one joint in up to 20% of cases.

Spondyloarthropathies typically cause an asymmetric oligoarthritis. Of these, reactive arthritis is most likely to present with acute onset of arthritis, and early in its course can be difficult to distinguish from disseminated gonococcal infection.

The use of four joints as a dividing line between oligoarthritis and polyarthritis is somewhat arbitrary, and there is overlap between disorders that cause oligoarthritis and polyarthritis. For example, rheumatoid arthritis can be oligoarticular in its early stages. Parvovirus B19 infection usually causes a true polyarthritis but on occasion produces an oligoarthritis. Conversely, many of the entities listed in Table 4–5 sometimes involve more than four joints.

A. LABORATORY EVALUATION

Complete blood cell count, serum electrolytes and creatinine, and urinalysis should be obtained. Analysis and culture of the synovial fluid are critical in the evaluation of acute oligoarthritis. The pharynx, urethra, cervix, and rectum—even when asymptomatic—should be cultured for *N gonorrhoeae,* and urethral and cervical swabs should be performed for *Chlamydia.* If bacterial endocarditis is a possibility, at least three blood cultures should be obtained, and a transesophageal echocardiogram may be indicated. Antibodies to streptococcal antigens (eg, streptolysin O) should be determined in cases of suspected acute rheumatic fever or poststreptococcal arthritis. The presence of antibodies to cyclic citrullinated peptides (CCP) is a strong predictor of evolution to rheumatoid arthritis but has limited sensitivity (~50%) in the early stages of the disease.

B. IMAGING STUDIES

Radiographs usually are of little help if the onset of the oligoarthritis is truly acute.

Differential Diagnosis

Disseminated gonococcal infection usually presents as a migratory tenosynovitis, often with characteristic skin lesions; meningococcemia can cause a similar syndrome but is much less common. Bacterial endocarditis can cause an oligoarthritis with either septic joints (due to hematogenous spread) or sterile inflammatory synovial fluid (likely due to immune complex disease); back pain is common, particularly in acute bacterial endocarditis. Reactive arthritis classically follows within 1–4 weeks of enteric or genitourinary infections, but the triggering infection is sometimes subclinical. In its presenting phase, reactive arthritis can be associated with significant constitutional signs and symptoms including prominent weight loss and fever. Most patients with the new onset of psoriatic arthritis either have, or have had, psoriasis, but in a minority (15%), the arthritis precedes the skin disease. Acute rheumatic fever produces a migratory arthritis in children; in adults, however, poststreptococcal arthritis is usually not migratory and is rarely associated with the other distinctive manifestations of rheumatic fever (eg, rash, subcutaneous nodules, carditis, and chorea) (see Chapter 52). Early disseminated Lyme disease can cause an acute oligoarthritis or monarthritis (especially of the knee), but more commonly presents as migratory arthralgias.

ACUTE POLYARTHRITIS

 ESSENTIAL FEATURES

- *Viral infections and rheumatoid arthritis are the leading causes of acute polyarthritis.*

- *Observation to distinguish persistent from self-limited polyarthritis is critical.*

Initial Clinical Evaluation

Viral polyarthritis typically resolves over days to a few weeks. Thus the longer polyarthritis persists, the less likely viral polyarthritis becomes. Rheumatoid arthritis usually has an insidious onset and presents to the physician after weeks or months of symptoms. Nonetheless, it begins abruptly in a sizeable minority of patients. Acute polyarthritis also can be the initial manifestation of SLE and a variety of uncommon entities, including systemic vasculitis (Table 4–6).

A. LABORATORY EVALUATION

The clinical setting should guide the decision to send tests for specific viral infections (eg, parvovirus B19 or hepatitis B). If viral polyarthritis is thought unlikely, then routine laboratory studies (including complete blood cell count, serum electrolytes and creatinine, liver function tests, and urinalysis), determinations of the ESR or CRP, and tests for serum rheumatoid factor, antibodies to CCP, and antinuclear antibodies (ANA) are indicated.

B. IMAGING STUDIES

Joint radiographs are rarely of value in acute polyarthritis and may be deferred until it is clear that the polyarthritis is persistent.

Differential Diagnosis

Many acute viral infections cause joint symptoms, with polyarthralgias being considerably more common than

Table 4–6. Differential Diagnosis of Acute Polyarthritis

- Common
    - Acute viral infections
    - Early disseminated Lyme disease
    - Rheumatoid arthritis
    - Systemic lupus erythematosus
- Uncommon or rare
    - Paraneoplastic polyarthritis
    - Remitting seronegative symmetrical synovitis with pitting edema (RS3PE)
    - Acute sarcoidosis, usually with erythema nodosum and hilar adenopathy
    - Adult-onset Still disease
    - Secondary syphilis
    - Systemic autoimmune diseases and vasculitides
    - Whipple disease

true polyarthritis. The prevalence of polyarthritis is high, however, in adults acutely infected with parvovirus B19. The pattern of viral polyarthritis often mimics that of rheumatoid arthritis. Adults acutely infected with parvovirus B19, the cause of "slapped cheek fever" in children, usually have only a faint rash on the trunk or no rash at all. IgM antibodies to parvovirus B19 are generally present at the onset of joint symptoms and persist for approximately 2 months. Acute hepatitis B causes an immune-complex–mediated arthritis, often with urticaria or maculopapular rash, during the preicteric phase of infection; tests for hepatitis B surface antigen are positive. Effective vaccination programs in the United States have substantially reduced the incidence of acute hepatitis B and have eliminated acute rubella infection, which also is associated with acute polyarthritis.

Acute-onset rheumatoid arthritis can be difficult to distinguish from virally induced acute polyarthritis, and many rheumatologists are hesitant to make a diagnosis of rheumatoid arthritis in the acute setting. Rheumatoid factor and anti-CCP have similar sensitivities (~50%) in early rheumatoid arthritis, but the specificity of anti-CCP antibodies is superior. The presence of anti-CCP antibodies is a strong predictor of progression to rheumatoid arthritis in patients with undifferentiated arthritis of recent onset (see Chapter 3).

Testing for ANA is essentially 100% sensitive for SLE but has low specificity. In a patient with polyarthritis or polyarthralgias, a positive assay for ANA should prompt a careful evaluation for other manifestations of SLE and additional serological tests (see Chapters 3 and 22).

CHRONIC MONARTHRITIS

 ESSENTIAL FEATURES

- *Distinguishing between inflammatory and noninflammatory arthritis is a key step toward establishing a diagnosis.*
- *Arthrocentesis and imaging studies are important diagnostic tests.*

Initial Clinical Evaluation

It is important to determine whether the symptoms and signs point to an inflammatory or noninflammatory process. Indolent infections are a concern with inflammatory monarthritis of weeks to even months in duration. The particular joint involved influences the differential diagnosis.

A. LABORATORY EVALUATION

A critical step is to determine whether the monarthritis is inflammatory or noninflammatory, preferably by analysis of synovial fluid. Synovial fluid should be sent for culture (for bacteria, mycobacteria, and fungus), cell count, and Gram stain, and should be examined for crystals by polarized light microscopy.

Routine laboratory studies (eg, complete blood cell count, serum electrolytes and creatinine, and urinalysis) and determinations of the ESR and CRP can provide helpful ancillary information. Patients with inflammatory monarthritis and negative bacterial cultures should be tested for Lyme disease and for reactivity to purified protein derivative.

B. IMAGING STUDIES

In contrast to acute monarthritis, radiographs can be helpful in the evaluation of processes present for weeks or more and can point to the correct diagnosis in cases of infection, osteoarthritis, osteonecrosis, neuropathic joints, and other entities.

Differential Diagnosis

A. INFLAMMATORY

A wide range of disease processes can cause inflammatory arthritis in a single joint for several weeks or longer (Table 4–7). Most patients with septic arthritis and gonococcal arthritis experience significant pain in the infected joint and seek medical attention within hours to days of the onset of symptoms. However, patients occasionally will present after a delay of several weeks, particularly if symptoms have been partially masked by the use of nonsteroidal anti-inflammatory drugs, antibiotics, or glucocorticoids (systemic or intra-articular).

Untreated indolent infections, on the other hand, commonly present after weeks or more of symptoms. These are associated with negative synovial fluid cultures for bacteria and require additional diagnostic tests and cultures to establish the correct diagnosis. Chronic Lyme disease can cause an inflammatory monarthritis, often of the knee, with synovial fluid WBC typically in the 10,000–25,000/mm^3 range. Tuberculous infection of a joint can present after days, weeks, or months of symptoms. Smears for acid-fast bacilli are positive in only 20% of cases; cultures for mycobacteria are positive in 80% but take weeks. Synovial biopsy can greatly expedite the diagnosis of tuberculous arthritis and is also indicated in suspected cases of fungal arthritis.

B. NONINFLAMMATORY

Osteoarthritis is the leading cause of chronic noninflammatory monarthritis, particularly when the hip, knee, first carpometacarpal joint, or acromioclavicular joint is

Table 4–7. Differential Diagnosis of Chronic Inflammatory Monarthritis

- Infection
  Nongonococcal septic arthritis
  Gonococcal
  Lyme disease and other spirochetal infections
  Mycobacterial
  Fungal
  Viral[a]
- Crystal-induced arthritis
  Gout
  Pseudogout
  Calcium apatite crystals[b]
- Monarticular presentation of an oligoarthritis or polyarthritis
  Spondyloarthropathy
  Rheumatoid arthritis
  Lupus and other systemic autoimmune diseases
- Sarcoidosis[a]
- Uncommon or rare
  Familial Mediterranean fever and other inherited periodic
    fever syndromes
  Amyloidosis[a]
  Foreign-body synovitis due to plant thorns, sea urchin
    spikes, wood fragments, etc
  Pigmented villonodular synovitis[c]

[a]Also can cause noninflammatory synovial fluid.
[b]Not detected by polarized light microscopy.
[c]Commonly associated with bloody, or blood-tinged
  brown, synovial fluid.

involved (Table 4–8). Internal derangements, such as a torn meniscus in the knee, often produce mechanical symptoms and characteristic findings on physical examination (see Chapter 12). Pain is frequently a prominent feature of osteonecrosis, which can produce large knee effusions when the distal femur is involved. Radiographs

Table 4–8. Differential Diagnosis of Chronic Noninflammatory Monarthritis

- Osteoarthritis
- Internal derangements (eg, torn meniscus)[a]
- Chondromalacia patellae[a]
- Osteonecrosis[a]
- Uncommon or rare
  Neuropathic (Charcot) arthropathy
  Sarcoidosis[a, b]
  Amyloidosis[a, b]

[a]Radiography of the affected joint often normal at
  presentation.
[a]Also can cause inflammatory synovial fluid.

are often normal early in the course of osteonecrosis, and diagnosis may require magnetic resonance imaging. Hip pain with a normal radiograph should raise the possibility of early osteonecrosis, particularly if the patient is relatively young and has a risk factor for osteonecrosis (see Chapter 58). Diabetes mellitus is the most common underlying cause of neuropathic arthropathy, which should be considered in a diabetic patient with foot, ankle, or knee arthritis. The involved joint may be warm and painful, but the joint fluid is typically noninflammatory. Radiographs usually show characteristic neuropathic changes.

CHRONIC OLIGOARTHRITIS

 ESSENTIAL FEATURES

- *Careful delineation of the arthritis and detection of extra-articular disease facilitate accurate diagnosis.*
- *Radiographs are often of diagnostic value.*

Initial Clinical Evaluation

Spondyloarthropathies are the most common cause of chronic inflammatory oligoarthritis (Table 4–9). For months or longer, however, it may be difficult to distinguish spondyloarthropathies from early-onset rheumatoid arthritis. Osteoarthritis commonly presents as a noninflammatory oligoarthritis of the hips or knees and usually does not present diagnostic difficulties.

A. Laboratory Evaluation

Synovial fluid should be analyzed for crystals and cultured. The distinction between inflammatory and noninflammatory chronic oligoarthritis often can be made on clinical grounds but is confirmed by the synovial fluid WBC count.

A positive test for serum rheumatoid factor, although not a specific test for rheumatoid arthritis, can help to establish the diagnosis in the proper clinical context. Antibodies to CCP have sensitivity similar to rheumatoid factor but greater specificity. Testing for HLA-B27 has utility in certain circumstances.

B. Imaging Studies

Radiographs can be of considerable value. An experienced radiologist or rheumatologist often can distinguish among the erosions of the spondyloarthropathies,

Table 4–9. Differential Diagnosis of Chronic Oligoarthritis

- Inflammatory causes
  - Common
    - Spondyloarthropathy
      - Reactive arthritis[a]
      - Ankylosing spondylitis[a]
      - Psoriatic arthritis[a]
      - Inflammatory bowel disease[a]
    - Atypical presentation of rheumatoid arthritis
    - Gout
  - Uncommon or rare
    - Subacute bacterial endocarditis
    - Sarcoidosis[b]
    - Behçet's disease
    - Relapsing polychondritis
    - Celiac disease[a]
- Noninflammatory causes
  - Common
    - Osteoarthritis
  - Uncommon or rare
    - Hypothyroidism
    - Amyloidosis

[a]Can be associated with involvement of the axial skeleton.
[b]Can be a migratory arthritis and have either inflammatory or noninflammatory synovial fluid.

rheumatoid arthritis, and gout. Radiographic demonstration of sacroiliitis points to a spondyloarthropathy and narrows the differential diagnosis considerably.

Differential Diagnosis

Although spondyloarthropathies typically cause an asymmetrical oligoarthritis and rheumatoid arthritis is usually a symmetrical polyarthritis, it can be difficult to differentiate these entities in patients with early disease. Several features are helpful in making this distinction. Ankylosing spondylitis always, and the other spondyloarthropathies often, produce inflammatory axial skeleton disease with sacroiliitis that causes pain and stiffness in the low back, particularly in the morning (see Table 4–9). Sacroiliitis is not a feature of rheumatoid arthritis, which involves the cervical spine but no other part of the axial skeleton. The prominent tenosynovitis of the spondyloarthropathies can produce dactylitis ("sausage digits") of the toes or fingers. Dactylitis is not seen in rheumatoid arthritis. (Dactylitis is not specific for the spondyloarthropathies; it also occurs in sarcoidosis and gout.) Reactive arthritis and the arthritis of inflammatory bowel disease have a predilection for the lower extremities. Rheumatoid arthritis invariably involves the hands, and >90% of cases eventually have wrist arthritis.

Many of the entities that cause chronic oligoarthritis have extra-articular manifestations that point to the correct diagnosis but that are easily overlooked. For example, psoriasis may be subtle, and the patient may be unaware of psoriatic lesions, particularly in the umbilicus, the external auditory canal, the scalp, and the anal cleft. The oral ulcers of reactive arthritis are painless and usually not detected unless specifically sought by the examining physician. Patients with inflammatory bowel disease may not volunteer that they have chronic diarrhea, particularly if bowel symptoms are intermittent. Antecedent anterior uveitis can be an important clue to the presence of a spondyloarthropathy, but patients generally do not associate ocular inflammation with arthritis and may not mention a past episode of anterior uveitis unless asked directly.

CHRONIC POLYARTHRITIS

 ESSENTIAL FEATURES

- *Rheumatoid arthritis and osteoarthritis are the leading causes of chronic polyarthritis.*
- *Careful delineation of the joints involved, particularly in the hands, can help point to the correct diagnosis.*

Initial Clinical Evaluation

Rheumatoid arthritis is the leading cause of chronic inflammatory polyarthritis, and osteoarthritis is the most common cause of chronic noninflammatory polyarthritis. Nonetheless, polyarthritis that persists for weeks or more has many possible etiologies and warrants careful diagnostic evaluation (Table 4–10). As is the case with other forms of arthritis, the distinction between inflammatory and noninflammatory processes is critical.

A. LABORATORY EVALUATION

If arthrocentesis is feasible, synovial fluid should be obtained and sent for cell count and analysis for crystals. Routine laboratory investigations (complete blood cell count, serum electrolytes and creatinine, and urinalysis) should be done. If the process appears inflammatory, studies also should include determinations of the ESR or CRP and tests for serum rheumatoid factor, anti-CCP antibodies, ANA, and hepatitis B and C.

B. IMAGING STUDIES

Radiographs are indicated in most cases of chronic polyarthritis of the hand. Radiographs of the hand usually

Table 4–10. Differential Diagnosis of Chronic Polyarthritis

Inflammatory polyarthritis
- Common
  Rheumatoid arthritis
  Systemic lupus erythematosus
  Spondyloarthropathies (especially psoriatic arthritis)
  Chronic hepatitis C infection
  Gout
  Drug-induced lupus syndromes
- Uncommon or rare
  Paraneoplastic polyarthritis
  Remitting seronegative symmetrical synovitis with
    pitting edema (RS3PE)
  Adult-onset Still disease
  Systemic autoimmune diseases and vasculitides
  Sjögren syndrome
  Viral infections other than hepatitis C
  Whipple disease

Noninflammatory polyarthritis
  Primary generalized osteoarthritis
  Hemochromatosis
  Calcium pyrophosphate deposition disease

show characteristic changes at the time of presentation of primary generalized osteoarthritis, hemochromatosis, calcium pyrophosphate deposition disease, and chronic tophaceous gout. In cases of rheumatoid arthritis and the spondyloarthropathies, however, the likelihood of radiographic joint erosions and other characteristic findings increases with the duration of the polyarthritis; hand radiographs may be normal, or demonstrate nonspecific changes only, for months or longer. Radiographs of the feet can reveal rheumatoid erosions even when hand films are unrevealing. The polyarthritis of SLE, drug-induced lupus, and chronic hepatitis C is usually non-erosive and does not produce characteristic radiographic findings.

Differential Diagnosis

Osteoarthritis and rheumatoid arthritis have different patterns of joint involvement in the hand. Osteoarthritis involves the distal interphalangeal (DIP) and proximal interphalangeal (PIP) joints and the first carpometacarpal joint. Rheumatoid arthritis, in contrast, involves the PIPs, the metacarpophalangeal (MCP) joints, and the wrists.

Osteoarthritis and rheumatoid arthritis typically spare certain joints. Osteoarthritis usually does not involve the MCP joints, wrists, elbows, glenohumeral joints, or ankles; degenerative arthritis of these joints raises the pos-sibility of antecedent trauma, calcium pyrophosphate deposition disease, underlying osteonecrosis, or neuropathic arthropathy. Rheumatoid arthritis usually spares DIP joints, the thoracic and lumbosacral spine, and sacroiliac joints.

In generalized osteoarthritis, interphalangeal joints, particularly the DIPs, may appear to be inflamed ("inflammatory osteoarthritis") and thus cause some diagnostic uncertainty. Radiographs, however, usually show typical degenerative changes (irregular joint space narrowing, sclerosis, and osteophytes). Psoriatic arthritis also commonly involves the DIP joints, usually with radiographic changes distinct from those of osteoarthritis. Psoriatic changes of the fingernail on the same digit often occur concomitantly with psoriatic involvement of a DIP joint.

Many diseases can mimic rheumatoid arthritis, but several warrant particular emphasis (Table 4–11). Features that distinguish rheumatoid arthritis and the spondyloarthropathies are discussed above. Chronic infection with hepatitis C is associated with a symmetrical polyarthritis and a positive test for rheumatoid factor (but not for anti-CCP antibodies). The polyarthritis of SLE is non-erosive but can lead to reducible swan-neck deformities of the fingers. On occasion chronic tophaceous gout is a remarkable mimic of rheumatoid arthritis, with tophi mistaken for rheumatoid nodules. Gout is not associated with rheumatoid factor (virtually all cases of nodular rheumatoid arthritis are seropositive), and the erosions of gout and rheumatoid arthritis have different radiographic characteristics. Analysis of synovial

Table 4–11. Some Mimics of Chronic Rheumatoid Arthritis

- Arthritis with radiographic erosions
  Spondyloarthropathies, especially psoriatic arthritis
  Gout
- Arthritis with positive rheumatoid factor
  Chronic hepatitis C infection
  Systemic lupus erythematosus
  Sarcoidosis
  Systemic vasculitides
  Polymyositis/dermatomyositis
  Subacute bacterial endocarditis
- Arthritis with nodules
  Chronic tophaceous gout
  Wegener granulomatosis
  Churg-Strauss syndrome
  Hyperlipoproteinemia (rare)
  Multicentric reticulohistiocytosis (rare)
- Arthritis of metacarpophalangeal joints and/or wrists
  Hemochromatosis
  Calcium pyrophosphate deposition disease

fluid for urate crystals is the definitive diagnostic test. Hemochromatosis and other causes of calcium pyrophosphate deposition disease lead to arthritis of the MCPs (especially the second and third) and wrists; radiographs often reveal hooklike osteophytes of the MCPs and degenerative changes, usually with chondrocalcinosis, of the wrist.

Although rheumatoid arthritis is the leading cause of chronic inflammatory polyarthritis, physicians must be certain that rheumatoid arthritis accounts for the full clinical picture. Rheumatoid arthritis is not a plausible explanation for the following: fever >38.3°C, substantial weight loss, significant adenopathy, rashes (apart from subcutaneous nodules), hematuria, and proteinuria. Failure to account for these additional clinical findings can lead to a failure to diagnose SLE, Still disease, subacute bacterial endocarditis, paraneoplastic syndromes, vasculitides, and the like.

REFERENCES

Baker DG, Schumacher HR. Acute monoarthritis. *N Engl J Med.* 1993;329:1013. (Thorough discussion of the differential diagnosis and evaluation of acute monarthritis.)

Pinals RS. Polyarthritis and fever. *N Engl J Med.* 1994;330:769. (Clinically useful guide to the important problem of fever in the setting of arthritis.)

van Gaalen FA, Linn-Rasker SP, van Venrooij WJ, et al. Autoantibodies to cyclic citrullinated peptides predict progression to rheumatoid arthritis in patients with undifferentiated arthritis: a prospective cohort study. *Arthritis Rheum.* 2004;50:709. (The presence of anti-CCP antibodies was the best predictor of progression to RA in this prospective study of a large cohort of patients with undifferentiated arthritis of recent onset.)

Approach to the Adolescent with Arthritis

5

Peggy Schlesinger, MD

 ESSENTIAL FEATURES

- *Inflammatory and noninflammatory conditions can cause joint pain in adolescents.*
- *Appropriate therapy for adolescents with arthritis requires attention to their developmental needs and discussion of school and vocational issues.*

GENERAL CONSIDERATIONS

There are many causes of joint pain occurring in childhood and adolescence (Table 5–1). Diagnostic accuracy is very important to ensure that the patient receives appropriate treatment.

The first step in evaluating a young patient who presents with musculoskeletal discomfort is to begin by distinguishing between **arthritis** with true synovitis and joint swelling and **arthralgia** or pain in and around joints. Pain in and around the joints without synovitis is usually caused by trauma, mechanical factors, or soft tissue syndromes. Excruciating joint pain and swelling, often with erythema, may indicate malignancy. A careful history of recent infections and exposures, as well as immunizations, can highlight possible infection-related causes of joint swelling and pain in the adolescent age group. Chronic childhood arthritis is one of the five most common chronic diseases of childhood, occurring with a frequency greater than diabetes or cystic fibrosis. Juvenile idiopathic arthritis (JIA), including psoriatic arthritis and the spondyloarthropathies of childhood, is the most common cause of chronic arthritis in childhood and adolescence.

EVALUATION

The initial evaluation of an adolescent with rheumatic disease includes a complete history and physical examination. In this age group, special attention should be paid to these issues:

- Age at menarche
- Is the patient skeletally mature? (A rough guide: is shoe size changing with every new pair?)
- Is the patient sexually active?
- Have there been prolonged or recurrent school absences?
- Are there barriers at school that make participation or attendance difficult?
- Has there been uninterrupted participation in physical education?
- Is there a history of participation in athletics?
- In what way does the patient make accommodations to compensate for arthritis symptoms (ie, wearing elastic waist sweat pants instead of jeans with buttons and zippers or avoiding going to the bathroom at school because of difficulty getting on and off the toilet)?
- Does the patient have a best friend with whom to share arthritis issues?
- Is there a receptive teacher or school counselor to contact if a Section 504 or individualized education plan is needed?
- Have vocational and career goals been identified?
- Has a disability/Supplemental Security Income application been filed?

JUVENILE IDIOPATHIC ARTHRITIS

Juvenile idiopathic arthritis (JIA) is a heterogeneous group of seven different disorders, all of which can cause persistent synovitis lasting 6 weeks or longer in patients younger than 17 years of age. The seven types of JIA are systemic onset (Still disease), enthesitis-related arthritis (ERA), psoriatic arthritis, oligoarticular arthritis, polyarticular seronegative arthritis, polyarticular seropositive arthritis, and "other." The systemic-onset, ERA and polyarticular seropositive subgroups are more commonly seen in the adolescent age group. The diagnosis of JIA is based on clinical criteria: the age of the child, the number and type of joints involved, and the presence of associated

Table 5–1. Differential Diagnosis of Arthritis in Adolescents

Infection-related	Metabolic/genetic
Lyme disease	Cystic fibrosis
Septic arthritis	Diabetes
Gonococcal arthritis	Sickle cell disease
Parvovirus	**Connective tissue**
Mononucleosis	**diseases**
Cytomegalovirus	Systemic lupus
Human immunodeficiency	erythematosus
virus	Dermatomyositis
Varicella	Mixed connective tissue
Endocarditis	disease
Streptococcal-associated	Sarcoid
arthritis	Vasculitis
Acute rheumatic fever	**Noninflammatory**
Hepatitis B and C	**conditions**
Toxic synovitis	Chondromalacia patella
Malignancy	Hypermobility syndrome
Bone tumors	Avascular necrosis
Leukemia	Skeletal dysplasias
Lymphoma	Slipped capital femoral
Neuroblastoma	epiphysis
Juvenile idiopathic	Osgood-Schlatter disease
arthritis (JIA)	Sever disease
Polyarticular JIA	Scheuermann disease
Systemic-onset JIA	Osteochondritis dissecans
Oligoarticular JIA	Synovial chondromatosis
(recurrent)	Synovial hemangioma
Psoriatic arthritis	Pigmented villonodular
Enthesitis-related	synovitis
arthritis (ERA)	
Arthritis of inflammatory	
bowel disease	
Reactive arthritis	
Juvenile-onset spondylitis	

symptoms such as rash, fever, or iritis. The subgroup of JIA is determined by the pattern of the illness during the first 6 months of symptoms. Laboratory and x-ray testing are helpful to rule out other possible causes of arthritis in children. There is no definitive lab test or x-ray finding that can confirm the diagnosis of JIA. For a detailed review of JIA, please see Chapter 21.

INFECTIONS

Rubella, mononucleosis, hepatitis B and C, and varicella infections have all been associated with transient joint swelling (<6 weeks) and should be considered in the differential diagnosis of arthritis in this age group (see Table 5–1). Immunization for varicella and the vaccine for measles, mumps, and rubella may be given to teenagers who did not receive their full complement of vaccinations as children. Vaccination with these attenuated viruses has also been associated with transient arthritis symptoms.

Parvovirus infection in the older child can cause fever and large joint polyarthritis with a morbilliform rash. Lyme disease, caused by *Borrelia burgdorferi,* can initially present with a rash followed by migratory, large joint arthritis. It is important to distinguish Lyme disease from JIA so that proper antibiotic therapy can be given. Although rheumatic fever is rarely seen anymore, the syndrome of streptococcal-associated arthritis is much more common and usually self-limited. Adolescents with antecedent streptococcal infection can develop true synovitis within 7–10 days as a result of the molecular mimicry involved in the immune response to their streptococcal infection. In streptococcal-associated arthritis, the chorea and carditis of rheumatic fever are absent, and joint symptoms resolve completely, but can recur with subsequent streptococcal infections.

Bloody diarrheal illnesses caused by *Campylobacter, Salmonella, Shigella, Yersinia,* and toxigenic *Escherichia coli* can be associated with postinfectious reactive arthritis in HLA-B27–positive teens. Sexually active teens may contract *Chlamydia* infection, which has also been associated with a reactive arthritis pattern, or gonococcal infection with immune complex–mediated vasculitis and arthritis.

MECHANICAL MIMICS

Noninflammatory conditions can cause joint pain and swelling in the adolescent patient that can mimic arthritis and be confusing diagnostically. The hallmark of this group of disorders is pain that worsens with activity in the absence of signs and symptoms of inflammation. Chondromalacia, Osgood-Schlatter disease, osteochondritis dissecans, Sever disease, Scheuermann disease, slipped capital femoral epiphysis, and hypermobility syndromes represent the most common causes of noninflammatory joint pain in this age group.

Chondromalacia patellae, or patellofemoral syndrome, is commonly seen in teenage girls as a cause of unilateral or bilateral knee pain that worsens with activity. Any activity that involves weight bearing on a bent knee can aggravate the pain of this condition. Climbing stairs, using the clutch in a car, standing up after prolonged sitting, participation in gym class, and competitive athletic activities can be particularly troublesome. A minority of girls with chondromalacia patellae (approximately 10%) will have knee swelling in addition to knee pain, and even fewer of these patients will have persistent knee swelling lasting more than 6 weeks. When this does occur, chondromalacia patellae is easily confused with JIA.

The diagnosis of chondromalacia patellae is confirmed by a positive patella inhibition test on examination

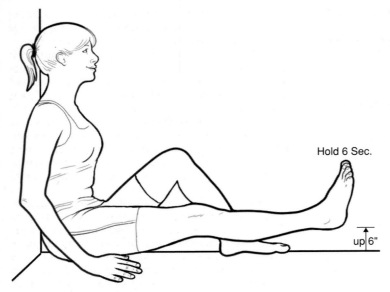

Hold 6 Sec.

up 6"

Figure 5–1. Isometric quadriceps-strengthening exercise.

in the setting of knee pain that worsens with activity, no morning stiffness, and no other affected joints, even in patients with prolonged knee swelling. Isometric quadriceps-strengthening exercises (Figure 5–1) will reduce pain and swelling and allow for a return to normal activity, even if this includes competitive athletics. Nonsteroidal anti-inflammatory drugs (Table 5–2), ice, and occasionally joint injection with 20 mg triamcinolone hexacetonide mixed with 2 mL of a long-acting local anesthetic will help manage the patient's pain and reduce swelling, allowing continued progress in an exercise program. Often knee pain with or without swelling returns when the patient becomes less compliant with the program of regular isometric quadriceps-strengthening exercises. The pain can be a good reminder to teens to make daily quadriceps exercises a part of their routine. Chondromalacia patellae is very common in adolescent girls and the symptoms can last for several years. Despite several years of knee pain as teenagers, the majority of these patients do not develop degenerative patellofemoral joint disease as adults.

Osteochondritis dissecans and Osgood-Schlatter disease are common causes of knee or ankle pain in adolescent boys. In osteochondritis dissecans, a piece of cartilage fractures producing pain and swelling in the affected joint. Knees (femoral condyles) and ankles (dome of the talus) are the most commonly affected joints. There is often a history of trauma to the affected joint, and the recommended treatment is orthopedic consultation. Osgood-Schlatter disease is caused by apophysitis at the patellar tendon insertion on the tibial tubercle with local-

ized pain in this area just below the knee. True synovitis is rare; however, the presence of painful swelling in close proximity to the knee joint can easily be confused with true arthritis.

Sever disease is a syndrome of similar etiology with epiphysitis occurring at the growth plate of the heel. This disorder is commonly seen in soccer players, and treatment may include the use of a heel cup, nonsteroidal anti-inflammatory drugs, and ice. Sever disease is self-limited and unrelated to any of the HLA-B27–related spondyloarthropathies, although the occurrence of heel pain in the adolescent male may be misleading to practitioners.

Joint hypermobility syndrome is familial and can be troublesome in the adolescent. Some teenagers are "double jointed," with ligamentous laxity and freely subluxing shoulders, patellae, and hips. The increased joint range of motion often leads to pain that is aggravated by continued use or repetitive activity, especially when they participate in competitive athletics. Weightlifting and strength training can help offset the tendency toward subluxation in these patients by using tight, bulky muscles to help provide internal stability to the joint. This is particularly helpful for shoulder and knee joints, where increasing muscle bulk and tone in the rotator cuff mechanism and the quadriceps can help reduce pain and bring useful joint excursion back to normal levels.

Slipped capital femoral epiphysis is a common cause of hip pain in teenage boys. Typically, the adolescent will complain of groin pain or referred pain in the knee that worsens with activity. Obesity is a predisposing factor in the development of this idiopathic disorder. Once the

Table 5–2. Nonsteroidal Anti-inflammatory Drugs (NSAIDs) Used in Pediatric Patients[a]

Drug	Dose	Formulation
Naproxen	20 mg/kg/d 10 mg/kg/dose bid up to 1000 mg/d	Liquid: 125 mg/5 mL Tablet: 220 mg, available over the counter Twice-daily dosing is convenient
Ibuprofen	40 mg/kg/d 10 mg/kg/dose qid up to 2400 mg/d	Liquid: 100 mg/5 mL Tablet: 200 mg, available over the counter
Tolmetin	30 mg/kg/d 10 mg/kg/dose tid up to 1800 mg/d	Tablets: 200, 400, and 600 mg
Indomethacin	1–3 mg/kg/d tid or qid up to 200 mg/d	Liquid: 25 mg/5 mL Approved for patients younger than 14 years old Used in younger patients with systemic-onset JIA or spondylitis
Meloxicam	0.125 mg/kg/d up to 7.5 mg/d	Liquid: 7.5 mg/mL Tablet: 7.5 and 15 mg Once-a-day dosing is convenient

[a] As of this writing, other NSAIDs have not been approved by the Food and Drug Administration for use in the pediatric age group. JIA, juvenile idiopathic arthritis.

diagnosis is made by x-ray, orthopedic consultation should be obtained.

Scheuermann disease, or vertebral apophysitis, can cause back pain in adolescents. It typically involves three contiguous vertebrae with involvement of the end-plates at each level; lower thoracic vertebrae are most commonly affected and thoracic kyphosis can develop in later life. This condition is easily confused with juvenile-onset spondylitis because both can be a cause of back pain in teenagers.

RHEUMATIC DISEASES & SYNDROMES

Other rheumatic syndromes that are well known in adults, such as Raynaud's phenomenon and fibromyalgia, can present initially in adolescence. The majority of teenagers who have Raynaud's phenomenon have no associated rheumatic disease and reassurance regarding the prognosis can be given liberally. Although a positive ANA may be present in these patients, it is not as useful as nail fold capillaroscopy in predicting which patients will go on to develop a systemic rheumatic disease. In young adults with Raynaud's phenomenon, abnormal nail fold capillaroscopy showing the typical pattern of dilation and dropout of capillary loops has been strongly correlated with the development of systemic disease, either progressive systemic sclerosis or juvenile dermatomyositis. Normal nail fold capillaries are seen in adolescents with Raynaud's phenomenon alone, and adolescents with Raynaud's phenomenon in association with other rheumatic diseases.

Treatment of Raynaud's phenomenon is directed at reducing the frequency of vasospastic episodes by keeping the hands and feet warm. Unfortunately, asking teenagers to wear socks and gloves to keep their extremities warm can be as effective as asking them to turn in homework early. Fortunately, treatment with biofeedback, solid fuel hand warmers, and medications such as extended-release niacin, diltiazem, and transdermal nitroglycerin can be used when needed, giving the patient better control over their symptoms.

Sleep issues loom large in adolescence. Teenagers seem to require much more sleep than adults, and also more than younger children do. The growth spurt and pubertal changes at this age are fueled by hormones such as growth hormone that are secreted in a circadian rhythm with the highest output during the night. Sleep disorders can present in early adolescence with fibromyalgialike arthralgias and myalgias. The good news is that these symptoms are amenable to therapeutic intervention. Treatment with low-dose amitriptyline at 10–30 mg qhs or cyclobenzaprine 10–30 mg qhs can correct a nonrestorative sleep pattern. Once the sleep cycle has been reset, a gradually increasing exercise program will help build specific muscle strength and improve endurance, thus allowing the patient to return to normal activity. As in adults, the disability from this fibromyalgialike syndrome can be extreme; however, with proper treatment the outlook for a return to normal activity is excellent.

Regional pain syndromes and soft tissue rheumatism present special challenges when they occur in the adolescent age group. Treatment is focused on returning the patient to normal activity as quickly as possible and addressing the accompanying psychosocial issues that can complicate recovery.

Systemic lupus erythematosus can present in adolescence and cause arthritis in this age group. The incidence of systemic lupus erythematosus is approximately 2:1 girls:boys before puberty, but 8:1 after puberty. The changing hormonal milieu of teenage girls can be incendiary, causing flares of this disease during these difficult years. Neuropsychiatric involvement with systemic lupus erythematosus can be particularly challenging to diagnose and treat in adolescent girls with frequent mood swings.

Vasculitis including Wegener granulomatosis, microscopic polyangiitis, polyarteritis nodosa, Henoch-Schönlein purpura, and leukocytoclastic vasculitis, among others, are also seen in the adolescent age group with signs and symptoms at presentation very similar to those of the adult form of the disease.

SCHOOL ISSUES

The goal of treatment should be to help the teenager return to normal function, which in most cases involves regular school attendance as well as participation in after-school activities. Under Public Law 94-142, students with disabling conditions are guaranteed access to an education in the public schools and modifications must be made to accomplish this. Modification of the school program may be needed to accomplish the goal of regular attendance. Examples of common modifications that can be done in public school include scheduling core classes later in the day to accommodate morning stiffness, arranging classes all on one level of the building to avoid stairs, offering an adaptive physical education program, and providing an extra set of textbooks to keep at home. The necessary changes can be made on an individual basis or by utilizing the Section 504 or individualized education planning process. Parent advocacy programs are in place in many states to help educate parents on the rights of disabled students, and how to work within the public school system to ensure a quality education for their child.

DEVELOPMENTAL STAGES OF ADOLESCENCE

During the teenage years, the adolescent begins to establish relationships outside the family, with the ultimate goal of achieving independence from the nuclear family. In the process, teenagers deconstruct and reconstruct their self-image, finding an identity that encompasses their new experiences. During this period, the parents' roles change from primary caregivers to advocates, allowing and encouraging more independence in their offspring.

It is important that these changes be incorporated into the medical setting as well. Adolescents want to be taken seriously in the physician-patient encounter. The adolescent may be more comfortable transitioning to an internal medicine physician for their primary care rather than their previous pediatric caregiver. They may prefer to see the practitioner by themselves, without a parent present. The physician can use this time alone with the young person to talk over feelings about many sensitive subjects such as body image concerns, sexuality, worries about the future, and the impact of their disability on everyday activities. Parents must be heard as well, often in a separate session, so that the physician has an accurate picture of the situation as a whole. Parental concerns can overwhelm both the patient and the physician; parents tend to be overprotective toward teens with chronic illnesses. Opportunities will arise when the physician can point out to parents how appropriately their teenager is responding to his or her illness. This will help parents begin to see their teenagers as capable managers of their illness. Camps for children of all ages with arthritis are another good place to encourage independence and appropriate self-care, while also building self-esteem.

The task of the adolescent is to put together a healthy self-concept as they near adulthood, ideally one that incorporates their illness but is not solely defined by it. They must also take on the responsibility of caring for themselves and their disease. The physician's role is to encourage this development in the adolescent patient, while helping parents evolve comfortably into a secondary role by pointing out examples when the patient is responding appropriately and by modeling encouragement for such behaviors. For a time it may feel as if there are two patients in the family—the adolescent and the parents—until such time as the adolescent can feel comfortable in the role of primary caregiver. This transition is absolutely necessary if the patient is to become an effective advocate for themselves and a responsible member of the healing partnership.

VOCATIONAL ISSUES

In addition to the transition from adolescence to adulthood, the teenager must navigate the road from high school to post-secondary education and the world of employment. There are approximately 200 transition-planning programs in this country that address the vocational needs of teens with chronic and potentially disabling conditions, but they cannot reach everyone who needs assistance. Vocational rehabilitation services can begin career counseling and the employment identification process with teens during their senior year in high school. Case management services may continue, depending on whether or not the patient qualifies for Social Security disability benefits. Working with the patient to identify specific career goals and individual abilities can help the adolescent focus their studies and make appropriate plans for their future. The assistance of the physician in this area is essential to making this transition to adulthood a success.

REFERENCES

Cassidy JT. *Textbook of Pediatric Rheumatology.* 4th ed. WB Saunders, 2001. (An excellent comprehensive text.)

Isenberg DA, Miller JJ, eds. *Adolescent Rheumatology.* Martin Dunitz, 1999.

McDonagh JE, Southwood TR, Ryder CAJ. Bridging the gap in rheumatology. *Ann Rheum Dis.* 2000;59:86–93.

Tucker LB, Cabral DA. Transition of the adolescent patient with rheumatic disease: Issues to consider. *Pediatr Clin North Am.* 2005;52:641–652. (Entire volume is devoted to childhood rheumatic disease.)

White PH. Success on the road to adulthood. Issues and hurdles for adolescents with disabilities. *Rheum Dis Clin North Am.* 1997;23:697–707.

White PH. Transition: a future promise for children and adolescents with special health care needs and disabilities. *Rheum Dis Clin North Am.* 2002;28:687–703, viii.

The Patient with Hand, Wrist, or Elbow Pain

E. Gene Deune, MD, & Daniel Most, MD

Hand pain is usually due to neurological, musculoskeletal, or vascular causes. An accurate history often distinguishes among these possibilities, and the physical examination frequently reveals findings that support the diagnosis. Diagnostic tests such as nerve conduction studies, electromyography, radiographs, computed tomography, and magnetic resonance imaging (MRI) may be needed to confirm the diagnosis.

TERMINOLOGY

As a general rule, the terminology for the hand and the finger hand should be descriptive rather than numerical. The fingers should be referred to by name: thumb, index finger, long finger, ring finger, and the small finger. Although it is obvious which finger is the fifth finger, it is not uncommon for people to refer to the index finger as the first finger, when the first finger is actually the thumb.

This practice should also be carried to the identification of the bones and joints of the fingers, so that the metacarpals should be referred to as the index metacarpal and the small finger metacarpal rather than the second and the fifth metacarpal. The first metacarpal is the thumb metacarpal. The phalanges of the fingers should be called the proximal, middle, or distal phalanges rather than P1, P2, or P3. The use of terminology with nonnumerical descriptors avoids confusion.

ASSESSMENT OF THE PATIENT

It is important to ascertain the quality of the pain and the presence or absence of other symptoms such as paresthesias. The history should determine the location of the discomfort within the hand and should identify any aggravating or alleviating factors. Other variables, such as the patient's age, occupation, medical and surgical histories, and a history of trauma can also point to the cause of pain.

The intensity of hand pain is subjective and often difficult to gauge. What one patient may perceive as very painful may be only slightly uncomfortable to another. Another difficulty is the absence of uniform vocabulary used by patients to describe discomfort. For example, a patient may use the term "pain" to refer to the absence of sensation rather than the word "numbness."

Cervical spine arthritis with proximal nerve root compression should always be kept in mind as a source of pain referred to the upper extremity (see Chapter 9). Conversely, severe pain in the hand may be referred proximally to the elbow, the axilla, or the neck. Ipsilateral cervical pain may represent protective muscle spasm secondary to the primary process in the hand or arm, or vice versa.

EXAMINATION OF THE HAND

The examination of the hand should be approached carefully, particularly when the patient is in pain. Much information can be gathered simply by observing the patient's hands while taking the history. Note the hand's posture. With the hand at rest, the fingers should be held in a normal cascade; the small finger is flexed slightly more than the ring finger, the ring finger slightly more flexed than the long finger, and the long finger slightly flexed more than the index finger (Figure 6–1). Mechanical processes such as tendon rupture, tendon laceration, or tendon inflammation with triggering can alter this repose cascade. Observe the spontaneous movements of the hands and note the presence or absence of swelling and the color of the hands. Always compare both hands, looking for evidence of asymmetry.

Although it is tempting to touch the part of the hand that is in pain first, it is sometimes more helpful to begin by examining the entire hand as a unit. Ask the patient to flex and extend the fingers and the wrist. Measure any limitations in the range of motion in the joints. Touching the hand gives the examiner a qualitative assessment of vascularity based on the temperature, moistness, and quality of the skin. A general sensory examination of the fingers can be conducted by using the cotton end of a swab for light touch and the snapped end of the wooden handle for sharp pain. Provocative tests (described below) can elicit signs of median nerve compression at the carpal tunnel.

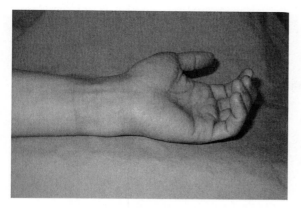

Figure 6–1. Normal repose cascade of the hand.

The Allen test assesses perfusion of the hand by the ulnar and the radial arteries. The examiner holds the patient's distal forearm at the wrist and applies pressure to the patient's radial and ulnar arteries with the thumb and fingers. The patient is asked to flex the fingers as hard as possible three times and then to extend the fingers. The hand should be completely pale. If it is not, the patient should be requested to squeeze once or twice more with continued pressure to both the ulnar and radial arteries. Next, the examiner releases the pressure on the radial artery while maintaining pressure on the ulnar artery. If the radial artery is functional, the fingers and hand will reperfuse and the hand will turn pink within two seconds. The ulnar artery is assessed in the same way, except that pressure is maintained on the radial artery while the pressure is released over the ulnar artery. To avoid confusion in the findings of the Allen test, it is better to describe the results in the patient's chart. "The Allen test was done and it shows the perfusion from the radial and the ulnar arteries to be intact" or "the Allen test was done and it shows poor perfusion by the ulnar artery." This description avoids the ambiguity of phrases such as "the Allen test is positive."

■ NEUROLOGIC CAUSES OF PAIN

External compression of a nerve or nerve roots is a common cause of pain in the hand. Peripheral nerve compression can present with varying symptoms, ranging from pure sensory abnormalities to pure motor paralysis or a combination of these. The level of compression determines the clinical symptoms. Proximal compression of nerve roots as they exit the vertebral bodies produces symptoms in a dermatomal distribution, whereas distal nerve compression causes symptoms in the defined region of the specific nerve. Symptoms of intrinsic peripheral nerve dysfunction, such as metabolic or demyelinating neuropathies, tend to manifest in multiple limbs and are more global within each limb. If the history and examination point to nerve compression, the next step in the work-up often is electrodiagnostic evaluation, which can elucidate the level and severity of compression and can determine the extent of muscle denervation due to the compression. Radiographic evaluation with plain radiographs, computed tomography, or MRI may be necessary. In the case of cervical compression due to cervical arthritis, plain radiographs and MRI are very helpful. Severe pain, weakness, or paresthesias due to peripheral nerve compression should warrant an evaluation and treatment by a hand surgeon because permanent changes can occur without timely intervention.

MEDIAN NERVE COMPRESSION AT THE WRIST (CARPAL TUNNEL SYNDROME)

 ESSENTIALS OF DIAGNOSIS

- *Paresthesias of the volar aspect of the thumb, index, and long fingers, and radial aspect of the ring finger.*
- *Positive Phalen maneuver and Tinel sign at the wrist.*
- *Thenar atrophy and weakened pinch with long-standing compression.*

Carpal tunnel syndrome is the most common nerve entrapment in the upper extremity. The syndrome refers to the symptoms due to the compression of the median nerve at the junction of the distal forearm and wrist.

The carpal tunnel lies within the proximal palm (Figure 6–2). The carpal bones form the radial, ulnar, and dorsal sides with the transverse carpal ligament forming the roof on the volar side. The transverse carpal ligament attaches on the radial side to the tuberosity of the trapezium distally and proximally to the tuberosity of the scaphoid and the styloid process of the radius. On the ulnar side, the ligament attaches to the hook of the hamate distally and the pisiform proximally. The nine flexor tendons to the fingers (flexor digitorum superficialis, flexor digitorum profundus, and the flexor pollicis longus) and the median nerve pass through the carpal tunnel. The transverse carpal ligament maintains the carpal arch and serves as a pulley for the flexor tendons. After it passes through the carpal tunnel, the median nerve divides into the digital sensory branches to the thumb, index, and

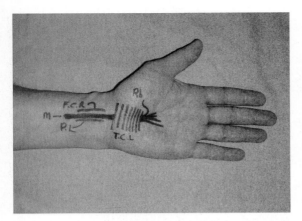

Figure 6–2. Surface anatomy of the carpal tunnel. The median nerve (M) becomes more superficial as it approaches the distal one-third of the forearm, but is still deep to both the palmaris longus tendon (P.L.) and the flexor carpi radialis (F.C.R.). As the median nerve continues distally into the hand, it enters the carpal tunnel. The roof of the carpal tunnel is formed by the transverse carpal retinaculum (T.C.L.). The recurrent branch (Rb) generally emerges at the distal edge of the transverse carpal ligament. Occasionally it will emerge through the fibers of the ligament. The median nerve continues through the proximal hand and then divides into its digital sensory branches.

long fingers, and the radial side of the ring finger. There is only one motor branch from the median nerve at this level of the wrist—the recurrent branch which provides the innervation to the majority of the thenar musculature. The recurrent branch has variable branching patterns, with the most frequent being the branch curling over the distal edge of the ligament (see Figure 6–2).

Carpal tunnel syndrome is most common in the fourth to the sixth decades of life and occurs more often in women than in men. Medical risk factors include diabetes mellitus, pregnancy, and hypothyroidism. It may also be associated with any activity that produces repetitive motion. There is controversy as to whether carpal tunnel syndrome is truly a work-related entity. Synovitis of the wrist due to rheumatoid arthritis and other forms of inflammatory arthritis can produce carpal tunnel syndrome. The most common cause of idiopathic carpal tunnel syndrome is the inflammation of the tenosynovium of the nine tendons within the carpal tunnel, resulting in the compression of the median nerve within the carpal tunnel. Occasionally, a tumor in the carpal tunnel can compress the median nerve. The most common tumors are giant cell tumors, lipomas, and ganglion cysts

(Figure 6–3). Acromegaly and amyloidosis are rare causes of carpal tunnel syndrome.

Clinical Findings

A. Symptoms and Signs

Classic signs of carpal tunnel syndrome include numbness and tingling in the thumb, index finger, long finger, and the radial side of the ring finger. These symptoms may be worse at night due to the wrist flexion that occurs with fetal positioning of the patient during sleep. Shaking or flicking the hand can sometimes relieve the pain (the "flick test"). Patients may incorrectly attribute their symptoms to vascular insufficiency because the hand "feels cold" and lowering the hand decreases the symptoms. Symptoms may be exacerbated during the day when the wrist is hyperflexed or hyperextended, such as with driving or typing. With longstanding compression there is grip and pinch weakness and complete loss of sensation in the affected fingers.

During the early stages of carpal tunnel syndrome, the hand examination may be normal. Two-point discrimination and grip and pinch strengths may be unaffected, and even provocative tests may not elicit signs of median nerve compression. As carpal tunnel syndrome progresses, however, tapping over the median nerve at the mid axis of the wrist elicits electric-shock–like discomfort at the site of the tap with paresthesias that radiate distally into the median nerve distribution (positive Tinel sign). Some patients may experience paresthesias that radiate proximally to the volar forearm. The Phalen maneuver provokes median nerve compression by active hyperflexion of the wrist; this test is considered positive if paresthesias in a median nerve distribution develop within 60 seconds. In the provocative Phalen test, the examiner exerts pressure over the median nerve at the distal forearm and passively flexes the patient's wrist. Some physicians use the cuff compression test, in which a blood pressure cuff is placed on the patient's forearm and inflated for 60 seconds to the midpoint pressure between the patient's systolic and diastolic pressures. It is positive if symptoms occur.

With advanced and severe compression of the median nerve in the carpal tunnel, there is thenar muscle atrophy (Figure 6–4) and occasionally, spontaneous fibrillations visible in the thenar eminence.

B. Imaging and Special Tests

If the diagnosis is in doubt or if symptoms persist despite conservative management, then electrodiagnostic testing should be performed. Imaging studies are not necessary unless a compressing mass or tumor is suspected, in which case an MRI should be ordered (see Figure 6–3). A diagnostic biopsy of the mass is done if required and followed by surgical resection.

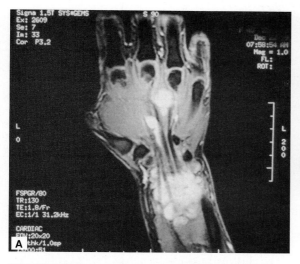

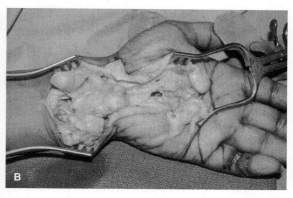

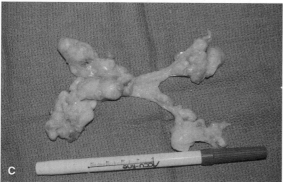

Figure 6–3. Median nerve compression due to a giant cell tumor in the carpal tunnel. **A:** Magnetic resonance image of the giant cell tumor spanning the carpal tunnel. **B:** Intraoperative view of the tumor within the carpal tunnel. **C:** The excised giant cell tumor.

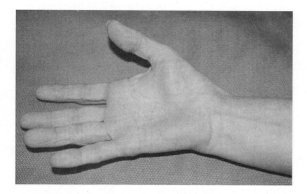

Figure 6–4. Thenar muscle atrophy due to long-standing carpal tunnel syndrome with extreme hand weakness.

Treatment

Conservative management for idiopathic carpal tunnel syndrome should aim at reducing the tenosynovial inflammation and swelling within the carpal tunnel. Splinting and the use of nonsteroidal anti-inflammatory drugs (NSAIDs) such as ibuprofen should be the first-line therapy. The splints should maintain the wrist at 5–10 degrees of extension and are available as prefabricated, over-the-counter "carpal tunnel splints." Splints can also be custom made by hand therapists. The patients should wear the splints during the most symptomatic times, particularly at night. Patients should also be instructed on proper ergonomics during the awake and sleeping hours to avoid any positions that cause compression of the median nerve. Approximately one-third of patients managed conservatively in this fashion will respond favorably.

Steroid injections into the carpal tunnel can also alleviate the symptoms but can cause median nerve injury if done incorrectly. The relief of symptoms by the steroid injection is often only temporary, because patients who require steroids usually have pathology severe enough to warrant surgical decompression. The injections are done by identifying the palmaris longus tendon at the distal forearm at the wrist. Triamcinolone or dexamethasone is mixed with 1% lidocaine without epinephrine, and the injection is given through a 30-gauge needle by inserting it into the forearm from the *ulnar* side of the palmaris longus tendon. Once inserted, the needle is gently advanced through the forearm fascia so the tip is just above the median nerve but below the level of the fascia. It is important that the patient is awake during the injection so that the patient can inform the operator of any electrical discharges that indicate that the needle tip is too far and is in the median nerve. If there are no paresthesias at that point, slowly administer the volume. If the steroid is injected into the correct plane, the patient will develop paresthesias in the median nerve distribution. If the needle is too superficial and is still above the forearm fascia, there will be a skin wheal and no paresthesias. The personal preference of the authors is to avoid steroid injections unless absolutely necessary.

If symptoms persist after a 2- to 3-month period of diligent splinting, NSAIDs, and perhaps a steroid injection, surgical intervention is indicated to avoid permanent damage to the median nerve and the muscles that it innervates. Surgical release can be done either through an open procedure or through the endoscopic approach.

COMPRESSION OF THE ULNAR NERVE AT THE WRIST (GUYON CANAL SYNDROME)

 ESSENTIALS OF DIAGNOSIS

- Paresthesias of the volar aspect of the ring and small fingers.
- Absence of paresthesias on the dorsal ulnar aspect of the hand.

The ulnar nerve and the ulnar artery pass from the forearm to the hand through the Guyon canal, which is located at the base of the hypothenar region. The canal is a small space and triangular in dimension. Its roof is defined by the volar palmar fascia. The lateral wall is formed by the hook of the hamate and the insertion of the transverse carpal ligament. The medial wall is formed by the pisiform bone.

Common causes of ulnar nerve compression in the Guyon canal are lipomas and ganglion cysts. Manual labor with repeated trauma to the hypothenar region can lead to scar adhesions of the ulnar nerve or to the development of an ulnar artery pseudoaneurysm that causes ulnar nerve compression and ischemia (the hypothenar hammer syndrome).

Clinical Findings

A. SYMPTOMS AND SIGNS

The ulnar nerve can be compressed either at the elbow or at the Guyon canal. Compression at the Guyon canal produces symptoms of numbness on the volar aspect of the small and ring fingers but not on the dorsal ulnar aspect of the hand. The absence of numbness on the dorsal ulnar aspect of the hand localizes the compression to the wrist rather than to the elbow, because the dorsal ulnar sensory nerve separates from the main trunk of the ulnar nerve 9 cm proximal to the Guyon canal. Therefore dorsal ulnar sensation is not affected by ulnar nerve compression within the Guyon canal. There may be weakness of the hypothenar muscles.

B. IMAGING AND SPECIAL TESTS

Electrodiagnostic studies may show slowing of the ulnar nerve impulses across the Guyon canal, but often are normal. However, it is important to confirm normal ulnar nerve conduction velocity at the elbow through the cubital tunnel. If hypothenar hammer syndrome is suspected an upper extremity vascular Doppler examination and an arteriogram should be ordered because vascular reconstruction of the ulnar artery may be required.

Treatment

The tortuosity of the Guyon canal precludes steroid injections, and splinting is usually ineffective. Surgical decompression is recommended. With mild ulnar nerve compression at the wrist in the presence of carpal tunnel syndrome, division of the transverse carpal ligament during the carpal tunnel surgery is often effective in decompressing the Guyon canal. If compression is more severe, a formal decompression of the Guyon canal is recommended.

COMPRESSION OF THE ULNAR NERVE AT THE ELBOW

ESSENTIALS OF DIAGNOSIS

- *Pain in the proximal forearm.*
- *Paresthesias of the volar and dorsal aspects of the small finger and of the ulnar side of the ring finger.*
- *Positive Tinel sign with percussion of the ulnar nerve at the elbow.*
- *Weakness and atrophy of the intrinsic muscles of the hand with long-standing compression.*

Proximal to the elbow, the ulnar nerve is located next to the medial head of the triceps and on the posterior surface of the medial intermuscular septum. As it approaches the elbow, it lies between the olecranon and the medial humeral epicondyle and enters the cubital tunnel. In the strictest definition, the cubital tunnel is defined by the elbow joint laterally, the flexor carpi ulnaris origin medially, and the medial epicondyle anteriorly. However, often the term "cubital tunnel" is used to include the region spanned by proximal fascial covering of the ulnar nerve proximal to the medial epicondyle and distal fascia between the two heads of the flexor carpi ulnaris. When this distal fascia is thickened, it is referred to as the Osborne band.

Clinical Findings

A. SYMPTOMS AND SIGNS

Compression of the ulnar nerve at the elbow produces an extreme aching or lancinating pain in the proximal forearm and paresthesias radiating distally to the small finger and the ulnar side of the ring finger. These symptoms are exacerbated by elbow flexion. Weakness and intrinsic muscular atrophy are usually late symptoms. Percussion of the ulnar nerve at the elbow will produce discomfort and paresthesia, a positive Tinel sign.

B. IMAGING AND SPECIAL TESTS

Electrodiagnostic studies help to establish the diagnosis and to determine the severity of the compression. Fibrillations noted on electromyography indicate neurologic compromise to the muscles.

Treatment

Conservative therapy is indicated in patients with minimal compression. NSAIDs are recommended. Patients are advised against maintaining postures that involve elbow flexion, such as arm crossing during awake hours and the fetal position during sleep. Elbow flexion causes ulnar nerve traction and compression as it traverses the cubital tunnel because the cubital tunnel is below the pivot point of the elbow flexion. To prevent excessive elbow flexion during sleep, patients should wear custom-made long arm splints to maintain the elbow at about 5 degrees of flexion. For those with coexisting carpal tunnel syndrome, the splint is extended beyond the wrist to keep the wrist at neutral. If both sides are affected, bilateral splints are made and patients are instructed to alternate the splints nightly, so that one arm is free to function in its normal capacity such as removing eyeglasses, turning the light off at night, and reaching for the clock. The patients are referred to occupational therapists for ergonomic exercises and posture modifications. If symptoms do not improve over 2–3 months or worsen, then surgical decompression may be indicated. In general, the symptoms can be relieved with surgery. Several surgical techniques have been proposed, and each has its own proponents.

COMPRESSION OF THE SUPERFICIAL RADIAL NERVE AT THE DISTAL FOREARM

ESSENTIALS OF DIAGNOSIS

- *Paresthesias of the dorsal aspects of the thumb, index, and long fingers.*
- *Nerve often compressed by a wristwatch or other constrictive band.*

The superficial branch of the radial nerve provides sensation to the dorsal thumb, index, and long fingers, and the radial dorsum of the hand and wrist. Its proximity to the bony prominence of the radius makes it vulnerable to extrinsic compression from a tight wristwatch or other constrictive band. Presenting symptoms often are numbness and paresthesias in the radial sensory distribution. Lancinating pain may indicate a traumatic etiology of the compression. The differential diagnosis includes de Quervain tenosynovitis and basilar joint arthritis of the thumb.

The initial treatment is to remove the offending constrictive band. If the symptoms persist after several weeks, the patient should be referred to a hand surgeon for potential exploration and neurolysis. Occasionally, radial sensory neuritis can be due to adjacent de Quervain tenosynovitis. In these cases injection of a short-acting local anesthetic into the area of most severe pain can be both diagnostic and therapeutic.

RADIAL NERVE COMPRESSION

 ESSENTIALS OF DIAGNOSIS

- *Idiopathic entrapment is uncommon.*
- *Aching pain in the extensor and supinator muscle masses in the proximal forearm.*
- *Difficult to distinguish from lateral epicondylitis.*

Traumatic compression of the radial nerve—such as occurs with a displaced fracture of the distal humerus—results in both motor findings (weakness of wrist extension) and sensory loss in the radial nerve distribution (decreased sensation on the radial aspect of the dorsum of the hand). Idiopathic entrapment of the radial nerve is uncommon, and when present, usually occurs after its bifurcation into a motor branch (posterior interosseus nerve) and sensory branch in the proximal forearm. Radial tunnel syndrome, the most common idiopathic entrapment of the radial nerve, results from compression of the motor branch in the region from the radius head to the supinator. Patients describe aching pain in the extensor and supinator muscle mass in the proximal forearm. There may not be significant weakness. When the superficial branch of the radial nerve is involved, there are dysesthesias and paresthesias that radiate to the dorsal radial surface of the forearm and the hand. Physical findings include tenderness of the radial nerve upon palpation along its path. Radial tunnel syndrome should be strongly suspected if the symptoms are reproduced by (1) resisted supination, (2) elbow flexion with the forearm in supination and the wrist in a neutral position, or (3) passive pronation with the wrist in full flexion. It can be very difficult to distinguish this rare condition from lateral epicondylitis, which is far more common. Therapeutic and diagnostic injections with lidocaine at the lateral epicondyle or within the radial tunnel can determine the etiology of the proximal forearm pain. Neurodiagnostic studies are usually not helpful unless there is evidence of muscle denervation, which is usually a late symptom of chronic compression.

Treatment

A 2- to 3-month course of NSAIDs, splinting, and muscle stretching exercises are often helpful; refractory cases should be referred for surgical exploration and decompression.

REFLEX SYMPATHETIC DYSTROPHY (SEE CHAPTER 63)

Reflex sympathetic dystrophy is a severe and often disabling condition that can occur after minor trauma, surgery, or stroke. Sometimes there is no identified precipitating event. Drucker described three sequential stages of reflex sympathetic dystrophy. In stage I, there is pain, edema, hyperhidrosis, and hypothermia, either immediately or several weeks after an injury to the limb. Stage II is characterized by skin pallor and coolness. The edematous tissues become indurated and the patient has constant pain. Fixed joint contractures, pain that limits the use of the extremity, proximal spread of pain, atrophic skin, and patchy radiographic osteoporosis characterize stage III. The diagnosis and treatment of reflex sympathetic dystrophy are reviewed in Chapter 63.

TENDINITIS AND TENOSYNOVITIS

Inflammation of the tenosynovium in the hand and wrist can cause pain and limitation of motion, typically in one or two fingers, which is worse upon awakening. Tenosynovitis can occur in any region where tendons traverse underneath a retinacular pulley. Trigger finger and de Quervain tenosynovitis are two classic examples. Findings on examination include thickened, tender volar tendon sheaths on palpation, with limited active but normal passive motion of the affected digit(s). Dorsal wrist tenosynovitis can produce an hourglass-shaped swelling, as soft tissues bulge on either side of the extensor retinaculum. Causes include rheumatologic disease, sports-related or occupational trauma, and repetitive motion injury, but many cases are idiopathic. Many patients respond to a 1- to 2-week course of NSAIDs and splinting. After the initial treatment, hand therapy may help to increase strength and range of motion. Refractory cases may require steroid injections into the tendon sheaths, or surgical decompression and synovectomy.

TRIGGER FINGER (STENOSING TENOSYNOVITIS)

ESSENTIALS OF DIAGNOSIS

- *Racheting motion during flexion of the affected finger.*
- *Locking of the finger.*

Clinical Findings

Triggering of the finger is caused by irritation and subsequent swelling of the flexor tendon tenosynovium at the proximal edge of the A1 pulley. The flexor tendons are unable to glide smoothly within the A1 pulley, resulting in pain and in the classic triggering or ratcheting motion during finger flexion. Further swelling results in locking of the finger, most commonly in flexion, as the swollen tendon can no longer glide through the A1 pulley. Once the finger is locked, the patient needs to passively extend or flex the finger to make it mobile. Acquired trigger fingers can be associated with rheumatoid disease and diabetes mellitus, but most cases are idiopathic and thought to be due to minor trauma such as that from repetitive motion or minor blunt force.

Congenital trigger thumb causes an inability to extend the thumb, which usually is not recognized until 2 or 3 years of age. The term is a misnomer: the thumb is locked in flexion but there is no actual triggering. In contrast to adult trigger finger, the thickening and the synovial inflammation are within the tendon rather than in the annular pulley. This palpable swelling of the flexor pollicis longus is referred to as "Notta nodule." There is often a familial history of congenital trigger thumb.

Treatment

Conservative therapy is initially indicated in acquired adult trigger finger. The patients are educated about possible etiology such as the preferential use of the finger during typing or forceful grasping of objects that causes minor direct blunt trauma to the proximal edge of the A1 pulley. Finger splints and NSAIDs are recommended as initial treatment for a trial of several weeks. If the patient has already tried this or if the triggering is severe, steroid injections are given into the potential space between the A1 pulley and the flexor tendon. Steroid injections may be repeated several times, but usually should not exceed three injections, unless there are medical contraindica-

tions to surgery. If triggering recurs, surgical release of the A1 pulley is indicated. This can be accomplished quite easily under local anesthetic, with low morbidity, although digital nerve laceration, stiffness, and infection with delayed wound healing have been reported. Congenital trigger thumb is treated with surgical release of the A1 pulley.

DE QUERVAIN TENOSYNOVITIS

ESSENTIALS OF DIAGNOSIS

- *Radial wrist pain.*
- *Pain with extension and abduction of the thumb.*
- *Positive Finkelstein sign.*

Clinical Findings

The dorsal compartments of the wrist act as pulleys for the wrist and finger extensors. A common cause of pain on the radial side of the wrist is de Quervain tenosynovitis: inflammation of the first dorsal extensor compartment which contains the tendons of the extensor pollicis brevis and the abductor pollicis longus (Figure 6–5). De Quervain tenosynovitis causes severe pain with thumb

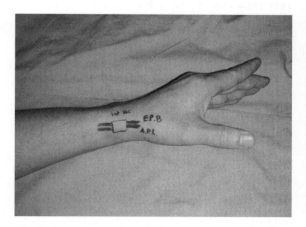

Figure 6–5. Surface anatomy of the left extensor pollicis brevis (E.P.B.) and the abductor pollicis longus (A.P.L.) tendons at the first dorsal extensor compartment (D.C.). Inflammation of this compartment gives rise to de Quervain tenosynovitis.

extension and abduction. There is usually pain on direct palpation of the compartment and pain when the patient "hitchhikes" the thumb against resistance. There can also be pain with passive ulnar deviation of the wrist with a clasped thumb (a positive Finkelstein test). Occasionally palpable crepitance is present in the compartment when the patient ranges the thumb, and a radial osteophyte may also be visible on radiographs. Differential diagnoses include thumb basilar joint arthritis and compression of the dorsal radial sensory nerve.

Treatment

Conservative treatment is the first-line therapy, consisting of NSAIDs, a thumb spica splint, and steroid injections into the first dorsal compartment. Care must be taken to infiltrate over both the extensor pollicis brevis and the abductor pollicis longus tendons, which are often separated by a septum within the first dorsal extensor compartment. Failure of conservative treatment may necessitate surgical first compartment release, which can be performed as an outpatient procedure with a very low rate of morbidity and a high rate of success.

MEDIAL & LATERAL HUMERAL EPICONDYLITIS

ESSENTIALS OF DIAGNOSIS

- *Pain and tenderness over the involved epicondyle.*
- *Wrist flexion exacerbates the pain of medial epicondylitis.*
- *Wrist extension exacerbates the pain of lateral epicondylitis.*

Clinical Findings

The forearm flexors originate from the medial humeral epicondyle, and the extensors originate from the lateral humeral epicondyle. Inflammation at the insertions of these muscles is referred to as either medial or lateral epicondylitis. The term "tennis elbow" refers to lateral epicondylitis, even though the great majority of patients who have this condition do not play tennis. Clinically there is pain at the epicondyle, and the pain worsens with contraction of the involved muscles. In lateral epicondylitis, the pain is worse with wrist extension and in medial epicondylitis with wrist flexion. There is also weakness of the

associated muscles. Epicondylitis is seen more commonly in the fourth and fifth decades of life. Younger patients should be examined for alternative causes of pain, such as elbow instability, tumors, or osteochondritis dissecans.

Treatment

A substantial majority (85–95%) of patients will respond to conservative therapy in the form of a 2- to 3-week course of rest, splinting, and NSAIDs, followed by a course of gentle strengthening exercises and the use of a commercially available forearm support band. Steroid injections (no more than three) are given for severe discomfort. Because of the risk of damage to the ulnar nerve, only experienced physicians should attempt injections of the medial epicondyle. Surgery is indicated if these conservative measures fail. Results of surgery can be good, but patients should expect a long period of physical rehabilitation afterward.

GANGLION CYSTS

ESSENTIALS OF DIAGNOSIS

- *Firm cystic masses adjacent to joints.*
- *Usually painless.*

Ganglion cysts are the most common masses in the hand or wrist. Despite the name, they are not related to nerves but rather arise from the herniation of synovium and joint fluid through a weakness in the joint capsule. The inciting factor may be a tear or localized degenerative change in the tenosynovium. A localized check-valve effect occurs at the base of the stalk, allowing ingress but not egress of synovial fluid from the joint into the protrusion. As fluid accumulates, a cyst forms. With partial resorption of the fluid by the cyst lining, the fluid inside becomes more concentrated, making aspiration of the fluid difficult. The most common location is at the dorsal wrist with the origin at the scapholunate joint. The second most common is at the volar radial wrist. Cysts can also occur in the fingers, elbow, and shoulder. Ganglion cysts are generally painless, but can cause pain due to compression of an overlying nerve or the joint space. An occult ganglion cyst is a very common cause of joint pain.

Treatment

Aspirating the ganglion cyst with a wide-gauge needle, such as an 18- or 20-gauge, is sometimes successful, but the recurrence rate is high. Surgical exploration is the most effective means of long-term control, if the entire cyst, check-valve, and underlying cause of the localized synovial degeneration (such as an osteophyte) are resected.

ARTHRITIS & OSSEOUS CAUSES OF PAIN

Hand and wrist pain can be due also to the underlying skeletal structures. The most common cause of pain in the middle aged to elderly population is osteoarthritis. Inflammatory arthritides that involve the hand, such as rheumatoid arthritis, psoriatic arthritis, gout, and pseudogout, are reviewed elsewhere (see Chapters 15, 19, 45, and 46).

Apart from arthritis, osseous causes of pain include minor trauma and bony tumors. These may produce only subtle abnormalities which may not be apparent on physical exam, but radiographs can detect hairline fractures and evidence of bone tumors.

BASILAR THUMB OSTEOARTHRITIS (THUMB CARPOMETACARPAL JOINT OSTEOARTHRITIS)

 ESSENTIALS OF DIAGNOSIS

- *Pain at the base of the thumb made worse by pinching activity.*
- *Pain and crepitance with passive rotation and compression of the thumb carpometacarpal joint.*
- *Degenerative changes of the thumb carpometacarpal joint on radiographs.*

Clinical Findings

The base of the thumb is the area in the hand most commonly affected by osteoarthritis. The thumb is a long lever, and the power of the thumb pinch can be more than 30 pounds. Pinch power at the tip of the thumb is amplified 25 times at the base of the thumb, because of the long lever arm (ie, up to 750 pounds of force). Persons who perform repeated pinching activities, such as sewing or knitting, commonly develop arthritis in the thumb carpometacarpal (CMC) joint. Physical exam findings include pain and crepitance on passive rotation and compression of the joint (the "grind test"). De Quervain tendinitis causes similar symptoms and must be excluded. With advanced thumb CMC joint arthritis, a palpable protrusion develops on the radial dorsal side of the thumb base that is visible when the thumb held in a slightly flexed and clasped position into the hand (a "shelf sign"). Radiographs show degenerative changes of the thumb CMC joint: irregular joint space narrowing, bony sclerosis, and osteophytes (Figure 6–6).

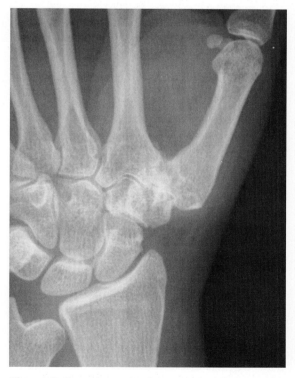

Figure 6–6. Radiograph of thumb basilar osteoarthritis. There is irregular loss of the joint space between the proximal thumb metacarpal and the trapezium bone, together with bony sclerosis and bony cysts. There is also proximal and radial subluxation of the thumb metacarpal, indicative of carpometacarpal joint ligament laxity, caused by the progressive arthritis.

Treatment

Osteoarthritis of the thumb CMC joint is treated initially with NSAIDs and a wrist-based thumb splint to immobilize the CMC joint. Should this not work, steroids can be injected into the joint to temporarily relieve the pain and the inflammation (generally, no more than three injections). The patients should be informed that the injections are given to relieve the pain and not to reverse the degenerative process. As the destruction of cartilage and joint progresses, pain and stiffness may eventually necessitate surgical intervention. Surgical options include tendon interpositional arthroplasty, with removal of both the proximal articular surface of the thumb metacarpal and the trapezium, followed by insertion of a tendon and ligament reconstruction of the joint. Silicone interposition arthroplasties have been performed in the past but are no longer advised because of prosthetic failure and silicone synovitis. Arthrodesis between the thumb metacarpal and the trapezium is another option in CMC joint arthritis but limits the range of motion in the thumb.

NODAL OSTEOARTHRITIS

ESSENTIALS OF DIAGNOSIS

- *Heberden and Bouchard nodes.*
- *Radiographic evidence of osteoarthritis at the distal and proximal interphalangeal joints.*

Nodal osteoarthritis is a common condition in patients over the age of 45 and affects the distal interphalangeal and proximal interphalangeal joints. The process may begin with redness and joint swelling ("erosive" or "inflammatory" osteoarthritis) that can be confused with inflammatory arthritides such as rheumatoid arthritis, psoriatic arthritis, and gout. As the disease progresses, patients develop permanent bony changes at the affected joints, known as Heberden nodes when they are at the distal interphalangeal joints and Bouchard nodes when they are at the proximal interphalangeal joints. It is important to note that osteoarthritis can coexist with the various inflammatory arthritides, making the diagnosis more challenging.

Treatment

NSAIDs are helpful in both the acute and chronic phases of osteoarthritis. Patients should be informed of the chronic, progressive nature of this illness, which in some

is extremely indolent, but in others can cause disabling loss of function. The latter are best referred to a hand surgeon, and can be offered a variety of palliative motion-sparing procedures.

VASCULAR CAUSES OF PAIN

Ischemic symptoms range from mild cold intolerance with decreased digital temperature and intermittent color changes to excruciating ischemic pain with fingertip ulceration or necrosis. The patient may also point out the presence of a mass that could represent an aneurysm or an arteriovenous malformation. Once vascular insufficiency is established as the explanation for hand symptoms, the cause of the insufficiency has to be determined. This may be due to an underlying medical condition such as thrombophilia, atherosclerosis, embolic disorder, Raynaud disease, connective tissue disease, malignancy, or diabetes mellitus. The patient should also be questioned about occupational and recreational exposure to vibration or other repetitive hand trauma that could cause hypothenar hammer syndrome. It is important to ask about exposure to tobacco and toxic chemicals such as epoxy resins that can cause distal capillary spasms. Symptoms affected by arm position or exacerbated by exercise may provide clues to the presence of thoracic outlet syndrome or proximal occlusive disease.

The upper extremity vascular examination begins with a thorough inspection of the skin for discoloration, scars, rashes, hair pattern, and ulceration. The fingernails may have chronic infections, hyponychial skin breakdown and scarring suggestive of chronic ischemia, or splinter hemorrhages from microemboli which have migrated distally from a proximal source. Careful palpation detects temperature differences between digits, the presence of vascular masses, thrills, and the presence and strength of brachial, radial, and ulnar pulses. Unilateral vascular findings suggest embolic disease.

Hand perfusion should be assessed with the Allen test, testing for perfusion through either the ulnar or the radial artery. Although there are false-positive and false-negative results, the Allen test is easy to perform and useful. Doppler can be used to evaluate the radial and ulnar arteries, as well as the digital arteries on both the ulnar and radial sides of the fingers. The magnetic resonance arteriogram, which is noninvasive, can image a vessel as small as 1 mm with good resolution. However, the arteriogram remains the gold standard for evaluating the vascular anatomy from the aortic root to the distal finger.

A comprehensive survey of the many vascular disorders of the upper extremity is beyond the scope of this chapter. Raynaud phenomenon, one of the more common etiologies of vascular hand pain, is reviewed in Chapter 25.

REFERENCES

Chumbley EM, O'Connor FG, Nirschl RP. Evaluation of overuse elbow injuries. *Am Fam Physician.* 2000;61:691–700.

Deune EG, Mackinnon SE. Endoscopic carpal tunnel release: the voice of polite dissent. *Clin Plast Surg.* 1996;23:487–505.

Drucker WR, Hubay CA, Holden WD, et al. Pathogenesis of post-traumatic sympathetic dystrophy. *Am J Surg.* 1959;97:454.

Ekstrom RA, Holden K. Examination of and intervention for a patient with chronic lateral elbow pain with signs of nerve entrapment. *Phys Ther.* 2002;82:1077–1086.

Foley AE. Tennis elbow. *Am Fam Physician.* 1993;48:281–288.

Goergen T, Dalinka MK, Alazraki N, et al. Chronic elbow pain. *Radiology.* 2000;215:339–343.

Green DP, Hotchkiss RN, Pederson WC. *Green's Operative Hand Surgery.* 4th ed. Churchill Livingstone, 1999.

Kalb RL. Evaluation and treatment of wrist and hand pain. *Hosp Pract.* 1998;33:129–132.

Mackinnon SE, Dellon AL. Ulnar nerve entrapment at the wrist. In: Mackinnon SE, Dellon AL, ed. *Surgery of the Peripheral Nerve.* Thieme, 1988:97–216.

Urbaniak JR, Roth JH. Office diagnosis and treatment of hand pain. *Orthop Clin North Am.* 1982;13:477–495.

Viegas SF. Atypical causes of hand pain. *Am Fam Physician.* 1987;35:167–172.

Watrous BG, Ho G Jr. Elbow pain. *Prim Care.* 1988;15:725–735.

Approach to the Patient with Ankle & Foot Pain

7

William M. Jenkin, DPM

Motion of the ankle and foot occurs primarily at the "essential" joints: the ankle (tibiotalar joint), the subtalar (talocalcaneal) joint, the midtarsal (talonavicular and calcaneal-cuboid) joints, and the metatarsophalangeal (MTP) joints (Figure 7–1). Each region of the distal lower extremity has its specific disorders. Therefore, the diagnostic approach to chronic pain in the foot and ankle begins with identifying the location of the problem (ie, the ankle, heel, midfoot, or forefoot).

■ ANKLE PAIN

The first step in the evaluation of a patient with ankle pain is to determine whether the pain is due to intra-articular or extra-articular causes. Intra-articular pain is often felt anteriorly, but some patients complain of a dull aching discomfort that is difficult to localize. Motion of the ankle joint (ie, dorsiflexion and plantar flexion of the foot) elicits pain. An ankle effusion may be present.

INTRA-ARTICULAR CAUSES OF ANKLE PAIN

 ESSENTIALS OF DIAGNOSIS

- *Ankle pain with dorsiflexion and plantar flexion of the foot.*
- *Tenderness and/or swelling of the ankle joint.*

Clinical Findings

A. SYMPTOMS AND SIGNS

Ankle effusions, if present, can be palpated anteriorly, just medial and lateral to the extensor tendons as they cross the joint line. The ankle joint allows the foot to dorsiflex and to plantarflex. Ankle motion may be limited and may demonstrate crepitation. An **ankle equinus** exists when there is inadequate dorsiflexion (less than 10 degrees) with the leg extended. If the process is isolated to the tibiotalar joint, the pain occurs with ankle motion (dorsiflexion and plantar flexion of the foot) but not with motion of the subtalar joint (inversion and eversion of the foot). Occasionally, determining whether the tibiotalar joint or the subtalar joint is the source of the discomfort is difficult; in these cases, symptomatic relief following injection of a local anesthetic into the tibiotalar joint defines it as the cause of symptoms.

B. IMAGING STUDIES

Radiographs of the ankle are obtained to evaluate for talar dome lesions, osteochondritis dissecans, loose bodies, and arthritic changes. Magnetic resonance imaging (MRI) provides information about the soft tissue around and within the joint such as ligament damage, synovitis, synovial impingement, and meniscoid bodies. Arthroscopic evaluation can provide definitive diagnosis.

Differential Diagnosis

The approach to acute onset of inflammatory arthritis in one ankle is the same as the approach to acute monarthritis elsewhere; infection and crystal-induced arthritis are leading causes, and the major priority is to exclude the possibility of septic arthritis (see Chapter 47). The spondyloarthropathies, particularly reactive arthritis, can cause acute or subacute onset of inflammatory arthritis of the ankle joint, usually as a component of an oligoarthritis. Sarcoidosis also can cause acute inflammatory arthritis of the ankles, often in association with erythema nodosum.

Rheumatoid arthritis and the spondyloarthropathies are the leading causes of chronic inflammatory arthritis of the ankles, almost always with evidence of arthritis in other joints.

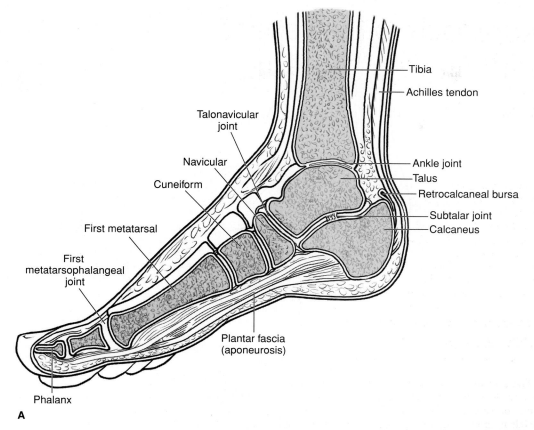

Figure 7–1. Anatomic relationships of the foot and ankle. **A:** Sagittal view at the level of the first metatarsal. (From Polley HF, Hunder GS. *Rheumatologic Interviewing and Physical Examination of the Joints.* 2nd ed. WB Saunders, 1978, Figure 14–5. With permission.)

Persistent ankle pain following an injury raises the possibility of a talar dome injury (eg, osteochondritis dissecans and transchondral "fractures"). Osteoarthritis of the tibiotalar joint is uncommon, and when present, is usually the result of significant trauma. Severe degenerative disease of the tibiotalar joint suggests neuropathic arthropathy, particularly if the patient is diabetic. Neuropathic changes in the subtalar and talonavicular joints usually accompany neuropathic arthropathy of the tibiotalar joint.

Treatment

In cases of acute ankle arthritis, symptomatic antiinflammatory measures should be instituted. If infection and trauma have been eliminated, an intra-articular glucocorticoid injection often provides lasting relief. Exterior support is helpful but must extend above the ankle.

Various types of prefabricated ankle braces can be used on a temporary basis.

In cases of chronic ankle arthritis, customized ankle-foot orthoses should be used for long-term management. Severe symptomatic chronic ankle arthritis is a therapeutic dilemma. Ankle arthrodesis provides pain relief, but the loss of ankle motion is disabling. Although the newer generation of prostheses shows some promise, ankle arthroplasty remains investigational.

EXTRA-ARTICULAR ANKLE PAIN

Extra-articular causes of ankle pain tend to localize to the posterior medial, the posterior lateral, or the anterolateral aspects of the ankle and produce characteristic findings depending upon which structures are involved (Table 7–1).

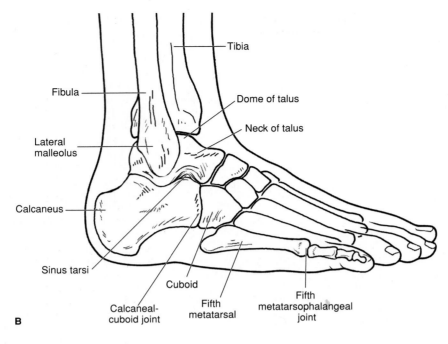

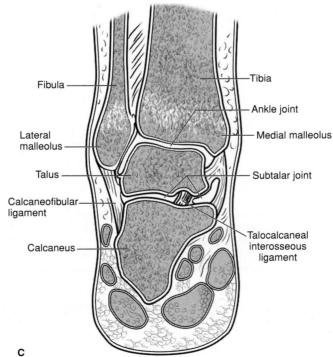

Figure 7–1. (Continued) **B:** Lateral view. **C:** Frontal section through the ankle and subtalar joint. (From Polley HF, Hunder GS. *Rheumatologic Interviewing and Physical Examination of the Joints.* 2nd ed. WB Saunders, 1978, Figure 14–1. With permission.)

Table 7–1. Extra-Articular Causes of Ankle Pain

Posterior medial ankle pain
Flexor hallucis longus dysfunction
Tibialis posterior tendon dysfunction
Tarsal tunnel syndrome

Posterior lateral ankle pain
Posterior talar impingement syndrome
Peroneal tendon dysfunction
Subtalar joint coalition
Sural nerve entrapment

Anterior lateral ankle pain
Sinus tarsi syndrome
Superficial peroneal nerve entrapment
Lateral ankle ligament pathology
Coalition of the talocalcaneal or calcaneal-navicular joints

POSTERIOR MEDIAL ANKLE PAIN

1. Flexor Hallucis Longus Dysfunction

ESSENTIALS OF DIAGNOSIS

- Pain with deep palpation of the flexor hallucis longus (FHL) posterior to the talus.

- Pain with ankle and hallux dorsiflexion.
- Triggering of the hallux.

Clinical Findings

A. SYMPTOMS AND SIGNS

FHL dysfunction is a repetitive use injury resulting in inflammation of the FHL tendon, and in more severe cases, stenosing tenosynovitis with nodule development and triggering of the great toe. FHL dysfunction occurs in both genders at all ages. Hypertrophy of the FHL muscle may contribute to development of the syndrome (placing ballet dancers at risk), but FHL dysfunction occurs in nonathletic persons as well.

FHL dysfunction causes pain or crepitation or both at the posterior medial ankle and is reproduced by passive or active motion of the FHL tendon. The pain may radiate along the medial arch and may be mistaken for distal plantar fasciitis. The pain improves with inactivity and may not be apparent when the patient first stands after sitting for a prolonged period. On examination, palpation of the FHL tendon at the posterior medial ankle (Figure 7–2) or the distal medial arch (or both) reproduces the pain, which is further exacerbated by dorsiflexion of the ankle and hallux.

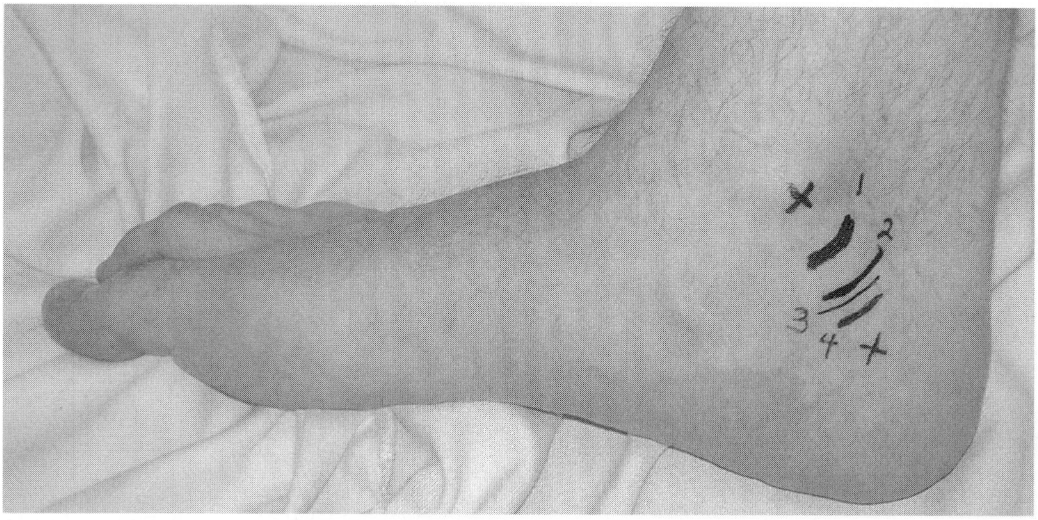

Figure 7–2. Photograph of the medial aspect of the foot demonstrating the relationships of the anatomic structures of the ankle and heel. The flexor retinaculum or laciniate ligament stretches between the medial malleolus (**X**) and the medial process of the tuberosity of the calcaneus (X). Passing below the flexor retinaculum are the tibialis posterior tendon (**1**), the flexor digitorum longus tendon (**2**), the neurovascular bundle containing the posterior tibial artery and nerve (**3**), and the flexor hallucis longus tendon (**4**).

B. IMAGING STUDIES

If the diagnosis is in doubt, tenography under fluoroscopy is the imaging study of choice.

Treatment

Initial measures include rest with avoidance of repetitive ankle motion, the use of nonsteroidal anti-inflammatory drugs (NSAIDs), and physical therapy. Recalcitrant cases should be treated with a glucocorticoid injection into the tendon sheath and a period of immobilization in a below-the-knee walker. If these measures fail, referral for surgical intervention in the form of a synovectomy and release of the retinaculum is indicated.

2. Tibialis Posterior Tendon Dysfunction

ESSENTIALS OF DIAGNOSIS

- *Early disease: pain and tenderness along the tibialis posterior tendon.*
- *Severe disease: ankle equinus, pes plano valgus.*

Clinical Findings

A. SYMPTOMS AND SIGNS

Progressive degenerative changes in the tibialis posterior tendon occur below the medial malleolus, producing posterior medial ankle pain and a series of foot deformities. In the early phase (stage 1), the patient complains of pain along the posterior tibial tendon either as it courses around and below the medial malleolus or at its insertion into the navicular bone. There is no gross deformity at this stage. Pain is reproduced with palpation and with resisted abduction of the foot. A gastrocnemius equinus (less than 10 degrees of ankle dorsiflexion with the leg extended while holding the foot neutral to supinated) is present. The tibialis posterior muscle and tendon are still functional, as evidenced by the patient's ability to lift the heel off the ground when standing on one foot (single heel raise) and to subtly invert the heel during the heel raise test. As the problem progresses, the tibialis posterior tendon becomes elongated, thin, and weakened and is no longer able to stabilize the midtarsal joint. The medial arch begins to sag as the forefoot begins to abduct upon the rearfoot, developing a pes plano valgus foot deformity (stage 2). This stage is associated with little to no muscle strength, depending on whether the tendon is weakened or ruptured. When the affected side is bearing weight and is viewed from behind, a maximum eversion (valgus) of the calcaneus is noted and more toes are visible as the forefoot abducts upon the rearfoot ("too many toes" sign) (Figure 7–3). The patient is unable to lift the heel off the ground when standing on one foot. The deformity is flexible and the arch can still rise as the hallux is dorsiflexed. In chronic situations, secondary problems, such as lateral sinus tarsi syndrome, hammer toe, and hallux valgus deformity result. Eventually, degenerative changes occur in the subtalar and midtarsal joints, resulting in pain in these joints and a nonreducible or fixed deformity that is severely disabling (stage 3).

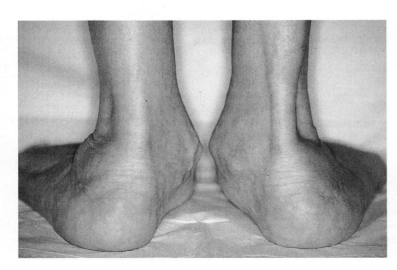

Figure 7–3. Pes planus. A posterior view of severely pronated feet reveals maximum eversion of the calcaneus (heel valgus). Abduction of the forefoot upon the rearfoot produces the "too many toes" sign.

B. IMAGING STUDIES

Weight-bearing anteroposterior and lateral radiographs of the foot aid in evaluating biomechanical relationships and detecting secondary arthritic changes.

Treatment

Early recognition of this problem improves the likelihood for success of nonoperative intervention in the form of custom rigid foot orthotics. Patients with stage 2 disease, however, should be referred to a foot and ankle surgeon for consideration of tendoachilles lengthening, tibialis posterior repair and augmentation, and medial column fusions as necessary. Triple arthrodesis is usually necessary for stage 3 disease. In the patient who is not a surgical candidate, a customized ankle foot orthosis is often beneficial. Regardless of stage, NSAIDs provide some symptomatic relief.

3. Tarsal Tunnel Syndrome

ESSENTIALS OF DIAGNOSIS

- *Entrapment of the posterior tibial nerve within the tarsal tunnel produces medial ankle pain and dysesthesias on the sole of the foot.*
- *Tapping over the tarsal tunnel just posterior to the medial malleolus elicits symptoms (Tinel sign).*

Clinical Findings

A. SYMPTOMS AND SIGNS

Entrapment of the posterior tibial nerve must be considered in the differential diagnosis of any plantar rearfoot or forefoot pain. The tarsal tunnel is a compartment located posteromedial to the ankle and bounded superficially by the laciniate ligament. In this compartment, the posterior tibial nerve lies just anterior to the tendon of the FHL (see Figure 7–2). The nerve can be compressed by a space-occupying lesion within the tunnel such as a ganglion (Figure 7–4), by inflammation of the tendons that pass through the tunnel, or by an os trigonum and trigonal process. Excessive pronation of the foot can stretch the nerve against the laciniate ligament and also result in an entrapment. If holding the foot in forced dorsiflexion and maximum eversion (pronation) for 15 seconds produces paresthesias on the sole, this is a positive sign for tarsal tunnel syndrome.

B. IMAGING STUDIES AND SPECIAL TESTS

Electromyography and nerve conduction studies should be performed but can be normal early in the entrapment. MRI provides excellent visualization of the tarsal tunnel and is indicated if there is suspicion of a space-occupying lesion within the tunnel (see Figure 7–4).

Treatment

Treatment consists of activity modification, antiinflammatory modalities, and if there is abnormal pronation, a trial of mechanical control with a custom foot orthotic. Supinating the foot to a neutral position ("depronating") reduces the pressure in the tarsal tunnel compartment and can diminish the irritation to the nerve

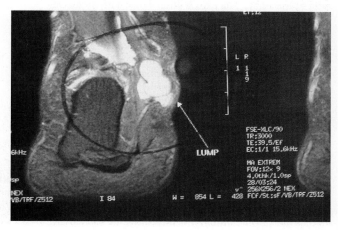

Figure 7–4. Coronal plane magnetic resonance image of a ganglion cyst within the tarsal tunnel. The cyst compresses the posterior tibial nerve, leading to symptoms of tarsal tunnel syndrome.

regardless of etiology. Recalcitrant cases or cases demonstrating abnormal electrodiagnostic testing should be referred for possible surgical intervention.

LATERAL ANKLE PAIN

1. Posterior Talar Impingement Syndrome

ESSENTIALS OF DIAGNOSIS

- *Pain with forced ankle plantar flexion.*
- *Radiographic demonstration of os trigonum, a trigonal process, or fracture of a trigonal process (Shepherd fracture).*

Clinical Findings

A. SYMPTOMS AND SIGNS

Posterior talar impingement syndrome is a painful symptom complex caused by impingement of the ankle joint capsule by the posterior lateral aspect of the talus. Os trigonum, trigonal process, and Shepherd fracture predispose the patient to posterior talar impingement (Figure 7–5). An os trigonum is a secondary ossicle attached to the posterior lateral tubercle of the talus by fibrous tissue. A trigonal process is an elongation of the posterior lateral tubercle. A fracture of the trigonal process (Shepherd fracture) can be difficult to distinguish radiographically from an os trigonum.

There may be a history of trauma. Symptoms consist of a dull aching pain localized to the posterior lateral aspect of the ankle. The pain is often worse with increased activity, especially forceful, repetitive plantar flexion at the ankle joint. The acute injury is of a plantar flexion inversion type. The patient often relates a history of an audible popping sound at the time of injury. In the chronic condition, the patient describes a history of repetitive plantar flexion associated with pain and swelling that increases with activities. Shepherd fracture should be suspected when there is acute onset of pain associated with trauma or when "ankle sprains" fail to respond to treatment after 6–8 weeks.

On examination, pain often can be reproduced by direct palpation laterally over the posterior process, just anterior to the Achilles tendon at the ankle/subtalar joint level. Pain is reproduced by the forceful plantar flexion of the foot at the ankle. Edema is common. When evaluating the chronic injury, it is imperative to also closely evaluate for FHL dysfunction.

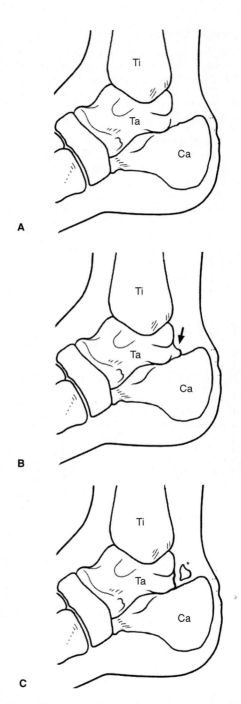

Figure 7–5. Trigonal process and os trigonum. Schematic representations of a lateral view of the tibia (Ti), talus (Ta), and calcaneus (Ca) of a normal foot (**A**), an elongated posterior lateral process of the talus or a trigonal process (arrow) (**B**), and an os trigonum (*) (**C**).

B. IMAGING STUDIES

Lateral radiographs of the ankle often reveal the presence of os trigonum, trigonal process, and Shepherd fracture. Computed tomography can detect fractures missed by plain radiography as well as other injuries to the lateral talus, including osteochondritis dissecans. An MRI of the area should be obtained if tendon involvement is suspected.

Treatment

Treatment of the Shepherd fracture consists of a weight-bearing, below-the-knee cast for 4–6 weeks. In the chronic condition, symptomatic anti-inflammatory therapies are instituted. If these treatments fail, it may be necessary to resort to night splints or injection of a glucocorticoid into the area in conjunction with casting. Recalcitrant cases should be referred for possible surgical excision.

2. Sinus Tarsi Syndrome

 ESSENTIALS OF DIAGNOSIS

- *History of inversion injury.*
- *Pain over the sinus tarsi and sensation of rearfoot instability.*
- *Relief of symptoms following injection of local anesthetic into the sinus tarsi.*

Clinical Findings

A. SYMPTOMS AND SIGNS

The sinus tarsi (a sulcus between the neck of the talus and the distal calcaneus) is located just anterior to, and slightly

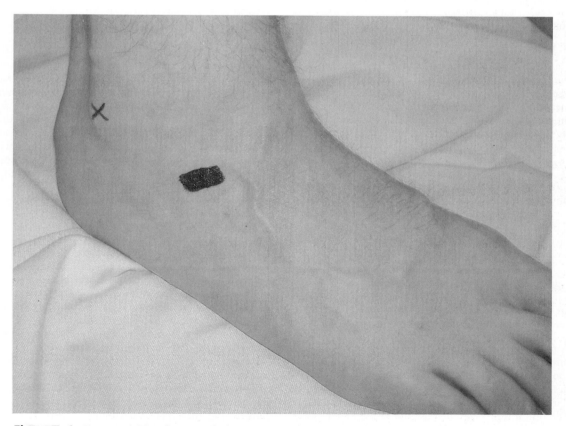

Figure 7–6. Sinus tarsi. The photograph demonstrates the location of the sinus tarsi (rectangle) anterior to, and slightly below, the lateral malleolus (**X**).

below, the lateral malleolus (Figures 7–1 and 7–6). Sinus tarsi syndrome is a result of damage to the tarsal canal ligaments. An inversion ankle injury is the most common cause, and sinus tarsi syndrome is often misdiagnosed as a chronic ankle sprain. Abnormal biomechanics induced by either pes planus or pes cavus can result in chronic strain on the lateral talocalcaneal interosseous ligament, also leading to sinus tarsi syndrome.

Patients complain of diffuse, deep aching pain on the dorsal-lateral aspect of the foot that increases on ambulation and is relieved by rest. There is a sensation of rearfoot instability, especially when walking on uneven terrain. The pain is reproduced by direct pressure over the sinus tarsi as well as with forced inversion and plantar flexion of the foot. Subtalar joint motion may be painful; despite the ligamentous injury and sensation of instability, the range of motion of the subtalar joint is not increased. Injection of local anesthetic deep into the sinus tarsi should cause transient relief of pain and is a helpful diagnostic tool. If care is taken to avoid skin anesthesia, a response to sinus tarsi injection excludes the possibility of entrapment of the superficial peroneal nerve, which can cause similar symptoms and can occur secondary to ankle sprain.

B. IMAGING STUDIES

Plain radiographs are normal but are indicated to rule out fractures and coalitions between the talus and calcaneus or calcaneus and navicular bones. MRI is a sensitive means for detecting disease in the sinus tarsi, but is only indicated in those cases in whom the diagnosis cannot be made on clinical grounds alone.

Treatment

Most cases respond to injection of glucocorticoid into the sinus tarsi. Recalcitrant cases may require immobilization for 3–4 weeks. If a biomechanical fault exists, the patient should be fitted with custom foot orthotics. If all other therapies fail, the patient should be referred for sinus tarsectomy.

■ HEEL PAIN

A range of disorders cause heel pain (Table 7–2). The initial approach to the patient with isolated heel pain should focus on the exact location of pain and tenderness within the heel. Heel pain is defined as infracalcaneal if it involves the plantar aspect of the calcaneus and retrocalcaneal if it involves the posterior and superior aspect of the calcaneus including the Achilles tendon.

Table 7–2. Causes of Heel Pain

Infracalcaneal pain
  Plantar fasciitis
  Infracalcaneal nerve entrapment
  Fat pad atrophy
  Infracalcaneal bursitis
  Calcaneal stress fracture
  Tarsal tunnel syndrome
  Radiculopathy
  Spondyloarthropathy
  Infection
  Tumor
Retrocalcaneal heel pain
  Achilles tendinitis
  Haglund deformity
  Pre-Achilles bursitis
  Retrocalcaneal bursitis
  Posterior lateral calcaneal exostosis
  Lateral calcaneal adventitious bursitis
Tenderness with lateral compression of the heel
  Stress fracture of the calcaneus
  Osteomyelitis (especially in children)
  Calcaneal apophysitis (especially in boys ages 8–15 years)

Identifying factors that exacerbate and ameliorate the pain is also helpful. Post-static dyskinesia (pain is worse on first standing and diminishes with walking) is characteristic of plantar fasciitis. The pain of Achilles tendinitis also subsides during activity. Conversely, patients with entrapment of the infracalcaneal nerve have pain that worsens with activity. Shoes with stiff counters exacerbate pain in patients with Haglund deformity (enlargement of the posterior superior aspect of the calcaneus), retrocalcaneal bursitis, pre-Achilles bursitis, and "pump-bump" deformity.

RETROCALCANEAL PAIN

For the evaluation of retrocalcaneal pain it is helpful to mentally superimpose a palpation grid in the form of a tic-tac-toe design on the posterior aspect of the calcaneus. The grid consists of three horizontal rows: upper (superior), middle, and lower (inferior), and three vertical rows: medial, central, and lateral squares (Figure 7–7).

In Haglund deformity the tenderness is most severe when palpating in the upper three horizontal squares (upper medial, upper central, upper lateral). In retrocalcaneal bursitis, tenderness is maximal in the upper medial and upper lateral squares with deep palpation just anterior to, and on either side of, the Achilles tendon. In pre-Achilles bursitis tenderness is created with light superficial palpation in the central middle and central lower squares of

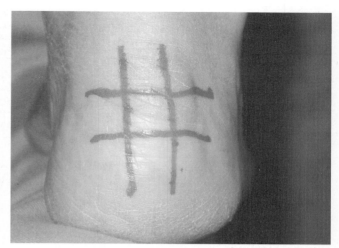

Figure 7–7. A tic-tac-toe grid on the posterior calcaneus. The grid helps determine the etiology of retrocalcaneal pain, as explained in the text. (From Chang TJ. *Master Techniques in Podiatric Surgery: the Foot and Ankle.* Lippincott Williams & Wilkins, 2005, Figure 22–2. Adapted with permission.)

the grid. Patients with Achilles tendinitis have tenderness when the tendon is squeezed from the sides along the tendon or at the insertion of the Achilles tendon in the central middle square with deep palpation. Ankle dorsiflexion often reproduces the pain of Achilles tendinitis. If Achilles insertional calcific spurring is present, then tenderness involves all three middle squares: medial, central, and lateral. "Pump-bump" deformities create pain in the lateral upper and lateral middle squares not involving the tendon and are associated with a superficial adventitious bursitis.

INFRACALCANEAL PAIN

To examine for causes of infracalcaneal pain, the plantar heel pad and plantar fascia should be placed on stretch by dorsiflexing the foot at the ankle and the toes and then should be palpated, noting the location and the extent of discomfort.

Tenderness with lateral compression of the heel suggests a stress fracture of the calcaneus in adults (Figure 7–8). In children and adolescents a painful response with lateral compression should raise the possibilities of

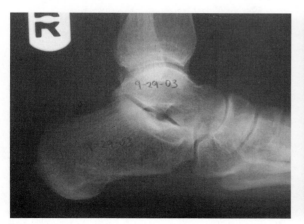

A

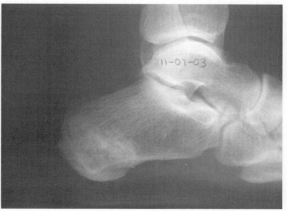

B

Figure 7–8. Insufficiency stress fracture of the calcaneus in a patient with osteoporosis. Lateral radiographs of the calcaneus reveal a stress fracture which is barely visible at the time of presentation (**A**) but which is readily apparent 4 weeks later (**B**).

calcaneal apophysitis (especially in boys aged 8–15 years) and osteomyelitis.

PLANTAR FASCIITIS

ESSENTIALS OF DIAGNOSIS

- *Heel pain on first arising that diminishes with walking.*
- *Pain and tenderness just anterior to the weight-bearing area of the heel.*

Clinical Findings

A. SYMPTOMS AND SIGNS

Plantar fasciitis is the most common cause of heel pain. It is the consequence of a biomechanical fault that causes tension of the intrinsic muscles and of the plantar fascia at its insertion to the calcaneus. Plantar fasciitis is aggravated by using flexible-soled shoes, by walking or standing on hard surfaces, and in the athlete by poor training.

Classically, the patient complains of heel pain on first arising and after a period of rest. Symptoms diminish with walking. Pain and tenderness are maximal at the point of insertion of the fascia into the medial tubercle just anterior to the weight-bearing area of the heel (proximal plantar fasciitis; Figure 7–9) or may extend distally along the fascia as it courses to the toes. If the plantar fascia is tender throughout its course along the medial arch, it is important to determine whether the pain decreases or increases when the fascia is relaxed as the foot is plantar flexed. This maneuver reduces pain in cases of plantar fasciitis. Increased pain suggests a deeper process, such as flexor tendinitis, joint ligament strain, or rarely, deep vein phlebitis. The foot usually appears to be normal; occasionally, pes planus or pes cavus is present.

B. IMAGING STUDIES

The diagnosis of plantar fasciitis is based on the history and examination. Radiographs are of little value in the diagnosis of plantar fasciitis but may be needed to rule out other disorders such as calcaneal stress fractures. The presence of infracalcaneal heel spurs on radiographs correlates poorly with symptoms.

Treatment

Treatment consists of activity modification, anti-inflammatory measures, Achilles and plantar fascial stretching, and addressing biomechanical faults. The pa-

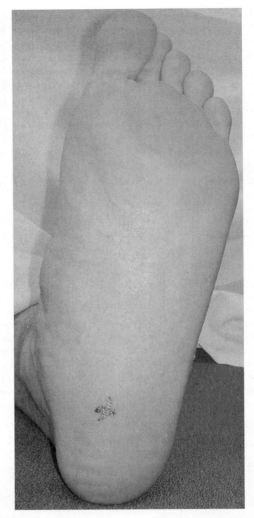

Figure 7–9. Plantar fasciitis. Photograph of the plantar aspect of the foot demonstrating the area of maximal tenderness for proximal plantar fasciitis.

tient is advised to avoid wearing slippers or walking barefoot. Tape immobilization, temporary over-the-counter supports, and custom foot orthotics are used to neutralize abnormal mechanical forces. After biomechanical control has been instituted, injections with a local anesthetic and glucocorticoid can be of benefit. The glucocorticoid can be mixed with a local anesthetic and delivered slowly via a 25-gauge, 1.25-inch needle from medially into the vault of the foot above the plantar fascial insertion into the medial calcaneal tubercle (Figure 7–10). Extracorporeal shock wave therapy administered while the patient is under anesthesia or surgical release of the plantar fascia are options in recalcitrant cases.

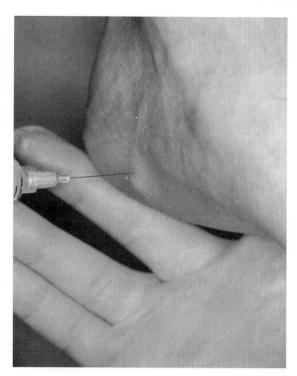

Figure 7–10. Therapeutic injection site on the medial heel for plantar fasciitis.

ENTRAPMENT NEUROPATHY OF THE INFRACALCANEAL NERVE (DISTAL TARSAL TUNNEL SYNDROME)

 ESSENTIALS OF DIAGNOSIS

- *Burning pain along the rim of the heel.*
- *Paresthesias with palpation medial to the insertion of the plantar fascia.*

Clinical Findings

A. SYMPTOMS AND SIGNS

Entrapment of the infracalcaneal nerve (a branch of the posterior tibial nerve) accounts for up to 20% of chronic infracalcaneal heel pain. It produces a sensation of burning along the rim of the heel that worsens with activity. There may be a history of post-static dyskinesia because the nerve entrapment is often the sequela of plantar fasci-itis. The point of maximal tenderness is medial and just dorsal to the insertion of the plantar fascia; palpation in this area can elicit paresthesias.

B. SPECIAL TESTS

Nerve conduction studies and electromyography are normal but help exclude proximal tarsal tunnel syndrome and radiculopathy.

Treatment

The initial treatment for this condition is the same as for plantar fasciitis. If symptoms persist after 6–12 months of treatment, neurolysis is performed.

FAT PAD ATROPHY

 ESSENTIALS OF DIAGNOSIS

- *Diffuse, central plantar heel pain aggravated by standing and activity on hard surfaces.*
- *Palpable atrophy of the heel pad.*

Clinical Findings

The fat pad of the heel consists of irreplaceable, specialized, separate hydraulic fat chambers designed to absorb shock and transmit mechanical forces to the calcaneus. The fat pad atrophies with age, certain rheumatologic diseases, vascular disease, multiple glucocorticoid injections, and trauma. The heel pain is central and diffuse. In severe cases, the underlying bone is palpable.

Treatment

The initial treatment consists of shoes and flexible heel cups that cushion and absorb shock.

HAGLUND DEFORMITY, RETROCALCANEAL BURSITIS, & PRE-ACHILLES BURSITIS

 ESSENTIALS OF DIAGNOSIS

- *The posterior superior aspect of the calcaneus is prominent, painful, and tender.*
- *Radiographic evidence of Haglund deformity of the calcaneus.*

Clinical Findings

A. Symptoms and Signs

Haglund deformity (posterior superior enlargement of the calcaneus) is an anatomic aberration that predisposes the posterior heel to shoe counter irritation, producing inflammation of the anatomic synovial-lined bursae located between the Achilles tendon and the calcaneus (retrocalcaneal bursitis). In some presentations, there is also an adventitious bursitis between the Achilles tendon and skin (pre-Achilles bursitis) as well as an insertional Achilles tendinitis. The patient typically complains of posterior heel pain and tenderness exacerbated by wearing shoes with enclosed stiff counters. Ankle dorsiflexion elicits pain with retrocalcaneal bursitis and Achilles insertional tendinitis. Due to its superficial location, pre-Achilles bursitis is sensitive to direct pressure. Pump-bump deformity (posterior lateral calcaneal exostosis with an overlying adventitious bursitis) is also associated with shoe counter irritation. Unlike Haglund deformity, only the lateral aspect of the calcaneus is prominent and the Achilles tendon is not involved.

B. Imaging Studies

Weight-bearing lateral radiographs reveal an enlarged retrocalcaneal bursal prominence if Haglund deformity is present. Erosions of the bone in the area of the retrocalcaneal bursae indicate chronic inflammation. There may be calcification of the Achilles tendon or its insertion. An MRI of the area gives information about all of the soft-tissue structures as well as the bone (Figure 7–11).

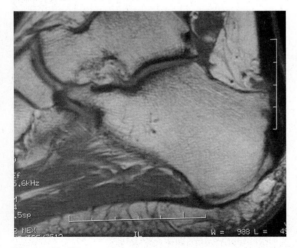

Figure 7–11. Magnetic resonance image of the calcaneus (sagittal view) demonstrating Haglund deformity, retrocalcaneal bursitis, cortical erosions, and Achilles tendinitis.

Treatment

Avoidance of shoes with stiff counters is mandatory. Soft-counter shoes with a heel lift or shoes without counters (eg, clogs or sandals) should be worn. NSAIDs, contrast baths, and ice massage can be used in the acute management. Pressure-off silicone sheet pads can be used long term when wearing shoes with counters. Glucocorticoid injections are to be used prudently and only as a last resort. With the exception of treating a superficial adventitious bursitis, glucocorticoid injection is best delivered in conjunction with cast immobilization. Pre-Achilles bursitis and pump-bump deformity usually respond to pressure off devices and shoe modifications. In recalcitrant cases involving Haglund deformity and retrocalcaneal bursitis, the patient should be referred for surgical intervention.

ACHILLES TENDINITIS

 ### ESSENTIALS OF DIAGNOSIS

- *Posterior heel pain with the initiation of activity and with ankle dorsiflexion.*
- *Tenderness at the insertion of the Achilles tendon onto the calcaneus (insertional tendinitis) or 4–5 cm proximal to the insertion (noninsertional tendinitis).*

Clinical Findings

A. Symptoms and Signs

Achilles tendinitis is usually mechanical in origin but can be a manifestation of reactive arthritis and the other spondyloarthropathies. Pain from Achilles tendinitis presents at the initiation of activity and often subsides during the activity, only to recur more intensely after the activity. Ankle dorsiflexion often reproduces the pain, and squeezing the Achilles tendon between the thumb and forefinger elicits discomfort. With insertional tendinitis, tenderness is maximal where the Achilles inserts onto the middle third of the calcaneus (central middle square of the palpation grid in Figure 7–7). When there is calcific spurring at the insertion of the Achilles, the area of discomfort involves the entire back of the calcaneus (all three middle squares of the palpation grid: medial, central, and lateral; Figure 7–7) and often is accompanied by a palpable prominence. Noninsertional tendinitis occurs 4–5 cm proximal to the insertion in an area where the tendon torques upon itself. Pain and palpable enlargement of the tendon is present. If the painful enlargement moves with tendon motion, then tendinosis or intratendinous linear tears and calcifications should be suspected (painful arc sign). The examination should determine whether there are any palpable defects within the tendon and whether ankle equinus is present.

B. IMAGING STUDIES

Radiographs (lateral weight-bearing and calcaneal axial views) can reveal insertional spurring and tendon calcifications (Figure 7–12). MRI can detect the extent and location of intratendinous linear tears and is essential prior to any surgical intervention.

Treatment

Treatment should begin with anti-inflammatory measures, stretching exercises, modification of activity (avoiding running and walking up hills and stairs), and biomechanical control in the form of temporary heel lifts, tape immobilization, and if abnormal pronation is present, custom foot orthotics. If the tendinopathy is not too far advanced, a 6- to 12-week program of muscle training supervised by physical therapy often obviates the need for further intervention. Immobilization in night splints or a cast for 4–6 weeks is indicated for recalcitrant cases. If the above measures fail, the patient should be referred for débridement and tendon lengthening.

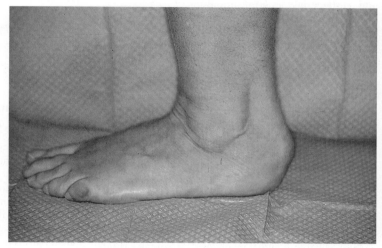

A

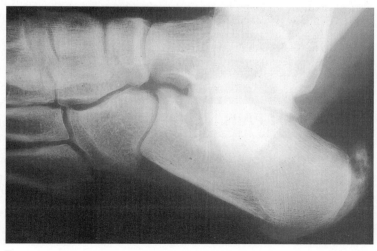

Figure 7–12. Achilles tendinitis. **A:** Photograph of a patient with a prominence in the area of the posterior superior aspect of the calcaneus. **B:** Lateral view radiograph of same patient demonstrating that an insertional calcific Achilles tendinitis, not Haglund deformity, is the cause of this deformity.   **B**

■ SUBTALAR JOINT & MIDFOOT DISORDERS

When a person is walking, subtalar joint motion correlates with hip motion and causes the foot to pronate with internal rotation of the hip and to supinate with external rotation of the hip. The motion of pronation unlocks the joints of the foot and occurs at heel contact as the foot strikes the ground, thereby absorbing shock and allowing the foot to adapt to uneven surfaces. Approaching mid stance (as the upper body moves over the foot), the hip externally rotates while the foot supinates. The motion of supination raises the arch, locks the joints of the foot, and creates a rigid lever for propulsion.

Inflammatory arthritis (eg, rheumatoid arthritis) and talocalcaneal coalitions can compromise subtalar motion.

A **pes planus** exists if the foot remains pronated beyond mid stance when subtalar joint motion produces maximal eversion of the heel. Pes planus often produces a heel valgus as the midtarsal joints unlock and collapse and as the forefoot abducts upon the rearfoot (see Figure 7–3). A pes planus is also often associated with an ankle equinus. Pes planus can be congenital or can be acquired as the result of rheumatoid arthritis, hypermobility syndromes, neuropathic arthropathy, and biomechanical disorders such as dysfunction of the tibialis posterior tendon.

Pes cavus is a rigid, excessively supinated foot that lacks shock absorption and has a high medial arch. Pes cavus can be congenital or the consequence of neuromuscular disorders such as Charcot-Marie-Tooth disease.

Biomechanical faults involving the subtalar, midtarsal, and MTP joints resulting in symptoms within the rearfoot, midfoot, and forefoot are treated with foot orthotics. While most of the information regarding the effectiveness of functional foot orthotics is anecdotal, several recent studies indicate that custom semi-rigid orthoses are effective and superior to off-the-shelf orthoses.

■ FOREFOOT PAIN

METATARSALGIA

Metatarsalgia, or pain in the region of the metatarsal heads and distal metatarsal shafts, can be generalized or localized to a single metatarsal and has many causes (Table 7–3). In all cases of metatarsalgia, it is important to rule out a metatarsal stress fracture as a cause of the discomfort.

Table 7–3. Causes of Central Metatarsalgia

Metatarsophalangeal joint stress syndrome
Intermetatarsal bursitis/neuritis
Morton neuroma
Stress fracture of the metatarsals
Freiberg disease (aseptic necrosis of the second metatarsal head)

METATARSAL STRESS FRACTURE

 ESSENTIALS OF DIAGNOSIS

- *"Central" metatarsalgia: pain over one or more of the central (second, third, or fourth) metatarsal shafts.*
- *Dorsal swelling.*
- *Positive "tuning fork" test.*

Clinical Findings

A. SIGNS AND SYMPTOMS

Metatarsal stress fractures are incomplete fractures of the diaphysis of the second, third, or fourth metatarsals. Fatigue stress fractures occur when abnormal, high energy, or repetitive forces—such as those generated by long-distance running—are placed on normal bone. Insufficiency or fragility stress fractures are a consequence of normal forces applied to abnormal bone. Most insufficiency stress fractures are associated with osteoporosis.

Stress fractures usually present as pain in the forefoot with weight bearing, accompanied by dorsal swelling. The onset of pain is acute but without a history of trauma. The pain is well localized and is reproduced by direct palpation dorsally along the involved metatarsal(s) shaft. Pain can also be localized to the fracture site by placing a vibrating tuning fork on the metatarsal shaft away from the area of discomfort.

B. IMAGING STUDIES

Plain radiographs (medial oblique, lateral, and anteroposterior views) should be obtained. Initially the fracture appears as a subtle break in the cortex of the distal metatarsal without bony callus formation (Figure 7–13). Early radiographs are often negative, and films should be repeated in 10 days if clinical suspicion warrants.

Treatment

Treatment consists of immobilization and rest. A rigid-soled fracture shoe or a prefabricated below-the-knee

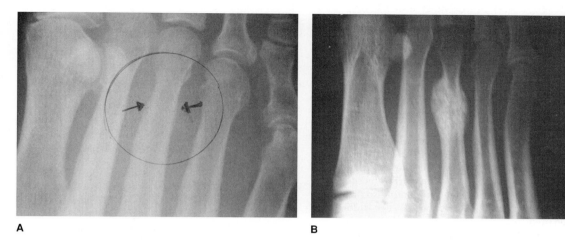

A   **B**

Figure 7–13. Radiographs demonstrating an insufficiency stress fracture of the third metatarsal. **A:** A cortical break at the metatarsal neck is barely visible at presentation. **B:** Four weeks later callus has formed at site of the stress fracture.

walking boot should be utilized for a period of 4–6 weeks. A fractured metatarsal can migrate dorsally, placing greater load on the adjacent metatarsals and leading to additional stress fractures.

METATARSOPHALANGEAL JOINT STRESS SYNDROME

 ESSENTIALS OF DIAGNOSIS

- *"Central" metatarsalgia: pain involving one or more of the central (second, third, or fourth) MTP joints.*
- *Positive luxation test for MTP joint instability.*
- *Central metatarsal heads palpable on the plantar surface.*

Clinical Findings

A. SYMPTOMS AND SIGNS

The MTP joint stress syndrome develops when there is transfer of stress from the load-bearing, flexible first and fifth MTPs to the fixed central MTP joints. Predisposing conditions include synovitis of the MTP joints due to rheumatoid arthritis or the spondyloarthropathies and biomechanical flaws, such as hallux limitus/rigidus and Morton foot (short first metatarsal). Initially (the pre-dislocation phase), there is inflammation of the MTP joints; dactylitis and minimal digital splaying may be

noted. Dislocation of the MTP joints occurs when there is rupture or attenuation of the plantar plate as it inserts into the base of the proximal phalanx. The second MTP joint is most often involved, but all of the central MTP joints can be affected. Digital deformities (hammer toe, claw toe, crossover toe) develop (Figure 7–14).

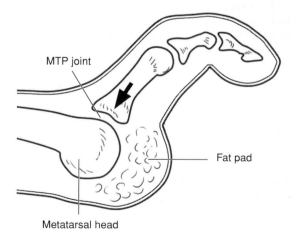

Figure 7–14. Diagram of a hammer toe deformity. There is dorsiflexion at the metatarsophalangeal joint and plantar flexion at the proximal interphalangeal joint. The protective fat pad normally beneath the metatarsal head displaces anteriorly. As the toe buckles, the retrograde digital force (arrow) places more stress upon the unprotected metatarsal head, creating metatarsalgia.

Eventually, the digital deformities cause anterior dislocation of the fat pad cushion of the forefoot and prolapse of the unprotected metatarsal heads, producing painful plantar callosity.

The pain is generally described as a dull ache in the ball of the forefoot, but in the predislocation phase, the pain sometimes has a burning quality similar to the symptoms of a neuroma. Pain occurs with weight bearing and increases with activities that place stress on the forefoot (eg, wearing high-heeled shoes). The pain is usually worse when walking barefoot. On examination, there may be plantar callosities and digital deformities such as splaying, hammering, clawing, and dactylitis. The involved metatarsal heads are tender when compressed between the examiner's thumb and forefinger. When dislocation has occurred, one or more of the metatarsal heads are readily palpable on the plantar surface. In less severe cases, the MTP joint luxation test (Lachman or vertical load test) assesses stability and integrity of the flexor plate and restraining ligaments. One hand stabilizes the metatarsal while the other lifts the proximal phalanx dorsally; findings of pain and ≥2 mm of dorsal displacement indicate an unstable MTP joint.

B. IMAGING STUDIES

Radiographs of the foot are not diagnostic but can help to exclude other conditions, such as a stress fracture.

Treatment

The involved digits should be held slightly plantar-flexed with tape or a digital splint in order to augment the flexor tendons and to reduce stress on the MTP joints. Patients should use supportive shoes with rigid soles and should avoid higher-heeled shoes. In more severe cases, the patient should be referred for biomechanical evaluation for custom foot orthotics or rocker-soled shoes, or both. Periarticular or intra-articular injection of a glucocorticoid can be given if the digit is splinted in plantar flexion to prevent dislocation.

MORTON NEUROMA

 ESSENTIALS OF DIAGNOSIS

- *Forefoot pain exacerbated by walking in shoes and often radiating to the third and fourth toes.*
- *Tenderness on palpation of the involved MTP interspace and Mulder click.*

Clinical Findings

Morton neuroma, a common cause of forefoot pain, is an entrapment neuropathy of an interdigital nerve, often associated with perineural fibrosis, that gives rise to a soft-tissue mass. The third MTP interspace is the most common location, although Morton neuromas are also found in the second, and rarely in the first or fourth interspaces. The patient describes burning, dull, or throbbing sensations that can radiate distally, transversely, or proximally, simulating a radiculopathy. The pain is intermittent and typically occurs while wearing shoes. Patients often remove their shoes and massage their feet in order to obtain relief. There is no pain with barefoot walking. There may be altered sensation on the sides or ends of the two toes adjacent to the involved interspace. Compression of the involved interspace with the thumb and forefinger of one hand while using the other hand to laterally compress the forefoot elicits pain. This maneuver also can cause the "neuromatous" mass to slip, producing a palpable click (Mulder click).

Treatment

Initial treatment consists of NSAIDs, contrast baths, and a lower-heeled, cushioned-soled shoe with a wide toe box. Using a dorsal approach, local anesthetic combined with a glucocorticoid can be injected into the involved distal interspace. Recalcitrant cases are referred for surgical neurolysis or neurectomy of the common digital nerve.

DEEP PERONEAL NERVE ENTRAPMENT

 ESSENTIALS OF DIAGNOSIS

- *Pain and dysesthesias of the first web and interspace.*
- *Nocturnal pain.*
- *Hypesthesia of the dorsal surfaces of the first interspace.*
- *Weakness of the extensor hallucis brevis in severe cases.*
- *Pain relief with nerve block.*

Clinical Findings

A. SYMPTOMS AND SIGNS

The patient with deep peroneal nerve entrapment presents with pain and abnormal sensation of the first

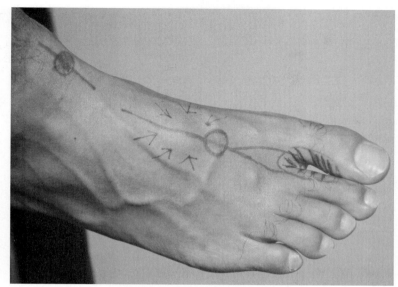

Figure 7–15. Peroneal nerve entrapment. Photograph illustrates the course of the peroneal nerve, the sites of proximal and distal entrapments (circles), and the region of abnormal sensation in the first web and interspace. In this case a dorsal exostosis of the second metatarsal cuneiform joint (arrows) contributed to distal entrapment.

web and interspace. The pain occurs with weight bearing but can continue into the evening at rest. Entrapment of the deep peroneal nerve occurs on the dorsal tarsus area in two separate locations (Figure 7–15).

Proximal entrapment (anterior tarsal tunnel syndrome) occurs in a tunnel that is formed under the extensor retinaculum where the nerve is bordered medially by the extensor hallucis longus tendon, laterally by the tendon of the extensor digitorum longus, and inferiorly by the tarsal bones. In this case pain is reproduced with palpation of the nerve under the extensor retinaculum over the instep. The pain is described as a deep aching to a burning sensation which radiates distally into the first web space. Pain is often aggravated at night in bed as the foot plantarflexes at the ankle, tensing the retinaculum and increasing pressure on the nerve. Late in the disease weakness of the extensor hallucis brevis may be noted.

Distal entrapment occurs where the nerve continues beyond the retinaculum at the second metatarsal cuneiform articulation. At this location the tendon of the extensor hallucis brevis crosses over the nerve as it exits from beneath the deep fascia. Degenerative changes of metatarsal cuneiform joints may contribute to the nerve entrapment. This area also corresponds to where the vamp of the shoe crosses the forefoot in certain shoe designs, such as pumps, and where lace-up shoes can cause irritation from lacing or the placement of an eyelet. The symptoms are the same as those of anterior tarsal tunnel syndrome except that plantar flexion does not increase symptoms.

Treatment

Symptomatic treatment in the form of rest, NSAIDs, modification of footgear (skip lacing, etc.), pressure-off pads, contrast baths, or ice massage is helpful. If plantar flexion increases symptoms, then immobilization in a below-the-knee walker should be instituted. Injections of glucocorticoids can be effective. Recalcitrant cases should be referred for consideration of surgery.

HALLUX LIMITUS & HALLUX RIGIDUS

 ESSENTIALS OF DIAGNOSIS

- *Limited or absent motion of the first MTP joint.*
- *Radiographic evidence of osteoarthritis of the first MTP joint.*

Clinical Findings

A. SYMPTOMS AND SIGNS

Hallux limitus and hallux rigidus are consequences of degenerative arthritis of the first MTP joint. Although a history of trauma (eg, ballet dancing) may be obtained, hallux limitus/rigidus usually is secondary to a biomechanical fault that leads to jamming of the first MTP

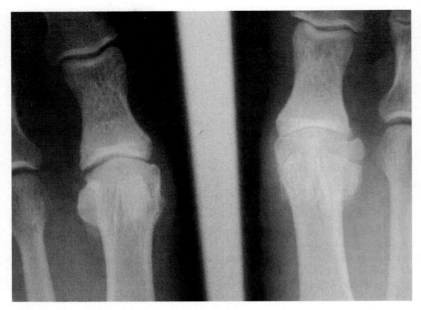

Figure 7–16. Radiographs of a patient with bilateral hallux limitus. On the left there is flattening of the metatarsal head and slight joint space narrowing. There is marked joint space narrowing on the more severely affected right first MTP joint.

joint. In hallux limitus, range of motion of the first MTP joint is decreased but not absent; pain is reproduced at the end points of motion. In hallux rigidus, joint motion is virtually absent, and what little there is creates pain and crepitation.

Patients complain of a deep, dull ache at the base of the great toe with weight bearing. The pain increases with any activity that places stress on the forefoot, such as walking barefoot, stooping, or wearing high-heeled shoes. Fragments of cartilage can shear off and become lodged in the synovium, triggering a detritic synovitis that is commonly mistaken for gout. Occasionally patients complain of numbness or burning in the first toe due to concomitant entrapment of the first dorsal digital nerve. The patient also may experience pain along the lateral column of the foot and lateral leg as he or she adducts the foot and uses the second through fifth MTP joints for propulsion in an attempt to walk without dorsiflexing the painful first MTP joint.

When the foot is examined while not bearing weight, hallux limitus is present if dorsiflexion of the first MTP joint is less than 65 degrees relative to the long axis of the first metatarsal. Occasionally, a first MTP joint exhibits normal range of motion when not bearing weight, but is functionally limited during gait. If dorsiflexion is less than 20 degrees as measured by the position of the hallux relative to the ground when standing, then a functional hallux limitus exists.

B. Imaging Studies

Radiographs of hallux limitus usually reveal flattening and dorsal spurring of the metatarsal head and an elevated first metatarsal (Figure 7–16). With time the degenerative changes of the first MTP joint worsen, creating hallux rigidus.

Treatment

Symptomatic treatment includes rest, contrast baths, and NSAIDs. Lower-heeled, rigid-soled shoes with soft uppers are advised. Injection of a local anesthetic and glucocorticoid into the first metatarsal interspace lateral to the joint or in the area of a nerve entrapment will usually quiet the symptoms. More severe cases benefit from rigid custom foot orthotics. Surgical intervention may be indicated if the above measures fail. Functional hallux limitus usually responds well to custom foot orthotics that load the central metatarsals.

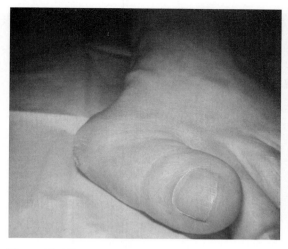

Figure 7–17. Severe hallux valgus.

HALLUX VALGUS

 ESSENTIALS OF DIAGNOSIS

- *Lateral deviation of the great toe.*
- *Medial bunion.*

Clinical Findings

A. SYMPTOMS AND SIGNS

Hallux valgus consists of medial deviation of the first metatarsal and a valgus deformity at the first MTP joint (Figures 7–17 and 7–18). It most likely results from the combination of a biomechanical fault, constrictive footgear, and walking on hard surfaces. Symptoms associated with the medial prominence of the first MTP joint usually are secondary to a pressure-induced bunion (an adventitious bursitis on the medial aspect of the joint), a nerve entrapment, or both. Sometimes the hallux valgus itself is asymptomatic but contributes to a painful forefoot deformity such as a hammer second toe or transfer metatarsalgia (see Figure 7–18).

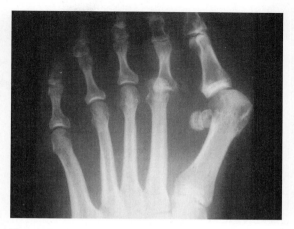

Figure 7–18. Weight-bearing radiograph of severe hallux valgus. Valgus deformity of the first MTP joint and medial deviation of the first metatarsal are readily apparent. The hallux valgus has led to dislocation of second MTP joint.

Treatment

Eliminating pressure from the bunion will minimize symptoms for patients with medial pain. Avoidance of high-fashion constrictive footgear is imperative. Bunion splints that attempt to correct the deformity are of little use, but custom shoes can benefit patients with severe deformity. Patients with continual symptoms or progression of deformity should be referred for surgical consultation.

REFERENCES

Oloff LM, Schulhofer SD. Flexor hallucis longus dysfunction. *J Foot Ankle Surg.* 1998;37:101. [PMID: 9571456]

Powell M, Seid M, Szer IS. Efficacy of custom foot orthotics in improving pain and function status in children with juvenile idiopathic arthritis: A randomized trial. *J Rheum.* 2005;32:943. [PMID:158683]

Woodburn J, Barker S, Helliwell PS. A randomized controlled trial of foot orthoses in rheumatoid arthritis. *J Rheum.* 2002;29:1377. [PMID:12136891]

Relevant World Wide Web Sites

[ProLab Orthotics/USA]
www.prolaborthotics.com

Approach to the Painful Shoulder   8

Robin V. West, MD, & Mark W. Rodosky, MD

There are many sources of shoulder pain, making the diagnosis and treatment of shoulder pain complex. A thorough patient interview is the starting point for establishing the diagnosis.

INTERVIEW

The quality of the pain should be documented and may include such characteristics as sharp, shooting, constant, burning, or aching. Features of the pain that need to be addressed include the date of onset, history of trauma, character of the pain, associated symptoms, and all aggravating and relieving factors. Associated symptoms may include numbness, weakness, instability, stiffness, redness, fevers, and weight loss.

Pain is a subjective complaint but needs to be documented in an objective manner. Questions that should be answered include the presence of night pain (often indicates rotator cuff pathology), analgesic requirements, degree of interference with work and activities of daily living, and an estimate by the patient of the amount of pain on a linear scale. Following the interview, the physical examination is the next step in the evaluation of a painful shoulder.

PHYSICAL EXAMINATION

The physical exam should be meticulous and can be mastered only by experience. A systematic approach should be used to avoid overlooking anything. The four basic steps of the exam include inspection, palpation, range of motion, and specialty tests.

Inspection

Observation is initially performed. How is the patient using the affected arm? Is he or she wearing a sling? Is the patient able to take off her or his coat without assistance? The initial impression is followed by inspection for scars, atrophy, muscle spasm, skin changes, or deformity (Figure 8–1). Scars provide information regarding trauma or previous surgery. Muscle wasting may be due to an underlying neurologic condition or to disuse atrophy. Paracervical spasm is common in patients with underlying cervical spine disease. Distal muscle wasting, like that of the interossei of the hand, may be found in cervical nerve root disorders. Deltoid wasting is best viewed over the anterior acromion and will produce a "squared-off" shoulder. Atrophy of the spinati will lead to a prominent scapular spine. Supraspinatus atrophy is more difficult to assess than infraspinatus atrophy since it is sheltered deep in the fossa under the trapezius.

Skin changes can aid in the diagnosis. Erythema, ecchymosis, or hair loss can indicate an infection, hemorrhage (seen with proximal biceps ruptures or fractures), or reflex sympathetic dystrophy. Deformities of the acromioclavicular joint may indicate previous trauma or underlying arthritis. Scapular winging is best assessed while the patient performs a wall push-up (Figure 8–2). Winging can be associated with thorax deformities, such as scoliosis, or with weakness of the major scapular stabilizers, including the trapezius, serratus anterior, or the rhomboids. Severe scapular winging is most commonly due to dysfunction of the long thoracic nerve and secondary serratus anterior palsy.

Palpation

Sites that should be palpated include the acromioclavicular and sternoclavicular joints, the biceps tendon (in the bicipital groove), the posterior joint line, and the rotator cuff at its insertion on the greater tuberosity. Deformities that may be tender along the course of the clavicle may be associated with either an acute or an un-united fracture. Tenderness over the superior surface of the acromion may indicate an os acromiale with underlying impingement. The acromioclavicular joint is best identified by following the clavicle and the spine of the scapula out laterally until they meet. Arthritis of the sternoclavicular and acromioclavicular joints is usually associated with tenderness. The greater tuberosity may be tender in patients with a fracture, rotator cuff tendinitis, or a tear. The bicipital groove is identified between the greater and lesser tuberosities. It can be palpated in thin patients as the arm is gently externally and internally rotated. The groove faces directly anterior when the arm is in about 10 degrees of internal rotation. Tenderness in the bicipital groove often indicates biceps tendinitis. Biceps tendinitis is seldom an isolated diagnosis, and is usually associated with underlying rotator cuff pathology. Glenohumeral joint arthritis may elicit posterior joint line tenderness.

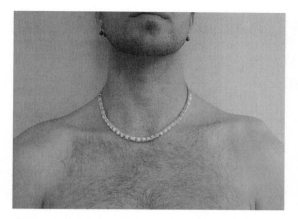

Figure 8–1. Inspection shows that there is a prominent acromioclavicular joint.

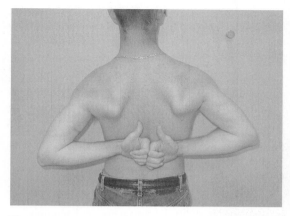

Figure 8–3. Document range of motion, checking internal rotation of both shoulders.

Range of Motion

Range of motion of the shoulder can be assessed in the upright or supine position. Active motion should always be compared to the contralateral side and documented. Passive motion only needs to be noted when active motion is incomplete. The motion of the opposite shoulder should also be documented. Because of the global nature of shoulder motion, a multitude of motions can be assessed. However, these various motions make documentation difficult. Therefore, the society of American Shoulder and Elbow Surgeons recommends recording the following arcs of motion. They have agreed that this list represents a standard protocol, which is simple and reproducible:

1. Total elevation
2. External rotation at side
3. External rotation in 90 degrees of abduction
4. Internal rotation

Total elevation represents a more functional measurement than forward flexion or abduction. With total elevation, the patient is allowed to find the most comfortable position in between the coronal and sagittal planes. Internal rotation is checked by having the patient scratch their back to the highest achievable point (Figure 8–3).

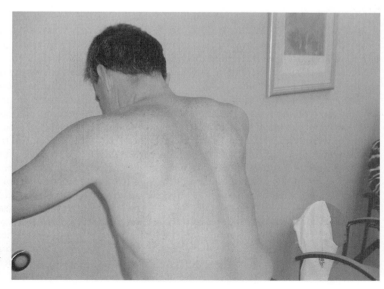

Figure 8–2. Have the patient do wall push-ups to check for scapular winging. This patient does not have evidence of scapular winging.

The point where the patient's thumb touches is recorded (ie, the gluteus, L4, or T7).

Neurologic Examination

Muscle strength should be assessed throughout all of the documented ranges of motion. Decreased strength may be seen in a patient with a rotator cuff tear, brachial plexus lesion, or cervical disk disease. Sensory testing should also be performed, along with evaluation of reflexes, to assess for central or peripheral nerve involvement.

Specialty Tests

Next, the exam becomes focused. Specialty tests are used to assess for instability, impingement, and acromioclavicular and bicipital pathology. Examination of the elbow and cervical spine should also be included in this part of the evaluation.

A. INSTABILITY

Laxity is asymptomatic, passive translation of the humeral head on the glenoid as determined by clinical examination. Laxity is not associated with pain and is necessary for normal glenohumeral joint motion. Laxity changes with position of the arm, as the static restraints tighten and decrease laxity at the extremes of motion.

Instability is a pathologic condition that manifests as pain or discomfort in association with excessive translation of the humeral head during active shoulder motion. Clinical and experimental studies demonstrate a wide range of normal laxity in the glenohumeral joint; therefore, it is the association of pain that separates instability from excessive laxity.

General ligamentous laxity is commonly associated with shoulder instability and should be assessed by evaluating the range of motion of several other joints. The degree of thumb hyperabduction and elbow and knee hyperextension should be documented as part of the instability portion of the exam.

The specific instability tests include the sulcus sign test, the load and shift test, the apprehension test, and the relocation test. These tests should be initiated on the unaffected shoulder first to obtain baseline data. Two components should be addressed during this part of the exam: (1) the amount of passive translation of the glenohumeral joint, and (2) the reproduction of symptoms of subluxation, dislocation, or apprehension by provocative testing.

The sulcus sign test establishes the presence of inferior laxity. This test is performed with the patient in the seated position. The arm is held at the side in neutral rotation. The examiner places a downward distraction force by grasping the distal humerus. The degree of the sulcus sign is determined by measuring the distance between the lateral acromion to the top of the humeral head. The contralateral shoulder is compared. An increased or symptomatic sulcus sign may indicate inferior instability and associated multidirectional instability.

The shift and load test is used to test for anterior and posterior translation. It is usually performed in the supine position but can also be performed in the upright position. To test for anterior translation of the patient's right shoulder, the examiner positions the patient's arm in the plane of the scapula, at about 45 degrees of abduction and neutral rotation. The examiner's right hand grasps the patient's arm and applies an axial load to the humeral head. This maneuver centers the humeral head in the glenoid. The examiner's right hand also controls the rotation of the patient's arm. The examiner uses her or his left hand, with the fingers placed anteriorly, to grasp the patient's upper arm. The examiner's left hand then shifts the humeral head anteriorly over the glenoid rim. The amount of translation can be determined by visual inspection and palpation. As the examiner maintains an axial load, the arm can be incrementally externally rotated. With progressive external rotation, the inferior glenohumeral ligament becomes taut, decreasing the anterior translation of the humeral head. The degree of translation can be graded. Grade I translation occurs when the center of the humeral head rides over the glenoid rim. Grade II occurs when the entire humeral head rides over the glenoid but reduces spontaneously. Grade III is defined as a complete dislocation, which requires a reduction maneuver to relocate the humeral head.

Posterior translation is evaluated in the same position as described for testing anterior translation. The patient is supine, with the arm held in the plane of the scapula. However, the exam is initiated with the arm in 45 degrees of external rotation. The examiner's hands are positioned as described for testing anterior translation. An axial load is applied, and the humeral head is translated posteriorly. The patient's arm is then sequentially rotated internally, and the exam is repeated. The posterior-inferior capsule becomes increasingly taut during internal rotation, decreasing the posterior translation of the humeral head. The posterior translation is graded the same as described for anterior translation.

The apprehension test places the shoulder in a provocative position of abduction and external rotation. This test should be performed in both the supine (Figure 8–4) and seated positions. The examiner abducts the patient's arm to 90 degrees and gently begins to externally rotate the arm. With increasing external rotation and controlled gentle forward pressure on the humeral head, the patient may have an apprehensive feeling of

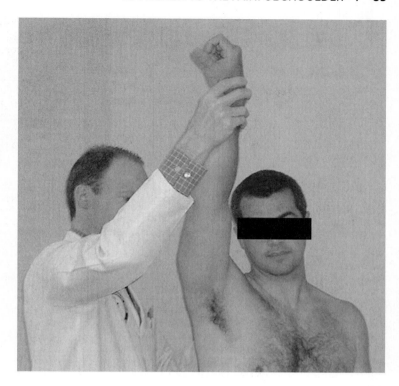

Figure 8–4. The apprehension test.

impending instability. Isolated pain is poorly correlated with instability, and a subjective feeling of apprehension by the patient has been shown to be more specific to the diagnosis of instability.

The relocation test should be performed in conjunction with the apprehension test. During this test, the examiner applies a posteriorly directed force on the humeral head with the patient's arm in the position that produces apprehension. This test reduces the humeral head, and a positive result is recorded if the symptoms of apprehension are eliminated.

B. IMPINGEMENT TESTS

Rotator cuff tendinitis has been termed shoulder impingement. The impingement sign and impingement test were described by Neer in 1977. The sign is considered positive when pain occurs with forcible elevation of the arm (Figure 8–5). This maneuver causes impingement of the inflamed supraspinatus tendon against the anterior inferior acromion. An alternative method for demonstrating impingement is to forward flex the arm to 90 degrees and then to forcibly internally rotate the shoulder (the Hawkins impingement sign; Figure 8–6).

The impingement test documents the patient's response to an injection of lidocaine into the subacromial space. After the injection is performed, the impingement maneuver is repeated. A significant reduction or abolition of the patient's pain constitutes a positive result and indicates a diagnosis of impingement.

C. ACROMIOCLAVICULAR DISORDERS

Acromioclavicular pain can be caused by degenerative changes or trauma. Associated tenderness and deformity are common after acromioclavicular trauma or with arthritis. The cross-arm adduction test may also be used to diagnose AC joint pathology. This test is performed with forced crossed-arm adduction in the 90-degree forward flexed position. Associated pain may indicate acromioclavicular joint pathology, usually degenerative arthritis.

D. BICEPS EVALUATION

Biceps pathology is seldom an isolated entity. It is usually a secondary diagnosis to impingement. However, it can be a primary diagnosis. Numerous tests have been described to test the biceps. However, their reliability is

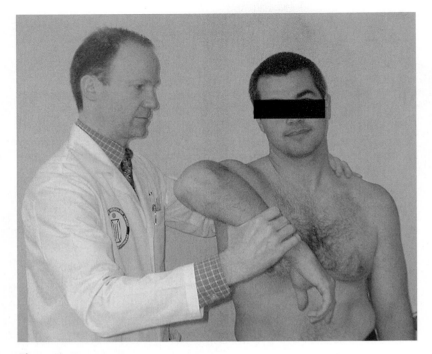

Figure 8–5. Neer impingement sign.

questionable. Tenderness in the bicipital groove, and Yergason and Speed are some of the tests that are used to assess biceps pathology. Tenderness in the bicipital groove may indicate inflammation of the long head of the biceps tendon. The Yergason test is performed with the elbow flexed to 90 degrees and the forearm pronated. The patient is then asked to actively supinate the arm against resistance as the examiner holds the patient's wrist. The Speed test is performed with the elbow extended and the forearm supinated. Forward elevation of the arm to 60 degrees is resisted. A positive result with either of these tests may indicate biceps inflammation.

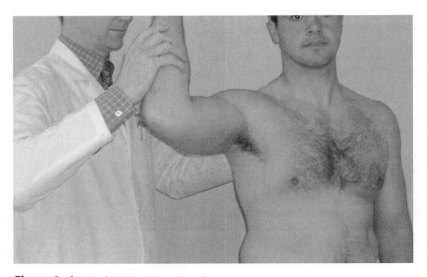

Figure 8–6. Hawkins impingement sign.

Vascular Examination

The vascular examination involves assessment of the entire upper limb. Skin texture, color, temperature, hair growth, pulses, and alterations in sensation should be documented and may relate to vascular problems. Vascular compression or thoracic outlet syndrome may cause shoulder pain. Thoracic outlet syndrome may cause a combination of neurologic and vascular signs. Several tests have been described to diagnose thoracic outlet syndrome. However, the reliability of these tests is not high.

A. THE ADSON MANEUVER

The examiner palpates the radial pulse. The patient's head is then rotated toward the affected shoulder. The involved shoulder is then externally rotated and extended. The patient takes a deep breath and holds it. A positive test occurs when there is a decrease in the pulse with this maneuver.

B. THE ROOS TEST (OR PROVOCATIVE ELEVATION TEST):

The arms are abducted to 90 degrees, the shoulders are externally rotated 100 degrees, and the elbows are flexed 90 degrees. The patient then opens and closes the hands slowly for 3 minutes. If the patient suffers from fatigue, cramping, or tingling before 3 minutes, the test is considered positive for thoracic outlet syndrome.

IMAGING

Plain radiographs are used to assess for fractures, arthritis, calcific tendinitis, destructive bone lesions, and the bony morphology of the acromion. There are multiple radiographic views that can be obtained to assess a painful shoulder.

The anteroposterior (AP) views in the plane of the scapula in neutral, internal, and external rotation are obtained to visualize the glenohumeral joint, and the greater and lesser tuberosities. Cysts on the greater tuberosity may indicate rotator cuff disease. Calcium deposits in the supraspinatus can also be visualized on these views and indicate calcific tendinitis.

The axillary view can be used to assess for subtle joint space narrowing (early arthritis; Figure 8–7), an os acromiale, or a glenohumeral dislocation. The West Point axillary view is a slight variation of the standard axillary view. It provides a better evaluation of the anteroinferior glenoid rim, which is especially important when assessing for a bony Bankart lesion (capsulolabral avulsion) or glenoid rim fracture.

The supraspinatus outlet view shows the coracoacromial arch, and is used to determine the acromial morphology. The acromion can be classified into three types, depending on the morphology. Type I acromions have a flat undersurface and have the lowest risk for impingement. Type II have a curved undersurface, and type III have a hooked undersurface. Type III acromions are associated with the highest percentage of rotator cuff tears.

The Stryker notch view demonstrates the posterolateral humeral head and is useful for identifying a Hill-Sachs deformity. A Hill-Sachs deformity is frequently found following an anterior shoulder dislocation and represents a compression fracture of the posterolateral humeral head.

Magnetic resonance imaging (MRI) can demonstrate rotator cuff pathology, labral disorders, and osseous

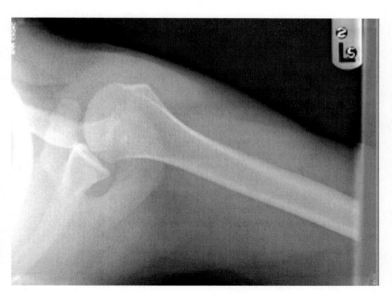

Figure 8–7. The axillary view radiograph is used to assess the glenohumeral joint for a concentric reduction or arthritis (joint space narrowing).

integrity. The advantages of MRI include the lack of ionizing radiation and the ability to detect small changes in soft-tissue composition without relying on an intravenous or an intra-articular injection of contrast material.

The accuracy in detecting full-thickness cuff tears has been reported to be between 93% and 100%. Partial-thickness tears are less accurately detected. The quality of the rotator cuff muscles, the size of the tear, and the involvement of the biceps tendon can be determined from the MRI. These MRI findings aid in the rehabilitation, surgical planning, and the postoperative planning following rotator cuff surgery.

An arthrogram can be used in addition to an x-ray or an MRI. The arthrogram in association with an x-ray has been shown to have a 95–100% accuracy rate for detecting full-thickness rotator cuff tears. An MRI arthrogram can aid in detection of partial-thickness tears.

DIAGNOSIS & TREATMENT

A working diagnosis needs to be established upon completion of the history, examination, and imaging. The following categories are the most common causes of shoulder pain:

- Cervical pathology
- Neurologic disorder
- Congenital anomaly
- Arthritis
- Trauma
- Instability
- Rotator cuff pathology
- Adhesive capsulitis
- Tumor

Cervical Pathology

Cervical spondylosis involves osteoarthritic changes of the joints of the cervical spine, including the facets and uncovertebral joints. Osteophytes may form and encroach upon the nerve root foramina. The cervical discs may also become desiccated and flattened.

Disc herniation consists of protrusion of the nucleus pulposus through a tear in the annulus fibrosis. The nerve root may become compressed within its foramen, producing cervical radiculopathy. Herniation can also occur in conjunction with cervical spondylosis.

Cervical radiculopathy and myelopathy may be caused by an acute, subacute, or insidious disc herniation. Subacute cervical radiculopathy is much more common than acute radiculopathy. Symptoms may include pain, paresthesias, and weakness. The dermatomal distribution of the pain, as well as weakness within certain muscles, may aid in differentiating the involved nerve root. The most commonly involved discs are C5–6 and C6–7.

Cervical myelopathy results from compression of the spinal cord. This compression may be caused by degenerative discs, facet or uncovertebral spondylosis, posterior vertebral osteophytes, or a hypertrophied ligamentous flavum. Symptoms of myelopathy may include weakness in the upper and/or lower extremities. Sensory complaints in the upper extremities are common. Global numbness is more common than the dermatomal symptoms that usually occur with radiculopathy. However, approximately 20% of patients do not have neck or upper extremity pain with cervical myelopathy.

Multiple radiologic techniques can be used to illustrate various aspects of cervical pathology. Besides plain radiographs, computed tomography (CT) and MRI scans can be used to evaluate the bony canal, epidural space, and the location and size of a disc herniation. Myelography is a dynamic study (flexion and extension) and provides good visualization of the intradural segments of the roots and cord. Combined CT and myelography offers the advantage of evaluating the bony and intradural architecture. Less volume of contrast is required with combined CT myelography than with myelography alone, resulting in fewer side effects. MRI is excellent for soft-tissue visualization.

The three main conservative treatment modalities for cervical disorders include: soft cervical collar immobilization, anti-inflammatory medications, and physical therapy modalities. Cervical traction may be helpful in young patients with isolated disc herniations but less helpful in patients with spondylosis. Epidural steroids, root injections, and facet blocks can be used for the treatment of spondylosis. Experienced physicians should perform these blocks to minimize the risk of complications. Surgical intervention is usually required in patients who fail medical management or those patients who have significant neurologic deficits, particularly weakness.

Neurologic Disorders

There are multiple neurologic disorders that can present with pain around the shoulder. Some of the more common disorders include serratus anterior nerve palsy, brachial plexus injury, and suprascapular nerve compression. Patients with long thoracic nerve palsy present with weakness of the serratus anterior muscle, which results in periscapular pain, winging of the scapula, and difficulty elevating the arm above shoulder level. The long thoracic nerve arises from C5, C6, and C7 and provides motor innervation to the serratus anterior muscle. The serratus anterior muscle originates from the upper nine ribs, inserts onto the inferior angle of the scapula, and provides upward rotation and protraction of the scapula. There are many causes of long thoracic nerve palsy, including blunt trauma, stretching of the nerve, viral infection, or iatrogenic trauma (during a mastectomy with axillary dissection). The palsy results in a loss of normal scapular stability and rotation. Winging of the scapula occurs with elevation of the arm. Electromyography is used to confirm the diagnosis and to follow nerve recovery. Most of the atraumatic palsies resolve over a 12- to 18-month period. Treatment in these patients with evidence of recovery includes observation and periscapular muscle strengthening. In patients with symptomatic scapular winging for longer than 1 year, who demonstrate no electromyographic or clinical evidence of recovery, surgical treatment may be considered. Multiple surgical procedures have been described, including a scapulothoracic fusion and dynamic muscle transfers. The goal of these procedures is pain reduction and improvement of scapular function.

Brachial plexus injuries can also cause shoulder pain. The most common causes of plexus injuries are traction caused by extreme movements, such as when the head is forced laterally during a football game or motorcycle accident. Direct trauma, with an associated clavicle fracture, can also result in a plexus injury. A thorough history, complete neurologic examination, and electrodiagnostic studies are essential in diagnosing the location, extent, and completeness of the injury. Poor prognosis is associated with supraclavicular lesions, complete injuries, and root avulsions. Patients with less severe injuries who demonstrate neural recovery or mild signs and symptoms are treated conservatively. Nerve reconstruction or repair is considered in more severe postganglionic lesions or open injuries.

Patients with suprascapular nerve entrapment often present with posterior shoulder pain, which radiates to the neck or down the arm. The suprascapular nerve arises from the upper trunk of the brachial plexus at Erb point. The nerve then courses posteriorly, deep to the trapezius, where it passes through the suprascapular notch. The notch is bounded by the transverse scapular ligament. After exiting the notch, the nerve innervates the suprascapular muscle and provides sensory branches to the AC joint, the rotator cuff, the glenohumeral joint, and the posterior capsule. The nerve then enters the spinoglenoid notch to finally reach the infraspinatus fossa, where it innervates the infraspinatus muscle.

Suprascapular nerve entrapment can occur from ganglion cysts arising from the glenohumeral joint, a hypertrophied spinoglenoid ligament, traction injuries, and microemboli which produce nerve ischemia. Ganglion cysts can cause entrapment at the suprascapular or spinoglenoid notch. Compression at the suprascapular notch causes weakness of both the supraspinatus and infraspinatus, while compression at the spinoglenoid notch causes isolated weakness of the infraspinatus. Physical examination may reveal atrophy of the spinati. Infraspinatus atrophy is more common and easier to identify than supraspinatus atrophy, since the supraspinatus muscle lies deep to the trapezius. Weakness in external rotation and forward elevation may also be noted. Routine shoulder radiographs rarely demonstrate pathology. Electromyographic and nerve conduction studies may localize the site of compression. An MRI of the shoulder can identify the ganglion cyst location and size. Initial treatment includes physical therapy and nonsteroidal anti-inflammatories. Physical therapy should concentrate on the scapular stabilizers, deltoid, and rotator cuff. Surgical intervention is recommended if more than 6 months of conservative treatment is unsuccessful. Surgery focuses on the source of the compression. The ganglion cyst can be excised through an open incision or decompressed arthroscopically.

Congenital Anomalies

Congenital anomalies are rare and can be the most difficult and perplexing problems of the shoulder girdle. The anomalies can be classified into disorders of the bones, muscles, or neurovascular system. A thorough discussion of congenital anomalies is out of the context of this chapter.

Arthritis

Arthritis can involve the glenohumeral, sternoclavicular (SC), or acromioclavicular (AC) joints. The arthritis can be degenerative, infectious, or inflammatory. Examination and radiographs can aid in the differentiation of the anatomic site and the type of arthritis. Examination findings may include decreased glenohumeral joint motion and tenderness to palpation over the posterior joint line in patients with glenohumeral arthritis. Tenderness over the AC joint, and pain with cross arm adduction may indicate AC joint arthritis. A long history of repetitive motion (manual labor or weightlifting) and chronic pain may lead to a diagnosis of degenerative arthritis. An insidious onset, with an associated family history, rashes, fevers, or involvement of multiple joints, may indicate an inflammatory arthritis. Infectious arthritis usually presents with an acute onset, fevers, redness, and warmth. The involved joint can be aspirated, and the synovial fluid can be analyzed to confirm the diagnosis. White blood cell counts over 100,000 cells/mL strongly suggest an infection.

Radiographs may also help differentiate the type of arthritis. Degenerative arthritis usually shows sclerosis, asymmetric joint space narrowing, and osteophytes. Inflammatory arthritis usually shows osteopenia, symmetric joint space narrowing, and lack of osteophytes. In the later stages, infectious arthritis often shows joint destruction, with a mixed pattern of sclerosis and osteopenia.

Degenerative and inflammatory arthritis can be treated conservatively with anti-inflammatories and physical therapy to maintain range of motion and strengthening. An intra-articular glenohumeral or acromioclavicular cortisone injection may also be used to relieve some of the symptoms. Surgical intervention is recommended for patients who have failed a course of conservative management. A distal clavicle excision can be performed for AC joint arthritis. A medial clavicle excision can be performed for SC joint arthritis. Degenerative glenohumeral joint arthritis can be treated with either a hemiarthroplasty or a total shoulder arthroplasty. Infectious arthritis is a surgical emergency and should be treated with surgical débridement and antibiotics.

Trauma

A traumatic event can result in a myotendinous injury, a fracture, or a dislocation. A thorough neurologic and vascular exam should be documented, and good radiographs are mandatory when evaluating a patient following an injury. Ecchymosis and deformity are common physical findings following a traumatic injury to the shoulder.

Most fractures can be treated in a sling initially, until further evaluation by an orthopedic surgeon is obtained. Open fractures, or ones that compromise the integrity of the skin, require emergent surgical intervention. Other injuries that should be treated urgently include posterior sternoclavicular and glenohumeral dislocations. Anterior SC dislocations are much more common and less dangerous, but posterior SC dislocations can compromise the underlying vessels and structures. These injuries are best assessed with a 40-degree cephalic tilt (serendipity) radiographic view (Figure 8–8) or a paraxial CT scan. An

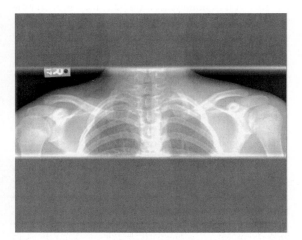

Figure 8–8. The serendipity view of both sternoclavicular joints. The left sternoclavicular joint shows a fracture dislocation of the medial clavicle.

urgent reduction of the posteriorly dislocated SC joint is often required.

Myotendinous injuries, including an acute rotator cuff tear, or a rupture of the pectoralis major or long head of the biceps, usually result in an acute onset of pain and weakness. Ecchymosis is a common finding. Initial treatment includes ice, rest, and NSAIDs. Surgical intervention is often required to perform a direct primary repair of the rotator cuff or pectoralis major acute ruptures.

Instability

The most common sequela of traumatic anterior shoulder dislocation is recurrence. Classic studies have documented a recurrence rate of 90% for patients under the age of 20. The recurrence rate is significantly lower in patients over the age of 40 years.

Patients with a traumatic dislocation will present with pain and guarding of their affected arm. Motion will be limited, and the shoulder contour may be disrupted. A neurovascular exam is important to document, since an associated axillary neuropraxia occurs in 5–35% of first-time anterior shoulder dislocations. Sensation testing over the lateral deltoid is the best place to assess the axillary nerve. Vascular injuries are rare but should be ruled out.

It is important to rule out a traumatic rotator cuff tear in older patients who sustain a shoulder dislocation. Associated cuff tears are common in older patients and can be confused with axillary neuropraxia during the clinical examination. Tears of the rotator cuff following dislocation have been reported to occur in 14–63% of patients. The incidence significantly increases in patients over the age of 50 years. Axillary neuropraxia will often present with weakness and numbness over the lateral aspect of the shoulder, while a rotator cuff tear presents only with weakness. An MRI can be performed to confirm the diagnosis of an associated rotator cuff tear.

Radiographic analysis should include a true AP in the plane of the scapula and an axillary view. The axillary view is mandatory to demonstrate an anterior or posterior glenohumeral dislocation. A West Point axillary view may better demonstrate an anterior-inferior glenoid rim fracture. Several recent studies correlating MRI arthrogram with surgical findings demonstrate an 88% sensitivity and 100% specificity in diagnosing inferior glenohumeral ligament tears.

Simple anterior dislocations without associated fractures can usually be reduced manually with sedation. Multiple reduction maneuvers have been described. The traction/counter traction technique is usually effective. From the contralateral side, an assistant holds a sheet that is wrapped around the patient's chest. The physician gently applies longitudinal traction to the injured side. A satisfying click is usually obtained with the reduction. The reduction should be confirmed with a true AP and axillary radiograph.

Following the reduction, a brief period of immobilization, activity modification, and a supervised rehabilitation program for rotator cuff and periscapular stabilizing exercises is used. Conservative treatment is usually the first line of treatment, with acute surgical stabilization being considered in young athletes returning to contact sports. Once recurrent episodes of instability have occurred, conservative treatment has failed; surgical intervention is then considered. Open and arthroscopic procedures that restore the normal glenohumeral anatomy are favored. The repair of the avulsed capsular-labral tissue (Bankart lesion) or reduction of the excessive capsular laxity is the goal of the reconstructive procedure.

Patients with multidirectional instability have symptomatic subluxation or dislocation in more than one direction: anterior, inferior, and posterior. The instability episodes are often atraumatic and painful. The primary cause is a loose redundant capsule. Swimmers, weightlifters, and gymnasts are particularly predisposed to multidirectional instability. The physical exam may demonstrate evidence of generalized ligamentous laxity, and a significant finding is usually the sulcus sign (described above). Once the diagnosis of multidirectional instability is established, a prolonged course of physical therapy is instituted. The therapy emphasizes deltoid, periscapular, and rotator cuff strengthening with the arm below the horizontal plane. Surgery is usually recommended after at least 6 months of supervised physical therapy. It is important to identify voluntary dislocators, because they are poor candidates for surgical stabilization. Surgical intervention includes a capsular shift, which decreases the glenohumeral joint capsular volume.

Rotator Cuff Pathology

Rotator cuff disorders represent a spectrum of disease, including inflammation, partial- or full-thickness tears, and cuff tear arthropathy. Mechanical impingement and intrinsic degenerative processes have been cited as factors underlying rotator cuff disease.

Impingement syndrome is one of the most common causes of shoulder pain. It is a clinical diagnosis, which is made on the basis of a careful history and physical examination. Radiographs, especially the outlet view, are helpful in demonstrating the presence of subacromial spurs and acromion morphology. A subacromial lidocaine injection is useful in verifying the diagnosis. In some patients, especially overhead athletes, it may be difficult to differentiate between functional subacromial impingement, subtle instability, and "internal impinge-

ment" of the undersurface of the rotator cuff on the posterior glenoid rim. Treatment of subacromial impingement initially includes a subacromial cortisone injection and a physical therapy program for rotator cuff strengthening to improve humeral head centering and stretching to improve stiffness. Refractory cases are treated with an arthroscopic acromioplasty.

An MRI or ultrasound can be obtained if there is concern that there is an associated rotator cuff tear. Plain MRIs have been found to have a sensitivity of 100% and specificity of 95% for diagnosing full-thickness rotator cuff tears and a sensitivity of 82% and specificity of 85% for partial thickness tears. Ultrasound is also an excellent tool for diagnosing full-thickness tears. Ultrasound has a sensitivity of 100% and specificity of 91% for full-thickness tears and a sensitivity of 80% and specificity of 98% for partial tears. Partial tears are best visualized with MRI arthrograms. Patients with a rotator cuff tear will often demonstrate weakness, recalcitrant pain, and night pain. Many partial-thickness tears can be managed nonsurgically. If a patient with a partial-thickness rotator cuff tear continues to have symptoms, arthroscopic surgery is recommended. This procedure usually entails an arthroscopic acromioplasty, débridement, and possible repair of the rotator cuff.

Factors to consider in the choice of treatment for full-thickness rotator cuff tears include the severity and duration of symptoms, functional limitations, patient demands and expectations, and tear size and location. Operative decisions are individualized and should not be based on MRI scans alone. There is a high prevalence of cuff tears in the asymptomatic population, with a direct correlation with increasing age. In a prospective study of 411 asymptomatic volunteers, rotator cuff tears were identified by ultrasound in 23% of patients. The incidence of tears was age-dependent. The prevalence increased to 31% and 51% in patients aged 70–79 years and over 80 years, respectively. These results provide evidence that patients with rotator cuff tears can exhibit relatively normal shoulder function. However, the natural history of rotator cuff tears remains unknown. A longitudinal analysis of asymptomatic cuff tears detected by ultrasonography was recently published. Fifty-eight patients with unilateral symptomatic rotator cuff tears and contralateral asymptomatic cuff tears were followed over a 5-year period. Twenty-three (51%) of the previously asymptomatic patients became symptomatic over a mean of 2.8 years. Twenty-three of the original patients returned for a repeat ultrasound, and nine of these patients had tear progression. No patient had a decrease in the size of the tear. These ultrasound findings in asymptomatic patients may represent an early phase of the pathologic process of rotator cuff tears in which symptoms have not yet developed.

The presence of a full-thickness rotator cuff tear is not necessarily an indication for surgery. As previously mentioned, MRI and cadaver studies have shown that a substantial number of asymptomatic patients have rotator cuff tears. The indications for rotator cuff repair are the presence of pain or functional deficits that interfere with activities or do not respond to conservative treatment. Early surgical intervention is usually recommended when there is an acute traumatic rotator cuff tear or when weakness is prominent or progressive.

Adhesive Capsulitis

Adhesive capsulitis or "frozen shoulder" is a poorly defined syndrome, in which both active and passive motion is lost because of soft-tissue contracture. Pain and limited motion are common complaints. The pain is typically worse at night, but progresses to a constant pain at rest. The syndrome is characterized by thickening and contracture of the joint capsule, which results in decreased glenohumeral joint volume. It is believed to be a benign, self-limited disorder, which tends to resolve over 1–2 years, although patients are often left with residual loss of motion. A variety of etiologies have been implicated in the disorder, including, trauma, inflammatory, and endocrine abnormalities. The inciting trauma is sometimes very mild and is often not recalled by the patient. It is common in patients with diabetes and is more frequently bilateral and resistant to treatment in this subset of patients.

Adhesive capsulitis is a clinical diagnosis and radiologic studies are not necessary to confirm the diagnosis. However, plain radiographs and an MRI should be ordered to rule out any underlying bony or soft-tissue problems.

Most patients with frozen shoulder respond to nonsurgical treatment with a supervised physical therapy program for stretching exercises. If the therapy program is unsuccessful, manipulation under anesthesia can be done to regain motion. An arthroscopic capsular release can be used in addition to the manipulation in treating cases of resistant adhesive capsulitis. An indwelling interscalene or intra-articular catheter can also be used in addition to the surgical treatment to facilitate early postoperative therapy.

Tumor

Radiographic abnormalities and bone or soft-tissue masses need to be evaluated in a well-organized and methodical fashion. The diagnostic work-up and treatment of bone and soft-tissue tumors about the shoulder is based on the principles of oncologic surgery. The work-up should be performed promptly to improve patient survival and functional outcome. The goals of treatment are first, preservation of life, followed by preservation of limb and function. Amputation was the primary treatment for primary bone tumors in the 1970s. However, successful limb salvage techniques have been developed for malignant and aggressive benign tumors.

The work-up of a tumor involves proceeding in a systematic fashion: clinical assessment, diagnostic studies, and biopsy in select cases. It is important to consult an orthopedic oncologist early in the work-up. Treatment should not be initiated until the oncologist has been consulted.

A thorough history should be documented. Patients often complain of associated symptoms including pain, fevers, and a mass. For example, an osteoid osteoma often causes night pain that is relieved by nonsteroidal anti-inflammatory medications. Patients with an Ewing sarcoma may have systemic signs and symptoms, such as fevers, sweats, and an elevated erythrocyte sedimentation rate.

Plain radiographs are the most useful and cost-effective study. Radiographs are relatively sensitive in detecting bony abnormalities, and they may show associated soft-tissue masses. Specific findings, including the anatomic location and the bony reaction, on the radiographs can be helpful in the diagnosis.

Certain tumors have a predilection for the epiphysis (chondroblastoma), the diaphysis (Ewing sarcoma), or the metaphysis (conventional osteosarcoma). Well-circumscribed lesions are usually associated with benign lesions, and a permeative appearance on the radiographs suggests an aggressive lesion. Periosteal reaction is a useful measure of lesion aggressiveness. Slowly expanding lesions, either benign or malignant, may produce a lamellar periosteal reaction ("onion skinning"). More rapidly growing tumors can expand beyond the periosteal sleeve and gives the appearance of a "sunburst" reaction.

In certain benign lesions, no further work-up is necessary after the radiographs. However, when treatment is indicated, other diagnostic studies are necessary. Technetium bone scans are helpful in determining polyostotic involvement or skip lesions. CT scans give excellent definition of bony structures, including cortical destruction, fractures, and soft-tissue calcification. MRI is useful is determining the osseous and soft tissue extension. Occasionally, other studies are required. These may include angiography to assess vascular involvement, a biopsy to aid in the diagnosis, or a CT scan of the chest to assess for metastatic disease.

Treatment is based on the diagnosis. Benign lesions (simple cysts) are usually treated nonoperatively. Aggressive-benign lesions (giant cell tumors) often require surgical intervention with curettage and bone grafting or cementation. Malignant lesions (Ewing sarcoma) usually require a combination of treatment modalities, including resection, chemotherapy, and radiation.

Injection Techniques

Prior to performing an injection, the patient should understand the risks and benefits of the procedure. The risks include an allergic reaction, infection, hypopigmentation of the skin, and poor blood glucose control in diabetics. The site should be thoroughly prepped with alcohol and povidone-iodine, and the injection should be performed under sterile conditions. The povidone-iodine is bacteriostatic when wet and only becomes bactericidal when it dries. The injection site can be injected with local anesthetic before the corticosteroid injection to help with pain control, or a combination of the local anesthetic and the corticosteroid can be injected together.

The choice of the corticosteroid is physician-dependent. Some physicians prefer to use more water-soluble agents for soft-tissue injections and less water-soluble ones for intra-articular injections. Use of the water-soluble agent in the soft tissue may result in fewer local effects, such as fatty atrophy and skin discoloration, while the less water-soluble agents may last longer for intra-articular injections and result in fewer systemic effects.

A. SUBACROMIAL SPACE

The subacromial space is most commonly injected in patients with impingement. The cortisone can serve as treatment, and the lidocaine can aid in the diagnosis (the impingement test). The injection is performed from the posterior aspect of the shoulder. The posterolateral corner of the acromion is palpated. The injection is placed into the subacromial space with a 22-gauge needle about 1 cm distal and 1 cm medial to the posterior corner.

B. GLENOHUMERAL

This space is seldom injected. It is more commonly aspirated to rule out an infection in patients who present with a fever and a painful, warm shoulder. A cortisone injection can be performed for the treatment of glenohumeral arthritis. The posterolateral corner of the acromion is the landmark for the injection. A 22-gauge needle is usually used for injection, and an 18-gauge needle is used for aspiration. A spinal needle is sometimes needed in larger patients. The entry site is about 2 cm distal and 2 cm medial to the corner of the acromion. The needle is directed towards the coracoid.

C. ACROMIOCLAVICULAR

The acromioclavicular joint can be injected in patients with arthritis or distal clavicle osteolysis. The acromioclavicular joint can be palpated by placing a finger in the corner formed by the transition of the scapular spine to the acromion. The acromioclavicular joint is just anterior to this transition. The joint should be visualized radiographically prior to the injection, as the distal clavicle is often sloped about 15 degrees in the coronal plane. This slope should be documented to aid in a smooth, correct insertion of the needle into the acromioclavicular joint. The injection is usually performed with a 22-gauge needle.

SUMMARY

Pain is the most common presenting symptom about the shoulder. The diagnosis is often challenging because of the many sources of shoulder pain. A thorough patient evaluation, including the interview, examination, and radiographic work-up is mandatory. An orthopedic consultation should be obtained early in the evaluation if there is concern about an infection, tumor, or traumatic injury that may require urgent surgical treatment. The injuries that may require early orthopedic intervention include a traumatic rotator cuff tear in a young patient, a displaced proximal humerus fracture, posterior SC joint dislocation, septic joint, clavicle fracture that compromises the skin, or an irreducible shoulder dislocation.

REFERENCES

Bottoni CR, Wilckens JH, DeBerardino TM, et al. A prospective, randomized evaluation of arthroscopic stabilization versus non-operative treatment in patients with acute, traumatic, first-time shoulder dislocations. *Am J Sports Med.* 2002;84:711–715. (This is a prospective, randomized clinical trial that was done to compare nonoperative treatment versus arthroscopic stabilization in acute, traumatic shoulder dislocations in young athletes.)

Chandnani VP, Gagliardi JA, Murnane TG, et al. Glenohumeral ligaments and shoulder capsular mechanism: Evaluation with MR arthrography. *Radiology.* 1995;196:27–32. (This is a retrospective study that compared MRI arthrogram with surgical observations in patients with instability, impingement, or pain.)

Cole BJ, Schumacher HR. Injectable corticosteroids in modern practice. *J Am Acad Orthop Surg.* 2005;13:37–46.

Goldberg BA, Nowinski RJ, Matsen FA. Outcome of nonoperative management of full-thickness rotator cuff tears. *Clin Orthop.* 2001;382:99–107. (This study documents the functional outcome of 46 patients with full-thickness rotator cuff tears who were treated nonoperatively.)

Iannotti JP, Zlatkin MB, Esterhai JL, et al. Magnetic resonance imaging of the shoulder: sensitivity, specificity, and predictive value. *J Bone Joint Surg (Am).* 1991;73:17–29.

McConville OR, Iannotti JP. Partial-thickness tears of the rotator cuff: Evaluation and MAnagement. *J Am Acad Orthop Surg.* 1999;7:32–43. (This is a review of the evaluation and management of partial-thickness rotator cuff tears.)

Milosavljevic J, Elvin A, Rahme H. Ultrasonography of the rotator cuff: a comparison with arthroscopy in one-hundred-and-ninety consecutive cases. *Acta Radiol.* 2005;46:858–865.

Morrison DS, Frogameni AD, Woodworth P. Non-operative treatment of subacromial impingement syndrome. *J Bone Joint Surg.* 1997;79A:732–737. (This is a retrospective analysis of 616 patients with subacromial impingement syndrome who were treated nonoperatively.)

Schenk TJ, Brems JJ. Multidirectional instability of the shoulder: Pathophysiology, diagnosis, management. *J Am Acad Orthop Surg.* 1998;6:65–72. (This is a review of the pathophysiology, diagnosis, and treatment of multidirectional instability of the shoulder.)

Tempelhof S, Rupp S, Seil R. Age-related prevalence of rotator cuff tears in asymptomatic shoulder. *J Shoulder Elbow Surg.* 1999;8:296–299. (This is a prospective study to determine the prevalence of rotator cuff tears in asymptomatic shoulders and to determine an age-dependent relationship.)

Warner JP. Frozen shoulder: Diagnosis and management. *J Am Acad Orthop Surg.* 1997;5:130–140. (This is a review of the diagnosis and management of adhesive capsulitis.)

Yamaguchi K, Tetro AM, Blam O, et al. Natural history of asymptomatic rotator cuff tears—A longitudinal analysis of asymptomatic tears detected sonographically. *J Shoulder Elbow Surg.* 2001;10:199–203. (This is a longitudinal study that evaluates the natural history of asymptomatic rotator cuff tears over a 5-year period to assess the risk for development of symptoms and tear progression.)

Approach to the Patient with Neck Pain

David Borenstein, MD

Neck pain is a common musculoskeletal symptom and accounts for a sizeable proportion of the 9.3 million physician visits that occur annually in the United States for soft-tissue disorders. Mechanical disorders cause 90% of episodes of neck pain. Mechanical neck pain may be defined as pain secondary to overuse of a normal anatomic structure or pain secondary to trauma or deformity of an anatomic structure (Figure 9–1). Mechanical disorders are characterized by exacerbation and alleviation of pain in direct correlation with particular physical activities. Neck pain due to mechanical disorders will decrease within 2–4 weeks in over 50% of patients; symptoms usually resolve within 2–3 months.

■ INITIAL EVALUATION

The goal of the initial evaluation is to differentiate patients with probable mechanical disorders from those with neck pain that requires more thorough immediate evaluation (Figure 9–2). A history should be taken and an examination should be performed in all patients with new-onset neck pain. The neurologic examination should determine whether there are any signs of cervical nerve root compression or evidence of cord compression (ie, spastic weakness, hyperreflexia, clonus, and positive Babinski signs).

Diagnostic radiographic or laboratory tests are not necessary during the initial evaluation of patients with probable mechanical neck pain. These tests, however, are indicated for those patients whose history and physical findings suggest persistent compression of the spinal cord or nerve roots or raise the possibility of neck pain as a component of an underlying systemic disease.

History

The history should establish the character, onset, location, radiation, aggravating and alleviating factors, intensity, and chronological development of the neck pain. Mechanical disorders cause pain that increases with ac-tivity. The end of the day is associated with more severe distress, and mechanical disorders improve with recumbency and rest. Tingling pain that radiates down an arm is suggestive of nerve impingement. Aching pain of slow onset that localizes to the base of the cervical spine suggests muscle or joint involvement. The history should determine whether the neck pain has unusual qualities that suggest a focal destructive process (due to infection or tumor) or pain referred from the heart or other viscera, whether there are symptoms of associated neurologic deficits, and whether there is an underlying systemic disease that could predispose to a serious neck problem (Table 9–1).

A few days to weeks is the duration of mechanical neck pain. Disc herniations may require 8–12 weeks to resolve. Medical conditions tend to cause persistent chronic pain.

Physical Examination

Abnormalities of the cervical spine may be observed while the spine is in motion or static. Observation of the spine from 360 degrees identifies any misalignments of the neck or shoulders. Pain in the neck may cause deviation that can be toward or away from the painful side.

Palpation can detect painful structures as well as increased paraspinous muscle tension. Posterior elements of the cervical spine are more easily identified than those located anteriorly. In general, midline tenderness is related to an intrinsic spinal disorder, while sensitivity to pressure in structures off the midline suggests soft-tissue pathology.

Active range of motion in all planes is helpful in documenting the extent but not the cause of cervical spine problems. Active and passive movement of the shoulders can help discriminate abnormalities of the appendicular skeleton from those of the cervical spine.

Neurologic evaluation, including reflex, sensory, and motor function both in the upper and lower extremities is essential to determine the extent of compromise of the central and peripheral nervous systems. The presence of long-tract signs is indicative of more severe spinal cord compression.

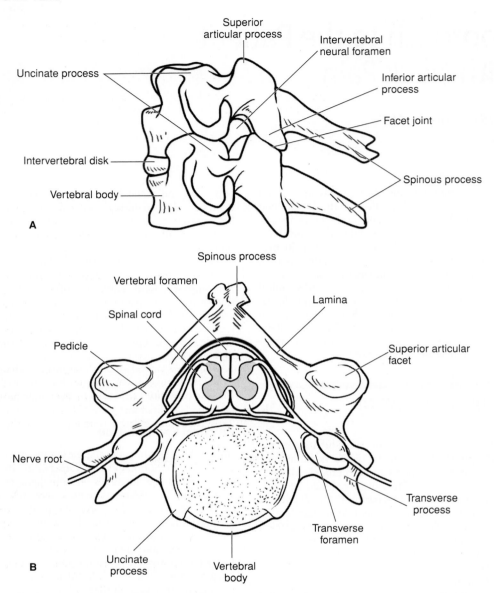

Figure 9–1. Schematic representation of a lateral view of the mid-cervical spine (**A**) and the superior aspect of C5 (**B**). The inferior articular processes from synovial-lined **facet joints** (also called **apophyseal joints**) with the superior articular processes of the vertebra below. The uncinate processes or posterolateral lips located on the superior aspect of the vertebral bodies interact with the inferolateral aspects of the vertebral body above, forming the small, non-synovial-lined **uncovertebral joints** (also referred to as the joints of Luschka). The spinal cord lies within the vertebral foramen formed by the vertebral body anteriorly, the pedicles laterally, and the laminae posteriorly. The cervical nerve roots course along "gutters" formed by the pedicles and exit through an intervertebral formen. The vertebral artery passes through the transverse foranen. (From Polley HF, Hunder GS. *Rheumatologic Interviewing and Physical Examination of the Joints.* 2nd ed. WB Saunders, 1978, Figure 11-1A. With permission.)

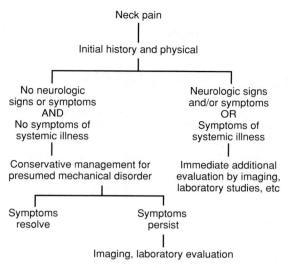

Figure 9–2. The initial evaluation of the patient with neck pain.

The Spurling maneuver is performed by extending the neck and rotating the head to one side and then the other. A positive result is the reproduction of radicular pain. This test is useful in confirming the presence of a cervical radiculopathy.

The Adson test for thoracic outlet obstruction is performed by palpating the pulse at the wrist while abducting, extending, and externally rotating the arm (Figure 9–3). The patient takes a deep breath and rotates the head to the affected side. If there is compression of

Table 9–1. Symptoms that Point to the Need for Urgent Evaluation in a Patient with Neck Pain

---

- Constitutional symptoms such as fever, night sweats, weight loss
- Unusual quality of the neck pain
  Greatest at night; exacerbated by recumbency
  Well-localized within the neck
  Occurring in a regular pattern and extending to structures outside the neck
- Neurologic symptoms
  Lower extremity weakness; difficulty walking
  Combination of upper and lower extremity symptoms
  Rectal and/or urinary incontinence
- Associated medical conditions
  Cancer, diabetes, AIDS, and injection drug use, for example

---

the subclavian artery, a marked diminution of the radial pulse is observed and is a positive test.

Laboratory Tests

Laboratory tests are not necessary for the diagnosis of mechanical neck pain. Determinations of the erythrocyte sedimentation rate and C-reactive protein are useful in the minority of patients with a systemic disorder causing neck pain.

Imaging Studies

Radiographic studies are needed for the small minority of patients who do not respond to a 6–8 week course of medical therapy, who demonstrate severe neurologic compromise, or who have signs or symptoms of a systemic illness.

Plain roentgenograms are easily obtained but offer few specific findings that identify the cause of neck pain. Many anatomic abnormalities are asymptomatic.

Magnetic resonance imaging (MRI) is a useful technique for individuals who fail medical therapy and who have clinical symptoms and signs of nerve compression. MRI is a sensitive means of identifying disc herniations, narrowing of the spinal canal, and increased inflammation in osseous and soft tissue structures. Computed tomography (CT) is a better technique for delineating bony structures. A disadvantage of CT is the exposure to ionizing radiation needed to obtain images of the spine.

Special Tests

Electrodiagnostic tests, electromyography, and nerve conduction tests are useful in the differentiation of central versus peripheral nerve compression (a more difficult distinction with cervical spine disorders as compared to lumbar spine problems). For example, electromyography and nerve conduction tests can help distinguish the individual who has median nerve compression at the wrist from the patient with a C6 or C7 spinal nerve compression from a herniated cervical disc.

■ DISORDERS REQUIRING URGENT EVALUATION

Suspected cervical myelopathy and neck pain in the setting of systemic disease require urgent evaluation in the form of imaging studies, laboratory investigation, and often referral to the appropriate specialist.

CERVICAL MYELOPATHY

 ESSENTIAL FEATURES

- *Symptoms of weakness in upper and lower extremities; urinary or rectal incontinence.*
- *Upper motor neuron signs on examination of the lower extremities.*

Cervical myelopathy occurs secondary to compression of the neural elements (spinal cord or nerve roots) in the cervical spinal canal. Cervical spondylitic myelopathy is the most common cause of spinal cord dysfunction in persons older than 55 years. The cause of the compression is usually a combination of osteophytes and degenerative disc disease that leads to a decrease in the volume of the spinal canal. The distribution and severity of symptoms depend on the location, duration, and size of the lesion.

Clinical Findings

A. SYMPTOMS AND SIGNS

The most frequent presentation of myelopathy is a combination of arm and leg dysfunction. Patients with cervical myelopathy may have symptoms in four limbs, difficulty walking, and urinary or rectal incontinence. Only one-third of patients with cervical myelopathy mention neck pain. Older patients may describe leg stiffness, foot shuffling, and a fear of falling. Physical examination reveals weakness of the appendages in association with spasticity; hyperreflexia, clonus, and a positive Babinski sign are findings in the lower extremities.

B. IMAGING STUDIES

MRI detects the extent of spinal cord compression and is the imaging test of choice for most cases. CT myelograms help distinguish between osteophytes and protruding discs. Plain radiographs reveal advanced degenerative disease with narrowed disc spaces, facet joint sclerosis, and osteophytes, but do not image neural compression.

C. TREATMENT

The natural history of cervical spondylitic myelopathy is gradual progression. Although some patients improve with conservative therapy, progressive myelopathy requires surgery to prevent further cord compression, vascular compromise, and myelomalacia. Outcomes are best when surgery is performed before severe neurologic deficits appear.

NECK PAIN ASSOCIATED WITH SYSTEMIC MEDICAL ILLNESS

 ESSENTIAL FEATURES

- *The history and examination help identify patients whose neck pain is not due to a mechanical disorder.*
- *The differential diagnosis and clinical context of each case determine the urgency and nature of the evaluation.*

Clinical Findings

A. SYMPTOMS AND SIGNS

Patients with neck pain require urgent evaluation if they have constitutional symptoms, symptoms that suggest either a focal process or referred pain, a history of cancer, or a condition that predisposes to infection (see Table 9–1). If present, signs or symptoms of radiculopathy or spinal cord compression add to the urgency of the situation. The differential diagnosis, clinical setting, and findings of the individual case dictate the use of imaging, laboratory investigations, and need for consultations.

B. DIFFERENTIAL DIAGNOSIS

Neck pain in the presence of fever, night sweats, weight loss, or a predisposing condition such as injection drug use, AIDS, or diabetes raises the possibility of **infection.** MRI and CT are indicated in cases of suspected vertebral osteomyelitis, discitis, and epidural abscess. In these conditions, radiographs of the cervical spine may demonstrate alterations of bone integrity, but especially early in the disease course, are often unrevealing.

Spinal cord infiltrative processes and vertebral column **tumors** tend to produce pain that is greatest at night or with recumbency. Patients with these symptoms and neurologic signs should undergo MRI of the central nervous system. Patients with nocturnal pain and with normal neurologic examinations may have a bone tumor. Benign bone tumors affect the posterior elements of vertebral bodies, while malignant lesions affect the vertebral bodies. If plain radiographs are unable to detect alterations in bone architecture, bone scan is a sensitive means to detect lesions over the entire axial skeleton. CT can clarify the nature of abnormalities seen on bone scan.

Pain localized directly over the bony structures of the cervical spine is usually associated with either **fracture** or **expansion of bone.** Any condition that replaces bone with abnormal cells or increases mineral loss from trabeculae causes fractures that occur spontaneously or with minimal trauma. Fractures cause pain in the area of the lesion. Physical examination identifies the maximum point of tenderness. A bone scan may identify the area of fracture if the radiograph is normal. MRI can identify the presence of malignancies, such as **myeloma,** that do not stimulate osteoblast activity and thus are not detected by bone scan.

The **spondyloarthropathies** and **rheumatoid arthritis** can cause early morning stiffness of the cervical spine lasting for hours. Patients with neck symptoms due to these diseases usually have extensive disease of other joints, but women with ankylosing spondylitis may have neck disease without low back pain. Flexion-extension views of the cervical spine can reveal the presence of C1–C2 subluxation in either the spondyloarthropathies or rheumatoid arthritis. MRI is an important technique to identify synovitis affecting the C1–C2 articulation in RA. MRI can also visualize the presence of bone marrow inflammation and edema in vertebral structures affected by AS.

Patients with **viscerogenic pain** (ie, neck pain secondary to cardiovascular, gastrointestinal, or neurologic disorders) have symptoms that recur in a regular pattern in structures that extend beyond the cervical spine. Pain with exertion raises the possibility of myocardial ischemia. Carotidynia is pain and tenderness over the carotid arteries. Esophageal disorders should be considered if neck pain occurs in association with eating. Posterior esophageal lesions, in particular, may affect the prevertebral space, causing neck pain. Disorders of the cranial nerves can cause cervical spine and facial pain.

Patients with **polymyalgia rheumatica** are over 50 years of age and have severe early morning muscle stiffness. Pain is localized to the proximal muscles of the shoulders and thighs. The erythrocyte sedimentation rate is elevated in most cases.

ACUTE NECK PAIN DUE TO A PROBABLE MECHANICAL DISORDER

 ESSENTIAL FEATURES

- *There are no signs or symptoms of systemic disease, and the neurologic examination is normal.*
- *A trial of nonoperative therapy is indicated.*

Patients with neck pain but without symptoms or signs of myelopathy or an associated systemic disorder should be treated with nonoperative therapy for 3–6 weeks. In general, imaging studies and laboratory investigations are not necessary unless the neck pain persists.

Nonoperative Therapy

Nonsteroidal anti-inflammatory drugs (NSAIDs) help decrease pain and inflammation that is associated with acute neck pain. Nonoperative management also includes muscle relaxants, non-narcotic analgesics, temperature modalities, local injections, and range-of-motion and strengthening exercises.

Medications that have rapid onset of action and are effective analgesics are preferred. In addition, drugs with sustained relief properties may offer more constant pain relief with fewer tablets each day. Muscle relaxants do not produce peripheral muscle relaxation but do offer additional pain relief for persons with increased paracervical muscle contractions. Patients must be informed of the potential sedative effects of these medications. Patients may use ice massage on painful areas for 10 minutes for additional analgesia. Some patients may find the application of heat to the neck improves range of motion by decreasing muscle tightness. A local injection with 10 mg of triamcinolone and 2–4 ml of lidocaine into the area of maximum tenderness in the paravertebral musculature or trapezia may decrease pain.

Because of the pain, patients often have difficulty complying with the recommendation of returning to normal motion of the cervical spine. Patients will limit motion and prefer to wear a cervical collar. Short-term immobilization is useful, particularly at night when motion during sleep increases neck pain. A soft collar that does not extend the neck is appropriate in most cases. Patients should understand that the eventual goal of therapy is a return to normal neck motion. Therefore, the collar should be used less frequently as neck pain improves.

PERSISTENT NECK PAIN

Most patients, including those with cervical radiculopathy, will improve within 2 months. If initial nonoperative treatment fails after 6 weeks, symptomatic patients are separated into two groups: patients with neck pain as the predominant complaint and patients with arm pain as the predominant complaint.

NECK PAIN PREDOMINANT

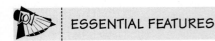

ESSENTIAL FEATURES

- *Osteoarthritis is a frequent cause of local neck pain.*
- *Muscle tightness is a common exacerbating factor.*

Differential Diagnosis & Treatment

Cervical strain causes pain in the middle or lower portion of the posterior aspect of the neck. The pain may cover a diffuse area or both sides of the spine. Physical examination reveals local tenderness in the paracervical muscles, decreased range of motion, and loss of cervical lordosis. No abnormalities are found on neurologic or shoulder examination. Laboratory tests are normal. Cervical spine roentgenograms of patients with cervical strain may be normal or demonstrate a loss of cervical lordosis. Therapy for chronic cervical strain includes modification of the choice or dose of NSAID, muscle relaxant, local injections, and neck exercises, including strengthening and range-of-motion.

Cervical spondylosis is associated with disc degeneration and the approximation of articular structures. This instability results in osteoarthritis with osteophyte formation in the uncovertebral and apophyseal joints. Neck pain is diffuse and may radiate to the shoulders, occipital area, or the interscapular muscles. Physical examination may reveal midline tenderness and pain at the limit of motion with extension and lateral flexion. Factors that exacerbate and alleviate neck pain help differentiate among the various causes of mechanical neck pain. Plain roentgenograms of the cervical spine demonstrate intervertebral narrowing and facet joint sclerosis. MRI of the neck reveals degenerative disc disease in over 50% of persons 40 years of age or older, many of whom are asymptomatic. The radiographic findings are significant only if they correlate with the clinical symptoms of the patient. Therapy for osteoarthritis of the cervical spine requires a balance between stability and maintenance of motion. Patient education is essential to maximize neck flexibility with range-of-motion exercises while decreasing pain by restricting neck movement with a cervical collar. NSAIDs and local injections may also diminish neck and referred pain. Most patients with cervical spondylosis have a relapsing course with recurrent exacerbations of acute neck pain.

Cervical hyperextension injuries (whiplash) of the neck are most often associated with rear-impact motor vehicle accidents, but diving, falls, and other sports injuries also cause whiplash. Whiplash is an acceleration-deceleration injury to the soft-tissue structures in the neck. Paracervical muscles are stretched or torn, and with severe injury, cervical intervertebral disc injuries occur. Severe whiplash also can damage the sympathetic ganglia, resulting in Horner syndrome, nausea, hoarseness, or dizziness. Symptoms of stiffness and pain on motion generally develop 12–24 hours after the accident. Patients may have difficulty swallowing or chewing. Physical examination reveals soreness of the neck with palpation, paracervical muscle contraction, and decreased range of motion. Neurologic examination is unrevealing, and radiographs demonstrate loss of cervical lordosis. Structural damage identified on radiographs occurs in patients with severe injuries that require immediate stabilizing therapy. Treatment of most whiplash injuries includes the use of a cervical collar for a minimal period of time. Longer use of collars may result in greater pain and decreased motion. Non-narcotic analgesics, NSAIDs, and muscle relaxants decrease pain and facilitate motion of the neck. Patients with persistent symptoms have pain secondary to apophyseal joint injury. Patients with persistent symptoms for more than 6 months rarely experience significant improvement.

If a patient with persistent neck pain does not have muscle tenderness and if the neurologic examination and imaging studies are unrevealing, the patient should have a complete psychosocial evaluation. Patients with neck pain who have psychiatric conditions may have conversion reactions or substance dependence as the cause of their symptoms.

ARM PAIN PREDOMINANT

ESSENTIAL FEATURES

- *Herniated intervertebral discs are a frequent cause of radicular pain.*
- *Cervical spinal stenosis is a cause of radicular pain in older persons.*

Differential Diagnosis & Treatment

Patients with arm pain refractory to nonoperative management frequently have symptoms and signs owing to mechanical pressure from a herniated disc or hypertrophic bone and secondary inflammation of the involved nerve roots. Cervical disc herniation occurs with the sudden exertion of heavy lifting. A **herniated cervical disc** causes radicular pain that radiates from the shoulder to the forearm and hand. The pain may be so severe that

Table 9–2. Characteristics of Radicular Pain Caused by Cervical Nerve Root Compression

Nerve Root	Area of Pain	Sensory Loss	Motor Loss	Reflex loss
C5	Neck to outer shoulder, arm	Shoulder	Deltoid	Biceps, supinator
C6	Outer arm to thumb, index finger	Index finger, thumb	Biceps	Biceps, supinator
C7	Outer arm to middle finger	Index, middle fingers	Triceps	Triceps
C8	Inner arm to ring and little fingers	Ring, little fingers	Hand muscles	None

the use of the arm is limited. Neck pain is minimal or absent. Physical examination reveals increased radicular pain with any maneuver that narrows the intervertebral foramen and places tension on the affected nerve. Compression, extension, and lateral flexion of the cervical spine (Spurling sign) cause radicular pain. Neurologic examination reveals sensory abnormalities, reflex asymmetry, or motor weakness corresponding to the damaged spinal nerve root and degree of impingement (Table 9–2). MRI is the best technique to identify the location of disc herniation and nerve root impingement. Electromyography and nerve conduction tests document nerve dysfunction and are able to differentiate nerve root impingement from peripheral entrapment syndromes (eg, carpal tunnel syndrome).

If arm pain occurs during exertion, vascular evaluation is indicated. Patients who complain of neck and arm pain that occurs with exertion should be evaluated for coronary artery disease, particularly if chest pain occurs in conjunction with arm pain. If the exertional pain is limited to the arm alone, an evaluation for thoracic outlet syndrome using the Adson test is also appropriate. Patients with thoracic outlet syndrome should be evaluated by appropriate imaging to rule out a Pancoast tumor (apical lung tumor). Patients with idiopathic thoracic outlet obstruction may benefit from isometric shoulder girdle exercises, improved posture, and limiting movements of the arm above the head. Surgery is helpful in a minority of patients.

REFERENCES

Bogduk N. The anatomy and pathophysiology of neck pain. *Phys Med Rehabil Clin N Am.* 2003;14:455. [PMID: 12948338] (A review of the structures causing pain in the cervical spine.)

Carette S, Fehlings MG. Cervical radiculopathy. *N Engl J Med.* 2005;353:392. [PMID: 16049211] (A review of the most current clinical data on the diagnosis and treatment of cervical radiculopathy.)

Mink JH, Gordon RE, Deutsch AL. The cervical spine: radiologist's perspective. *Phys Med Rehabil Clin N Am.* 2003;14:493. [PMID: 12948340] (An atlas of the radiographic abnormalities affecting the cervical spine.)

Rao R. Neck pain, cervical radiculopathy, and cervical myelopathy: Pathophysiology, natural history, and clinical evaluation. *J Bone Joint Surg.* 2002;84A:1872. [PMID: 12690874] (Myelopathy is discussed as an entity that causes a wide variety of clinical symptoms and signs.)

Swenson RS. Therapeutic modalities in the management of nonspecific neck pain. *Phys Med Rehabil Clin N Am.* 2003;14:605. [PMID: 12948344] (An evidence-based review of the therapies utilized in the care of neck pain patients.)

Relevant World Wide Web Sites

[The American College of Rheumatology]
http://www.rheumatology.org

[American Academy of Orthopaedic Surgeons]
http://www.aaos.org

[Hospital for Joint Diseases Orthopaedic Institute]
http://www.hjd.org

[Dr. David Borenstein America's Back Doctor]
http://www.drborenstein.com

Approach to the Patient with Low Back Pain

Rajiv K. Dixit, MD

ESSENTIAL FEATURES

- *Most patients with acute low back pain improve spontaneously within 4 weeks.*
- *Degenerative change in the lumbar spine is the most commonly identified cause of low back pain.*
- *Diagnostic testing is rarely indicated unless symptoms persist beyond 4 weeks.*
- *The presence of imaging abnormalities should be carefully interpreted since they are frequently seen in asymptomatic persons.*
- *Most patients respond to a program that includes analgesia, education, aerobic conditioning, and physical therapy. Surgery is rarely needed.*

Low back pain (LBP) is the most common musculoskeletal complaint and a leading cause of work disability; an estimated 80% of the population will experience it during their lifetime.

LBP affects the area between the lower rib cage and gluteal folds and frequently radiates into the thighs. Most LBP is benign and self-limited. Ninety percent of patients with acute LBP improve spontaneously within 4 weeks, although low-grade symptoms may persist in some. Approximately half of the patients with acute LBP will experience one or more episodes of LBP over the next few years, but these too will generally be self-limited. Less than 1% of the patients with acute LBP have true sciatica, which is defined as pain in the distribution of a lumbar nerve root often accompanied by sensory and motor deficits (Table 10–1 and Figure 10–1).

Risk factors that have been associated with LBP include heavy lifting, driving motor vehicles, jogging, weaker trunk strength, obesity, pregnancy, psychosocial factors, and cigarette smoking.

Clinical Findings

A. History

An important aspect of history-taking in a patient with LBP is to ensure that conditions that require early diagnostic testing are identified (Table 10–2).

Mechanical LBP increases with physical activity and upright posture and is relieved by rest and recumbency. Severe and acute mechanical LBP in a slender and elderly woman is suspicious for a vertebral compression fracture secondary to osteoporosis. **Nonmechanical LBP,** especially when accompanied by nocturnal pain, suggests the possibility of underlying infection or neoplasm.

Inflammatory LBP, as seen in the spondyloarthropathies, typically worsens with rest, improves with activity, and is accompanied by morning stiffness that lasts half an hour or longer. Sciatica and pseudoclaudication suggest neurologic involvement. **Sciatica** results from nerve root compression, generally from a herniated disc, and produces lancinating pain in a radicular distribution. Sciatica should be differentiated from nonneurogenic **sclerotomal** pain, which arises from pathology within the disc, facet joint, or lumbar paraspinal muscles and ligaments. Like sciatica, sclerotomal pain is often referred into the lower extremities, but unlike sciatica, sclerotomal pain is nondermatomal in distribution, is dull in quality, and pain usually does not radiate below the knee or have associated paresthesias.

Persistence of LBP may be associated with depression, job dissatisfaction, and pursuit of disability compensation or litigation.

B. Physical Examination

Examination of the back usually does not lead to a specific diagnosis. A general physical examination, including a neurologic examination, may help identify those few, but nevertheless important, cases of LBP that are secondary to a systemic disease or those in which there is neurologic involvement.

Inspection may reveal the presence of **scoliosis.** Scoliosis can be either **structural** or **functional.** A structural scoliosis is associated with structural changes of the

Table 10–1. Neurologic Features of Lumbosacral Radiculopathy

Disc Herniation	Nerve Root	Motor	Sensory (Light Touch)	Reflex
L3–4	L4	Dorsiflexion of foot	Medial foot	Knee
L4–5	L5	Dorsiflexion of great toe	Dorsal foot	None
L5–S1	S1	Plantar flexion of foot	Lateral foot	Ankle

Table 10–2. Indications for Early Diagnostic Testing

Spinal fracture
  Significant trauma
  Prolonged glucocorticoid use
  Age >50 years
Infection or cancer
  History of cancer
  Unexplained weight loss
  Immunosuppression
  Injection drug use
  Nocturnal pain
  Age >50 years
Cauda equina syndrome
  Urinary retention
  Overflow incontinence
  Fecal incontinence
  Bilateral or progressive motor deficit
  Saddle anesthesia
Spondyloarthropathy
  Morning stiffness in the back
  Low back pain that improves with activity
  Age <40 years

vertebral column and sometimes the rib cage as well. As the patient bends forward (flexing the spine), structural scoliosis persists whereas functional scoliosis usually disappears. Paravertebral muscle spasm and leg length discrepancy are leading causes of functional scoliosis.

Palpation can detect paravertebral muscle spasm that often leads to loss of the normal lumbar lordosis. Point tenderness over the spine has sensitivity but not specificity for vertebral osteomyelitis. A palpable step-off between adjacent spinous processes indicates spondylolisthesis.

Limited spinal motion (flexion, extension, lateral bending, and rotation) is not associated with any specific diagnosis since LBP due to any cause may limit motion. Range-of-motion measurements, however, can help in monitoring treatment.

The hip joints should be examined for any decrease in range of motion because hip arthritis, which normally causes groin pain, may occasionally present as LBP. Tenderness over the greater trochanter of the hip is seen in trochanteric bursitis, which can be confused with LBP. The presence of more widespread tender points, especially in a female patient, suggests the possibility that LBP may be secondary to fibromyalgia.

A **straight-leg raising test** should be performed on all patients with sciatica or pseudoclaudication. Straight-leg raising places tension on the sciatic nerve and thereby stretches the sciatic nerve roots (L4, L5, S1, S2, and S3). If any of these nerve roots is already irritated, such as by impingement from a herniated disc, further tension on the nerve root by straight-leg raising will result in radicular pain that extends below the knee. The test is done by the examiner cupping the patient's heel in his or her hand and flexing the hip while keeping the knee extended. The test is positive if radicular pain (not merely back or hamstring pain) is produced when the leg is raised less than

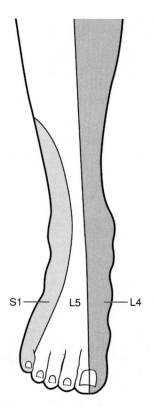

Figure 10–1. Lower extremity dermatomes.

60 degrees. The straight-leg raising test is very sensitive (95%) but not specific (40%) for clinically significant disc herniation at the L4–5 or L5–S1 level (the sites of 95% of disc herniations). False-negative tests are more frequently seen with herniation above the L4–5 level. The straight-leg raising test is usually negative in patients with spinal stenosis. The crossed straight-leg raising test (with sciatica reproduced when the opposite leg is raised) is insensitive (25%) but highly specific (90%) for disc herniation.

The neurologic examination (see Table 10–1) should always include motor testing with focus on dorsiflexion of the ankle (L4), great toe dorsiflexion (L5), and foot plantar flexion (S1); determination of knee (L4) and ankle (S1) deep tendon reflexes; and tests for dermatomal sensory loss (see Figure 10–1). The inability to toe walk (mostly S1) and heel walk (mostly L5) may indicate muscle weakness. Muscle atrophy can be detected by circumferential measurements of the calf and thigh at the same level bilaterally.

C. LABORATORY FINDINGS

Laboratory studies play a minor role in the investigation of LBP. They are used mostly in identifying patients with systemic causes of LBP. A patient with normal blood cell counts, erythrocyte sedimentation rate, and radiographs of the lumbar spine is unlikely to have an underlying systemic disease (infection, malignancy, or spondyloarthropathy) as the cause of LBP.

D. IMAGING STUDIES

Diagnostic tests should be done early for patients who have evidence of a major or progressive neurologic deficit and those in whom an underlying systemic disease is suspected (see Table 10–2). Otherwise, diagnostic tests are not required unless symptoms persist for more than 4 weeks. Because 90% of patients with LBP recover spontaneously within 4 weeks, this approach avoids unnecessary early testing.

A major problem with imaging studies is that many of the anatomic abnormalities seen are common in asymptomatic persons. These abnormalities are often the result of age-related degenerative changes and are frequently present after the age of 30. Making causal inferences based on imaging abnormalities can be hazardous in the absence of corresponding clinical findings and can lead to unnecessary and costly interventions with a potential for iatrogenic complications.

Plain radiographs of the spine do not usually help in determining the cause of LBP. Abnormalities such as single disc degeneration, facet joint degeneration, Schmorl nodes (intraspongy disc herniation), spondylolysis, mild spondylolisthesis, transitional vertebrae (lumbarization of S1 or sacralization of L5), spina bifida occulta, and mild scoliosis are equally prevalent in persons with and without LBP. Plain radiography should be limited to patients with clinical findings suggestive of infection, cancer, spondyloarthropathy, or trauma, or those who continue to have LBP after 4–6 weeks of conservative care. It is noteworthy that radiation exposure to the female gonads from standard views of the lumbar spine is equivalent to that of a daily chest radiograph for several years.

Computed tomography and magnetic resonance imaging (MRI) should be reserved for patients in whom there is a strong clinical indication of underlying infection or cancer, or for the evaluation of patients with significant or progressive neurologic deficits. MRI is the preferred modality for the detection of spinal infection and cancers, herniated discs, and spinal stenosis. When interpreting the results of MRI and computed tomography, it is important to remember that most asymptomatic adults above age 30 will have evidence of either disc bulges (symmetric and diffuse extension of the disc) or disc protrusion (focal or asymmetric extension of the disc). Therefore when these findings are seen in a patient they may not necessarily be the cause of LBP. MRI with the intravenous contrast agent gadolinium is useful for the evaluation of patients with prior lumbar spine surgery (with no hardware present) to help in the differentiation of scar tissue from recurrent disc herniation.

The significance of a focal high signal (high-intensity zone) in the posterior annulus on a T2-weighted image is controversial. It is thought to represent annular tears and to correlate with positive findings on provocative discography (which itself is a controversial procedure). **Discogenic LBP** has been diagnosed in patients with these high-intensity zones, and spinal fusion surgery is often recommended. The high prevalence of high-intensity zones in asymptomatic individuals, however, calls this approach into question.

Bone scanning is used primarily to detect infection, bony metastases, and occult fractures. Bone scans have limited specificity due to poor spatial resolution, and thus abnormal findings often require confirmatory imaging, such as MRI.

E. SPECIAL TESTS

Nerve conduction studies and electromyography are unnecessary when a patient has an obvious radiculopathy or isolated LBP. Electrodiagnosis, however, may be helpful in differentiating the limb pain of peroneal nerve palsy from that of L5 radiculopathy or in evaluating possible factitious weakness. Electromyographic changes depend on the development of muscle denervation following nerve injury and cannot be detected until a few weeks after the injury.

Table 10–3. Causes of Low Back Pain

Originating from spine
Mechanical
Neoplastic
Infectious
Inflammatory
Metabolic
Originating from viscera

Table 10–4. Mechanical Causes of Low Back Pain

Lumbar spondylosis[a]
Disc herniation[a]
Spondylolisthesis[a]
Spinal stenosis[a]
Diffuse idiopathic skeletal hyperostosis
Fractures
Idiopathic (sprain and strain, lumbago)

[a]Related to degenerative changes.

Differential Diagnosis

LBP usually originates from the lumbar spine or associated muscles and ligaments (Table 10–3). Rarely, pain is referred to the back from visceral disease. Over 95% of LBP is mechanical (Table 10–4). Mechanical LBP is due to an anatomic or functional abnormality without underlying inflammatory or neoplastic disease. Degenerative change (also referred to as lumbar spondylosis or lumbar osteoarthritis) is by far the most common disorder seen within the spine and the most important cause of mechanical LBP. Degenerative changes occur in both the intervertebral disc and facet joint (Figure 10–2).

A precise pathoanatomic diagnosis cannot be made in most patients with acute LBP. The focus of the initial diagnostic evaluation, therefore, is to identify the small proportion of patients with systemic disease (infection, neoplasm, and spondyloarthropathy together account for

only 1% of patients with LBP) or with neurologic involvement that requires urgent or specific intervention.

A. LUMBAR SPONDYLOSIS

Lumbar spondylosis, or osteoarthritis of the lumbar spine, is the most commonly identified cause of LBP. Symptomatic patients complain of mechanical LBP. Recurrent attacks of acute LBP may occur in some patients while chronic LBP may develop in others. In patients with facet joint osteoarthritis, the pain may radiate into the posterior thigh and be exacerbated by bending ipsilateral to the involved joint (**facet syndrome**).

Imaging evidence of degenerative changes (facet joint or disc space narrowing, osteophytosis, and subchondral sclerosis) increases with age and is common. However, the relationship between these changes and back pain is complex. Patients with severe LBP may have minimal

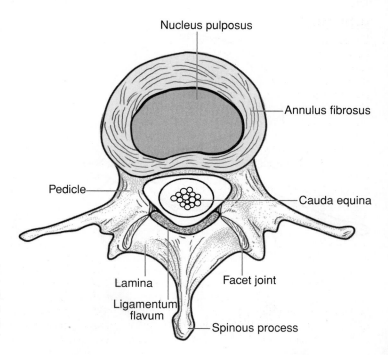

Figure 10–2. Schematic drawing showing a cross-sectional view through a normal lumbar vertebra. The facet joints are formed by the articulation between the superior facet of the vertebra below and the inferior facet of the vertebra above.

Nucleus pulposus

Annulus fibrosus

Pedicle

Cauda equina

Lamina

Facet joint

Ligamentum flavum

Spinous process

radiographic changes, and conversely, patients with advanced changes may be asymptomatic.

Spinal instability (in the absence of fractures or spondylolisthesis) remains a controversial diagnosis. Spinal instability is identified by demonstrating abnormal vertebral motion (anteroposterior displacement or excessive angular change of adjacent vertebrae) on flexion-extension radiography. However, such spinal motion may be seen in asymptomatic persons, and its relationship to the causation of pain is unclear.

B. Disc Herniation

The nucleus pulposus in a degenerated disc may prolapse and push out the weakened annulus, usually posterolaterally. Imaging evidence of disc herniation (bulging or protrusion) is commonly seen, even in asymptomatic adults. Occasionally, however, disc herniation results in a nerve root impingement syndrome (Figure 10–3). This accounts for less than 1% of patients with LBP but is nevertheless important to identify. Such disc herniation may be precipitated by a wide range of activities from heavy lifting to trivial movement.

Ninety-five percent of lumbar disc herniations involve either the L4–5 or L5–S1 disc. In general, the more caudal nerve root is impinged, that is, the L5 nerve root with L4–5 herniation and the S1 nerve root with L5–S1 herniation. Nerve root impingement results in sciatica. Indeed, sciatica has such a high sensitivity (95%) that its absence makes clinically significant lumbar disc herniation unlikely.

The natural history of disc herniation is favorable. Studies using sequential MRI testing reveal that the herniated portion of the disc tends to regress with time. In most patients, the radicular pain resolves over a period of weeks, and fewer than 10% of patients with nerve root impingement will require surgical decompression.

Rarely, a massive midline disc herniation compresses the cauda equina, causing **cauda equina syndrome**—a surgical emergency. Patients usually present with bilateral sciatica and motor deficits. Sensory loss in a saddle distribution is common, and urinary retention with overflow incontinence is usually present. Fecal incontinence may also occur.

Internal disc disruption is a controversial disorder diagnosed by provocative discography. Following contrast injection into the disc, the radiographic appearance and induced pain are assessed. Discographic anatomic abnormalities and induced pain are, however, frequently seen in asymptomatic persons, and more importantly the discogenic pain attributed to disc disruption frequently improves spontaneously.

C. Spondylolisthesis

Spondylolisthesis is the anterior displacement of a vertebra on the one beneath it. This displacement is usually the result of degenerative changes in the disc and facet joints (**degenerative spondylolisthesis**) but also can be due to a developmental defect in the pars interarticularis of the vertebral arch that produces **isthmic spondylolisthesis** (Figure 10–4).

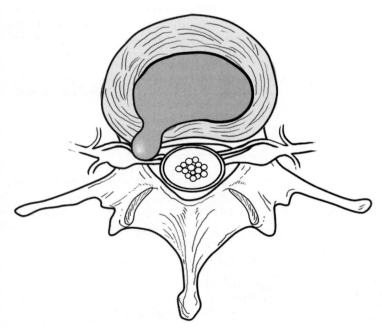

Figure 10–3. Schematic drawing showing posterolateral disc herniation resulting in nerve root impingement.

A

B

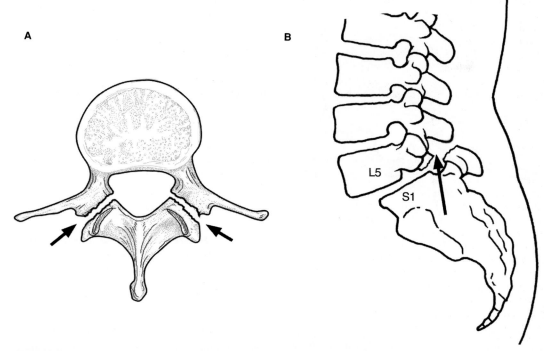

Figure 10–4. **A:** Spondylolysis with bilateral defects in the pars interarticularis (arrows). **B:** Spondylolysis of the L5 vertebra (arrow) resulting in isthmic spondylolisthesis at L5–S1.

Most patients with a minor degree of spondylolisthesis are asymptomatic, although some patients may have mechanical LBP. Greater degrees of spondylolisthesis occasionally cause nerve root impingement (usually L5) or spinal stenosis. Rarely, extreme slippage results in cauda equina syndrome.

D. Spinal Stenosis

Lumbar spinal stenosis is defined as a narrowing of the spinal canal, its lateral recesses, and neural foramina that may result in a compression of lumbosacral nerve roots. Lumbar stenosis can be asymptomatic; up to 20% of asymptomatic adults over age 60 have evidence of spinal stenosis on imaging. Spinal stenosis can occur at one or more levels and the narrowing can be asymmetric.

Degenerative changes are the cause of spinal stenosis in an overwhelming majority of cases (Table 10–5). The intervertebral disc loses vertical height as it degenerates; this results in a bulging of the now redundant and often hypertrophied ligamentum flavum into the posterior part of the canal. Any herniation of the degenerated disc narrows the anterior part of the canal while hypertrophied facets and osteophytes may compress nerve roots in the lateral recess or intervertebral foramen (Figure 10–5).

The hallmark of spinal stenosis is **pseudoclaudication** (neurogenic claudication). The symptoms of pseudoclaudication are usually bilateral. The patient complains of pain and discomfort together with weakness or paresthesias in the buttocks, thighs, and legs.

Table 10–5. Causes of Lumbar Spinal Stenosis

Congenital
Idiopathic
Achondroplastic
Acquired
Degenerative
Hypertrophy of facet joints
Hypertrophy of ligamentum flavum
Disc herniation
Spondylolisthesis
Scoliosis
Iatrogenic
Postlaminectomy
Postsurgical fusion
Miscellaneous
Paget disease
Fluorosis
Diffuse idiopathic skeletal hyperostosis

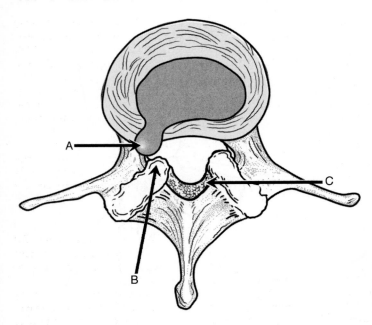

Figure 10–5. Spinal stenosis secondary to a combination of disc herniation (**A**), facet joint hypertrophy (**B**), and hypertrophy of the ligamentum flavum (**C**).

Unsteadiness of gait is a frequent complaint. The lumbar component of pain is frequently mild. Pseudoclaudication is induced by standing or walking and relieved by sitting or flexing forward. In fact, the most important finding may be a history of no pain when the patient is seated with the spine flexed. This forward flexion increases the canal diameter and may lead to the patient adopting a simian stance. It has been hypothesized that a diminished supply of arterial blood to the cauda equina is the cause of neurogenic claudication. Recent evidence, however, suggests that direct pressure on the nerve roots is the major mechanism. Factors that favor a diagnosis of pseudoclaudication over vascular claudication include the preservation of pedal pulses, provocation of symptoms by standing just as readily as by walking, and location of the maximal discomfort to the thighs rather than the calves.

The physical examination of a patient with lumbar spinal stenosis is often unimpressive. Severe neurologic deficits are rarely seen. Lumbar range of motion may be normal or reduced and the result of straight-leg raising is usually negative. Deep tendon reflexes and vibration sense may be reduced. Mild weakness is seen in some. The significance of these findings is often difficult to determine in elderly patients. The diagnosis of spinal stenosis is most often suspected when a history of pseudoclaudication is elicited and is best confirmed by MRI.

Spinal stenosis is an indolent condition, and the symptoms evolve gradually. Most patients remain stable, although some gradually worsen over a period of years.

E. DIFFUSE IDIOPATHIC SKELETAL HYPEROSTOSIS

Diffuse idiopathic skeletal hyperostosis is characterized by florid hyperostosis of the spine. Marginal bony proliferation leads to the formation of anterior osseous ridges that fuse and give the appearance of flowing wax on the anterior bodies of the vertebrae on radiography. Ossification of paraspinous ligaments such as the anterior and posterior longitudinal ligaments may be seen. The thoracic spine is most commonly involved, although the cervical and lumbar regions may also be affected. Lesions are most prominent anteriorly and along the right lateral aspect of the spine. Involvement of the left lateral aspect in patients with situs inversus has led to speculation that the descending thoracic aorta plays a role in the location of calcification. Intervertebral disc spaces are preserved and sacroiliac and facet joints appear normal. This helps differentiate diffuse idiopathic skeletal hyperostosis from spondylosis and the spondyloarthropathies. Extraspinal manifestations include irregular new bone formation ("whiskering") and large bone spurs that are often seen at the olecranon process and calcaneus. Severe ligamentous calcification may be seen in the patellar, sacrotuberous, and iliolumbar ligaments.

Diffuse idiopathic skeletal hyperostosis is usually seen in the middle-aged and the elderly. In spite of the extensive radiologic abnormalities, pain is often minimal or absent with only moderate limitation of spinal motion. Stiffness, which may be generalized, is a common complaint. Rarely, dysphagia or cervical myelopathy can occur secondary to extensive ossification of the anterior or posterior longitudinal ligaments, respectively. An association with diabetes mellitus has been noted.

F. IDIOPATHIC LOWER BACK PAIN

A definitive pathoanatomic diagnosis cannot be made in 80% of patients with LBP, largely because of the weak association between symptoms and the results of imaging. Thus, nonspecific terms such as lumbago, strain, and sprain have come into use. Strain and sprain have never been anatomically or histologically characterized. Therefore idiopathic LBP is a more accurate label for these patients who have a mostly self-limited syndrome of back pain.

G. NEOPLASTIC

Cancer is an unusual cause of LBP. Most cases result from involvement of the spine by metastatic carcinoma (especially prostate, lung, breast, thyroid, or kidney) or multiple myeloma.

Patients are usually older than 50 years and may give a history of weight loss or cancer in the past. Recumbency often does not improve the LBP and nocturnal pain is common. Missing the diagnosis can lead to irreversible neurologic compromise, ranging from cord compression to cauda equina syndrome.

Radiographs can reveal a compression fracture or lytic or blastic lesions that may be present in one or several vertebral bodies with sparing of the disc space. MRI is the test of choice to confirm bony metastases.

Patients with neurologic involvement may need urgent radiation therapy or surgical decompression.

H. INFECTIOUS

Vertebral osteomyelitis, epidural abscess, and septic discitis are infrequent but important causes of LBP. Osteomyelitis usually results from hematogenous spread from a distant source of infection and can lead to the formation of an epidural abscess. The most common organism is *Staphylococcus aureus,* followed by streptococci and gram-negative bacteria. Tuberculosis and nontubercular granulomatous infections (blastomycosis, cryptococcosis, actinomycosis, coccidioidomycosis, and brucellosis) of the spine are rare but should be considered in the appropriate clinical setting. Risk factors for osteomyelitis and epidural abscess include immunosuppression, diabetes, intravenous drug abuse, alcoholism, renal failure, and urinary tract infections. Septic discitis generally results from a procedure, such as disc excision, that inoculates the disc space.

Back pain that is not relieved by rest or recumbency, spine tenderness over the involved segment, and an elevated erythrocyte sedimentation rate are the most common findings. Fever may only be seen with abscess formation, and the white blood cell count is often normal. An untreated epidural abscess can result in spinal cord com-

pression or cauda equina syndrome. Radiographs may show a narrowed disc space with erosion of adjacent vertebrae, but these changes often take weeks to appear. MRI is the most sensitive and specific imaging technique to detect spinal infections. A biopsy for culture is recommended, especially if blood cultures are negative. Treatment consists of intravenous antibiotics for 6 weeks and surgical decompression if an epidural abscess is present.

I. INFLAMMATORY

The spondyloarthropathies (see Chapters 17–19) cause inflammatory LBP characterized by prolonged early morning stiffness of the back that improves with activity and worsens with rest.

J. METABOLIC

The major consideration is the occurrence of acute LBP secondary to a vertebral compression fracture in a patient with osteoporosis (see Chapter 57). Most patients are postmenopausal women.

Paget disease of bone is often detected in an asymptomatic patient by the incidental finding of either an elevated alkaline phosphatase or characteristic radiographic abnormality. Back pain secondary to involvement of the spine is most common in the lumbar area. The pain may be due to the pagetic process itself, to secondary osteoarthritis in the facet joints, or rarely to a pathologic fracture of a vertebra. Spinal cord and cauda equina compression secondary to Paget disease have been seen on rare occasions.

K. VISCERAL

Disease in organs that share segmental innervation with the spine can cause pain to be referred to the spine. In general, pelvic diseases refer pain to the sacral area, lower abdominal diseases to the lumbar area, and upper abdominal diseases to the lower thoracic spine area. Local signs of disease, such as tenderness to palpation, paravertebral muscle spasm, and increased pain on spinal motion, are absent.

A partial list of causes includes a contained rupture of an abdominal aortic aneurysm, pyelonephritis, ureteral obstruction due to renal stones, chronic prostatitis, endometriosis, ovarian cysts, inflammatory bowel disorders, colonic neoplasms, and retroperitoneal hemorrhage (usually in a patient taking anticoagulants).

Treatment

Specific treatment is available only for the small fraction of patients with LBP who either have major neural compression or have an underlying systemic disease (infection, malignancy, or spondyloarthropathy). In the vast majority of patients with LBP, either the precise cause cannot be determined, or when the cause is determined, no specific treatment is available. These patients are managed with a conservative program centered on analgesia, education, and physical therapy. Less than 1% of patients with LBP need surgery.

One should be wary of the proliferation of unproven medical, surgical, and alternative therapies. Most have not been rigorously tested in randomized controlled trials; uncontrolled studies can produce a misleading impression of efficacy due to the favorable natural history of LBP.

For management purposes, patients with LBP are considered to have either **acute LBP** (duration less than 3 months), **chronic LBP** (duration greater than 3 months), or a **nerve root compression syndrome.**

A. Acute Lower Back Pain

Patients often seek medical attention for sudden onset of severe mechanical LBP. Examination usually reveals paravertebral muscle spasm and severe decrease in range of motion secondary to pain.

Patients with acute LBP are advised to stay active and continue ordinary daily activities within the limits permitted by pain. Bed rest of more than 1 or 2 days is discouraged.

Medications are used for symptomatic relief. Aspirin, acetaminophen, and nonsteroidal anti-inflammatory drugs are effective analgesics. Some patients, however, may need short-term narcotic analgesia. Muscle relaxants, used for a few days, may help some patients. Oral glucocorticoids are of no benefit in patients with acute LBP, including those with sciatica.

Back exercises are not helpful in the acute phase, and a physical therapy referral is usually unnecessary in the first month. Later, a program of regular back exercises including stretching exercises, aerobic conditioning, and loss of excess weight are used to prevent recurrences. The purpose of back exercises is to stabilize the spine by strengthening the trunk muscles. Flexion exercises strengthen the abdominal muscles and extension exercises strengthen the paraspinal muscles. Various exercise programs have been developed and appear to be equally effective. Educational booklets that include back exercises and safe lifting techniques are helpful. Back school may be effective for worksite-specific patient education but has not been shown to be effective in nonoccupational settings.

There is no evidence that spinal manipulative therapy is superior to other standard treatments for patients with acute or chronic LBP.

There is limited evidence to support the use of epidural glucocorticoid injections for short-term relief of radicular pain. Epidural injections are not recommended for LBP without radiculopathy. Injections of trigger points, ligaments, sacroiliac joints, and facet joints with anesthetic agents or glucocorticoid are of unproven efficacy and are not recommended in the management of LBP.

Nerve root blocks are also not recommended for therapeutic or diagnostic purposes.

Self-application of heat or cold is an easy and inexpensive option. Shoe lifts are considered only when the leg length inequality is more than 1 inch.

Modalities such as ultrasound, cutaneous laser treatment, shortwave diathermy, electrical stimulation, and transcutaneous electrical nerve stimulation are not effective in the treatment of LBP. Other treatments such as lumbar braces, traction, acupuncture, dry-needling, biofeedback, and massage are also largely ineffective and not recommended.

LBP is common in pregnancy and although it frequently starts before the twelfth week it is rarely progressive. Back pain can be reduced in most pregnant patients by the use of an inelastic low sacroiliac belt that does not compress the abdomen.

Kyphoplasty (Figure 10–6) and vertebroplasty (percutaneous injection of bone cement into a fractured vertebral body through bone biopsy needles) are two technically demanding procedures that are gaining popularity for the treatment of pain associated with new osteoporotic compression fractures that do not respond to conventional treatment. Kyphoplasty may improve the height of the fractured vertebra and the related kyphosis in some patients. Complications include cement leakage that may result in neurologic compromise and cement embolus to the lungs. There are no randomized, placebo-controlled trials to support the use of these procedures. There is also a concern about the mechanical strength of adjacent vertebrae following these procedures.

B. Chronic Lower Back Pain

In most patients, the cause of chronic LBP is unclear. The clinical spectrum is wide. Some patients complain of severe unremitting pain, but most have a nagging mechanical LBP that may radiate into the buttocks. Patients with chronic LBP may experience periods of acute exacerbation. Treatment is centered on relief of pain and restoration of function. Results are often unsatisfactory, and complete relief of pain is unrealistic for most. However, the large majority of patients with chronic back pain continue working.

Acetaminophen and nonsteroidal anti-inflammatory drugs may provide some degree of analgesia but the evidence for their efficacy is not compelling. Long-term use of narcotic analgesics should be avoided, but this is not always possible. Antidepressants are useful in the one-third of patients who have associated depression. Low-dose tricyclic antidepressants (eg, amitriptyline 10–75 mg at bedtime) may help some patients without depression, but anticholinergic side effects are common.

Back exercises (see section on Acute Lower Back Pain, above), aerobic conditioning, loss of excess weight, and patient education are effective in managing chronic LBP.

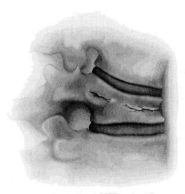

Fractured Vertebra

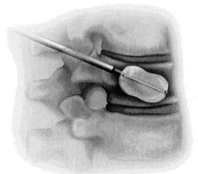

Balloon Inflation

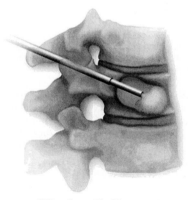

Filling the void with cement

Figure 10–6. Balloon kyphoplasty. The first illustration is of a fractured osteoporotic vertebra. In the next illustration an orthopedic balloon has been percutaneously guided into the fractured vertebral body and inflated, reducing the fracture and elevating the superior endplate. The balloon is then deflated and removed, thereby creating a void. The final illustration shows filling of the void with cement. (Reproduced from Kyphon Pictures with permission.)

Multidisciplinary pain centers offer a combination of drug therapy, behavioral therapy, physical therapy, and patient education. These therapies may be helpful in selected patients as long as the center is not procedure-oriented and avoids the use of unproven and expensive therapies including invasive procedures.

Massage, when combined with exercise and education, may be beneficial for patients with chronic LBP and the benefit may continue for at least a year after the course of massage is over. As with patients with acute LBP, there is no evidence to support the use of injection therapies and modalities for chronic LBP.

Prolotherapy is an injection-based treatment that has been used for chronic LBP. Proponents of prolotherapy hypothesize that back pain in some patients stems from weakened ligaments. Repeatedly injecting the ligaments with an irritant sclerosing agent is believed to strengthen the ligaments and reduce pain. However, there is no evidence that prolotherapy injections are more effective than control injections.

Radiofrequency denervation of the small nerves to the facet joints is sometimes recommended for patients with the facet syndrome. There is no evidence of benefit beyond a few weeks following this procedure.

Spinal cord stimulation is yet another modality used for the relief of chronic LBP. An electrical generator delivers pulses to a targeted spinal cord area through leads implanted via laminectomy or percutaneously. The mechanism of action is poorly understood, and there are insufficient data to support its use. The use of intraspinal drug infusion systems for intrathecal delivery of analgesics (usually morphine) is also not supported by adequate data.

The exact pathophysiology of pain in degenerative disease of the lumbar spine remains elusive. It is therefore not surprising that as a general principle, the results of back surgery are disappointing when the goal is relief of back pain rather than relief of radicular symptoms resulting from neurologic compression. The role of surgical treatment of chronic disabling LBP without neurologic involvement remains controversial. The most common surgical treatment in these patients with degenerative changes is spinal fusion. The rationale for fusion is based on its successful use at painful peripheral joints. A growing body of clinical evidence now suggests that functional restoration through a cognitive-behavioral therapy–based intensive rehabilitation program can generate improvements similar to spinal fusion.

Intradiscal electrothermal annuloplasty is another unproven procedure for the relief of chronic LBP in patients with positive discography. A wire-containing catheter is inserted into the disc, positioned against the posterior annulus, and then heated. This presumably shrinks collagen fibrils and cauterizes granulation and nerve tissue.

Table 10–6. Indications for Surgical Referral

Disc herniation
   Cauda equina syndrome (emergency)
   Severe neurologic deficit
   Progressive neurologic deficit
   Greater than 6 weeks of sciatica (elective)
   Persistence of significant neurologic deficit beyond
     6 weeks (elective)
Spinal stenosis
   Severe neurologic deficit
   Progressive neurologic deficit
   Persistent and disabling pseudoclaudication (elective)
Spondylolisthesis
   Significant or progressive neurologic deficit

The use of lumbar artificial discs for spinal arthroplasty, in patients with degenerative disc disease at one level from L4–S1 and no spondylolisthesis, has recently been approved in the United States. Approval was based on data showing efficacy equal to that of spinal fusion. This may be faint praise given the lack of evidence for the effectiveness and safety of spinal fusion. Few data support the hypothetical advantage that, unlike spinal fusion, artificial discs will protect adjacent levels from further degeneration by preserving motion.

C. Nerve Root Compression Syndromes

1. Disc herniation—Patients with radicular pain in whom a disc herniation with nerve root compression is suspected should be treated nonsurgically, as described in the section on Acute Lower Back Pain, for the first 6 weeks unless they have a severe or progressive neurologic deficit. Most patients (approximately 90%) will respond. Elective surgery may be considered in the few patients who have a significant persistent neurologic deficit or severe sciatica after 6 weeks of conservative care (Table 10–6).

Laminotomy with limited discectomy is generally the procedure of choice. A microdiscectomy is the same procedure but with the use of a microscope. Percutaneous techniques, including microendoscopic discectomy, are less effective.

2. Spinal stenosis—The symptoms of spinal stenosis remain stable for years in most patients and may actually improve in a few. Even when symptoms progress, there is little likelihood of irreversible neurologic impairment. Therefore, nonoperative treatment is a rational choice for most patients. Analgesics, nonsteroidal anti-inflammatory drugs, loss of excess weight, physical conditioning, exercises (including those that reduce lumbar lordosis), and epidural glucocorticoids may provide symptomatic relief.

Patients with a progressive or severe neurologic deficit are surgical candidates (see Table 10–6). Elective surgery may be considered in patients with severe and disabling pseudoclaudication. Surgical treatment is aimed at decompression of the neural elements. This is accomplished by laminectomy or laminotomy with excision of the ligamentum flavum and medial aspect of the hypertrophied facet joints and removal of any protruding disc material. If spinal instability is present (as with spondylolisthesis) or results from surgical decompression, fusion of vertebral segments may be required.

3. Spondylolisthesis—The vast majority of patients are treated conservatively. Rarely, a patient may need decompression surgery with fusion if a significant or progressive neurologic deficit develops from nerve root impingement or as a result of spinal stenosis. Surgical fusion for spondylolisthesis with chronic disabling pain but no neurologic deficit may yield better results than nonsurgical treatment. Unfortunately, long-term follow-up shows that this benefit is not sustained.

REFERENCES

Bigos S, et al. Acute low back problems in adults. Agency for Health Care Policy and Research, Public Health Service, U.S. Department of Health and Human Services. Clinical Practice Guideline No. 14. Report No. 95-0642. December 1994. (A classic, comprehensive, and critical evaluation of the published literature with recommendations for managing acute LBP.)

Carragee EJ. Persistent low back pain. *N Engl J Med.* 2005;352:1891–1898. [PMID: 15872204] (An overview of chronic low back pain.)

Deyo RA, Weinstein JN. Low back pain. *N Engl J Med.* 2001;344:363. [PMID: 2945917] (Concise overview of the clinical features, diagnostic evaluation, and treatment.)

Jarvik JG, Deyo RA. Diagnostic evaluation of low back pain with emphasis on imaging. *Ann Intern Med.* 2002;137:586. [PMID: 12353946] (A detailed review of the different imaging techniques.)

Relevant World Wide Web Sites

[American Academy of Orthopaedic Surgeons]
   http://www.aaos.org

[Institute for Clinical Systems Improvement]
   http://www.ICSI.org

[National Guideline Clearinghouse]
   http://www.guideline.gov

The Patient with Hip Pain

Ilksen Gurkan, MD, & Simon Mears, MD, PhD

Hip pain is a common complaint of patients presenting for medical care. Most patients have a broad definition of the hip, which includes the thigh, back, and groin areas. The clinician must be aware of common referred pain patterns from spinal stenosis and trochanteric bursitis. The hip joint and its periarticular structures are relatively inaccessible to evaluation by palpation for possible tenderness. Therefore accurate evaluation of patients with "hip" pain depends on the identification of specific historical features of the symptoms, the determination of the exact cause of the pain (through careful medical history and appropriate physical examination), a basic understanding of common radiographic findings, and a thorough understanding of the potential differential diagnosis. The particular cause of hip pain often correlates with the age of the patient. This chapter reviews the important general features in the history, physical examination, and imaging modalities and presents a list of differential diagnoses with a detailed profile of findings and diagnostic clues for each cause.

Clinical Findings

A. SYMPTOMS AND SIGNS

1. History—The location of the pain and activities associated with that pain frequently are the most reliable indicators of the cause. Pain located primarily in the groin and associated with weight-bearing or range of motion is most typically related to intra-articular hip abnormalities. Hip pain beginning in the low back and radiating down the buttock and back of the leg to the side of the calf and lateral side of the foot is more likely to be referred radiculopathy than an intra-articular hip abnormality. Pain localized to the side of the hip is most likely to be greater trochanteric bursitis.

The characteristics and timing of hip pain help determine diagnosis. Patients with severe hip pain that is generalized, constant, or worse at night may have a malignancy or an infection affecting the hip. To differentiate between acute and chronic hip pain, patients should be asked about the onset of symptoms. A sudden traumatic event associated with the onset of pain strongly suggests fracture or injury to the soft tissues about the hip. Repetitive loading activities can result in a femoral stress fracture. Pain that develops slowly over time is common in

arthritic conditions. For example, a person with hip osteoarthritis experiences a gradual onset of slowly worsening hip pain and decreasing range of motion. It becomes progressively harder to walk normally, especially going up and down stairs. Factors that aggravate the pain also need to be scrutinized carefully. For example, pain that is reproduced with palpation, lateral in nature, and worse with lying on the affected hip usually is trochanteric bursitis. Questions regarding what type of activities exacerbate the pain can reveal important abnormal mechanics during running, such as the feet crossing the midline (increased adduction), wide pelvis and genu valgum, or running on oval tracks that lack banks. Such activities can cause trochanteric bursitis.

The age of the patient is important in helping determine the cause of pain. Children are susceptible to particular hip problems such as slipped capital femoral epiphysis and Perthes disease. Adolescents and young adults commonly have avascular necrosis, hip dysplasia, or femoroacetabular impingement. Middle-aged and older patients often have hip arthritis, low back pain, or trochanteric bursitis.

Associated symptoms are helpful in differentiating pain from the hip and other sources. Extra-articular findings can be important in helping identify the type of arthritis (eg, tophi in gout, nodules in rheumatoid arthritis, or pustular rash in gonococcemia). Patients who report snapping in and around the hip may have one of the "snapping hip syndromes," which are divided into internal and external causes. Internal snapping can be caused by the iliopsoas tendon slipping over the osseous ridge of the lesser trochanter or the anterior acetabulum or by the iliofemoral ligament riding over the femoral head. Acetabular labral tears or loose bodies can cause intra-articular snapping associated with sharp pain in the groin and anterior thigh. External snapping results from a tight iliotibial band or gluteus maximus tendon riding over the greater tuberosity of the femur. These types of snapping occur during hip flexion and extension, especially during internal rotation. Radiation of pain down the leg or in conjunction with back pain may represent a spine abnormality as a primary cause, or if the pain radiates from the lateral hip to the knee, trochanteric bursitis. In rare instances, an intrapelvic, intra-abdominal, or retroperitoneal abnormality (ranging from uterine fibroids to a sports hernia to a retroperitoneal hematoma or infection) may be the cause of hip symptoms.

2. Physical Examination—A basic understanding of hip anatomy and biomechanics is the cornerstone of an accurate physical examination of the patient with hip pain. The hip is formed by the proximal femur and the articulation with the pelvis. The bony anatomy of the proximal femur includes the femoral head, the femoral neck, and the greater and lesser trochanters. The acetabulum, the mating socket for the femoral head, is coated with articular cartilage, and a rim of fibrocartilage (the labrum) adds to the stability of the hip and circumscribes the outer edge of the acetabulum. The main abductors of the hip are the gluteus medius and minimus, which attach to the greater trochanter, and the primary hip flexor is the iliopsoas tendon, which inserts on the lesser trochanter. The iliotibial band originates along the brim of the iliac wing (along the anterior and posterior margins), consolidates over the greater trochanter, travels laterally along the thigh, and inserts in the proximal leg. These tendinous insertions have an associated bursa where the tendon crosses a bony protuberance. Friction is decreased between the gluteus maximus and the greater trochanter by the trochanteric bursa, between the gluteus maximus and the vastus lateralis origin by the gluteofemoral bursa, and between the ischial tuberosity and gluteus maximus by the ischial bursa. The muscles around the hip can be classified into four main groups (Figure 11–1).

a. Inspection of the hip—Inspection of the hip begins with the careful observation of the patient's gait. Two phases of gait need to be observed: stance phase (when the foot is on the ground and bears weight) and swing phase (when the foot moves forward and does not bear weight). Most of the problems appear during the weight-bearing stance phase.

The width of the gait, the shift of the pelvis, and flexion of the knee should be observed as well as the lumbar portion of the spine. With the patient in the supine position, the lumbar spine reflects a slight lordosis. Loss of lordosis may reflect vertebral spasm, and excess lordosis may suggest a flexion deformity of the hip. Therefore this observation should always be followed with the assessment of leg-length symmetry. Leg shortening and external rotation with pain suggest hip fracture. The anterior and posterior surfaces of the hip should be inspected for areas of muscle atrophy or bruising related to a traumatic event or neuromuscular disease.

Pain is a common cause of limp. The characteristic of an antalgic limp is shortened standing time on the affected side. When pain arises in the hip joint, the trunk also shifts toward the painful side. Moving the body's center of gravity toward the painful hip decreases the moment arm of body weight to hip joint, reducing total force on the hip. This maneuver should not be confused with a Trendelenburg gait, which is secondary to a weakened medius muscle. In the Trendelenburg gait pattern, the opposite side of the pelvis tilts downward during the stance phase on the weakened side, and in an effort to compensate for the weakness, the trunk lurches toward the weakened side during the same walking cycle phase. This action moves the center of gravity nearer the fulcrum on the weak side and shortens the moment arm from the center of gravity to the hip joint to produce the characteristic waddle.

A limp is common in patients with substantial hip arthritis or disease in other joints of the lower extremity. The limp may be caused by pain, shortening of the leg, flexion contracture, or weakness in the pelvic girdle muscles and/or in other parts of the lower limb, such as in a paralyzed quadriceps gait pattern, triceps surae gait pattern, and dorsiflexor gait pattern. Therefore a thorough evaluation of lower extremity muscle strength is essential for diagnosing the cause of the limp. Manual muscle testing is useful for evaluating flexors (iliopsoas and rectus femoris), extensors (gluteus maximus and hamstrings), abductors (gluteus medius and minimus), and adductors (adductor longus, magnus, and brevis; pectineus and gracilis). Muscle testing should be performed on the lower leg muscles (ankle and toe dorsiflexors and plantar flexors) to evaluate for weakness due to a radiculopathy.

b. Palpation—With the patient supine, the clinician should ask the patient to place the heel of the leg being examined on the opposite knee. This position facilitates palpation along the inguinal ligament. Bulges along the ligament can be inguinal hernias or aneurysms, which can be secondary causes of hip pain outside the hip joint (eg, ischemia secondary to vascular disease or compression of an aneurysm). From lateral to medial, a sequence of nerve, artery, vein, and lymph nodes can be palpated. Enlarged nodes suggest infection. Tenderness over the femoral greater trochanter indicates local bursitis rather than arthritis. With the patient lying on the nonaffected side and the hip flexed and internally rotated, the trochanteric bursa over the greater trochanter can be palpated (Figure 11–2). The ischiogluteal bursa cannot be palpated unless it is inflamed (Figure 11–3). When it is inflamed, this bursitis can mimic sciatica. Bursitis is one of the major causes of tenderness around the hip joint, but other causes of such tenderness include synovitis of the hip joint or psoas abscess. Tenderness without swelling on the posterolateral surface of the greater trochanter suggests localized tendinitis or muscle spasm from referred hip pain. Crepitus, or a grating sensation in the joint, felt by the patient or determined by the examiner, is a late manifestation of an arthritic condition and is not a sensitive or specific indicator.

c. Range of motion—Motions of the hip include flexion, extension, abduction, adduction, and rotation.

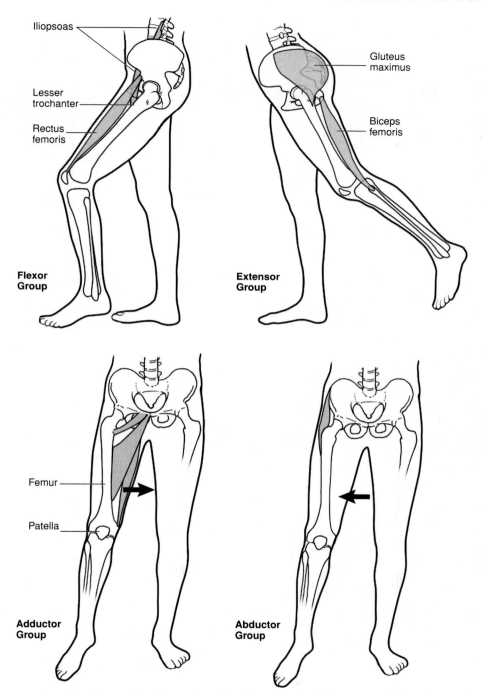

Figure 11–1. Four powerful muscle groups that move the hip are shown with their attachments to the femur and pelvis. (From Bickley LS, Szilagyi PG. The musculoskeletal system. In: *Bates' Guide to Physical Examination and History Taking.* 8th ed. Lippincott Williams & Wilkins, 2003:479. With permission.)

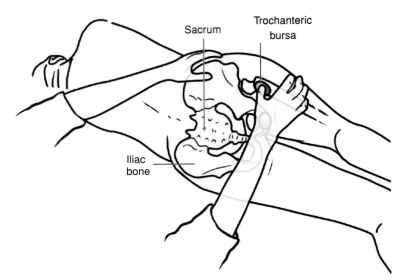

Figure 11–2. With the patient lying on the unaffected side and the affected hip flexed and internally rotated, the trochanteric bursa over the greater trochanter can be palpated. Swelling with tenderness suggests trochanteric bursitis. Tenderness without swelling along the posterolateral aspect suggests localized tendinitis. (From Bickley LS, Szilagyi PG. The musculoskeletal system. In: *Bates' Guide to Physical Examination and History Taking.* 8th ed. Lippincott Williams & Wilkins, 2003:508. With permission.)

The hip can flex further when the knee is also flexed. In the case of a hip with a flexion deformity, flexion of the unaffected hip prevents full leg extension of the affected hip, which appears flexed (Figure 11–4). With the patient supine, the examiner places one hand on the patient's iliac crest. As the patient attempts to extend the hip to neutral, the clinician can detect pelvic movement that might be mistaken for hip movement. Flexion deformity may be masked by an increase in lumbar lordosis and an anterior pelvic tilt. Assessment of the extension can be aided by positioning the patient face down and extending the

thigh toward the clinician in a posterior direction. Stabilizing the pelvis by pressing down on the opposite anterior superior iliac spine with one hand, grasping the ankle with the other, and abducting the extended leg marks the limit of hip abduction (Figure 11–5). Restricted abduction (normal range, 45–50 degrees) is common in hip osteoarthritis. In the same manner, moving the leg medially across the body and over the opposite extremity marks the adduction limit. Flexing the leg to 90 degrees at hip and knee, stabilizing the thigh with one hand, grasping the ankle with the other, and rotating the lower

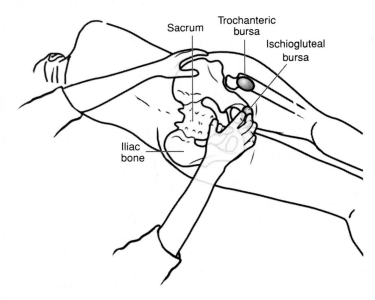

Figure 11–3. Unless inflamed, the ischiogluteal bursa cannot be palpated. Shown are the location of (directly over the ischial tuberosity) and the palpation technique for the ischiogluteal bursa. (From Bickley LS, Szilagyi PG. The musculoskeletal system. In: *Bates' Guide to Physical Examination and History Taking.* 8th ed. Lippincott Williams & Wilkins, 2003:508. With permission.)

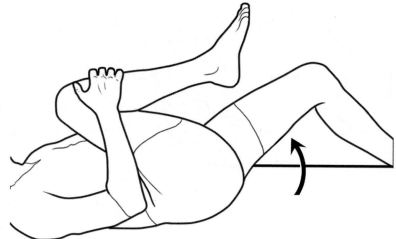

Figure 11–4. In flexion deformity of the hip, the affected hip does not allow full leg extension when the opposite hip is flexed. Therefore the affected hip appears flexed. (From Bickley LS, Szilagyi PG. The musculoskeletal system. In: *Bates' Guide to Physical Examination and History Taking*. 8th ed. Lippincott Williams & Wilkins, 2003:509. With permission.)

extremity externally (normal, 45 degrees) and internally (normal, 35 degrees) identifies the hip's rotation limits (Figure 11–6). These maneuvers usually demonstrate any existing loss of internal rotation (often the earliest change and therefore an especially sensitive indicator of hip disease), flexion, extension, or abduction. As the disease progresses, prolonged joint stiffness and limitations of movements become more evident. Limitation of joint movement may be secondary to flexion contractures or mechanical obstructions.

   d. Symmetry and other joint involvement— Joint involvement in rheumatoid arthritis, ankylosing spondylitis, or systemic lupus erythematosus is usually symmetrical, though often one side is more affected than the other. Hip disease in osteoarthritis, psoriatic arthritis, or reactive arthritis is often unilateral. Involvement of other joints may provide clues about the primary disease that affected the hip. For example, metacarpophalangeal and proximal interphalangeal deformity and involvement indicate rheumatoid arthritis, whereas distal interphalangeal involvement can indicate osteoarthritis.

B. LABORATORY FINDINGS

Additional evaluation is indicated when the diagnosis remains uncertain, response to therapy is not as expected, or substantial clinical changes occur. Certain problems require immediate attention and prompt treatment. For

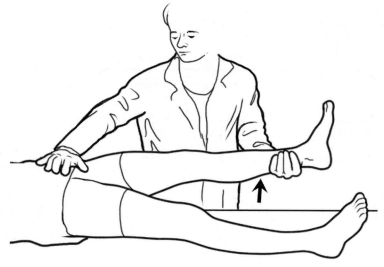

Figure 11–5. The limit of hip abduction is determined by stabilizing the pelvis with one hand pressing down on the opposite anterior superior iliac spine and with the other hand grasping the ankle and abducting the extended leg. (From Bickley LS, Szilagyi PG. The musculoskeletal system. In: *Bates' Guide to Physical Examination and History Taking*. 8th ed. Lippincott Williams & Wilkins, 2003:510. With permission.)

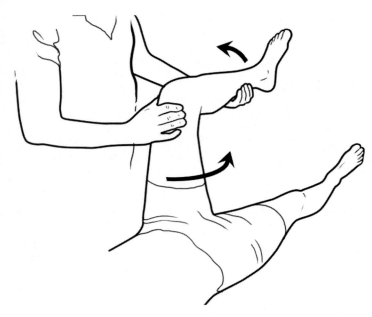

Figure 11–6. Establishing the rotation limits of the hip is done by flexing the leg to 90 degrees at the hip and knee, stabilizing the thigh with one hand, and with the other hand grasping the ankle and rotating the lower extremity externally (normal, 45 degrees) and internally (normal, 35 degrees). (From Bickley LS, Szilagyi PG. The musculoskeletal system. In: *Bates' Guide to Physical Examination and History Taking.* 8th ed. Lippincott Williams & Wilkins, 2003:511. With permission.)

example, joint fluid examination is essential for the diagnosis of acute monarthritis. Hemorrhagic joint fluid suggests fracture, bleeding diathesis, or malignancy. Intensely inflammatory effusions (see Chapter 2) suggest pyogenic infection requiring immediate antibiotic therapy and aspiration or other drainage to establish the diagnosis and prevent joint destruction.

When rheumatoid systemic diseases are suspected, clinically indicated laboratory work may include tests for erythrocyte sedimentation rate and rheumatoid factor. Blood tests are useful in diagnosing some specific types of arthritis (for specific tests, see the chapters for each disease).

Synovial fluid analysis, which may help exclude other diagnoses, allows most effusions to be classified as normal, inflammatory, noninflammatory, infectious, or hemorrhagic (Table 11–1). Each type of effusion suggests certain joint diseases. So-called noninflammatory effusions are actually mildly inflammatory but tend to suggest diseases with less inflammatory mechanisms. If infection is suspected, a portion of the synovial fluid sample should be sent to the laboratory for Gram stain and culture. Synovial fluid analysis provides a definitive diagnosis for infections and crystal arthropathies that rarely affect hip joints. However, aspiration of the hip joint for hip pain based on factors other than evidence of an

Table 11–1. Analysis of Synovial Fluid in the Hip

Parameter	Normal	Inflammatory	Noninflammatory	Infectious	Hemorrhagic
Color	Clear	Clear	Opaque	Opaque	Sanguineous
Viscosity	High	High	Low	Variable	Variable
White blood cell counts/mm³	<200	<2000	>2000	>50,000	Variable
Percentage of polymorphonuclear neutrophils	<25%	<25%	>25%	>50%	Variable
Examples		Traumatic, osteoarthritis, neuropathic, hypertrophic arthropathy	Seropositives, seronegatives, crystal arthropathies	Septic arthritis	Trauma, hemophilia

underlying infection is uncommon. Therefore imaging modalities are always preferred as the first-line diagnostic tools.

C. IMAGING STUDIES

1. Plain radiography—Plain radiographs of the hip and pelvis should be ordered as the first diagnostic test for patients with hip pain. Plain radiographs can delineate the alignment, bone mineralization, articular cartilage, and soft tissue. Alignment abnormality may indicate a fracture, a dislocation, or secondary causes of osteoarthritis such as congenital dislocation of the hip or slipped capital femoral epiphysis. Bone mineralization indicates osteoporosis or osteopenia as the underlying cause of pain. An anteroposterior pelvic radiograph and a "frog-leg" lateral hip radiograph may reveal fractures, provide a better view of the anterolateral femoral head, and help evaluate for osteonecrosis. For patients in the later stages of osteonecrosis, radiographs show a break in the cortex and a rim sign (a subcortical black lucent line) characteristic of femoral head collapse. A 40-degree cephalad anteroposterior view is useful for elucidating subtle femoral neck and pubic fractures. On plain radiographs, joint-space narrowing is indicative of articular cartilage loss, spurs or osteophytes are indicative of arthritic change, segmental radiolucency or sclerotic changes of the femoral head are indicative of avascular necrosis, calcifications are indicative of synovial chondromatosis, and soft-tissue calcification is indicative of calcific tendinitis. Figure 11–7 shows the changes associated with certain disorders, as seen on the anteroposterior pelvic view.

2. Arthrography—Arthrography, which involves obtaining images after a contrast agent has been injected into the hip, is a useful tool for showing labral abnormalities, especially when it is performed in conjunction with magnetic resonance imaging (MRI). Magnetic resonance arthrography is the most sensitive and specific test for labral tear of the hip. Injection with local anesthetic agents during the arthrogram can be a powerful tool for the diagnosis of hip abnormalities: if the injection does not reduce the pain (however transiently), other diagnoses should be ruled out. Arthrography continues to have a role in the diagnosis of infection and loosening of the prosthesis in the patient with a painful total joint arthroplasty.

3. Computed tomography—Computed tomography (CT) of the hip and pelvis is most useful in the assessment of fractures, particularly complex fractures. Pelvic and acetabular fractures, osseous sequelae of hip dislocation, and intra-articular osseous fragments are better visualized by CT than by plain radiographs. CT also is useful in characterizing calcifications secondary to tumor matrix within bone or soft tissue or to ossification, and CT is the best modality for imaging cortical bone.

4. Magnetic resonance imaging—MRI provides excellent visualization of medullary bone and soft tissues.

The diagnosis of osteonecrosis of the femoral head is made earlier by MRI than by any other technique, including bone scintigraphy, CT, and plain radiographs. MRI also is the method of choice for the diagnosis of occult hip fracture in the elderly, and despite its expense, can be cost-effective for this purpose. MRI is the most accurate method for the diagnosis of stress fractures around the hip and pelvis, and it is the best test for the diagnosis of transient osteonecrosis of the hip. It is also the most valuable test for the staging of bony and soft tissue tumors around the hip. MRI is frequently helpful in documenting synovitis of the hip joint by revealing effusion (eg, in pigmented villonodular synovitis). Magnetic resonance arthrography is useful in defining labral abnormalities.

5. Bone scans—Bone scans are useful for detecting metastatic disease (when suspected), avascular necrosis, arthritis, and Paget disease of bone. Scintigraphy delineates regions of increased metabolic activity ("hot-spots") by increased uptake of a radioactive tracer.

6. Electromyography and nerve conduction velocity studies—Electromyography and nerve conduction velocity studies are used in the differential diagnosis of hip pain to evaluate referred lumbosacral plexopathies and to assess local nerve entrapment or nerve damage from trauma, surgery, or other disease states.

7. Injections—Differential block of the hip joint can be a valuable adjunct in differentiating the source of intra-articular hip joint pain. This procedure is best undertaken in the fluoroscopy suite, with arthrography used to confirm the location of the injection. The technique may be particularly useful in distinguishing intra-articular hip abnormalities from referred lumbosacral radiculopathy and possible soft-tissue conditions. Dye injection along the iliopsoas tendon sheath under fluoroscopy sometimes reveals the snapping of the iliopsoas tendon over the pelvic brim, and when accompanied by lidocaine or corticosteroid injection, may help prove that the tendon condition is the pain generator.

D. SPECIAL TESTS

1. Stinchfield test—The Stinchfield resisted hip flexion test evaluates the pain response caused by an increase in hip joint reactive force and is a valuable tool for distinguishing between intra-articular and extra-articular hip abnormalities causing groin, thigh, buttock, and even pretibial leg pain. The patient in supine position is asked to elevate the leg while the examiner applies gentle manual resistance to the ankle with the knee extended. Reproduction of pain in a typical pattern related to the sensory innervation of the hip (groin, thigh, buttock, or knee) makes the test positive for a hip abnormality.

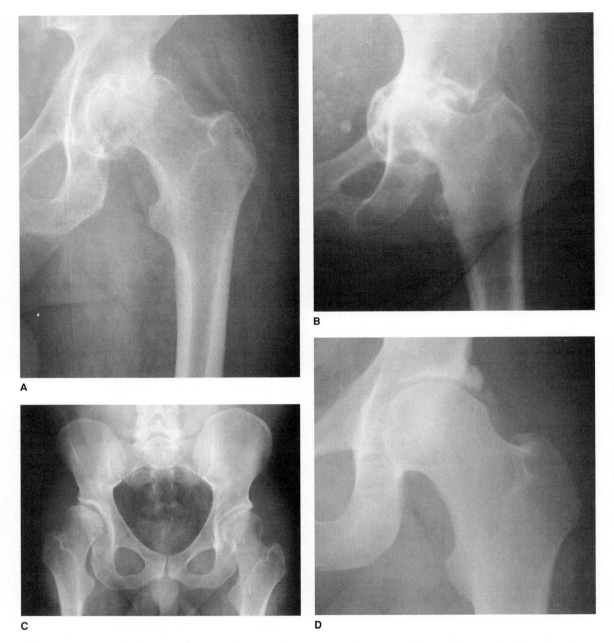

Figure 11–7. Common radiographic findings. **A:** Osteoarthritis: asymmetric joint space narrowing, joint sclerosis, osteophytes, and subchondral cysts. **B:** Rheumatoid arthritis: symmetrical joint space narrowing and protrusio acetabuli. **C:** Dysplasia: acetabular uncovering and increased acetabular slope. **D:** Femoroacetabular impingement: peripheral osteophytes.

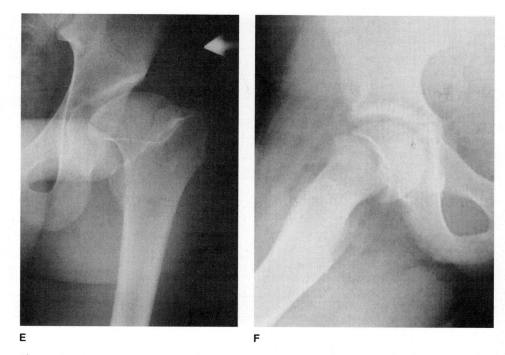

E

F

Figure 11–7. (Continued) E: Perthes disease: incongruent joint and misshapen femoral head.
F: Slipped capital femoral epiphysis: fracture through the epiphyseal growth plate.

2. Patrick test—In the Patrick test, the patient lies supine and the clinician holds the affected leg and rotates it externally. Pain so elicited suggests sacroiliitis, hip abnormality, or an L4 nerve root lesion.

E. DIFFERENTIAL DIAGNOSIS

The age of the patient is critical in diagnosing the cause of hip pain. Figure 11–8 shows a helpful timeline for this diagnosis and Table 11–2 provides a guide to treatment of common hip conditions.

1. Children—Neonates are susceptible to hematogenous infection and can present with an acute septic joint. Children 3–10 years old who have hip pain most commonly have an infection, acute transient synovitis, or Perthes disease (also known as Legg-Calvé-Perthes disease). A normal radiograph and hip pain is most commonly associated with a self-limiting condition termed acute transient synovitis of the hip. If the child has a fever or sign of infection, hip aspiration should be performed to rule out an acute septic joint. Sepsis should be treated with identification of the organism and appropriate intravenous antibiotics, with consideration for surgical washout. Perthes disease is a condition that causes a portion of the femoral head to develop ischemic necrosis

and collapse. Radiographs will reveal evidence of Perthes disease (see Figure 11–7E). The hip then gradually remodels, but later in life up to 50% of patients develop early hip arthritis. Children are treated symptomatically and may require realignment surgery if substantial collapse occurs.

The most common diagnosis in children aged 11–16 years old who have hip pain is slipped capital femoral epiphysis. This condition represents a fracture through the growth plate or epiphysis of the femoral neck (see Figure 11–7F). In 50% of the cases, slipped capital femoral epiphysis occurs bilaterally and is treated surgically to prevent additional slippage, osteonecrosis, and chondrolysis. Fractures occur in different patterns in adolescent patients than in adults. Sudden muscular exertion can cause avulsion injuries and injury at the bony insertion of the tendons around the hip.

Children also develop a different set of oncologic problems than do adults, including primary osteosarcoma and Ewing sarcoma, whereas adult and elderly patients most commonly have metastatic disease. Tumors seen on radiographs should be further evaluated with MRI scanning.

2. Adults—Young adults may develop stress fractures of the femoral neck in response to an increase in exercise.

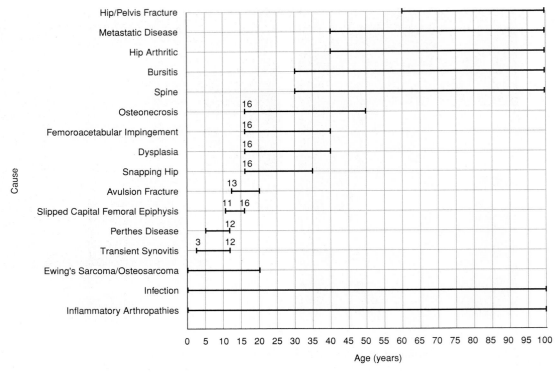

Figure 11–8. Timeline of causes of hip pain.

Table 11–2. Interventions for Common Hip Conditions

Condition	Intervention
Degenerative arthritis (osteoarthritis)	Physiotherapy, NSAIDs, activity modification, surgery
Inflammatory arthritis (rheumatoid arthritis)	NSAIDs, disease-modifying anti-rheumatic medications, corticosteroids, synovectomy, joint replacement
Infection	Surgical drainage, intravenous antibiotics
Pelvic fracture	Pain medications, ambulatory aid
Hip fracture	Surgical fixation
Avulsion fracture	Ice, NSAIDs, activity modification, rarely surgery
Tumor (metastatic)	Chemotherapy/radiation therapy, surgery to strengthen bone with prophylactic nailing or replacement
Tumor (Ewing sarcoma/osteosarcoma)	Surgical resection of tumor with or without joint replacement, chemotherapy, radiation therapy
Osteonecrosis	Early stages: decompression or bone grafting; late stages: hip replacement
Soft-tissue injuries (iliopsoas bursitis)	Muscle stretching, steroid injection, physiotherapy
Trochanteric bursitis	Ice, NSAIDs, muscle stretching, steroid injection, physiotherapy
Spine dysfunction	NSAIDs, physiotherapy, cortisone injections, surgery for decompression/fusion
Snapping syndromes	Muscle stretching, ice, NSAIDs, physiotherapy
Dysplasia	NSAIDs, activity modification, surgery for realignment or hip replacement
Femoroacetabular impingement	NSAIDs, activity modification, surgery for hip reshaping or hip replacement
Slipped capital femoral epiphysis	Surgical fixation
Perthes disease	Activity modification, possible surgery

NSAID, nonsteroidal anti-inflammatory medication.

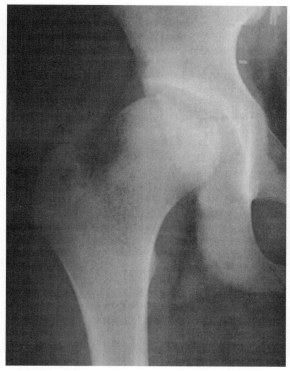

A

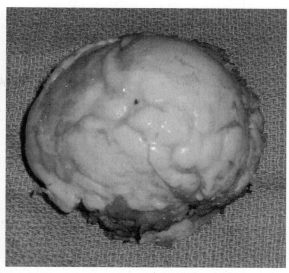

B

Figure 11–9. Osteonecrosis. **A:** The radiographs reveals subchondral lucency and collapse of a segment of femoral head. **B:** At the time of hip replacement, the collapsed bone has delaminated from the cartilage.

Adults up to the age of 40 may develop hip pain from several patterns of disease that gradually lead to early hip arthritis. The first is hip dysplasia, which occurs when the acetabulum does not develop correctly over the femoral head (see Figure 11–7C). The severity of this process ranges from mild changes to full dislocation. In mild forms, hip dysplasia causes excessive anteversion of the acetabular cup, which leads to gradual wear on the labrum with labral tearing. Wear then begins to occur at the edge of the joint, causing early arthritis. It is possible to reorient the acetabulum surgically with a periacetabular osteotomy to prevent later hip arthritis.

The second condition that can lead to early arthritis and hip pain in the young adult is femoroacetabular impingement. The upper lateral portion of the femoral neck gradually impinges on the acetabulum, leading to labral tearing, osteophyte formation around the hip (see Figure 11–7D), and ultimately hip stiffness and arthritis. It is possible to treat impingement surgically by removing the impinging osteophytes or reshaping the femoral head.

Young adults may develop osteonecrosis of the femoral head. This condition can be associated with prednisone use, heavy alcohol use, deep sea diving, or coagulopathies. Osteonecrosis, which can develop in multiple joints (but especially the hips and knees), can cause

subchondral bone in the femoral head to die. The cartilage above the necrotic bone collapses, and arthritis ensues (Figure 11–9). MRI scans are the most sensitive test for osteonecrosis and are positive before radiographic changes appear. In mild cases, bone grafting procedures may be successful, but in advanced cases, hip replacement surgery is required.

Middle-aged patients commonly have hip pain from osteoarthritis of the hip, trochanteric bursitis, or spinal causes. Osteoarthritis of the hip is generally unilateral, and the pain is worse with weight-bearing and twisting motions of the hip (see Figure 11–7A). Typically the pain is in the groin and leads to gradual hip stiffness and limp. Trochanteric bursitis presents with lateral pain that is often worse at night when the patient lies on the affected side. Spinal problems present with radiculopathy or pain that starts in the lower back and radiates down the leg to the foot. Weakness or numbness may occur with nerve compression in the back.

The hip pain in elderly patients (>60 years old) typically comes from osteoarthritis, metastatic disease, trochanteric bursitis, spinal stenosis, or fracture. Radiographs that reveal lytic lesions of the femoral neck or hip in these patients typically are the result of metastatic disease. Often surgery is needed to strengthen or replace the bone. Osteoporotic elderly patients are also at high risk for fracture of the femoral neck or the pelvis. All elderly patients with acute hip pain should be ruled out for fracture because fractures in this population may occur with mild trauma, such as a fall, or with no precipitating event and an insidious onset (insufficiency fractures). Fractures causing hip pain are located in the proximal femur, the acetabulum, or the pelvis. If radiographs are negative, an MRI scan should be performed.

3. All ages—Patients of all ages may develop infections in the hip joint. Immunosuppressed patients and those who use intravenous drugs are particularly vulnerable and often do not show systemic signs of infection. Joint infections cause unrelenting pain and fevers and should be diagnosed by hip aspiration. Treatment should be intravenous antibiotics and surgical débridement of the hip. Patients of all ages also are susceptible to a range of inflammatory arthritides, from juvenile rheumatoid arthritis in the young patient to rheumatoid arthritis, ankylosing spondylitis, or psoriatic arthritis in the adult patient. Rheumatoid arthritis often is bilateral and generally affects both hips as well as other joints throughout the body (see Figure 11–7B).

REFERENCES

Bird PA, Oakley SP, Shnier R, et al. Prospective evaluation of magnetic resonance imaging and physical examination findings in patients with greater trochanteric pain syndrome. *Arthritis Rheum.* 2001;44:2138. [PMID: 11592379] (These researchers evaluated patients with greater trochanteric pain syndrome via magnetic resonance imaging for the prevalence of gluteus medius tendon abnormalities.)

Byrd JW, Jones KS. Diagnostic accuracy of clinical assessment, magnetic resonance imaging, magnetic resonance arthrography, and intra-articular injection in hip arthroscopy patients. *Am J Sports Med.* 2004;32:1668. [PMID: 15494331] (Magnetic resonance arthrography was much more sensitive than magnetic resonance imaging at detecting various lesions, but it had twice as many false-positive interpretations. Response to an intra-articular injection of anesthetic was a 90% reliable indicator of intra-articular abnormality.)

Hedger S, Darby T, Smith MD. Unexplained hip pain: look beyond the obvious abnormality. *Ann Rheum Dis.* 1998;57:131. [PMID: 9640126] (This study presents a case and emphasizes the underestimation of the incidence of bursitis as a cause of hip pain.)

Jackson SM, Major NM. Pathologic conditions mimicking osteonecrosis. *Orthop Clin North Am.* 2004;35:315. [PMID: 15271539] (Magnetic resonance imaging has become increasingly helpful in establishing an early diagnosis of avascular necrosis. Avascular necrosis often shows a classic pattern on such imaging; findings earlier in the course of the disease are less specific. Many pitfalls can complicate interpretation, and a number of pathologic conditions can share features of early avascular necrosis on magnetic resonance imaging and plain radiographs.)

Rossi F, Dragoni S. Acute avulsion fractures of the pelvis in adolescent competitive athletes: prevalence, location and sports distribution of 203 cases collected. *Skeletal Radiol.* 2001;30:127. [PMID: 11357449] (Rossi and Dragoni reviewed the distribution of this common injury among athletes according to the sports activities in which they participated. Avulsion fractures were most common in the pelvis during soccer and gymnastics.)

Tanzer M, Noiseux N. Osseous abnormalities and early osteoarthritis: the role of hip impingement. *Clin Orthop Relat Res.* 2004;429:170. [PMID: 15577483] (This article reviews the role of femoroacetabular impingement as a common cause of early hip arthritis. A pistol-grip deformity of the hip is shown to be associated with labral tears and early degenerative arthritis of the hip.)

Troum OM, Crues JV III. The young adult with hip pain: diagnosis and medical treatment, circa 2004. *Clin Orthop Relat Res.* 2004;418:9. [PMID: 15043086] (Troum and Crues review the diagnosis and treatment of common hip problems in the young adult.)

Zacher J, Gursche A. 'Hip' pain. *Best Pract Res Clin Rheumatol.* 2003;17:71. [PMID: 12659822] (Zacher and Gursche review the common causes of hip pain and give recommendations for treatment.)

Approach to the Patient with Knee Pain

Carl A. Johnson, MD

Knee pain may result from trauma, overuse, internal derangement, osteoarthritis, or inflammatory arthritis. In addition, pain about the knee may be due to vascular or neurologic conditions. Hip disease may also refer pain to the knee, distal thigh, or both. The initial evaluation of a patient with knee pain should provide sufficient information to determine whether the pain is the result of intra-articular or periarticular knee pathology, or whether it may be produced by or referred from another source. In addition, the initial history and physical examination must identify specific conditions, such as septic arthritis or arterial occlusion, that may require urgent surgical intervention, other conditions that are amenable to nonoperative treatment, and those that may require further specialized evaluation or treatment (Table 12–1). The initial evaluation should provide clues to enable the examiner to formulate a provisional differential diagnosis, which may then be confirmed or refined through use of imaging studies or laboratory findings.

Initial Clinical Assessment

 ### ESSENTIAL FEATURES

- *Conditions such as septic arthritis or vascular occlusion may require acute intervention.*
- *Knee pain may be referred from ipsilateral hip disease or may be due to a neurologic condition resulting from degenerative arthritis of the lumbosacral spine, lumbar disc herniation, or spinal stenosis.*

History

The significant features of the history should include the onset and history of the pain as well as any prior history of similar problems in the knee or other joints. A history of trauma, whether recent or remote, should be noted. The nature of the onset of pain, including the location of the pain, whether the pain began suddenly, or whether symptoms began gradually and insidiously should be determined. The examiner should seek information about the response of pain to activity; whether the pain is constant or intermittent; and whether it is present only with weight-bearing, at rest, or both. The history should elicit information about whether activities such as negotiating stairs or inclines, weather changes, rest, or position exacerbate the symptoms, and whether rest, moving about, stretching, or other factors may relieve them. Specific questions to determine whether the onset of symptoms may have been associated with any specific activity or change in activity, such as recreational exercise, physically demanding work, or hobbies, may be helpful.

A history of swelling as well as its location should be sought. A history of stiffness, locking, catching, snapping, grinding, and crepitus should be obtained (Table 12–2). Locking symptoms must be further characterized as either true mechanical locking or nonmechanical locking due to apprehension or reluctance to move the knee because of pain or anticipation of pain. Similarly, symptoms of giving way should also be further investigated to determine whether they are the result of mechanical instability, weakness, or possible neurologic problems. A history of change in sensation, low back pain, radicular symptoms, feelings of leg weakness or heaviness, muscle cramps, and claudication may alert the examiner to the possibility of neurologic or vascular problems. Fevers, chills, or a history of infection elsewhere should also be noted.

A more comprehensive past medical history may be required in selected cases. A history of prior glucocorticoid use or alcohol abuse should alert the examiner to the possibility of avascular necrosis of the hip, which may initially present with thigh pain, knee pain, or both. Diabetes, systemic glucocorticoid use, HIV, and other conditions that may compromise immune function should similarly raise the clinician's index of suspicion to the possibility of septic arthritis.

Table 12–1. Diagnoses to be Excluded as a Cause of Knee Pain

- Critical exclusionary diagnoses
  - Septic arthritis
  - Arterial occlusion
- Mimics of knee pain
  - Ipsilateral hip disease (osteoarthritis, osteonecrosis, fracture)
  - Neuropathic conditions (lumbar disc disease, spinal stenosis, saphenous nerve entrapment)

Physical Examination

The physical examination should include observation and characterization of the patient's gait, when possible, specifically seeking abnormal gait features such as antalgic limp, Trendelenburg gait, and ataxic gait (Table 12–3). An antalgic gait is characterized by shortened stance phase of gait on the affected side, as the patient avoids weight-bearing on the painful limb. An unsteady walk, generally wide-based, with the feet thrown outward due to impaired coordination, is a feature of an ataxic gait. A Trendelenburg gait is characterized by listing of the trunk toward the affected side with each step. Overall limb alignment should be assessed for varus or valgus deformity. Extensor mechanism alignment is measured by the Q angle (normally 15 degrees valgus ±5 degrees), determined by the angle between the orientation of the quadriceps tendon and the patellar ligament (Figure 12–1). Excessive Q-angle valgus correlates with increased likelihood of patellar subluxation. Muscle atrophy, abnormal joint contours, and patellar tracking should be assessed. Abnormalities of the skin, including old scars, color, or temperature changes, should be noted. Swelling should be characterized as diffuse or localized and by whether it represents an intra-articular ef-

Table 12–2. History for Evaluation of Knee Pain

Onset and history
History of trauma, prior problems, or similar problems with other joints
Response to activity and rest
Factors that exacerbate symptoms
Factors that improve symptoms
History and nature of swelling
Stiffness, locking, catching, grinding, or crepitus
Symptoms of giving way or instability
Changes in sensation or muscle strength
Muscle cramps, claudication
Fevers or chills
Hip, groin, or thigh pain
Pertinent general medical conditions

Table 12–3. Physical Examination for Evaluation of Knee Pain

Observation of gait, alignment, deformities
Presence and location of warmth
Presence and location of swelling
Active and passive range of motion
Patellar tracking, mobility, apprehension
Collateral and cruciate stability
Meniscal tests
Tenderness to palpation and localization
Hip pain or stiffness
Vascular examination (pedal pulses, skin, hair distribution)
Neurologic examination (sensation, muscle strength, straight leg raise)

fusion or soft-tissue swelling. Localized swelling may also be specifically described as medial, lateral, popliteal, or prepatellar.

Active and passive range of motion should be measured and compared with the contralateral knee, noting flexion contractures, hyperextension, and any extension lag. Crepitus should be noted and localized, and patellar tracking should be observed. A sudden lateral deviation of the patella occurring as the knee approaches full extension, described as a positive "J-sign," may indicate patellar subluxation. The patellar apprehension sign, in which the examiner attempts to subluxate the patella laterally with the knee slightly flexed, often provokes the quadriceps to contract in response to the sensation of impending pain or patellar dislocation in patients with patellar tracking problems.

Medial and lateral stability should be examined at full extension and 30 degrees of knee flexion. Anterior cruciate ligament stability is determined by the Lachman test (Figure 12–2), the anterior drawer sign (Figure 12–3), and the flexion rotation drawer test or pivot shift. The posterior drawer test is used to assess posterior cruciate ligament integrity. Ligament stability findings should be compared with those of the contralateral knee to evaluate whether any perceived laxity is pathologic. In persons with apparent generalized laxity conditions, it may be helpful to examine the elbow and wrist joints for hyperextensibility and ability to touch the thumb to the ipsilateral forearm. The McMurray and Appley meniscal compression tests may detect meniscal tears, although the sensitivity and specificity of these tests are not sufficient to rely entirely on those findings alone. Palpation about the knee can provide substantial information by localizing tenderness to a specific area or anatomic structure, such as the medial or lateral joint lines, patellar facets, pes anserine bursa, tibial tubercle, tendons, ligaments, or bony structures.

The hip joint must be examined to exclude the possibility that knee pain may be referred from ipsilateral hip

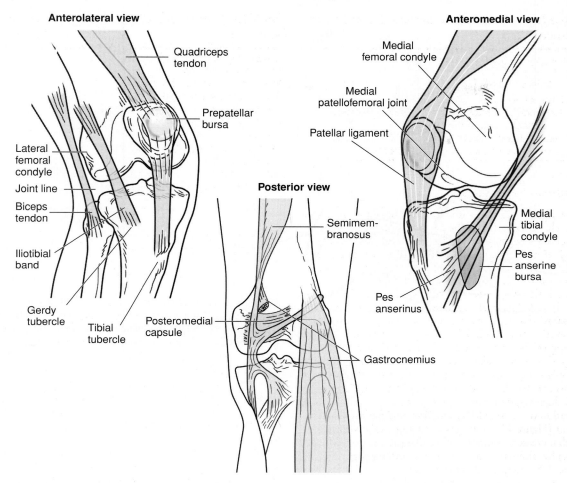

Anterolateral view

Quadriceps tendon

Prepatellar bursa

Lateral femoral condyle

Joint line

Biceps tendon

Iliotibial band

Gerdy tubercle

Tibial tubercle

Anteromedial view

Medial femoral condyle

Medial patellofemoral joint

Patellar ligament

Medial tibial condyle

Pes anserine bursa

Pes anserinus

Posterior view

Semimembranosus

Posteromedial capsule

Gastrocnemius

Figure 12–1. Functional anatomy of the knee.

disease. If pain is produced in the groin or thigh by active straight-leg raising against resistance or if significant limitation of hip range of motion is detected, further evaluation, including radiographic imaging of the hip, may be indicated. Pedal pulses, skin quality and pigmentation, and hair distribution on the feet and legs provide information about vascular status. When indicated, motor and sensory testing, examination of reflexes, and straight-leg raise testing may help identify pain from lumbosacral spine pathology.

Oberlander MA, Shalvoy RM, Hughston JC. The accuracy of the clinical knee examination documented by arthroscopy. A prospective study. *Am J Sports Med.* 1993;21:773. [PMID: 8291625] (Discusses the accuracy of clinical examination findings in diagnosing intra-articular knee pathology.)

Shybut GT, McGinty JB. The office evaluation of the knee. *Orthop Clin North Am.* 1982;3:497. [PMID: 7099586] (Describes a systematic approach to the clinical examination of the knee.)

SEPTIC ARTHRITIS

 ESSENTIAL FEATURES

- *Early recognition and treatment of septic arthritis is essential to minimize articular cartilage destruction and potentially life-threatening infection.*
- *Joint aspiration and synovial fluid analysis are the most helpful diagnostic tests.*

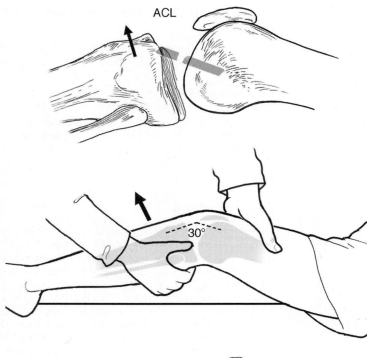

Figure 12–2. The Lachman test for anterior cruciate ligament (ACL) tear is at 30 degrees of flexion. The extremity does not have to be lifted or the foot stabilized.

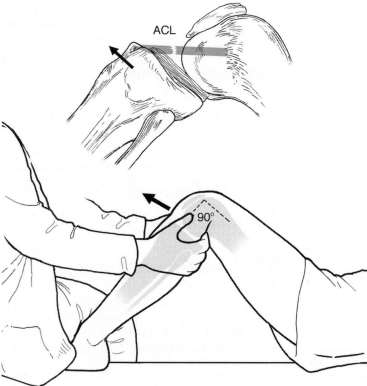

Figure 12–3. The anterior drawer test determines anterior cruciate instability. Flex the knee to 90 degrees and stabilize the foot. Note the forward shift of the tibia. ACL, anterior cruciate ligament.

Clinical Findings

A. SYMPTOMS AND SIGNS

Septic arthritis of the knee is generally associated with a history of severe, unremitting pain of recent onset exacerbated by motion and weight-bearing and with swelling, fevers, chills, or infection elsewhere. Pain is improved at rest. Physical findings include limited range of motion, associated with pain. Erythema, warmth, and diffuse tenderness are present about the knee. Swelling and an effusion are also present. Septic arthritis is unlikely when pain is intermittent, when range of motion is normal, and in the absence of warmth or effusions.

B. LABORATORY FINDINGS

Joint aspiration and synovial fluid analysis should be performed in all cases of suspected septic arthritis of the knee. Analysis of the synovial fluid for cell count with differential, Gram stain, and polarized light microscopy analysis for crystals should be performed. Cultures should be evaluated for bacteria, mycobacteria, and fungi. A complete review of the results of synovial fluid analysis can be found in Chapter 2. Routine peripheral blood tests including a complete blood cell count with differential, erythrocyte sedimentation rate, C-reactive protein, and blood cultures should also be obtained, both to help establish the diagnosis of septic arthritis and to assist in monitoring the effectiveness of subsequent treatment.

C. IMAGING STUDIES

Radiographs generally provide little information to establish the diagnosis of septic arthritis of the knee. However, radiographs may confirm the presence of preexisting osteoarthritis, which may predispose patients to the development of septic arthritis. Baseline radiographs may also be useful as a reference to assess possible future joint destruction and osteomyelitis, which may result from septic arthritis.

Differential Diagnosis

The clinical presentation of septic arthritis may be virtually indistinguishable from that of a crystal-induced arthritis, yet the diagnosis must be made without delay in order to minimize the likelihood of articular cartilage destruction and potentially life-threatening sepsis. Synovial fluid analysis is essential to differentiate between the diagnoses of gout, pseudogout, or septic arthritis. Other entities that may present as an inflammatory monarthritis are outlined in Chapter 4.

ARTERIAL OCCLUSION

 ESSENTIAL FEATURES

- *Prompt recognition of acute arterial occlusion is essential to prevent gangrene and possible loss of limb.*
- *Absent pulses with loss of sensation and strength should alert the examiner to the possibility of arterial occlusion.*

Clinical Findings

A history of acute and constant pain, unrelieved by any means, and associated with altered sensation and strength should suggest the possibility of arterial occlusion. Acute arterial occlusion generally produces diffuse leg pain not localized to the knee alone. Physical findings including absent pedal pulses, objective motor weakness, cyanosis, and decreased skin temperature may also be evident. The knee examination is often normal. The consequences of delayed recognition and treatment of acute vascular occlusion include paralysis, compartment syndrome, contractures, gangrene, and amputation. When suspected on the basis of the physical findings above, vascular consultation should be obtained without delay.

ANTERIOR KNEE PAIN

 ESSENTIAL FEATURES

- *Pain provoked or exacerbated by climbing stairs, squatting, and arising from a chair associated with peripatellar tenderness are common features of the syndrome of anterior knee pain.*
- *Laboratory and imaging studies are not generally indicated in the initial evaluation.*

Clinical Findings

The syndrome of anterior knee pain refers to a constellation of symptoms and physical findings that generally localizes to the patellofemoral articulation and the surrounding structures. Patellofemoral arthralgia, historically known as "chondromalacia patellae," usually begins insidiously without a specific provocative injury or incident.

A. SYMPTOMS AND SIGNS

Climbing or descending stairs or inclines generally exacerbates the pain. Symptoms are also provoked by squatting, kneeling, or arising from chairs. On closer questioning, there is frequently an identifiable activity in which the patient participates, or may have participated, that may have contributed to precipitating the symptoms. Exercise programs that include leg presses, full arc knee extensions, squatting, or high-impact loading (such as running or jogging) may generate extremely high patellofemoral joint reaction forces and can often precipitate the syndrome. Other activities such as housework, gardening, and hiking can provoke patellofemoral pain. Although the pain is usually most apparent with activity, patients with patellofemoral arthralgia often experience pain when sitting for prolonged periods with the knee flexed. This symptom, commonly noted when driving a car or sitting in a movie theatre, is referred to as a positive "movie sign" or a positive "theatre sign." Crepitus, nonmechanical locking, and sensations of giving way are common. True mechanical locking is rare.

On palpation, there is often tenderness over the articular surface of the patella. The medial and lateral aspects of the patellar articular surfaces, referred to as the medial and lateral facets, respectively, may be examined by manually subluxing the patella medially or laterally and palpating under the edges of the patellar facets. The knee must be fully extended and the quadriceps must be fully relaxed in order to allow the patella to be subluxed sufficiently to palpate its articular aspect. Tenderness associated with patellofemoral arthralgia is frequently noted over the medial patellar facet and often in the soft tissues adjacent to the patella. In patients with patellar tracking problems, the patellar apprehension sign, in which the examiner attempts to subluxate the patella laterally with the knee slightly flexed, often provokes the quadriceps to contract in response to a sensation of impending pain or patellar dislocation. Patients with increased generalized laxity, joint hypermobility, and relative dysplasia of the vastus medialis portion of the quadriceps musculature may be at increased risk for patellofemoral arthralgia, although these are not essential findings for the diagnosis. Similarly, abnormalities of lower extremity alignment including genu valgus, internal femoral torsion, and external tibial torsion may increase the likelihood of developing the syndrome, although these findings are not universal. Excessive tightness or contracture of the peripatellar retinaculum is noted in some cases, determined by measuring the amount of mediolateral patellar excursion possible in the fully extended knee with the quadriceps muscles relaxed. Normally, there should be at least 2 cm of side-to-side passive patellar movement. Excessive retinacular tightness may produce pain in the peripatellar tissues and potentially further increase patellofemoral pain by increasing joint pressures. The anterior knee pain syndrome is generally not associated with swelling, fevers or chills, erythema, instability, loss of motion, sensory changes, or muscle weakness.

B. LABORATORY FINDINGS

No laboratory studies are generally indicated for the syndrome of anterior knee pain. In cases presenting with an effusion, or if there is significant prepatellar bursal swelling, aspiration may be considered. Fluid obtained at aspiration should be examined for crystals if gout or pseudogout is suspected. Blood tests are rarely helpful in this setting.

C. IMAGING STUDIES

When the history and physical findings strongly support the diagnosis of anterior knee pain, radiographic assessment may be deferred. In such cases, a therapeutic trial of activity modification, avoidance of patellar loading activities (using stairs, squatting, or running), a home exercise program, analgesics, and nonsteroidal anti-inflammatory medications (unless contraindicated) may be initiated. The response of symptoms to such a trial may be useful from a diagnostic perspective. If symptoms continue, formal physical therapy may be prescribed for isometric quadriceps sets; straight-leg raising; short arc extensions; and stretching of the hamstrings, quadriceps, and calf muscles. Retinacular stretching and passive patellar mobilization should be prescribed when retinacular tightness has been noted.

Radiographs should be obtained when symptoms have persisted for 6 weeks despite the above measures. In addition to routine anteroposterior and lateral radiographs of the knee, patellar sunrise or Merchant views, which specifically demonstrate the axial representation of the patellofemoral articulation, should be obtained. The sunrise or Merchant views often demonstrate degenerative arthritic changes involving the patellofemoral articulation better than anteroposterior and lateral views, and may also demonstrate patellar subluxation or tilt with respect to the femoral trochlea. The length of the patellar ligament, as measured from the distal pole of the patella to its insertion on the tibial tubercle, and the length of the patella should be approximately equal (±20%). If the length of the patellar ligament exceeds the patellar length by more than 20%, patella alta is present, a condition that is also frequently seen in association with patellar tracking abnormalities. Patella baja, defined as the condition when the length of the patellar ligament is less than 80% of the length of the patella, may indicate fibrosis and contracture of the infrapatellar tissues following injury or surgery and may be associated with anterior knee pain. Magnetic resonance imaging (MRI) is rarely indicated in the initial evaluation of anterior knee pain.

Table 12–4. Differential Diagnosis of Anterior Knee Pain

Patellofemoral arthralgia
Osteoarthritis
Patellar tendinitis
Quadriceps tendinitis
Prepatellar bursitis
Synovial plica
Osgood-Schlatter disease
Sinding-Larsen-Johansson disease
Internal derangement of the knee
Saphenous nerve entrapment (Hunter canal syndrome)

Differential Diagnosis

The differential diagnosis of anterior knee pain includes patellofemoral arthralgia, osteoarthritis, patellar tendinitis, quadriceps tendinitis, prepatellar bursitis, synovial plica, Osgood-Schlatter disease, Sinding-Larsen-Johansson disease, internal derangement of the knee, and saphenous nerve entrapment (Table 12–4). Radiographs, particularly the patellar sunrise view, provide the best means of differentiating between osteoarthritis and anterior knee pain without arthritis. Precise anatomic localization of the pain and tenderness usually enables the examiner to differentiate patellofemoral arthralgia from tendinitis of the quadriceps or patellar ligaments. The tenderness in patellofemoral arthralgia is usually most pronounced in the area of the medial patellar facet, whereas the most common site of tenderness due to quadriceps or patellar tendinitis is at the tendon-bone insertion. Osgood-Schlatter disease also presents with pain and tenderness, usually accompanied by swelling at the tibial tubercle in an adolescent. Prominence of the tibial tubercle and bony ossicles adjacent to the tubercle are frequently seen on radiographs in Osgood-Schlatter disease. In Sinding-Larsen-Johansson disease, similar pain, tenderness, and radiographic changes are localized to the distal pole of the patella. Prepatellar swelling, present in cases of prepatellar bursitis, is absent in patellofemoral arthralgia. Plica syndrome, often associated with a history of repetitive overuse or minor direct trauma to the anteromedial aspect of the knee, is characterized by pain and tenderness localized specifically to a palpable fold or thickening of the synovium over the edge of the medial femoral condyle, adjacent to the patella. The patient may also note a snapping sensation in this area. Internal derangement of the knee may mimic anterior knee pain and should be considered in cases refractory to initial treatment. The clinical assessment of internal derangement of the knee is discussed later in this chapter.

Another uncommon condition, which may also present with pain localized to the anteromedial aspect of the knee, results from compression or irritation of the saphenous nerve in the region of the Hunter adductor canal in the medial aspect of the distal thigh. The symptoms may mimic the pain of patellofemoral arthralgia, although the tenderness in this condition usually extends well proximal to the knee joint to the area of the Hunter canal in the thigh and often extends distally along the course of the saphenous nerve medially in the calf.

Fulkerson JP, Shea KP. Disorders of patellofemoral alignment. *J Bone Joint Surg Am.* 1990;72:1424. [PMID: 2229126] (Comprehensive discussion of chondromalacia patellae, anterior knee pain, and patellar alignment.)

Jacobson KE, Flandry FC. Diagnosis of anterior knee pain. *Clin Sports Med.* 1989;8:179. [PMID: 2665950] (Presents a systematic approach to the clinical evaluation and differential diagnosis of anterior knee pain.)

Patel D. Plica as a cause of anterior knee pain. *Orthop Clin North Am.* 1986;17:273. [PMID: 3714211] (Review of the anatomy and clinical presentation of symptomatic synovial plicae.)

BURSITIS OR TENDINITIS

 ESSENTIAL FEATURES

- *The most helpful diagnostic information is the precise localization of the pain and tenderness.*
- *Laboratory and imaging studies are generally not indicated in the initial evaluation.*

Clinical Findings

A. SYMPTOMS AND SIGNS

Pain due to bursitis or tendinitis about the knee is usually related to activity, although the onset is generally spontaneous and atraumatic. Symptoms improve with rest. Physical findings include localized extra-articular swelling and point tenderness, directly related to the anatomic location of a bursa or tendon. Common sites for bursitis are the bursa of the pes anserine, located between the anteromedial tibial metaphysis and the tendons of the pes anserine near their insertion, and the prepatellar bursa, located subcutaneously directly anterior to the patella. Frequent sites for tendinitis include the quadriceps tendon at or near its insertion on the proximal patellar pole, the patellar ligament at its origin on the distal pole of the patella, and the iliotibial band in the area of the lateral femoral epicondyle. Since these structures are extra-articular, there is no joint effusion and swelling is localized to the involved bursa or tendon. Range of motion is not restricted except for guarding due to the pain itself. Instability, locking, and other mechanical symptoms are not present.

Infection may occasionally present in the setting of bursitis. A history of fevers, extreme pain and tenderness localized to the bursa, and local erythema should alert the examiner to the possibility of septic bursitis.

B. Laboratory Findings

Routine laboratory studies are not indicated except in the rare setting in which septic bursitis may be suspected. In such cases, the bursa should be aspirated and the fluid analyzed using Gram stain and cultures. The fluid should be tested for crystals and cell count.

C. Imaging Studies

Radiographs are of little value in the evaluation of a patient with bursitis or tendinitis. However, since the pain and tenderness are extra-articular and often overlying the bony structures, anteroposterior, lateral, and sunrise view radiographs may be indicated in selected cases to exclude the possibility of stress fracture, tumor, or other osseous conditions that may produce pain in the same area.

Differential Diagnosis

The differential diagnosis of bursitis or tendinitis about the knee includes the syndrome of anterior knee pain or patellofemoral arthralgia, meniscal disease, and osteoarthritis (Table 12–5). Precise clinical localization of the pain and tenderness is usually sufficient to determine the most likely diagnosis, and radiographs may help exclude such possibilities as fractures or other bony abnormalities. In refractory cases with normal radiographs, bone scans may help exclude other occult bony pathology such as stress fractures, osteonecrosis, or neoplasms. Similarly, MRI may identify soft tissue lesions such as cysts, ganglions, and tumors. Bursitis may also be confirmed by a diagnostic injection of local anesthetic into the bursa.

Table 12–5. Differential Diagnosis of Bursitis or Tendinitis

Anterior knee pain syndrome
Meniscal pathology
Osteoarthritis
Occult bony pathology (stress fracture, osteonecrosis, tumor)
Soft tissue lesions (cysts, ganglions)

INTERNAL DERANGEMENT OF THE KNEE

 ESSENTIAL FEATURES

- *Symptoms and physical findings of internal derangement of the knee are primarily mechanical.*
- *Radiographs and MRI are the most helpful diagnostic tools.*

Clinical Findings

A. Symptoms and Signs

Internal derangement of the knee refers to a group of disorders involving the intra-articular structures of the knee joint. Symptoms of locking, snapping, or popping suggest an internal derangement of the knee. The onset of symptoms is often sudden and may be associated with a specific provocative event or injury. The symptoms are generally intermittent, mechanical in nature, and associated with and exacerbated by activity. They improve with rest. Crepitus is frequently present but may be intermittent. The patient should be asked specifically about a history of prior knee injuries or episodes. Prior injuries, often temporally remote and sometimes seemingly trivial or even forgotten by the patient, may provide clues to the diagnosis.

On physical examination, there is often an effusion, which may fluctuate in size, swelling localized to the joint line, mechanical restriction of motion, and joint line tenderness. Palpation about the knee, including the suprapatellar, medial, and lateral synovial recesses, may reveal evidence of an intra-articular loose body, a fragment of bone or cartilage (also commonly referred to as a "joint mouse") that may move freely about the knee resulting in intermittent pain, popping, and locking. When extension is restricted by an apparent mechanical obstruction, gentle passive pressure may be applied to attempt to obtain further extension. If such pressure produces pain and the knee returns to its previously flexed position, this represents a positive "Spring sign," usually indicative of a displaced meniscal tear. Meniscal compression tests may be positive, although the sensitivity and specificity of these tests are limited and the findings must be considered in the context of the remainder of the history and examination.

Collateral and cruciate ligament testing should be performed. Medial and lateral stability should be assessed by varus and valgus stress of the knee at full extension and with the knee flexed 30 degrees. Instability resulting from an injury of the anterior cruciate ligament may be detected by the anterior drawer test, Lachman test, or flexion rotation drawer test. The posterior drawer test is used to assess the integrity of the posterior cruciate ligament. Stability findings should be compared with those of the contralateral knee to assess their significance and to identify those persons in whom generalized laxity conditions may exist. The patellofemoral joint should also be examined for tenderness and possible tracking abnormalities. A positive apprehension test or other abnormal evidence of patellar subluxation may be indicative of patellar instability, which may mimic other disorders of internal knee derangement.

B. LABORATORY FINDINGS

Laboratory testing is rarely indicated in the evaluation of suspected internal knee derangement. Aspiration of the knee may be considered in the setting of an acutely painful knee with a significant effusion. Although it is not always necessary to obtain a laboratory analysis of the fluid, the nature of the fluid may be helpful diagnostically. An acute hemarthrosis may suggest a tear of the anterior cruciate ligament, patellar dislocation, or synovial impingement. Hemarthrosis may also occur in patients taking anticoagulation medications or in the setting of other coagulation disorders. A hemarthrosis with associated fat globules may indicate the presence of an intra-articular fracture. Dark brown serosanguineous synovial fluid may suggest the possibility of pigmented villonodular synovitis, a disorder characterized by proliferation of synovium with formation of brown villous and nodular projections. Although uncommon, this disorder may also present as a chronic inflammatory arthritis, most frequently involving the knee joint. A clear or amber effusion with high viscosity, a white blood cell count <2000/mL, and no crystals suggests a noninflammatory etiology. An inflammatory etiology may be suspected when the fluid is yellow to cloudy, turbid, and of low viscosity, and the white blood cell count exceeds 3000/mL. Crystals, when present, also denote an inflammatory process.

C. IMAGING STUDIES

Radiographs including anteroposterior, lateral, and patellar sunrise or Merchant views (axial views of the patellofemoral articulation) should be obtained when internal derangement of the knee is suspected. Plain films may reveal fractures, arthritic changes, bony loose bodies, and chondrocalcinosis. Additional views such as femoral notch or tunnel views may be necessary to reveal loose bodies, osteochondritis dissecans, or spontaneous osteonecrosis of the femoral condyles. An anteroposterior radiograph angled 15 degrees caudally may reveal an occult fracture of the tibial plateau, and occult fractures of the femoral condyles or tibial plateau may be demonstrated on oblique radiographs obtained in 45-degree internal and 45-degree external rotation. Weight-bearing views may be necessary to demonstrate joint space narrowing due to osteoarthritis. Standing anteroposterior views may be sufficient in many cases, although posteroanterior standing views obtained with the knees flexed 45 degrees may be necessary in those instances in which arthritis is suspected but not demonstrated on routine standing views (Figures 12–4 and 12–5).

Bone scans may reveal occult fractures not seen on plain radiographs, particularly stress fractures or insufficiency fractures associated with osteoporosis. Avascular necrosis and spontaneous osteonecrosis may also present with normal radiographs, yet may be evident on bone scan and MRI. A bone bruise or bone marrow edema, also seen on MRI, may be seen following trauma or in association with osteoarthritis, even in the absence of plain radiographic abnormalities. MRI is also sensitive in detecting meniscal tears and may reveal useful information about the condition of the articular cartilage, ligaments, and other periarticular soft tissue structures. The presence of a Baker cyst on MRI in an adult knee is indicative of intra-articular disease that results in increased production of synovial fluid, which accumulates in the medial aspect of the popliteal fossa, distending the synovium posteriorly through the interval between the medial head of the gastrocnemius and the semimembranosus tendon. Seen frequently in association with degenerative arthritis and posterior medial meniscal tears, the finding of a Baker cyst in an adult should prompt further evaluation for intra-articular disease, if none has previously been apparent.

Differential Diagnosis

Conditions that result in symptoms and physical findings characteristic of internal knee derangement include meniscal pathology, loose bodies, osteochondritis dissecans, ligamentous instability, synovial impingement, arthritis, and bony abnormalities ranging from fracture to osteonecrosis (Table 12–6). Symptomatic meniscal tears may be suspected when there is a history of locking,

Table 12–6. Differential Diagnosis of Internal Derangement of the Knee

Meniscal pathology
Loose bodies
Osteochondritis dissecans
Ligamentous instability
Synovial conditions (plica, impingement, pigmented
   villonodular synovitis)
Arthritis
Bony abnormalities (fracture, osteonecrosis)

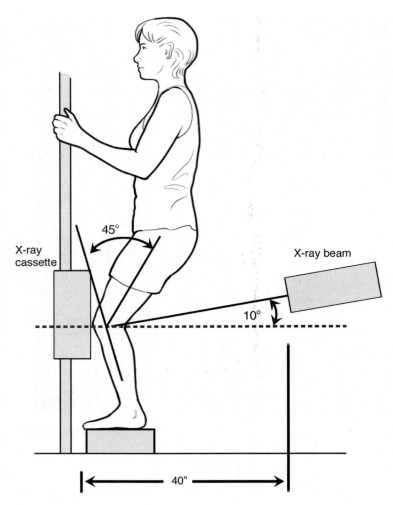

X-ray
cassette

45°

X-ray beam

10°

40"

Figure 12–4. Technique for positioning the patient and x-ray equipment
to obtain the 45-degree posteroanterior
weight-bearing radiograph of the knee.

crepitus, and positive McMurray or Appley meniscal compression tests. The most reliable finding on examination is tenderness localized specifically to the joint line, particularly in the absence of significant radiographic evidence of degenerative arthritis. Although MRI is quite sensitive in the detection of meniscal tears, it should be noted that approximately one-third of asymptomatic individuals over 50 years of age would be found to have a torn meniscus on MRI. Thus the mere presence of a torn meniscus on MRI in an older person does not necessarily indicate that the symptoms are attributable to the tear, and further clinical correlation is indicated. Congenital or developmental meniscal abnormalities, such as discoid lateral meniscus, may present in a fashion similar to a torn meniscus, although radiographic findings of abnormal widening and squaring of the lateral compartment joint space should lead to suspicion of a discoid

meniscus. MRI is also helpful in firmly establishing the diagnosis.

Loose bodies are often suspected on the basis of the patient's perception of something moving about within the knee, with episodes of mechanical locking, and often a palpable fragment of bone or cartilage on examination. Radiographs may reveal the presence and location of bony loose bodies, although cartilaginous loose bodies will not be evident on radiographs and are often not seen on MRI. Osteochondritis dissecans, which most often occurs during adolescence, may also present in adulthood with mechanical symptoms of pain, crepitus, popping, and locking. The radiographic appearance usually reveals fragmentation, irregularity, or a lucent defect of the articular surface of one of the femoral condyles, most often involving the lateral aspect of the medial femoral condyle. The fragment may partially or completely

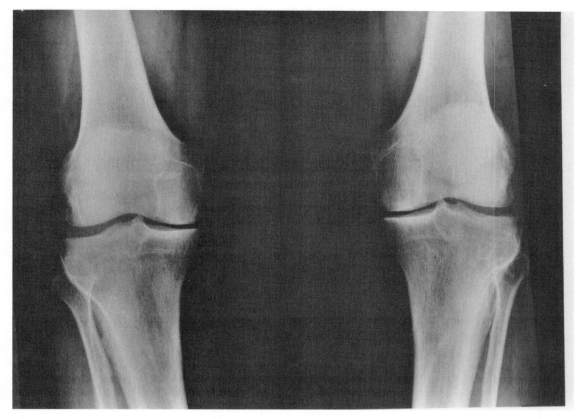

Figure 12–5. **A:** Weight-bearing anteroposterior radiograph reveals sclerosis of the medial compartments of both knees, although the joint space appears to be only mildly narrowed.

separate from the condyle, causing symptoms of a loose body. Loose bodies and the condylar lesion seen in osteochondritis dissecans are often better seen radiographically on a tunnel view or femoral notch view than on routine anteroposterior and lateral radiographs.

Ligamentous instability is generally suspected or diagnosed on the basis of the history and physical findings. Laxity on one or more of the tests previously described for the collateral and cruciate ligaments is often sufficient to make the diagnosis. Increased side-to-side motion of the knee may also be seen when performing the collateral ligament examination in patients with osteoarthritis of the medial and/or lateral compartments. This "pseudolaxity" is the result of thinning or absence of articular and meniscal cartilage associated with the arthritic process, in contrast to true laxity resulting from incompetence of the ligament itself. The age of the patient as well as other information from the history and examination, especially a varus or valgus deformity, may help differentiate between laxity or instability due to ligamentous injury and

pseudolaxity associated with arthritis. Radiographs will generally reveal the presence of joint space narrowing if pseudolaxity is the result of medial or lateral compartment arthritis. If significant arthritis is suspected and not evident on standing anteroposterior and lateral radiographs, 45-degree flexed standing posteroanterior radiographs (see Figure 12–1) should be obtained to look further for joint space narrowing. MRI may be helpful in documenting the diagnosis of a ligament injury when in doubt and may also reveal associated pathology such as meniscal or osteochondral injuries.

Synovial plicae, intra-articular folds of synovium, and portions of the infrapatellar fat pad may occasionally become pinched or entrapped between the articular surfaces of the patella and femur or between the femur and tibia. Such impingement may cause sharp localized pain, swelling, and popping. In some cases, locking or loss of motion may also be seen. Localization of the area of tenderness can help distinguish this entity from meniscal pathology, and in some cases, the plica or fold of

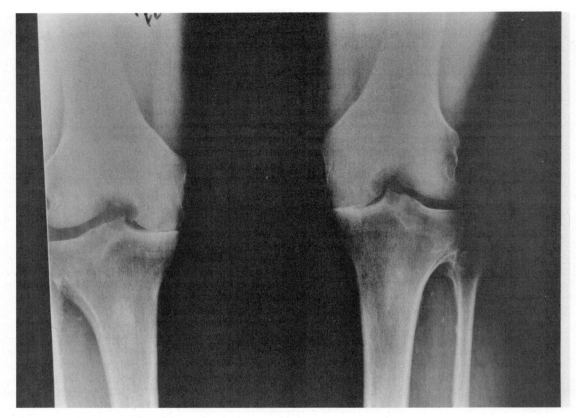

Figure 12–5. (***Continued***) **B:** The 45-degree posteroanterior radiograph of the same patient reveals complete loss of joint space in the medial compartments of both knees. Osteophytes of the tibial spines and intercondylar notch of the femur are also more apparent on the 45-degree flexion posteroanterior view.

tender synovium may be palpable. Synovial nodules associated with pigmented villonodular synovitis may also produce similar mechanical symptoms. Aspiration of the characteristically dark brown serosanguineous fluid associated with pigmented villonodular synovitis is helpful in the diagnosis. Radiographic studies, although not usually helpful with other disorders of synovial plicae or impingement, may reveal juxta-articular subchondral erosions involving both sides of the joint in pigmented villonodular synovitis, with preservation of the articular cartilage. MRI may also reveal hemosiderin deposition, with low signal intensity, in the synovium of pigmented villonodular synovitis.

Arthritis may be associated with several other intra-articular abnormalities such as meniscal tears, loose bodies, synovial impingement, and ligamentous laxity or pseudolaxity that may produce symptoms of internal derangement of the knee. In some cases, the arthritis may

otherwise be relatively asymptomatic, although its presence may greatly influence the choice of treatment. The possibility that arthritis may be presenting with symptoms of internal knee derangement should be considered in older persons, patients with a past history of meniscectomy or long-standing instability, patients with significant obesity, and patients with a family history of arthritis. (See the following sections on osteoarthritis and inflammatory arthritis for discussion of clinical features.)

Fowler PJ, Lubliner JA. The predictive value of five clinical signs in the evaluation of meniscal pathology. *Arthroscopy.* 1989;5:184. [PMID: 2775390] (Compares the relative accuracy of various clinical examination findings in diagnosing a torn meniscus.)

Hughston JC, Hergenroeder PT, Courtenay BG. Osteochondritis dissecans of the femoral condyles. *J Bone Joint Surg Am.* 1984;66:1340. [PMID: 6501330] (Review of the etiology, clinical findings, and management of osteochondritis dissecans.)

OSTEOARTHRITIS OF THE KNEE

 ESSENTIAL FEATURES

- *Pain due to osteoarthritis of the knee is generally increased with activity and improved with rest.*
- *Weight-bearing radiographs are the most useful diagnostic study.*

Clinical Findings

A. SYMPTOMS AND SIGNS

Patients who seek medical attention for pain due to osteoarthritis of the knee often describe long-standing pain that began insidiously and worsened gradually. Symptoms are generally chronic, as opposed to episodic, and are exacerbated by activity and weight-bearing, particularly during stair climbing and when arising from a seated position. Although pain is usually improved at rest, it may sometimes persist after activity and may also be influenced by weather changes. Mechanical symptoms such as locking and popping may occur due to coexistent meniscal pathology or loose bodies, although such symptoms are otherwise not commonly associated with the arthritis alone. Physical findings frequently include crepitus, deformity, fixed contractures, and decreased range of motion. When present, tenderness is usually greatest over the joint lines but may also be noted over osteophytes and occasionally over the juxta-articular aspect of the tibial metaphysis and/or the femoral condyles. Periarticular osteophytes may be palpable. An effusion and slight increase in warmth about the knee may also be seen intermittently in osteoarthritis due to the inflammatory response of the synovium to the products of cartilage degradation. However, localized swelling, erythema, fevers, and chills are not characteristic of osteoarthritis.

B. LABORATORY FINDINGS

Routine laboratory studies are rarely necessary in the initial evaluation of suspected osteoarthritis. However, if inflammatory arthritis is suspected, arthrocentesis should be performed and the synovial fluid analyzed for cell count and crystals. See Chapter 4 for a discussion of laboratory studies in osteoarthritis.

C. IMAGING STUDIES

The most useful imaging studies in the evaluation of a patient with suspected osteoarthritis of the knee are plain radiographs, specifically anteroposterior weight-bearing, lateral, and patellar sunrise views of the knee. Early radiographic features of osteoarthritis include spurring of the

tibial spines and squaring of the edges of the femorotibial compartments. Irregularity of the articular surfaces, marginal osteophytes, and subchondral cyst formation may be seen later. Joint space narrowing reflects the loss of articular cartilage, which may be underestimated on non–weight-bearing films. Standing anteroposterior films may also fail to demonstrate joint space narrowing in some cases, and the lateral view should be closely scrutinized to assess the distance between the medial and lateral femoral condyles and their respective tibial articulations. In addition, weight-bearing posteroanterior radiographs taken with the patient standing with both knees flexed 45 degrees (see Figures 12–4 and 12–5) may reveal significant narrowing of the femorotibial compartments not seen on the previous views. In addition, as this view also resembles a femoral tunnel or notch view, the 45-degree flexed standing view may also reveal loose bodies, osteochondritis dissecans lesions of the femoral condyle, and femoral notch osteophytes better than routine anteroposterior and lateral views. Patellofemoral arthritis may be evident on the lateral radiograph, although the severity of joint space narrowing and presence of subluxation are usually better visualized on patellar sunrise views.

MRI is rarely necessary in the initial assessment of suspected osteoarthritis of the knee, particularly in advanced disease. In early arthritis, MRI may demonstrate coexistent meniscal pathology, which may sometimes produce symptoms of internal derangement. It must be remembered, however, that asymptomatic meniscus tears are frequently seen on an MRI of persons over age 50. The finding of a torn or degenerative meniscus on MRI in an older individual must be correlated with the history and physical findings before attributing the symptoms to the meniscal pathology. Similarly, effusions and cruciate ligament abnormalities are often seen on MRI in older individuals in the absence of symptoms. The presence of a Baker cyst on MRI in an adult is highly suggestive of intra-articular disease, usually degenerative arthritis, meniscal pathology, or synovitis. Bone marrow edema seen on MRI may correlate with the pain of arthritis, although the pathophysiology of this process is not yet known.

Differential Diagnosis

The differential diagnosis of osteoarthritis of the knee includes inflammatory arthritis, osteonecrosis, and internal derangement of the knee (Table 12–7). The syndrome of anterior knee pain may also mimic the clinical presentation of patellofemoral arthritis. Clinically, the pain in osteoarthritis is exacerbated by activity and relieved at rest, whereas inflammatory arthritis is associated with stiffness after rest, which improves with activity. Synovial fluid analysis and the distinguishing radiographic features of both conditions are discussed elsewhere in

Table 12–7. Differential Diagnosis of Osteoarthritis of the Knee

Inflammatory arthritis
Osteonecrosis
Internal derangement
Anterior knee pain syndrome

this chapter and in Chapter 4. Anterior knee pain from other sources may be distinguished from patellofemoral arthritis on the basis of the presence or absence of patellar osteophytes, sclerosis, articular irregularity, subchondral cysts, and joint space narrowing, usually seen best on patellar sunrise views.

Felson DT. Clinical practice. Osteoarthritis of the knee. *N Engl J Med.* 2006;354:841. [PMID: 16495396]

Lotke PA, Ecker ML. Osteonecrosis of the knee. *J Bone Joint Surg Am.* 1988;70:470. [PMID: 3279040] (Discusses the presentation, evaluation, etiology, and treatment of osteonecrosis of the knee.)

Rosenberg TD, Paulos LE, Parker RD, Coward DB, Scott SM. The forty-five degree posteroanterior flexion weight-bearing radiograph of the knee. *J Bone Joint Surg Am.* 1988;70:1479. [PMID: 3198672] (Describes a supplementary radiographic technique that is more sensitive in detecting osteoarthritic changes in some patients.)

INFLAMMATORY ARTHRITIS OF THE KNEE

 ESSENTIAL FEATURES

- *Prompt recognition and treatment of septic arthritis are essential.*
- *Synovial fluid analysis is the most helpful test.*

Clinical Findings

A. Symptoms and Signs

The pain due to inflammatory arthritis of the knee is frequently associated with stiffness after rest and improvement after activity. Patients may also experience similar problems in other joints as well as fevers, chills, or other systemic symptoms. Mechanical symptoms such as locking or popping are uncommon. Physical findings include presence of an effusion, synovial thickening, warmth, and decreased range of motion. Tenderness is diffuse rather than localized.

B. Laboratory Findings

Joint aspiration and synovial fluid analysis provide the most helpful diagnostic information in the assessment of suspected inflammatory arthritis of the knee. Synovial fluid that is yellow or cloudy, turbid, with low viscosity, and in which the white blood cell count is >3000/mL is consistent with inflammatory arthritis. Crystals may also be present in association with gout or pseudogout. Gram stain and cultures of the synovial fluid should be obtained in the setting of presumed inflammatory arthritis to exclude the possibility of septic arthritis. Blood studies including complete blood cell count, erythrocyte sedimentation rate, and serum uric acid level may also be helpful. Further information outlining the laboratory findings associated with inflammatory arthritis can be found in Chapter 4.

C. Imaging Studies

Radiographic findings in early inflammatory arthritis are usually normal. Diffuse, symmetric joint space narrowing, juxta-articular osteopenia, and periarticular erosions may be seen within weeks of the onset of acute inflammatory arthritis. Radiographs may also be helpful in distinguishing inflammatory arthritis from osteoarthritis, osteonecrosis, and neuropathic arthritis. Although no radiographic abnormalities may be evident in early osteonecrosis, a radiolucent lesion and flattening of the femoral condyle may be seen later. In addition, bone scans reveal intense uptake in the femoral condyle in osteonecrosis. MRI in osteonecrosis may be extremely helpful, with T2-weighted images demonstrating a low-signal area in the central portion of the lesion in the femoral condyle, surrounded by high-intensity signal around the periphery, most likely due to edema. MRI may also help determine the size of the lesion, which determines treatment and prognosis. However, MRI changes may not be seen early in the course of osteonecrosis and may persist long after clinical symptoms have resolved.

Differential Diagnosis

The differential diagnosis of inflammatory arthritis includes septic arthritis, crystal-induced arthritis, osteoarthritis, osteonecrosis, neuropathic arthropathy, and pigmented villonodular synovitis (Table 12–8). Analysis of the synovial fluid is key to establishing the diagnosis. The clinical presentation of fever and elevated peripheral white blood cell count is suggestive of infection but may also occur in crystalline arthropathy. Conversely, some cases of septic arthritis may present without fever and with a normal peripheral white blood cell count. See Chapter 4 for additional information about synovial fluid analysis and peripheral blood studies in inflammatory arthritis.

Table 12–8. Differential Diagnosis of Inflammatory Arthritis of the Knee

Septic arthritis
Crystal-induced arthritis
Osteoarthritis
Osteonecrosis
Neuropathic arthropathy
Pigmented villonodular synovitis

Osteonecrosis involving the distal femur may present suddenly and is often associated with an effusion. This condition may be distinguished from an acute inflammatory arthritis by tenderness localizing to the bone rather than diffuse synovial tenderness. Radiographs, nuclear bone scans, and MRI may also confirm the diagnosis of osteonecrosis.

The presentation of neuropathic arthropathy or Charcot joint may resemble that of an inflammatory arthritis, with a severe effusion, diffuse tenderness, and warmth. Once again, however, the synovial fluid in this process is characteristically noninflammatory and the radiographic features of neuropathic arthropathy are quite diagnostic, with severe joint destruction and shards of fragmented bone.

Pigmented villonodular synovitis may also present as an inflammatory arthritis. Although this disorder is relatively uncommon, the knee is more frequently involved than other joints. Aspiration of dark brown serosanguineous synovial fluid should raise suspicion of this disease. Juxta-articular subchondral erosions involving both sides of the joint may be seen on radiographs. Articular cartilage is preserved, despite extensive marginal erosions. MRI may also be helpful, revealing hemosiderin deposition in the synovium with characteristic low signal.

Lee YU, Sartoris DJ. Imaging of the knee. *Curr Opin Orthop.* 1995;6:56. (Thorough review of the applications of imaging modalities including conventional radiography, arthrography, radionuclide imaging, computed tomography, ultrasound, and MRI to the knee.)

The Patient with Diffuse Pain

13

John B. Winfield, MD

FIBROMYALGIA

ESSENTIALS OF DIAGNOSIS

- *Consider fibromyalgia when a patient complains of the following:*
  - *Widespread pain for longer than 3 months.*
  - *Fatigue associated with usual daily activities.*
  - *Sleep disturbances.*
  - *Changes in personality and mood.*
  - *Multiple symptoms that cannot be easily explained.*
- *Consider alternative explanations to a diagnosis of fibromyalgia. Conversely, if an alternate diagnosis is present, ask: "Which symptoms are due to concomitant fibromyalgia?" Specifically, assess the following:*
  - *Onset, location, and nature of pain, together with ameliorating and exacerbating factors.*
  - *Sleep quality.*
  - *Current and past stressors.*
  - *Adverse experiences during childhood, such as physical, emotional, or sexual abuse.*
  - *How the patient deals with the usual stresses of daily life, feelings of anxiety, and feelings of depression.*
  - *The presence of regional pain syndromes, such as temporomandibular joint pain, irritable bowel syndrome, and chronic pelvic pain. These disorders overlap with fibromyalgia and very frequently coexist in the same patient.*
- *Physical and neurologic examinations will be normal unless there are coexisting diagnoses.*

General Considerations

Chronic pain and fatigue that have no clear organic cause are extremely prevalent in the general population, especially among women and persons of lower socioeconomic status: regional pain, 20%; widespread pain, 11%; fibromyalgia by American College of Rheumatology criteria, 3–5% in females and 0.5–1.6% in males; and chronic fatigue, ~20%. Fibromyalgia may develop in both children and older persons.

Although there continues to be debate about whether fibromyalgia is a discrete illness or simply the extreme end of a spectrum of pain and distress in the general population, abnormal central nociceptive processing is now established as the basis for a generalized decrease in thresholds for pain perception and pain tolerance. Fibromyalgia frequently coexists with systemic lupus erythematosus ($> \frac{1}{3}$), rheumatoid arthritis ($\sim \frac{1}{4}$), and other systemic disorders. In addition, fibromyalgia overlaps with chronic fatigue syndrome, irritable bowel syndrome, and multiple other regional pain syndromes. Associated psychiatric conditions, especially depression, anxiety, posttraumatic stress disorder, and personality disorders, are common among patients with fibromyalgia.

The American College of Rheumatology classification criteria for selecting fibromyalgia subjects for research studies are not diagnostic criteria and should not be used as such in clinical settings. Pain elicited by manual pressure at designated tender points included in these criteria (Figure 13–1) may be present in only a minority of these typical regions.

In assessing patients with fibromyalgia, a detailed social and behavioral history, identification of current and past stressors, and recognition of depression are essential. The physician should validate the patient's complaints. Failure to do so, or a dismissive attitude taken toward the complaints, may become an important perpetuating factor in this illness. Therapy must be individualized in this very heterogeneous population, combining pharmacologic treatment of pain, depression, and sleep disturbances with nonpharmacologic approaches, including education, graded aerobic exercise, and promotion of self-efficacy for control of pain through self-management, rather than health care–seeking behavior. The therapeutic goal is *care* not *cure*.

Pathogenesis

The multifactorial etiology and pathogenesis of pain in fibromyalgia is not fully understood. Nevertheless, a

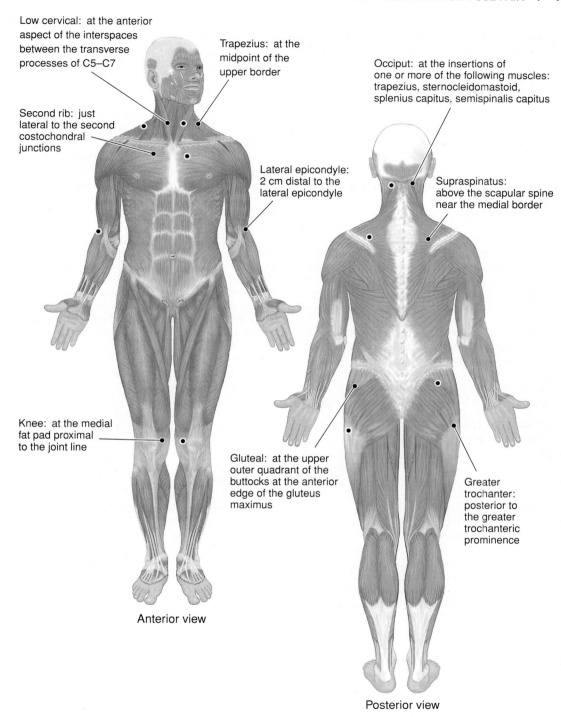

Low cervical: at the anterior aspect of the interspaces between the transverse processes of C5–C7

Trapezius: at the midpoint of the upper border

Occiput: at the insertions of one or more of the following muscles: trapezius, sternocleidomastoid, splenius capitus, semispinalis capitus

Second rib: just lateral to the second costochondral junctions

Lateral epicondyle: 2 cm distal to the lateral epicondyle

Supraspinatus: above the scapular spine near the medial border

Knee: at the medial fat pad proximal to the joint line

Gluteal: at the upper outer quadrant of the buttocks at the anterior edge of the gluteus maximus

Greater trochanter: posterior to the greater trochanteric prominence

Anterior view

Posterior view

Figure 13–1. Eighteen tender points used in the American College of Rheumatology classification criteria for fibromyalgia.

clinically useful conceptual basis for understanding the nature of pain is provided by the International Association for the Study of Pain definition: Pain is "an unpleasant sensory and emotional experience associated with actual or potential tissue damage, or described in terms of such damage." The pain *experience* involves simultaneous parallel processing of sensory-discriminative elements of nociception (twisting one's ankle), afferent input from somatic reflexes (sweating and heart rate acceleration), and major contributions from pathways and regions of the brain concerned with cognition (Is my ankle broken?) and emotional aspects of pain. Collectively, these determine the subjective intensity of pain. Negative psychological factors (depression and anxiety, loss of control, or unpredictability in one's environment) and certain cognitive aspects (negative beliefs and attributions or catastrophizing) amplify perceived pain.

Recent research has identified many of the central mechanisms that underlie abnormal nociceptive processing in fibromyalgia, including recognition of discrete abnormalities in pro-nociception and anti-nociception pathways, serotonin- and dopamine-related genes, and dysregulation of the stress response system. The principal effectors of the stress response system (hypothalamic-pituitary-adrenocortical axis and the sympathetic nervous system) become activated in pain states. Although these effectors are normally adaptive, they may become maladaptive in chronic pain syndromes, thereby contributing to diffuse aching pain, fatigue, poor sleep, low mood and anxiety, and flulike illness.

Psychological variables clearly operative in fibromyalgia include pain beliefs and attributions; hypervigilance (expectancy); active and passive coping strategies; perceived self-efficacy for pain control; mood, depression, and anxiety; personality traits and disorders; and pain behaviors. Certain environmental and sociocultural variables also contribute to chronic diffuse pain, such as a history of poor health in parents; parental pain history; poor family environment; and childhood abuse, particularly sexual abuse. Other environmental and sociocultural variables that can serve to perpetuate symptoms in fibromyalgia include lack of spousal and family support, poor work environment and job dissatisfaction, focus on definable causes, media hype, primary and secondary gain, diagnostic "waffling" and inappropriate diagnostic testing, and prescription of long courses of physical therapy by well-meaning physicians.

Clinical Findings

A. SYMPTOMS AND SIGNS

The hallmark of fibromyalgia is widespread pain (above and below the waist and on both sides of the body) for longer than 3 months. Pain is described as "exhausting," "miserable," or "unbearable." The pain often radiates dif-

fusely from the axial skeleton over large areas of the body, primarily in muscles. Arthralgias may be present together with a subjective sense of joint swelling. Synovitis is not confirmed by physical examination unless another co-existing rheumatic disease is present. Morning stiffness may be prominent. The patient may complain that a light touch or even a breeze is unpleasant (allodynia, defined as pain with stimulation that should not be painful). The skin may "burn." Nondermatomal paresthesias are common.

Regional pain syndromes, such as headache, temporomandibular joint pain, irritable bowel syndrome, and chronic pelvic pain overlap with fibromyalgia and very frequently coexist in the same patient. Indeed, the diagnostic label applied often is determined by which specialist the patient sees first.

Marked fatigue with usual activities is almost universal and may dominate the clinical picture. As with diffuse pain, physical and laboratory examinations fail to define abnormal findings other than deconditioning. Associated symptoms are subjective muscle weakness not confirmed by loss of muscle power or elevated creatinine kinase levels, hypersomnolence during the day, and exhaustion after mild exercise. Pain and fatigue may be intermittent, with "good days and bad days." On good days, the patient may overexert herself or himself, leading to a subsequent increase in pain and fatigue over ensuing days. Exercise often is feared and avoided.

Poor sleep almost always is present, and the patient awakens unrefreshed. Specific sleep abnormalities may be demonstrable, particularly a-wave intrusion into slow d-wave non-REM sleep, restless legs syndrome, and sleep apnea. Formal sleep testing should be sought in patients whose sleep does not improve with hypnotics and proper sleep hygiene.

Current and past stressors and adverse experiences should be explored. Persons with fibromyalgia often carry huge psychological burdens of stress and distress that may precede chronic pain.

Patients often report difficulty dealing with the usual stresses of daily life, feelings of anxiety, and feelings of depression. A majority of patients have current or lifetime depression. Recognition of mood disorders, anxiety, and insomnia is the essential first step in developing approaches for improving chronic pain and fatigue.

Reporting of multiple symptoms that cannot be explained ("diffusely positive" review of systems) is very common. Many patients meet the criteria established in the fourth edition of the *Diagnostic and Statistical Manual of Mental Disorders* for somatoform disorder (Figure 13–2). When physical and neurologic examinations are normal, it is important that the physician not pursue unnecessary diagnostic laboratory or imaging evaluations for each symptom. Conversely, it should be recognized that fibromyalgia and somatoform disorders

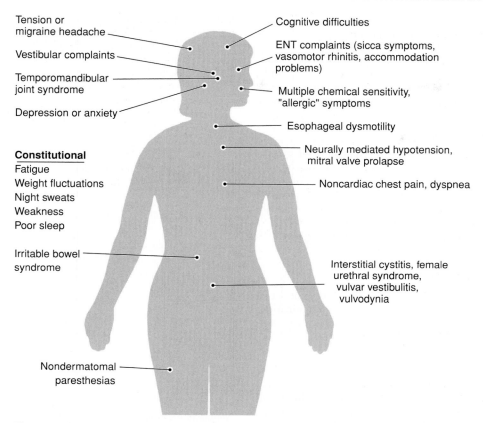

Tension or migraine headache

Vestibular complaints

Temporomandibular joint syndrome

Depression or anxiety

Constitutional
Fatigue
Weight fluctuations
Night sweats
Weakness
Poor sleep

Irritable bowel syndrome

Nondermatomal paresthesias

Cognitive difficulties

ENT complaints (sicca symptoms, vasomotor rhinitis, accommodation problems)

Multiple chemical sensitivity, "allergic" symptoms

Esophageal dysmotility

Neurally mediated hypotension, mitral valve prolapse

Noncardiac chest pain, dyspnea

Interstitial cystitis, female urethral syndrome, vulvar vestibulitis, vulvodynia

Figure 13–2. Symptoms in fibromyalgia in addition to "pain all over" and tender points. ENT, ear, nose, and throat.

are extremely common in primary care, and therefore frequently coexist with other significant illnesses. Optimum care requires recognition and treatment of both fibromyalgia and any comorbid illnesses present.

Cognitive impairment ("fibro-fog") manifests as difficulty finding the right word, decreased short-term memory, forgetting names, or difficulty concentrating, and is extremely common. In some cases, this is exacerbated by central effects of psychotropic medications.

Many patients exhibit functional impairment in multiple activities of daily living, such as performing household chores, shopping, or working an 8-hour day. Patients with fibromyalgia suffer frustration with respect to their perceived poor states of health and the apparent inability of the medical profession to help them. Not infrequently there are fixed beliefs that minor traumatic events, viruses (Epstein-Barr), chemical sensitivities ("sick building syndrome"), or other physical agents (silicone breast implants or "black mold") caused their illness. Such false beliefs may lead to litigation and can

be a barrier to recovery. The physician should be aware of pending litigation regarding causation of fibromyalgia, disability determination, or worker's compensation claims. Therapy is unlikely to be effective until such issues are resolved.

B. Laboratory Findings

There are no characteristic laboratory findings in fibromyalgia. The results of routine testing are normal unless a coexisting or alternative diagnosis is present. Additional laboratory tests are unnecessary unless there is a specific indication from the history and physical examination. Antinuclear antibodies, complete blood cell count, erythrocyte sedimentation rate, C-reactive protein levels, urine dipstick, thyroid-stimulating hormone levels, creatine kinase, aspartate aminotransferase, and alanine aminotransferase are useful screening tests for autoimmune diseases, hematologic problems, systemic inflammatory states, hypothyroidism, myopathies, and occult liver disease. Illnesses in these categories can present with chronic pain and fatigue.

C. IMAGING STUDIES

Radiographs of the spine or other joints may be indicated to confirm the presence of conditions that serve as "pain generators," such as osteoarthritis or degenerative spondylosis.

D. SPECIAL EXAMINATIONS

Several tender points should be palpated with manual pressure of ~4 kg (just enough pressure to cause blanching of the thumbnail). Pressure on the characteristic tender points shown in Figure 13–1 elicits pain, not just tenderness, and usually is accompanied by pain behaviors, such as withdrawal, grimacing, or groaning. Do not attempt to apply pressure to all tender points because this is unnecessary and causes distress.

Differential Diagnosis

The diagnoses listed in Table 13–1 should be considered. Objective signs on physical or neurologic examinations should be present before the clinician embarks on extensive diagnostic evaluations.

Treatment

Much of the current treatment of fibromyalgia is empiric, based on proposed rather than on established models of pathophysiology. To date, no drug has been specifically approved by the U.S. Food and Drug Administration for treatment of fibromyalgia. Pain, poor sleep, low mood and depression, anxiety, and fatigue usually are amenable to pharmacologic therapy, but the treatment plan should be both individualized and multifaceted, incorporating pharmacologic, physical, psychological, and behavioral approaches. The goal is palliation of symptoms, not cure.

Special approaches are required for treatment of diffuse pain in older persons and in children. Most common in preadolescent to adolescent girls, unexplained diffuse or localized pain may be associated with incongruent affect and disproportional functional impairment. Psychological distress in the child or the family is common. Elements of therapy include discontinuation of all medications, a psychological evaluation and psychotherapy if necessary, and a program of aerobic exercise and cognitive-behavioral approaches. Most children do well.

A. PHARMACOLOGIC

Peripheral pain generators, such as osteoarthritis, inflammatory arthritis, neuropathic pain, herniated discs, and spinal stenosis, should be identified and treated using nonsteroidal anti-inflammatory drugs and analgesics.

Table 13–1. Differential Diagnosis of Fibromyalgia

Rheumatologic disorder	SLE,[a] rheumatoid arthritis, Sjögren syndrome[a]
	Polyarticular osteoarthritis, degenerative spondylosis
	Polymyalgia rheumatica[a]
	Polymyositis, statin myopathy
	Regional pain syndromes[a]
	Osteomalacia
	Hypermobility syndromes
Neurologic disorder	Carpal tunnel syndrome[a]
	Cervical radiculopathy[a]
	Metabolic myopathies
	Multiple sclerosis[a]
	Cervical cord compression
Chronic infection	SBE, brucellosis, hepatitis C, HIV, for example
Endocrine disorder	Hypothyroidism[a]
	Non-IDDM
	Hyperparathyroidism
Neoplastic disorder	Myeloma; metastatic breast, lung, and prostate cancer
Psychiatric disorder	

[a]Diagnoses commonly encountered.
SLE, systemic lupus erythematosus; SBE, subacute bacterial endocarditis; Non-IDDM, non-insulin-dependent diabetes mellitus.

Such medications are effective in peripheral nociceptive pain but are less useful in the central pain of complex etiology in fibromyalgia. Their use should be based on a stepwise approach using nonopioid and opioid analgesics either singly or in combination, as determined by pain intensity: acetaminophen, 325–650 mg every 4–6 hours or 1000 mg 3 or 4 times daily, not to exceed 4 g/d; nonsteroidal anti-inflammatory drugs; tramadol, 50–100 mg every 4 hours in association with acetaminophen; or for severe pain not responsive to the above, opioids. Depending on the specific musculoskeletal disorder, various combinations of glucocorticoid injections, activity modification, splints, counterforce bracing, local heat or cold, and in some cases surgical procedures may also be indicated for pain generators.

For treatment of the chronic pain of complex etiology in fibromyalgia, use a multidisciplinary therapeutic approach incorporating various adjuvant medicines, graded aerobic exercise, and psychological and behavioral interventions to reduce distress and promote self-efficacy and self-management. Antidepressant drugs are especially useful in fibromyalgia because of the high prevalence of comorbid depression and because many antidepressants exhibit efficacy for pain control.

A well-established first-line agent is the tricyclic antidepressant amitriptyline, 10–50 mg at bedtime, often in combination with a selective serotonin reuptake inhibitor (eg, 10–40 of fluoxetine every morning) or one of the newer dual serotonin/norepinephrine reuptake inhibitors, such as venlafaxine (150–225 mg daily) or duloxetine (30–60 mg daily), which have been shown to improve many symptoms in fibromyalgia regardless of comorbid depression. Carefully monitor the patients for worsening depression or emergence of suicidal thoughts. While muscle relaxants generally provide only short-term benefit, the tricyclic cyclobenzaprine, 10–20 mg at bedtime, may provide added benefit.

Many patients also require an antiepileptic drug, particularly when marked allodynia and hyperalgesia are present. Antiepileptic drugs ameliorate both pain sensitivity and serve as adjunctive medications for disturbed sleep and depression. Escalate gabapentin weekly by 300-mg increments from 300 mg at bedtime to 600 mg 3 times daily; weight gain is a troublesome side effect at higher doses. Topiramate, escalating at weekly intervals from 25–50 mg at bedtime to 100–200 mg twice daily, is also useful for migraine prophylaxis and may facilitate weight loss. Tiagabine, escalating weekly from 2–4 mg at bedtime to 16–32 mg/d in divided doses or recently released pregabalin (150–450 mg daily in 3 divided doses) are useful alternatives.

Topical capsaicin as a general measure can be very useful when applied twice daily to painful areas with gentle massage; the patient should be informed that perceived benefit may require 3–4 weeks of therapy. Anxiety disorders are common in fibromyalgia, thus anxiolytics of different durations of action are frequently useful adjuncts. Many choices are available, including: clonazepam (long half-life), escalate after 3 days from 0.25 mg twice daily to a maximum of 4 mg/d; lorazepam (medium half-life), 2–3 mg/d given 2 or 3 times daily; temazepam (medium half-life), 7.5–30 mg at bedtime; alprazolam (short half-life), 0.25–0.5 mg 2 or 3 times daily; or buspirone, start at 7.5 mg twice daily (the usual dose is 15 mg twice daily). In considering the choice of an anxiolytic drug, it should be remembered that certain antidepressants also have indications for anxiety disorders.

Several other drugs play a role in special circumstances. Clonidine, 0.1 mg orally 3 times daily, is useful in neuropathic pain and to decrease withdrawal symptoms

when tapering opioids. Pramipexole, a dopamine-3 receptor agonist, in an evening dose of 4.5 mg has been demonstrated in a randomized controlled trial to improve pain scores, fatigue, and function in a subset of patients requiring opioids for pain control.

Treat disturbed sleep aggressively. When institution of good sleep hygiene, recognition and treatment of associated medical conditions known to disturb sleep, and sleep medications are ineffective, request a formal sleep study to identify sleep apnea and restless legs syndrome (particularly common in fibromyalgia) or other specific sleep disorders. Useful drugs to improve sleep in fibromyalgia are a single *low* bedtime dose of a tricyclic antidepressant (eg, doxepin), cyclobenzaprine, trazodone, or temazepam, either singly or in combination with a non-benzodiazepine hypnotic (zolpidem, 5–10 mg at bedtime; zaleplon, 5–10 mg at bedtime; or newly released eszopiclone, 2–3 mg at bedtime). Benzodiazepines such as triazolam probably are unsuitable in fibromyalgia because of associated daytime sedation and cognitive impairment. Clonazepam, 0.5–1.5 mg at bedtime, may be effective for restless legs syndrome.

Preliminary data suggest that sodium oxybate, a naturally occurring neuromodulator/neurotransmitter, reduces pain and fatigue and improves sleep abnormalities (a-intrusion and decreased slow-wave sleep) in fibromyalgia. Currently approved by the Food and Drug Administration for cataplexy associated with narcolepsy, this oral solution is diluted in water and taken in two 2.2-g doses nightly 2.5–4 hours apart.

Depression must be treated aggressively; without improvement in depression, other treatment approaches will fail. Encourage formal or informal counseling and treat pharmacologically with one of the following: a tricyclic antidepressant; a selective serotonin reuptake inhibitor (fluoxetine, 10–40 mg every morning, maximum 80 mg/d; citalopram, start at 20 mg/d, maximum 60 mg/d); a dual reuptake inhibitor (duloxetine, 20–60 mg daily; venlafaxine, start at 37.5–75 mg/d divided twice daily, maximum 375 mg/d); fluvoxamine, start at 50 mg at bedtime, maximum 150 mg twice daily; paroxetine, start at 20 mg every morning, maximum 50 mg/d; or sertraline, start at 50 mg every morning, maximum 200 mg/d); a serotonin antagonist (mirtazapine, start at 15 mg at bedtime, usual effective dose 15–45 mg/d); bupropion, start at 100 mg twice daily, increase to 100 mg 3 times daily after 1 week; or trazodone, start at 50 mg twice daily, usual effective dose 200–300 mg twice daily.

Fatigue generally improves with effective treatment of pain, depression, and sleep disturbances in combination with a graded aerobic exercise program. Modafinil (approved by the Food and Drug Administration for narcolepsy), 100–200 mg/d, or tropisetron (5-HT$_3$ receptor antagonist, not currently available in the United States) may benefit those patients in whom overwhelming fatigue is a persistent complaint.

B. NONPHARMACOLOGIC

When nonpharmacologic treatments have been compared with pharmacologic treatments alone, nonpharmacologic treatments generally have been of greater benefit. A meta-analysis of 49 fibromyalgia outcome treatment studies concluded that "the optimal intervention for fibromyalgia would include non-pharmacologic treatments, specifically exercise and cognitive-behavioral therapy (CBT), in addition to appropriate medication management as needed for sleep and pain symptoms." Various forms of exercise, strengthening and stretching, biofeedback and relaxation, CBT, hypnotherapy, or combinations of such treatments have all been shown to be of benefit.

Biofeedback alone or combined with relaxation therapy, CBT, and various forms of exercise significantly improves physical status and self-reported fibromyalgia symptoms, but not daily functioning. However, whether biofeedback/relaxation training plus exercise training maintains improvement over the long term is less certain.

Graded aerobic exercise, especially aquatherapy, is effective in fibromyalgia with respect to overall well-being, tender point count, self-reported pain, depression, state-trait anxiety, and self-efficacy, at least over the short term. The degree of response is significantly determined by the patient's capacity to effectively cope with her or his illness. High-intensity fitness programs should be avoided because they are associated with increased pain and fatigue, with consequent poor compliance.

Not all experts agree that CBT in fibromyalgia syndrome is cost-effective and provides additional benefit over other interventions. Other psychological interventions, such as guided imagery, may improve self-reported pain over the short term.

Many widely used nonpharmacologic treatments are of uncertain benefit. Although trigger point injections are commonly used by some health care practitioners for treatment of myofascial pain, the definition and reliability of "trigger points," "taut bands," and "muscle twitch" responses upon which myofascial pain syndromes are based are open to question. Randomized controlled clinical trials examining dry needling, saline injections, anaesthetic injections, botulinum toxin, acupuncture, and sham acupuncture as therapies have not shown significant benefit beyond nonspecific, placebo-related effects. Ultrasound treatment of myofascial "trigger points" is no more effective in reducing pain than sham ultrasound. Similarly, low-level laser therapy and sphenopalatine blocks have no place in the treatment of fibromyalgia.

Almost all patients with fibromyalgia use complementary and alternative medicine, at least in part because of distrust of physicians and frustration with the limited efficacy of much traditional care. While such approaches to treatment as hypnotherapy, relaxation techniques (eg, yoga, Tai Chi, or meditation), and osteopathic manipulation may have efficacy, others, such as vegetarian diets and exposure to static magnetic fields have no demonstrable benefit. Properly designed controlled trials have not been reported for most other complementary and alternative medicines. The physician should inquire about self-administered herbs and other substances because many are potent pharmacologic agents with potential for interaction with conventional medicines.

C. EDUCATION AND LIFESTYLE MEASURES

Although time consuming, educational efforts validate symptoms, inform regarding the nature of fibromyalgia and the role of stress, lessen fear regarding outcome, promote self-efficacy, and provide a rationale for the treatment program. Begin education at the first visit, emphasizing that an *active* role for the patient in the treatment plan is essential, particularly with respect to compliance with a regular *graded* (go slow and not overdo) aerobic exercise program. Advise the patient regarding the effects of stress and counsel regarding approaches to reduce current stressors. Encourage self-efficacy (the belief that the patient can control pain and fatigue through self-management).

Complications

The adverse impact of fibromyalgia on the patient, on family, and on society is high. Scores on the Rand 36-item Health Survey (SF-36), a self-report questionnaire measuring functional impairment and well-being, usually are in the severely impaired range in all areas (physical functioning, pain, role limitations, emotional well-being, social functioning, energy/fatigue, and general health perception). More than 25% of patients seen in academic medical centers receive some type of disability or other compensation payment.

When treating patients with fibromyalgia, two other potential complications should be kept in mind. First, be alert for dependence on opioids, benzodiazepines, and muscle relaxants, recognizing that drug-seeking behavior ("pseudoaddiction") often means that chronic pain is not being controlled adequately. Abrupt cessation of such medications may be associated with withdrawal symptoms. Second, use of the term "posttraumatic" fibromyalgia by physicians may unwittingly contribute to the development of chronic pain in patients with acute pain following minor injury. The current consensus of experts in this area is that this term not be used.

When to Refer to a Specialist

Referral to a rheumatologist familiar with fibromyalgia is appropriate when the diagnosis is unclear, when response to therapy is inadequate, and when comorbid musculoskeletal or autoimmune conditions are present. Psychiatric referral is indicated when significant psychiatric comorbidity is present and is essential for severe depression with suicidal ideation and for comorbid psychosis. Psychotherapeutic counseling is helpful for many patients.

Prognosis

Most patients will improve with respect to self-reported pain, disturbed sleep, and fatigue, but daily functioning often remains impaired. The goal of therapy is care, not cure. Distinct subsets of patients vary in their prognosis: "Adaptive copers" do well clinically, whereas "dysfunctional" patients with high levels of pain, anxiety, and opioid dependence and those with pending litigation do poorly. While it is not possible to entirely reverse the allodynia and hyperalgesia in fibromyalgia, quality of life can be improved for many patients in response to therapy if ongoing stressors are relieved and if self-efficacy for control of pain can be achieved.

REFERENCES

Adler GK, Geenen R. Hypothalamic-pituitary-adrenal and autonomic nervous system functioning in fibromyalgia. *J Rehabil Med.* 2003;41(Suppl):89–94.

American Geriatrics Society Panel on Chronic Pain in Older Persons, 1998.

Baker K, Barkhuizen A. Pharmacologic treatment of fibromyalgia. *Curr Pain Headache Rep.* 2005;5:301–306.

Benca RM, Ancoli-Israel S, Moldofsky H. Special considerations in insomnia diagnosis and management: depressed, elderly, and chronic pain populations. *J Clin Psychiatry.* 2004;65(Suppl 8): 26–35.

Bradley LA. Psychiatric co-morbidity in fibromyalgia. *Curr Pain Headache Rep.* 2005;9:79–86.

Henriksson KG. Fibromyalgia—from syndrome to disease. Overview of pathogenetic mechanisms. *Rheum Dis Clin North Am.* 2005;31:187–202.

Kroenke K. Patients presenting with somatic complaints: epidemiology, psychiatric co-morbidity and management. *Int J Methods Psychiatr Res.* 12:34–43, 2003.

Rossy LA, Buckelew SP, Dorr N, et al. A meta-analysis of fibromyalgia treatment interventions. *Ann Behav Med.* 1999;21:180. [PMID: 10499139]

Turk DC, Okifuji A, Sinclair JD, Starz TW. Differential responses by psychological subgroups of fibromyalgia syndrome patients to an interdisciplinary treatment. *Arthritis Care Res.* 1998;11:397. [PMID: 9830884]

Winfield JB. Psychological determinants of fibromyalgia and related syndromes. *Curr Rev Pain.* 2000;4:276. [PMID: 10953275]

Relevant World Wide Web Sites

[American College of Rheumatology]
http://www.rheumatology.org/public/factsheets/fibromya_new.asp

[Arthritis Foundation]
http://www.arthritis.org/conditions/DiseaseCenter/Fibromyalgia/fibromyalgia.asp

[Fibromyalgia.com]
http://www.fibromyalgia.com

[Health information for the whole family from the American Academy of Family Physicians]
http://Familydoctor.org

[Medlineplus Health Information: A service of the U.S. National Library of Medicine and the National Institutes of Health]
http://www.nlm.nih.gov/medlineplus/fibromyalgia.html

[The American Fibromyalgia Syndrome Association]
http://www.afsafund.org/

[University of Missouri Health Care: Fibromyalgia Self-Help Course]
http://www.muhealth.org/~information/fibromyalgiaselfhelp.shtml

Pregnancy & Rheumatic Diseases

Pin Lin, MD, Phyllis Bonaminio, MD, & Rosalind Ramsey-Goldman, MD, DrPH

SYSTEMIC LUPUS ERYTHEMATOSUS

 ESSENTIAL FEATURES

- *Systemic lupus erythematosus (SLE) increases risk of spontaneous abortion, intrauterine fetal death, intrauterine growth restriction, and prematurity.*
- *Patients should not become pregnant when SLE is active.*
- *Pregnancy should be planned.*
- *Distinguishing SLE flare from preeclampsia is difficult.*
- *A multidisciplinary approach to patient care is essential for optimal outcome.*

General Considerations

SLE primarily affects women of childbearing age. Typical clinical symptoms include fatigue, fever, arthralgias, arthritis, photosensitive rash, pleuritic chest pain (serositis), Raynaud phenomenon, periorbital and leg swelling (glomerulonephritis), limb or visceral pain (vasculitis), and bruising or generalized weakness (hematologic abnormalities) (see Chapter 22).

SLE increases the risk of spontaneous abortion, intrauterine fetal death, preeclampsia, intrauterine growth restriction, and preterm birth. SLE not only affects pregnancy outcome, but the pregnancy can potentially affect disease activity. Optimizing care of the mother and fetus requires a coordinated team approach among internists, rheumatologists, obstetricians specializing in high-risk pregnancies, and in some instances, nephrologists and neonatologists.

Family Planning

Since SLE does not decrease fertility and since both maternal and fetal outcomes improve when maternal disease activity is quiescent for at least 6–12 months before pregnancy, great emphasis should be placed on contraception and timing of conception.

A. CONTRACEPTION

Barrier methods, such as condoms and foam or a diaphragm with spermicidal jelly, are the safest means of preventing conception because these strategies do not increase the risk of causing an SLE flare. However, the efficacy of these methods depends on the attentiveness of the woman and her partner.

Many patients may already be taking a combination pill when SLE is first diagnosed. Estrogen has been associated with an increased risk of an SLE flare developing or thromboembolic events. Combined oral contraceptive medications containing a low dose of estrogen do not generally cause flares of SLE in patients with mild to moderate SLE. In those patients, a pill with the lowest estrogen dose could be considered as long as there is no history of hypercoagulable risk. If there is a risk of thromboembolism, then a combination hormone pill containing estrogen and progesterone is contraindicated.

An alternative hormonal medication for contraception is a single agent, progesterone, which is available in an oral or injectable form. Progesterone alone has not been associated with precipitating SLE flares or thromboembolic events. However, women often complain of breakthrough bleeding while on the progesterone-only preparation, thus limiting compliance. Fortunately, irregular bleeding usually subsides after the patient has been taking this medication for a few months.

Since SLE patients may be at increased risk for infection, an intrauterine device is not a preferred method of contraception. However, if the woman is not taking immunosuppressive drugs (including prednisone) and does not have a history of frequent genitourinary infections, then the intrauterine device may be considered.

B. RISKS

There is still debate about whether pregnancy increases SLE activity. On the one hand, most studies suggest that the chance of flare during pregnancy and postpartum is minimal if the patient has controlled or inactive disease at the time of conception. On the other hand, women with active disease at conception appear more likely to have a disease flare during or after pregnancy. For instance, women with active nephritis at conception have approximately a 50–60% chance of having a renal flare during pregnancy or postpartum; however, they only have a 7–10% chance of a renal flare if they conceive during a period of inactive disease.

Women with established SLE have approximately an 80% chance of having a live birth. However, women with SLE should also be counseled about the increased risk of adverse fetal outcome risks such as preterm birth, pregnancy loss, and intrauterine growth restriction. The risk of preterm birth, birth before 37 weeks of gestation, is approximately 33% compared with 5–15% in the general population. Risk factors for preterm birth include increased maternal SLE activity, nephrotic range proteinuria, maternal hypertension, and premature rupture of membranes. Women with SLE have a higher incidence of pregnancy loss, including spontaneous abortion and intrauterine fetal death (stillbirths). The risk of spontaneous abortion—spontaneous termination of pregnancy before the 20th week of gestation—is approximately 15%, compared with 7–13% in the general obstetric population. The risk of intrauterine fetal death—spontaneous termination of pregnancy after the 20th week of gestation—is approximately 4%. The risk of intrauterine growth restriction—weight below the 10th percentile for gestational age—is approximately 17% in women with SLE, compared with 10% in the general obstetric population. Active maternal lupus, nephritis or renal impairment, the presence of anti-Ro/SS-A antibodies which can cause neonatal lupus erythematosus (NLE), and antiphospholipid antibodies have all been associated with fetal loss.

C. Contraindications

Women with active disease or a flare within the last 6 months should delay becoming pregnant for at least 1 year, while women with newly diagnosed SLE should delay becoming pregnant for at least 2 years.

Women with new, recurrent, or persistent renal disease indicated by an active urinary sediment, proteinuria >3 g/24 h, moderate to severe hypertension, and creatinine levels >2 mg/dL should be discouraged from becoming pregnant.

Women with pulmonary hypertension (pulmonary artery pressure >40 mm Hg) or decreased cardiac output may not be able to tolerate the increase in intravascular volume that occurs during pregnancy, and should be discouraged from becoming pregnant.

Women with lupus who have active central nervous system disease such as cerebritis, uncontrolled seizure activity, and active psychosis and a history of cerebrovascular accidents should also be counseled against getting pregnant.

Patients who are taking cyclophosphamide, methotrexate, warfarin, leflunomide, angiotensin-converting enzyme inhibitors (captopril, lisinopril, or equivalent), angiotensin receptor blockers (valsartan or losartan), or anticonvulsants (diphenylhydantoin, valproic acid, and carbamazepine) must be discouraged from becoming pregnant until these medications have been discontinued at least 3–6 months before conceiving because the risk is high for drug-associated fetal abnormalities. The same restriction should apply to male lupus patients taking methotrexate and leflunomide who desire to have children. Alternative medications that can be used during pregnancy are discussed later.

Leflunomide requires a special drug elimination procedure once a woman has discontinued the medication and desires to become pregnant. The elimination procedure involves administering cholestyramine at 8 g 3 times a day for 11 days (the days do not have to be consecutive unless there is a need to rapidly lower the plasma levels). Afterward, plasma levels must be verified by two separate tests at least 14 days apart. Levels should be <0.02 mg/L; if the levels are not at the required level, additional cholestyramine should be considered.

Cyclophosphamide can cause infertility in both male and female patients by causing azoospermia and premature ovarian failure, respectively. In women, this risk increases with her age, the severity of SLE, and high cumulative dose of the medication. In contrast, men receiving this medication can have azoospermia with even one exposure. The use of gonadotropin-releasing hormone analogue in women and testosterone in men during treatment with cyclophosphamide may be protective. Banking ova and sperm prior to starting cyclophosphamide can also be considered.

Prenatal Evaluation

A. History

The physician should begin by closely reviewing the patient's presenting symptoms of SLE, frequency and severity pattern of flare signs and symptoms, and any laboratory abnormalities since presentation. Knowing how a disease flare manifested in the past may help the physician distinguish an SLE flare from changes that normally occur during pregnancy.

Medications should be reviewed; those with teratogenic potential must be stopped and alternatives should be selected.

B. Physical Examination

The physical examination should include height, weight, blood pressure, and a general physical examination with

Table 14–1. Suggested Laboratory Evaluation Schedule for Monitoring Pregnancy in a Patient with Systemic Lupus Erythematosus

Laboratory Evaluation on Initial Visit	Frequency After Initial Visit
CBC with differential and platelets	Every 1–3 months
Liver function tests including albumin	Initial visit
Chemistry panel including BUN, creatinine, and glucose	Every 1–3 months
Urinalysis with microscopic examination	Monthly
Spot or 24-hour urine for protein and creatinine	Each trimester
C3, C4, and CH50	Each trimester
dsDNA antibody	Each trimester
Antiphospholipid antibodies and lupus anticoagulant	Initial visit
Anti-SS-A/Ro and anti-SS-B/La antibodies	First trimester

CBC, complete blood cell count; BUN, blood urea nitrogen.

a special focus on the heart, lungs, joints, oral ulcers, lymphadenopathy or rash, and the presence of edema.

C. Laboratory Findings

The recommended initial work-up is detailed in Table 14–1. A few of the tests deserve further comment. If the spot urine ratio of protein to creatinine is abnormal (>0.3), then perform a 24-hour urinalysis for protein, creatinine, and creatinine clearance. If a woman has had poor obstetric outcomes in the past, usually defined as three prior fetal losses, the presence of antiphospholipid antibodies should be suspected, and antibody testing should be ordered.

Anti-SS-A/Ro and anti-SS-B/La antibodies help determine whether a woman's infant is at risk for NLE including congenital heart block (CHB) (see section on Special Circumstances, below).

Monitoring for disease activity by general examination and laboratory values should be continued until 3–6 months postpartum. The SS-A/Ro and SS-B/La antibodies need only be tested at the initial visit.

D. Fetal Monitoring

Women with SLE are at increased risk for intrauterine growth restriction and preterm births (<37 weeks of ges-

tation dated from the last menstrual period). Therefore, it is important to confirm menstrual dating with ultrasonography at the first prenatal visit to accurately estimate gestational age.

During the first trimester, fetal heart tones should be auscultated by Doppler or ultrasonogram at each office visit, starting as early as 10 weeks.

During the second trimester, a level 2 ultrasonogram should be done between 16 and 20 weeks of gestation to assess fetal anatomy, with a special focus on cardiac function to assess for the presence of CHB if the mother is SS-A/SS-B-antibody–positive. A study is underway to assess occurrence and treatment of CHB in SSA/Ro- and/or SSB/La-positive mothers. During this time, the obstetrician continues monitoring fetal heart tones and fundal height. A delay in fundal height growth may indicate growth restriction and require more frequent monitoring.

At 24 weeks of gestation, the fetus has reached an age of potential viability. Therefore, any evidence suggesting imminent fetal demise may require delivery.

During the third trimester, monitoring of fundal height is continued and an ultrasonogram should be done frequently if the mother is SS-A/Ro- or SS-B/La-antibody–positive. At 28 weeks of gestation, a weekly biophysical profile, consisting of a nonstress test and an ultrasonogram examination that assesses amniotic fluid volume, fetal body movements, fetal tone, and breathing movements should be performed. Low amniotic fluid volume may indicate decreased placental perfusion. A Doppler or pulse wave of the umbilical artery should be done if placental abnormalities are suspected. If any of these test results are abnormal, early delivery may be indicated.

E. Special Circumstances

Mothers who have SS-A/Ro and/or SS-B/La antibodies have a 2–5% risk of having a baby with NLE, with half of these having CHB. The NLE syndrome includes photosensitivity, rash, cytopenias, and hepatomegaly or splenomegaly, and these are usually transient manifestations. CHB is a rare manifestation of this syndrome, but accounts for a majority of the mortality in NLE. In many cases, CHB is permanent, and the infant may require a pacemaker. Unfortunately, in some instances, CHB may result in fetal or neonatal demise.

Special Problems

A. SLE Flare versus Normal Changes of Pregnancy

A particular challenge facing physicians who care for patients with SLE is how to distinguish an SLE flare from the normal changes of pregnancy (Table 14–2).

Table 14–2. Lupus Manifestations Versus the Normal Changes of Pregnancy

System	SLE	Normal Pregnancy
Cutaneous	Raised inflammatory rash often sparing the nasolabial folds	Irregular, hyperpigmented, and patchy rash (chloasma)
Musculoskeletal	True arthritis	Arthralgias, bland knee effusions
Cardiovascular	Pericarditis	Increased resting heart rate, low blood pressure, murmur
Renal	Increased creatinine or proteinuria compared with baseline or active urinary sediment	Decreased BUN, increased CrCl, slight increase in proteinuria
Pulmonary	Pleuritic chest pain	Shortness of breath, hyperventilation
Hematologic	Cytopenias	Anemia (iron deficient), decreased platelets, elevated WBC without a left shift
Serologic	Unchanged or decreasing C3 and C4 levels, rising dsDNA	Increased ESR
Constitutional	Fever not due to infection	Fatigue

BUN, blood urea nitrogen; CrCl, creatinine clearance; WBC, white blood cell count; ESR, erythrocyte sedimentation rate.

1. Musculoskeletal and cutaneous manifestations— Normal pregnancy is associated with alopecia, facial or palmar erythema, arthralgias, and edema. Low back pain and pelvic pain are common complaints and are usually due to the softening and stretching of the ligaments from hormonal changes in preparation for delivery and from the added weight gain straining the lower back. Women may experience bland knee effusions, which must be distinguished from true arthritis that may be attributed to an SLE flare.

Skin changes associated with normal pregnancy can often be mistaken for SLE exacerbations. Alopecia is due to a fluctuation in the amount of estrogen. Whereas alopecia associated with pregnancy tends to be diffuse and usually occurs postpartum when the level of estrogen is at its lowest, hair loss associated with SLE can be either diffuse or occur in patches and occur at any time during pregnancy. The pregnancy facial mask called chloasma or melasma gravidarum is irregular, hyperpigmented, and patchy in appearance; located on the forehead, cheeks, and the bridge of the nose; and is due to increased melanin deposition in skin macrophages. In SLE, the malar or butterfly rash extends over the cheeks and can involve the bridge of the nose. This rash can be macular but is usually erythematous and raised and can have papules or plaques.

2. Cardiovascular, renal, and pulmonary systems— The normal physiologic effects on the cardiovascular system in pregnancy include an increase in resting heart rate up to 90 beats per minute, lower blood pressure, and a crescendo-decrescendo systolic murmur. In contrast, pericardial chest pain may be associated with an SLE flare.

The renal system also undergoes normal physiologic alterations in the pregnant patient including a lowering of the blood urea nitrogen and creatinine with an increase in creatinine clearance. There may also be a slight increase in proteinuria due to the increase in glomerular filtration rate that normally accompanies pregnancy. Hematuria or red cell casts in the urine do not occur in a normal pregnancy. If the serum creatinine increases compared with baseline instead of decreasing and the urinary sediment is active (red or white cell casts or hematuria), then an SLE flare should be considered.

Finally, the pulmonary system changes in pregnancy are manifested as shortness of breath and hyperventilation. These are common complaints and are secondary to the increased level of progesterone. Pleuritic chest pain or pain with deep inspiration can be a sign of active SLE.

3. Hematologic and immunologic changes— An increase in intravascular volume of up to 50% causing mild anemia with a hematocrit ranging from 30–35% occurs during pregnancy. Iron deficiency may also contribute to anemia due to increased demand for iron stores by both the mother and fetus. Thrombocytopenia ranging from 100,000–150,000/mL can develop and is believed to be due to increased platelet turnover. Other hematologic abnormalities occurring during a normal pregnancy include an elevated white blood cell count without a left shift ranging from 10,000–15,000/mL. On the contrary, during SLE flare, leukopenia (WBC <4000/mL) usually occurs. Cytopenias must be considered in the context of other symptoms and laboratory data before attributing them to an SLE flare.

The erythrocyte sedimentation rate increases in normal pregnancy and cannot be used to detect SLE disease activity. The erythrocyte sedimentation rate can reach >40 mm/h by the Westergren method during normal pregnancy, and the elevated erythrocyte sedimentation rate is due to an increase in protein, especially fibrinogen, in pregnancy and should not be mistaken as an acute phase reactant supporting an SLE flare.

Serum complement levels normally increase during pregnancy. Levels of C3, C4, or both that are unchanged or begin to fall may indicate an SLE exacerbation.

An SLE flare can therefore be suggested when a raised inflammatory rash, arthritis, lymphadenopathy, fever not due to infection, or pleuritic chest pain is present. Laboratory tests that have been helpful in distinguishing a flare include leukopenia, hematuria and red cell casts, falling C3 or C4 or both complement levels, and rising titers of dsDNA antibody.

B. Lupus Nephritis versus Preeclampsia

Preeclampsia is defined as the abrupt onset of hypertension and proteinuria after 20 weeks of gestation and is most commonly found in the primagravida. Pregnant patients with SLE are at increased risk for preeclampsia, especially if the patient has a prior history of renal disease or hypertension, or has positive antiphospholipid antibodies. The risk of developing preeclampsia in a woman with lupus nephritis is as high as 38% versus 0.5–10% of the general obstetric population. Consequently, there is an increased risk for preterm delivery and fetal death if active nephritis or preeclampsia is present.

Distinguishing between a lupus nephritis flare and preeclampsia is a challenging clinical problem during pregnancy (Table 14–3). During the second half of pregnancy, significant proteinuria and hypertension develop in up to 25% of women with SLE, but this may be due to either preeclampsia or lupus nephritis. By definition, normal blood pressure excludes preeclampsia. However, both lupus nephritis and preeclampsia can have hypertension, proteinuria, or edema. Thrombocytopenia and hemolytic anemia can be seen in an SLE flare; however, both are also features of the HELLP syndrome (*h*emolytic anemia, *e*levated *l*iver enzymes, and *l*ow *p*latelets), which is a variant of preeclampsia.

The laboratory features that suggest an SLE flare include the development of proteinuria before the third trimester; active urinary sediment with red blood cell or white blood cell casts or both, a fall or failure to increase complement levels (C3, C4, or CH50), and a rise in titer of dsDNA antibodies. Two other tests that may be used because they are more indicative of preeclampsia are impaired calcium excretion (levels below 11.5 mg/dL by spot urine testing or below 195 mg in a 24-hour urine test) and elevated uric acid levels.

Distinguishing between lupus nephritis and preeclampsia is important because treatment options are

Table 14–3. How to Differentiate Between Lupus Nephritis and Preeclampsia

Manifestation	Lupus Nephritis	Preeclampsia
Gravidity	Any pregnancy	Usually prima-gravida
Hypertension	Present/absent	DBP >90 mm Hg
Proteinuria	Before third trimester	After third trimester
Active urinary sediment (RBC or WBC casts)	Present	Absent
C3, C4	Low or failure to rise	Normal or rising
Anti-dsDNA antibodies	Rising	Absent
Uric acid levels	Normal	High
Impaired calcium excretion	Absent	Present

RBC, red blood cell; WBC, white blood cell; DBP, diastolic blood pressure.

completely different. A lupus nephritis flare is treated with glucocorticoids and possibly remittive drugs, whereas preeclampsia is treated with antihypertensive medication to control the blood pressure and immediate delivery.

Managing the SLE Flare

A general guideline in choosing a medication to use during pregnancy is that the risk of lupus flare and the risk of adverse maternal and fetal outcome must outweigh the risk of the drug toxicity to the fetus. The U.S. Food and Drug Administration (FDA) has developed a classification system for the safety of drugs used during pregnancy (Table 14–4).

A. Glucocorticoids

Any signs of an SLE flare should be aggressively treated with the lowest possible dose of glucocorticoids (prednisone or methylprednisolone) needed to control the disease (Table 14–5). For most patients, this may be as little as 10 mg/d of prednisone, but for active disease the dose of glucocorticoids may be as high as 1 mg/kg/d.

The FDA regards glucocorticoids as category B drugs (see Table 14–4).

Table 14–4. FDA Categories of Drug Safety During Pregnancy

Category	Description
A	Adequate, well-controlled studies in pregnant women have not shown an increased risk of fetal abnormalities.
B	Animal studies have revealed no evidence of harm to the fetus; however, there are no adequate and well-controlled studies in pregnant women.
	or
	Animal studies have shown an adverse effect, but adequate and well-controlled studies in pregnant women have failed to demonstrate a risk to the fetus.
C	Animal studies have shown an adverse effect and there are no adequate and well-controlled studies in pregnant women.
	or
	No animal studies have been conducted and there are no adequate and well-controlled studies in pregnant women.
D	Studies, adequate well-controlled or observational, in pregnant women have demonstrated a risk to the fetus. However, the benefits of therapy may outweigh the potential risk.
X	Studies, adequate well-controlled or observational, in animals or pregnant women have demonstrated positive evidence of fetal abnormalities. The use of the product is contraindicated in women who are or may become pregnant.

(From http://www.fda.gov/fdac/features/2001/301_Preg.html#categories, with permission.)

Glucocorticoids have not been found to be teratogenic in humans, although there have been reports of cleft palate in rabbits and mice. The fetus is protected from the effect of prednisone or hydrocortisone because of the placental enzyme 11-β-dehydrogenase, which oxidizes these glucocorticoids into the inactive form. In contrast, dexamethasone and betamethasone cross the placenta and are used for fetal indications if preterm delivery is imminent. The transplacental property of dexamethasone makes it the drug of choice for treating NLE. Fetal risks associated with glucocorticoid use include premature rupture of membranes, intrauterine growth restriction or low birth weight, and preterm delivery. Maternal complications from these medications include maternal gestational diabetes mellitus, hypertension, osteoporosis, and infection. However, if maternal disease is uncontrolled, the benefits of using glucocorticoids outweigh the drug toxicity risks to the mother and fetus.

The use of glucocorticoids as prophylactic treatment to prevent SLE exacerbations is generally not accepted as routine practice. However, if a woman has been taking glucocorticoids within the last year, then stress dose glucocorticoids at delivery are required. The usual recommended dose of hydrocortisone is 100 mg intravenously every 8 hours (or equivalent) for a period of 24 hours. Pre-delivery dosages of glucocorticoids, if any, may be started day 1 postpartum if normal oral intake resumes. Up to 20% of the glucocorticoid dose is secreted in the breast milk. Although breast-feeding is generally safe, SLE patients taking more than 20 mg of glucocorticoids may consider nursing 4 hours after the last dose.

B. HYDROXYCHLOROQUINE

The antimalarial hydroxychloroquine may be administered to control SLE disease activity. The usual dose is between 200 and 400 mg/d or up to 6 mg/kg/d. The exact mechanism of action is unclear. Although regarded as an FDA category C medication with animal studies showing fetal effects and no controlled human studies, there are only rare reports of congenital malformations or ophthalmologic abnormalities in babies born to mothers while taking this medication.

Hydroxychloroquine is a long-acting drug and remains in the body for from 2 to 4 months following its discontinuation. If a woman becomes pregnant while taking hydroxychloroquine, there is no rationale to stop the medication since therapeutic levels remain in the body for 2–4 months, which is during the period of organogenesis for the fetus. However, discontinuation of this medication may cause a subsequent SLE exacerbation. Therefore, if a mother conceives while on this medication, the benefit of continuing hydroxychloroquine throughout the pregnancy and preventing a flare outweighs the very minimal risk to the fetus. The decision to continue hydroxychloroquine should be based on a discussion between the specialist and the patient

Table 14–5. Medications Used to Treat Rheumatic Diseases During Pregnancy

Drug	FDA Risk Category	Fetal Effects	Use in Lactation	Other Comments
Glucocorticoids (prednisone, methylprednisolone, hydrocortisone)	B	Premature rupture of membranes, intrauterine growth restriction, preterm delivery in human studies. No congenital defects in humans. Animal studies show cleft palate.	Yes	Watch for maternal gestational diabetes, elevated blood pressure, and osteoporosis; women may need stress doses at delivery.
Sulfasalazine	B	Increased risk of neonatal jaundice during third trimester	Yes	Folic acid supplementation recommended.
Heparin	C	Thrombocytopenia and osteoporosis	Yes	Calcium supplementation is recommended.
NSAIDs including selective COX-2 inhibitors	C	Premature closure of the ductus arteriosus, prolongation of labor and delivery; and hemorrhage when used during the third trimester	Some	Low-dose aspirin (<325 mg/d) has no adverse effects on fetal renal function, ductus arteriosus, or hemorrhage risk.
Hydroxychloroquine	C	Very rare congenital anomalies attributed to this drug.	Yes	Long acting. Discontinue at least 3 months before conception if patient does not want this medication.
Cyclosporine A	C	Preterm delivery, low birth weight, hypertension, and pregnancy-induced hypertension	No	Monitor maternal blood pressure and renal function.
Mycophenolate mofetil	C	Limited information indicates no fetal abnormalities.	No	Limited information available in the renal transplant literature.
Azathioprine	D	Rare neonatal immunosuppression	No	Used if major organ involvement or as a glucocorticoid-sparing agent to control disease
TNF-α inhibitors	B	Limited information in animals indicates no fetal abnormalities.	No	Limited information in humans.
Interleukin-1 receptor antagonists (IL1-Ra)	B	Limited information in animals indicates no fetal abnormalities.	No	Limited information in humans.

COX-2, cyclooxygenase 2; NSAID, nonsteroidal anti-inflammatory drugs; TNF, tumor necrosis factor.

and her partner. Although about 2% of the maternal hydroxychloroquine dose can be found in breast milk, breast-feeding while taking the medication is generally safe.

C. Azathioprine

Azathioprine is a medication used for the treatment of SLE associated with major organ involvement or as a glucocorticoid-sparing drug. The usual dose of this medication ranges between 1 and 2.5 mg/kg/d. Azathioprine is a prodrug that gets converted to 6-mercaptopurine. Both azathioprine and 6-mercaptopurine interfere with the synthesis of purine nucleotides, resulting in cytotoxicity and decreased cell proliferation. Folic acid supplementation at 1 mg/d is recommended while taking azathioprine and 6-mercaptopurine.

Azathioprine and 6-mercaptopurine are FDA category D drugs. The fetal liver lacks the enzyme inosinate phosphorylase, which converts azathioprine to its active metabolite, 6-mercaptopurine. Although azathioprine readily crosses the placenta, only trace amounts of 6-mercaptopurine are found in cord blood. Therefore, this fetal enzyme deficiency should protect the fetus from the adverse effects of azathioprine. The rare adverse effects that have been reported in infants exposed to azathioprine in utero include neonatal immunosuppression characterized by leukopenia, lymphopenia, absence or decreased levels of immunoglobulins, and intrauterine growth restriction. Azathioprine is contraindicated during breast-feeding.

D. Nonsteroidal Anti-Inflammatory Drugs

Nonsteroidal anti-inflammatory drugs (NSAIDs) are FDA category C agents. NSAIDs variably inhibit the enzyme cyclooxygenase and decrease prostaglandin production. Adverse fetal effects observed following third-trimester ingestion of NSAIDs include premature closure of the ductus arteriosus, which can lead to primary pulmonary hypertension and prolongation of gestation and labor. Other potential fetal side effects include excessive maternal and neonatal hemorrhage during delivery because of the antiplatelet effects of NSAIDs. Oligohydramnios may occur due to the effect of NSAIDs on the fetal renal output. It is generally recommended that NSAIDs be discontinued during the last trimester of pregnancy; if treatment is needed, low-dose prednisone can be used as a safer alternative. Low-dose aspirin, which is used for the treatment of antiphospholipid antibody syndrome, is the exception and should be continued throughout pregnancy.

Cyclooxygenase-2 inhibitors, including celecoxib and meloxicam, are FDA category C drugs. Their risks are similar to those of traditional NSAIDs, and they should be discontinued during the last trimester of pregnancy.

E. Cyclosporine A

Cyclosporine A is an FDA category C drug. The usual dose is 2.5 mg/kg/d, with the maximum dose not exceeding 5 mg/kg/d. The mechanism of action involves the inhibition of cytotoxic T cells, thus decreasing the production of interleukin-2. Most of the information regarding cyclosporine and pregnancy comes from data on pregnant renal transplant patients. Cyclosporine has been associated with the risk of preterm delivery, low birth weight, hypertension, and pregnancy-induced hypertension. This medication has not been found to be teratogenic in animals or humans; however, there was one isolated case of proximal renal damage in fetal rat kidney. Cyclosporine A is secreted in breast milk and is contraindicated during breast-feeding.

F. Mycophenolate Mofetil

Mycophenolate mofetil is a prodrug that is enzymatically broken down into the active metabolite mycophenolic acid. Mycophenolic acid is a purine synthesis inhibitor that causes a decrease in lymphocyte production and adhesion.

This medication has been used in renal transplant patients and was most recently incorporated into the treatment of lupus nephritis. Mycophenolate mofetil has shown efficacy comparable to that of cyclophosphamide

in treating diffused proliferative glomerulonephritis in small series of SLE patients for at least 1 year. However, the long-term efficacy of mycophenolate mofetil for treating lupus renal disease is still unknown. This medication is regarded as a category C medication by the FDA. While no large series have been conducted on its safety during pregnancy, cases of malformations in infants exposed in utero have been reported in transplant patients. We suggest that this medication should be avoided during pregnancy and while breast-feeding, and if needed, azathioprine should be substituted.

G. Other Disease-Modifying Medications

Medications such as cyclophosphamide, leflunomide, penicillamine, methotrexate, and chlorambucil are not recommended for use during pregnancy, due to their FDA category D or X rating because of their teratogenic potential (Table 14–6). Occasionally, these cytotoxic medications are used in life-threatening instances during the second or third trimester of pregnancy, but a qualified specialist should determine appropriate dosages of these medications. Women should continue folic acid even after discontinuation of methotrexate to prevent the occurrence of folate deficiency.

H. Nonrheumatic Medications Needed During Pregnancy

1. Antihypertensives—Antihypertensive medication may be required during pregnancy to control blood pressure. Methyldopa (FDA category B) and hydralazine (FDA category C) have been used by obstetricians for many years and are considered safe to use during pregnancy (Table 14–7).

β-Blockers such as atenolol, labetalol, or metoprolol, and thiazide diuretics have been shown to cause decreased placental perfusion leading to fetal growth restriction. Despite this concern, qualified physicians have used both medications in high-risk pregnant patients. Ultrasonographic assessment for fetal growth while taking this medication is recommended.

Calcium channel blockers are generally considered safe during pregnancy.

Angiotensin-converting enzyme inhibitors and angiotensin receptor blockers are contraindicated during pregnancy because of the association with fetal renal abnormalities.

2. Anticonvulsants—All anticonvulsants have teratogenic potential. A qualified physician should decide whether use of these medications is essential for maternal health.

3. Antidepressants—Antidepressants may be required for symptoms of depression or chronic pain. Tricyclic antidepressants such as amitriptyline and imipramine are FDA category C drugs. There have been animal studies

Table 14–6. Rheumatic Disease Medications Contraindicated During Pregnancy

Drug	FDA Risk Category	Fetal Effects	Use in Lactation	Other Comments
Cyclophosphamide	D	Myelosuppression	No	May be used if maternal disease is life-threatening.
Leflunomide	X	May increase risk of fetal death or have teratogenic effects.	No	Need cholestyramine washout prior to conception. Check the serum level after washout.
Penicillamine	D	Cutislaxa	No	Discontinue 6 months before conception.
Chlorambucil	D	Unknown	No	Discontinue 6 months before conception.
Methotrexate	X	Myelosuppression, desquamating fibrosing alveolitis, chromosome abnormalities in clinically normal infants	No	Discontinue 3–6 months before conception. Continue folic acid supplementation after this medication is discontinued.

involving amitriptyline given at higher than normal human doses showing teratogenic effects in mice and hamsters. There were also studies in rats that showed delayed ossification of fetal vertebral bodies. Therefore tricyclic antidepressants should only be used if necessary.

Selective serotonin reuptake inhibitors such as sertraline, fluoxetine, and citalopram are FDA category C drugs. Reproduction studies in rats have generally shown an increase in stillborn pups, a decrease in pup weight, and an increase in pup deaths during the first few days postpartum following maternal exposure to higher than normal human doses of these selective serotonin reuptake inhibitors. Only sertraline showed evidence of delayed ossification when pregnant rats were exposed to higher than normal human doses of this medication during organogenesis.

Buyon JP, Clancy RM. Neonatal lupus: basic research and clinical perspectives. *Rheum Dis Clin North Am.* 2005;31:299.

Buyon JP, Kalunian KC, Ramsey-Goldman R, et al. Assessing disease activity in SLE patients during pregnancy. *Lupus.* 1999;8:677.

Chang E, Ramsey-Goldman R. Managing systemic lupus erythematosus during pregnancy. *Womens Health.* 2001;1:53.

Clowse ME, Magder LS, Witter F, Petri M. The impact of increased lupus activity on obstetric outcomes. *Arthritis Rheum.* 2005;52:514.

Katsifis GE, Tzioufas AG. Ovarian failure in systemic lupus erythematosus patients treated with pulse intravenous cyclophosphamide. *Lupus.* 2004;13:673.

Parke AL. Anti-rheumatic drugs in pregnancy. *Bull Rheum Dis.* 2002;51:9.

Petri M, Kim MY, Kalunian KC, et al. Combined oral contraceptives in women with systemic lupus erythematosus. *N Engl J Med.* 2005;353:2550. [PMID: 16354891]

Somers EC, Marder W, Christman GM, Ognenovski V, McCune WJ. Use of a gonadotropin-releasing hormone analog for protection against premature ovarian failure during cyclophosphamide therapy in women with severe lupus. *Arthritis Rheum.* 2005;52:2761.

Temprano KK, Bandlamudi R, Moore TL. Antirheumatic drugs in pregnancy and lactation. *Semin Arthritis Rheum.* 2005;35:112.

ANTIPHOSPHOLIPID ANTIBODY SYNDROME

 ESSENTIAL FEATURES

- *May be a primary syndrome or secondary to SLE or other underlying disorders.*
- *Includes the anticardiolipin antibodies, lupus anticoagulant, and occasionally b_2 glycoprotein I antibodies.*
- *Antiphospholipid antibody syndrome has been linked to recurrent fetal loss, intravascular clotting with venous or arterial thrombosis, and thrombocytopenia.*

General Considerations

Antiphospholipid antibody syndrome (APS) can occur as a primary syndrome with no previous diagnosis of a

Table 14–7. Nonrheumatic Disease Medications Used During Pregnancy

Drug	FDA Risk Category	Fetal Effects	Other Comments
Antihypertensives			
Methyldopa	B	Reproduction studies performed in rats revealed no evidence of harm to the fetus. There are no well-controlled human studies, but published reports of the use of this drug during all trimesters of pregnancy indicate that the likelihood of fetal harm is remote.	Considered safe to use during pregnancy.
Hydralazine	C	Teratogenic effects observed in studies involving mice and rabbits using higher than normal human doses included cleft palate and malforma-tions of facial and cranial bones. There are no well-controlled human studies.	Despite the animal studies, this medication is considered safe to use during pregnancy.
β-Blockers	C	Decreased placental perfusion leading to fetal growth restriction.	Use only if necessary.
Calcium channel blockers (nifedipine)	C	Studies using various animals including rats, mice, and rabbits showed anomalies such as cleft palate, rib deformities, fetal death, and prolonged pregnancy.	Despite animal studies this medication is considered safe to use during pregnancy.
Angiotensin-converting enzyme inhibitors (captopril or lisinopril) and angiotensin receptor blockers (valsartan or losartan)	D	Renal effects.	Contraindicated.
Anticonvulsants (all)		Teratogenic.	Use only if necessary.
Tricyclic antidepressants (amitriptyline or imipramine)	C	Teratogen in animal studies. Delayed ossification of fetal vertebral bodies.	Use only if necessary.
Selective serotonin reuptake inhibitors (sertraline, fluoxetine, or citalopram)	C	Animal studies showing increase in stillbirth, decreased weight, and increased death.	Use only if necessary.

connective tissue disorder and includes a history of recurrent arterial or venous thrombosis, recurrent fetal loss, or thrombocytopenia (50,000–100,000 platelets/mL). Secondary APS is associated with an underlying connective tissue disorder such as SLE or rheumatoid arthritis (RA). Both primary and secondary APS also include the an-

tibodies anticardiolipin antibodies, lupus anticoagulant (LAC), or b_2 glycoprotein I (see Chapter 24).

Patients with APS may have recurrent arterial or venous thrombotic events including deep venous thrombosis, pulmonary emboli, transient ischemic attacks, cerebrovascular accident, and myocardial infarction.

Thrombocytopenia and livedo reticularis, a lacy-looking rash over the trunk and extremities, are also common findings in patients with APS. The presence of these antibodies during pregnancy may increase the risk of fetal loss, including spontaneous miscarriages that typically occur after 10 weeks of gestation, midpregnancy fetal distress, intrauterine growth restriction, prematurity, and preeclampsia. APS-related pregnancy morbidity and mortality was originally thought to be caused by thrombosis in the uteroplacental circulation, which resulted in abnormal placental function. Recent experimental models implicate complement activation as a required mediator of antiphospholipid antibody–induced pregnancy loss and thrombosis.

Laboratory Findings

Healthy women with no history of SLE, thrombosis, thrombocytopenia, repeated fetal loss during any gestational period, or preeclampsia do not need to be screened for APS.

Laboratory tests positive for anticardiolipin antibodies and LAC support the diagnosis of APS in the appropriate clinical setting.

The enzyme-linked immunosorbent assay for anticardiolipin antibodies is widely available and standardized. Normal levels are usually less than 16 GPL U/mL and IgM less than 10 MPL U/mL. (GPL is the abbreviation for immunoglobulin G and phospholipid, and MPL is the abbreviation for immunoglobulin M and phospholipid.) High positive values are above 80 GPL U/mL or 40 MPL U/mL.

The presence of LAC may initially be indicated by an elevated activated partial thromboplastin time or a false-positive rapid plasma reagin test for syphilis. Abnormal results in either test should warrant further investigation. In patients with the presence of circulating LAC, the activated partial thromboplastin time will not correct when normal plasma is added in a 1:1 mix. The activated partial thromboplastin time will normalize in patients with a factor deficiency. Another test to aid in the recognition and confirmation for LAC is the dilute Russell viper venom time.

Patients in whom both anticardiolipin antibodies and LAC are negative but who have a clinical history consistent with APS should be screened using enzyme-linked immunosorbent assay for β_2 glycoprotein I antibody.

Treatment

Treatment of APS depends on the patient's history. Prophylactic use of heparin or aspirin in asymptomatic women with no history of thrombosis or pregnancy loss is not recommended. However, a baby aspirin may occasionally be used if antibody titers are elevated in an asymptomatic woman who has no prior history of pregnancy complications.

A combination of low-dose aspirin (80 mg/d) and unfractionated heparin (5000 IU every 12 hours) or low-molecular-weight heparin (enoxaparin or dalteparin) has been successful in preventing APS-induced fetal loss. Based on mouse models, the primary effect of heparin may be to inhibit complement activation induced by antiphospholipid antibody, as opposed to anticoagulation. Treatment should commence once conception is confirmed and be continued until delivery. Anticoagulation should be continued for 6 weeks postpartum, using either form of heparin or switching to warfarin. Glucocorticoids are reserved for the treatment of inflammatory-based symptoms such as thrombocytopenia or an SLE flare and are generally not recommended for use in the treatment of APS when anticoagulation or antiplatelet agents are used.

Low-molecular-weight heparin and heparin are FDA category B and C drugs, respectively. These medications do not cross the placenta, and therefore do not cause harm to the fetus. However, both medications have been associated with maternal thrombocytopenia. Heparin, more than low-molecular-weight heparin, has been associated with osteoporosis in women who used them during pregnancy. Supplementation with 1500 mg/d of calcium is highly recommended to prevent bone loss.

Chang E, Ramsey-Goldman R. Antiphospholipid antibodies and RA: barriers to successful pregnancy? *Womens Health.* 2001;1:97.

Cuadrado MJ, Hughes GRV. Hughes (antiphospholipid) syndrome. Clinical features. *Rheum Dis Clin North Am.* 2001;27:507.

Girardi G, Redecha P, Salmon JE. Heparin prevents antiphospholipid antibody-induced fetal loss by inhibiting complement activation. *Nat Med.* 2004;10:1222.

Lockshin MD, Erkan D. Treatment of the antiphospholipid syndrome. *N Engl J Med.* 2003;349:1177.

Pettila V, Leinonen P, Markkola A, Hiilesmaa V, Kaaja R. Postpartum bone mineral density in women treated for thromboprophylaxis with unfractionated heparin or LMW heparin. *Thromb Haemost.* 2002;87:182.

RHEUMATOID ARTHRITIS

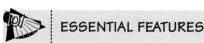

ESSENTIAL FEATURES

- *Arthritis usually improves during pregnancy.*
- *Adverse pregnancy outcomes are not increased.*
- *Postpartum joint flares are common.*

General Considerations

Pregnancy is associated with improvement of clinical signs and symptoms of RA in up to 75% of patients. Most women with RA see a reduction in disease activity by the end of the first trimester. Approximately 20–30% of pregnant patients with RA will need medications to control disease activity. However, it is important to monitor all postpartum patients with RA closely because there is approximately a 90% risk of flare by 3–6 months after delivery.

Women with RA do not have decreased fertility compared with the general obstetric population. RA does not increase adverse pregnancy outcomes including, stillbirth, prematurity, or low birth weight.

Special Problems

Special care must be taken in patients with cervical spine disease who need surgical delivery by cesarean section if general anesthesia is needed because of the risk associated with atlantoaxial subluxation. Women may require cervical bracing to prevent hyperextension or nasotracheal intubation instead of orotracheal intubation.

Women with severe hip disease or hip replacement may not have adequate range of motion to allow normal vaginal delivery, and thus will require surgical delivery. The patient with an artificial joint who requires surgical delivery may need antibiotics to prevent bacterial seeding to the joint.

Management of the RA Flare

Treatment of a patient with RA who is having a flare depends on the type of complaint, either localized or systemic symptoms and signs. If only one or two joints are involved, intra-articular injections with glucocorticoids may be the best option. If a woman requires systemic treatment for multiple joint complaints or extra-articular manifestations, oral glucocorticoids are among the safest alternative medications. As mentioned previously in the SLE section, the lowest possible dose of glucocorticoids to control symptoms is recommended. Other medications, such as NSAIDs, hydroxychloroquine, and azathioprine, may also be used and are discussed in the SLE section above and in Table 14–4.

Sulfasalazine is another alternative medication safely used during pregnancy. The preferable dose is usually <3 g/d. Sulfasalazine is classified as an FDA category B drug. However, there is a theoretical risk of the infant developing kernicterus during the neonatal period. Despite this risk, sulfasalazine is often continued during pregnancy if indicated. There is no evidence that sulfasalazine causes congenital malformations. Sulfasalazine can cause azoospermia in men. This is reversible upon discontinuation of the medication, and should be discussed with male patients who desire to have children.

This medication is safe during breast-feeding. Folic acid supplementation is recommended because sulfasalazine may cause folate deficiency.

The biologic agents approved for the treatment of RA include tumor necrosis factor-a inhibitors and interleukin-1 receptor antagonists. Although the FDA regards the tumor necrosis factor agents etanercept, infliximab, and adalimumab and the interleukin-1 receptor antagonist anakinra as category B drugs, there are minimal human data to reassure safety of their use during pregnancy. Data from the infliximab safety database, which is maintained by the drug's manufacturer, suggest that infliximab exposure during pregnancy resulted in outcomes similar to those in the U.S. population of pregnant women. A survey of practicing North American rheumatologists on the safety of tumor necrosis factor inhibitors during pregnancy suggested that this class of drugs did not increase maternal-fetal complications compared with published data on pregnancy in healthy women. Despite these findings, caution should be taken when using these medications during pregnancy. Safety in breast-feeding with the biologic medications is also unknown and should be avoided if possible (Table 14–8).

Rituximab has been studied in RA, SLE, diabetes mellitus, and certain types of vasculitis. It is a monoclonal antibody against the CD20 antigen on the B-lymphocyte surface. It is classified as a class C medication by the FDA. It should be avoided during pregnancy and breast-feeding if possible until more data on its safety are available.

Within the first 3–6 months postpartum, flares are common in mothers with RA. If the mother is nursing, then glucocorticoids at the lowest dose necessary to control symptoms are recommended. However, the mother should be encouraged to resume her prepregnancy therapeutic regimen as soon as possible to minimize joint damage.

Katz JA, Antoni C, Keegan GF, et al. Outcome of pregnancy in women receiving infliximab for the treatment of Crohn's disease and rheumatoid arthritis. *Am J Gastroenterol.* 2004;99:2385.

Temprano KK, Bandlamudi R, Moore TL. Antirheumatic drugs in pregnancy and lactation. *Semin Arthritis Rheum.* 2005;35:112. [PMID: 16194696]

SPONDYLOARTHROPATHIES

 ESSENTIAL FEATURES

- *Disorders including psoriatic arthritis, ankylosing spondylitis, reactive arthritis, and arthritis secondary to inflammatory bowel disease (IBD).*

Table 14–8. Medications Used in Various Rheumatic Diseases

Drug	Systemic Lupus Erythematosus	Rheumatoid Arthritis	Spondyloarthropathy	Antiphospholipid Antibody Syndrome
Glucocorticoids	X	X	X	X
NSAIDs	X	X	X	X
Hydroxychloroquine	X	X		
Sulfasalazine	X	X	X	
Azathioprine	X	X	X	
Cyclosporine A	X	X		
Mycophenolate mofetil	X			
TNF-α blockers		X	X	
IL-1-Ra		X		
Gold		X		
Cyclophosphamide	X	X		
Leflunomide	X	X	X	
Methotrexate	X	X	X	
Chlorambucil	X (rare)			
Heparin/LMWH				X

NSAIDs, nonsteroidal anti-inflammatory drugs; TNF-α, tumor necrosis factor-α; IL-1-Ra, interleukin-1 receptor antagonist; LMWH, low-molecular-weight heparin.

- *Patients with psoriatic arthritis often improve symptomatically during pregnancy; however, patients with ankylosing spondylitis may have flares.*

General Considerations

There is limited information regarding these diseases and pregnancy. Women with ankylosing spondylitis often get an exacerbation of spinal symptoms or peripheral arthritis mid-gestation. However, 80% of women with psoriatic arthritis tend to improve beginning in the first trimester and then continuing throughout pregnancy. Women with IBD, regardless of arthritic disease, are at increased risk for preterm birth and lower birth weight independent of disease activity. Patients with active bowel symptoms are at increased risk for spontaneous abortion, stillbirth, and developmental defects; therefore, active IBD must be treated aggressively during pregnancy. There is no information regarding reactive arthritis and pregnancy outcome in the literature.

Managing a Spondyloarthropathy Flare

Since women with psoriatic arthritis improve, most joint flares will involve patients with ankylosing spondylitis and IBD. Symptoms of pain and stiffness may be treated with NSAIDs or glucocorticoids with similar precautions as mentioned previously. Women with active bowel symptoms must be treated aggressively with glucocorticoids for the acute flare. Sulfasalazine, azathioprine, or 6-mercaptopurine may be used for maintenance. Higher doses of folic acid are needed in the pregnant patient with IBD.

SCLERODERMA

 ESSENTIAL FEATURES

- *Pregnancy risks are chiefly seen with diffuse scleroderma.*
- *Pregnancy risks are small with limited scleroderma.*

General Considerations

There are two types of systemic scleroderma: limited and diffuse. The limited form is characterized by cutaneous changes with some internal organ involvement, while diffuse scleroderma not only affects the skin but is more likely to have life-threatening internal organ involvement (see Chapter 26). Women with scleroderma do not have decreased fertility compared with the general obstetric population.

Pregnancy does not seem to affect the course of scleroderma in women with limited disease; however, some women with diffuse disease have increased skin thickening postpartum. Gastrointestinal reflux, constipation, and arthralgias were the most common complaints that worsened during pregnancy; however, Raynaud phenomenon often improved. There is evidence that women with both limited and diffuse scleroderma are at increased risk for preterm birth; however, the risk of miscarriage was increased in women with long-standing diffuse disease only. The reported cases of renal crisis during pregnancy occurred in women with early diffuse disease. Therefore, women with diffuse scleroderma should wait until their disease is stable before getting pregnant to decrease the risk of renal crisis. Women with pulmonary hypertension (pulmonary artery pressure >40 mm Hg) should be discouraged from becoming pregnant.

Managing the Symptoms Caused by Scleroderma

There are no medications proven to be effective in modifying the course of scleroderma. Most complaints are symptomatic in nature and management is directed toward relieving the symptoms. Raynaud disease can be treated conservatively with avoidance of cold temperatures. If symptoms persist, vasodilators such as nifedipine have been successfully used during pregnancy. Gastroesophageal reflux disease is treated with lifestyle modifications such as avoiding lying down within 3 hours after meals, elevating the head of the bed, avoiding acidic food such as coffee or spicy food, and avoiding foods that relax the lower esophageal sphincter such as fatty foods, peppermint, alcohol, and chocolate. Medications such as antacids may also be considered if lifestyle modifications are not successful. Proton pump inhibitors are FDA category B drugs and include lansoprazole, pantoprazole, rabeprazole, and esomeprazole. The only FDA category C drug is omeprazole because high doses in rabbits resulted in embryo lethality, fetal resorptions, and pregnancy disruptions. Since there are no adequate or well-controlled studies in pregnant women regarding proton

pump inhibitors, these medications should be used only if necessary during pregnancy. Angiotensin-converting enzyme inhibitors are contraindicated during pregnancy unless there is a life-threatening situation such as a renal crisis.

Lautenbach GL, Petri M. Women's health. *Rheum Dis Clin North Am.* 1999;25:539.

Steen VD. Pregnancy in women with systemic sclerosis. *Obstet Gynecol.* 1999;94:15.

OTHER RHEUMATIC DISEASES
Dermatomyositis & Polymyositis

There are few data regarding pregnancy outcome in women with these diseases because the pregnancy experience for women during the reproductive years is minimal. As with other rheumatic diseases, conception should be planned during a period of remission. Both the woman's age at polymyositis and dermatomyositis onset, and disease activity influence the outcome of the fetus. Fetal outcome is better in women with childhood onset inflammatory myositis than in those with adult onset. Fetal prognosis is worse if a woman develops dermatomyositis or polymyositis during pregnancy, especially if the onset is during the first trimester. However, pregnancies in most women with established disease resulted in live births. The most common complications of pregnancy in women with established disease were intrauterine growth restriction or preterm birth.

Dermatomyositis or polymyositis flares during pregnancy should be treated promptly since fetal complications occur frequently during periods of active disease. Corticosteroids are the mainstay of treatment, aiming at normalizing muscle enzymes. Azathioprine is considered if corticosteroids are insufficient.

Doria A, et al. Pregnancy in rare autoimmune rheumatic diseases: UCTD, MCTD, myositis, systemic vasculitis and Behcet disease. *Lupus.* 2004;13:690.

Vasculitis

There are few data regarding pregnancy outcome, since vasculitis tends to affect men more than women, and this disease tends to occur in female patients after their childbearing years. Patients with active disease at the time of conception and during pregnancy seem to have higher rates of maternal and fetal complications than patients whose disease is in remission. Flares should be managed depending on the severity of the disease with corticosteroids as the mainstay of treatment.

SECTION II

Rheumatoid Arthritis & Spondyloarthropathies

Rheumatoid Arthritis: The Disease—Diagnosis and Clinical Features

15

James R. O'Dell, MD

ESSENTIALS OF DIAGNOSIS

- *Symptoms generally start in proximal interphalangeal (PIP), metacarpophalangeal (MCP), and metatarsophalangeal (MTP) joints.*
- *Joint symptoms must persist for at least 6 weeks.*
- *Diagnostic criteria include morning stiffness, arthritis in three joint areas, arthritis in hands, symmetric arthritis, rheumatoid nodules, serum rheumatoid factor, and radiographic changes.*

General Considerations

Rheumatoid arthritis (RA) is the second most common form of chronic arthritis and affects approximately 1% of the adult population worldwide. This potentially crippling disease shortens survival, and most importantly, significantly compromises quality of life in most affected patients. RA is an inflammatory disease of unknown etiology, and most patients have systemic features such as fatigue, low-grade fevers (up to 38 °C), anemia, and elevations of acute phase reactants (erythrocyte sedimentation rates and C-reactive protein levels). Despite these systemic features, the primary target of this disease is the synovium. Some clinicians have likened RA to a cancer of the synovial tissues because these proliferate in an uncontrolled fashion, resulting in excess fluid production, erosion of surrounding bone, and damage to tendons and ligaments.

The good news is that current therapeutic strategies will result in substantial clinical benefit for the majority of patients, particularly if the disease is diagnosed and treated early (see Chapter 16). Over the last decade there has been a dramatic change in how clinicians think about and treat RA.

Clinical Findings

A. SYMPTOMS AND SIGNS

RA may present at any age in any patient. However, it is more common in women (3:1) (Table 15–1). The typical age of onset in women is the late childbearing years, while men are often in their sixth to eighth decade. Although RA has a significant genetic component, most patients

Table 15–1. Classic Manifestations

- Gender: Female (3:1 ratio)
- Age: Late childbearing years in women (sixth to eighth decade in men)
- Onset: Insidious (builds up over several weeks to months)
- Distribution: Symmetric small joints—MCP, PIP, and MTP (spares DIP) joints
- Systemic: Fatigue, possible weight loss, occasional low-grade fevers
- Symptoms: Joint stiffness (worse in morning), pain, swelling
- Laboratory: Anemia, elevated ESR or CRP or both, thrombocytosis, positive rheumatoid factor in 60–80%

MCP, metacarpophalangeal; PIP, proximal interphalangeal; MTP, metatarsophalangeal; DIP, distal interphalangeal; ESR, erythrocyte sedimentation rate; CRP, C-reactive protein.

will have no significant family history. The onset may be fulminant, coming on almost overnight, but is more commonly insidious, building up over several weeks to months.

The distribution of involved joints is a critical clue to the underlying diagnosis (Figure 15–1). Most patients report involvement of small joints first, classically the PIP, MCP, and MTP joints, with involvement of large joints occurring later. Symptoms include pain, swelling, and stiffness, with stiffness often dominating, particular in the mornings. Routine activities like brushing teeth and combing hair may be very difficult early in the morning, and patients often report running warm water over their hands to "get them working." Patients with early disease often complain that rings no longer fit and that they have pain on the balls of the feet while walking to the bathroom in the morning.

1. Articular manifestations—RA can affect any of the synovial joints (see Figure 15–1). Most commonly, the disease starts in the MCP, PIP, and MTP joints followed

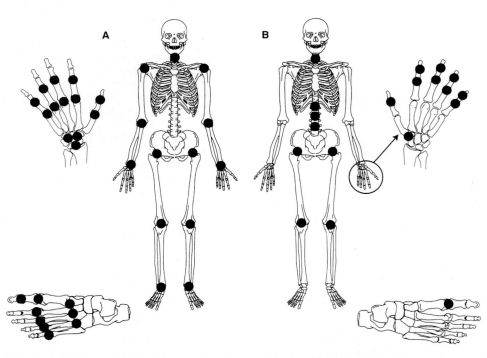

Figure 15–1. The joint distribution of the two most common types of arthritis are compared: rheumatoid arthritis (**A**) and osteoarthritis (**B**). Rheumatoid arthritis involves almost all synovial joints in the body. Osteoarthritis has a much more limited distribution. Importantly, rheumatoid arthritis rarely, if ever, involves the distal interphalangeal joints, but osteoarthritis commonly does.

by the wrists, knees, elbows, ankles, hips, and shoulders in roughly that order. Early treatment helps limit the number of joints involved. Of particular importance, RA almost always spares the distal interphalangeal (DIP) joints (in contrast, these joints are often involved in osteoarthritis and psoriatic arthritis). Less commonly, and usually only in more advanced cases, RA may involve the temporomandibular, cricoarytenoid and sternoclavicular joints. RA may involve the upper part of the cervical spine, particularly the C1–C2 articulation, but unlike the spondyloarthropathies, rarely if ever involves the rest of the spine. Patients with RA are, however, at an increased risk for osteoporosis, and this risk should be considered and dealt with early.

The **hands** are a major site of involvement in almost all patients with RA; hand involvement is responsible for a significant portion of the disabilities caused by RA. Typical early disease is shown in Figure 15–2A with the swelling of the PIP joints easily seen. The DIP joints are almost always spared unless the patient also has osteoarthritis; both diseases are common and can coexist, particularly in elderly patients. Radiographs can detect evidence of articular damage early in the course of disease and long before the appearance of joint deformities (Figure 15-3). Late established disease all too commonly causes ulnar deviation of the fingers at the MCPs and swan-neck deformities (hyperextension of the PIP joints; Figure 15–2B). Boutonnière (or buttonhole) deformities of the fingers result from hyperextension of the MCP joints. If the clinical disease remains active, hand function will slowly deteriorate.

Wrists are involved in most patients with RA. Early in the course of the disease, synovial proliferation in and around the wrists can compress the median nerve, causing carpal tunnel syndrome. Chronic synovitis can lead to radial deviation of the wrist, and in severe cases, to volar subluxation. Synovial proliferation of the wrist can invade extensor tendons, leading to rupture and abrupt loss of function of individual fingers.

The **feet,** particularly the MTP joints, are involved early in almost all cases of RA and are second only to hand involvement in terms of the problems they cause. Radiographic erosions occur at least as early in the feet as in the hands. Subluxation of the toes at the MTP joints is common and leads to the dual problem of skin ulceration on the top of the toes and painful ambulation because of loss of the cushioning pads that protect the heads of the metatarsals. Symptoms from MTP subluxation can respond to orthotics but may require surgery.

Involvement of **large joints** (knees, ankles, elbows, hips, and shoulders) is common but generally occurs somewhat later than small joint involvement. Characteristically, the entire joint surface is involved in a symmetric fashion. Therefore RA is not only symmetric from one side of the body to the other, but is also symmet-

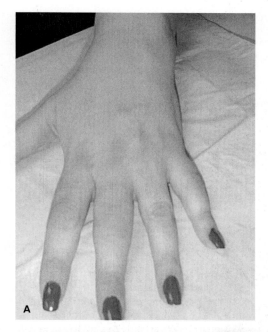

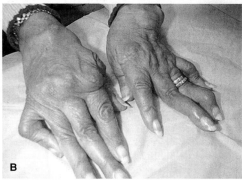

Figure 15–2. **A:** A patient with early rheumatoid arthritis. There are no joint deformities, but the soft tissue synovial swelling around the third and fifth proximal interphalangeal (PIP) joints is easily seen. **B:** A patient with advanced rheumatoid arthritis with severe joint deformities including subluxation at the metacarpophalangeal joints and swan-neck deformities (hyperextension at the PIP joints).

ric within the individual joint. In the case of the knee (Figure 15–4A), the medial and lateral compartments are both severely narrowed in RA, whereas osteoarthritis usually involves only one compartment (Figure 15–4B). Total joint replacements of hips and knees can dramatically improve function and quality of life and

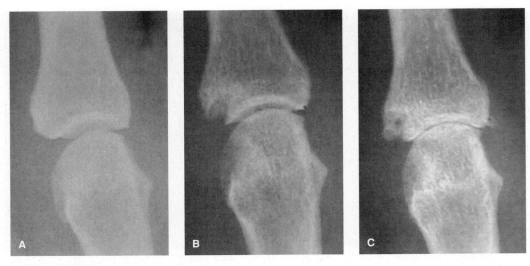

Figure 15–3. Progressive destruction of a metacarpophalangeal joint by rheumatoid arthritis. Shown are sequential radiographs of the same second metacarpophalangeal joint. **A:** The joint is normal 1 year prior to the development of rheumatoid arthritis. **B:** Six months following the onset of rheumatoid arthritis, there is a bony erosion adjacent to the joint and joint space narrowing. **C:** After 3 years of disease, diffuse loss of articular cartilage has led to marked joint space narrowing.

should be considered in patients with severe mechanical damage.

Synovial cysts present as fluctuant masses around involved joints (large or small). Synovial cysts from the knee are perhaps the best examples of this phenomenon. The inflamed knee produces excess synovial fluid that can accumulate posteriorly because of a one-way valve effect between the knee joint and the popliteal space (popliteal or **Baker cyst**). Baker cysts cause problems by compressing the popliteal nerve, artery, or veins; by dissecting into the tissues of the calf (usually posteriorly); and by rupturing into the calf. Dissection usually produces only minor symptoms such as a feeling of fullness. Rupture of a Baker cyst, however, leads to extravasation of the inflammatory contents into the calf, producing significant pain and swelling that may be confused with thrombophlebitis (the so-called pseudothrombophlebitis syndrome). Ultrasonography of the popliteal fossa and calf is useful to confirm the diagnosis and to rule out thrombophlebitis, which may be precipitated by popliteal cysts. Short-term treatment of popliteal cysts usually involves injecting the knee with glucocorticoids to interrupt the inflammatory process.

Although most of the spine is spared in RA, the **cervical spine** (especially the C1–C2 articulation) is not. As with RA elsewhere, bony erosions and ligament damage can occur in this area and can lead to subluxation. Most often, subluxation is minor, and patients and caregivers need only be cautious and avoid forcing the neck into positions of flexion. Occasionally, C1–C2 subluxation is severe and requires complex surgical intervention in an attempt to prevent compromise of the cervical cord, and in some cases, death.

Wherever synovial tissue exists, RA may cause problems; the temporomandibular, cricoarytenoid, and sternoclavicular joints are examples. The cricoarytenoid joint is responsible for abduction and adduction of the vocal cords. Involvement of this joint may lead to a feeling of fullness in the throat, to hoarseness, or rarely to a syndrome of acute respiratory distress with or without stridor when the cords are essentially frozen in a closed position. In this latter situation, emergent tracheotomy may be life-saving.

2. Extra-articular manifestations—RA is a systemic disease in all patients and features such as fatigue, weight loss, and low-grade fevers ($< 38 \,^{\circ}$C) occur frequently, and like all the other extra-articular features, tend to be more common in those patients with rheumatoid factor.

Rheumatoid nodules are seen in approximately one-quarter of patients with RA, almost exclusively in those patients who are seropositive for rheumatoid factor. Indeed, patients with nodules but without rheumatoid factor should be carefully evaluated for an alternative diagnosis, such as chronic tophaceous gout. Rheumatoid nodules are usually subcutaneous and typically occur on extensor surfaces and other pressure points (particularly forearms [Figure 15–5]) or over joints. Rarely they

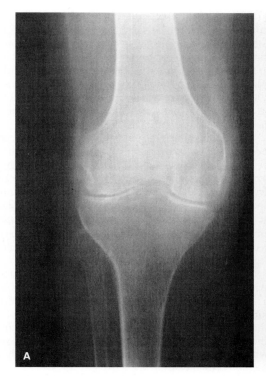 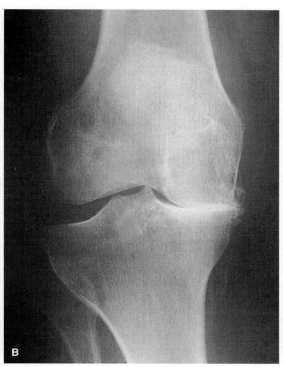

Figure 15–4. The radiographic features of rheumatoid arthritis and osteoarthritis are compared with regard to large joint involvement. **A:** Symmetric loss of cartilage space that is typical of inflammatory arthritis such as rheumatoid arthritis. Note that both the medial and lateral compartments are severely narrowed. Despite this severe narrowing, there is very little in the way of subchondral sclerosis or osteophyte formation since these repair mechanisms are generally shut off in active rheumatoid arthritis. **B:** Complete loss of the cartilage in the medial joint compartment with significant subchondral sclerosis and osteophyte formation. The lateral compartment in this patient is not involved. These features are typical of osteoarthritis.

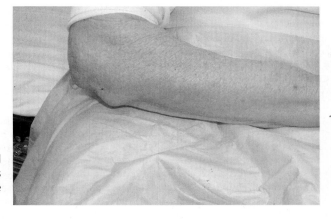

Figure 15–5. A rheumatoid nodule in a typical location on the extensor surface of the forearm is apparent in this patient with seropositive, erosive rheumatoid arthritis.

develop in viscera (lungs and heart, for example) or in the sclera of the eye. Rheumatoid nodules are firm and nontender (unless traumatized), have a characteristic histologic picture, and are thought to be triggered by small vessel vasculitis. Methotrexate therapy can trigger a syndrome of increased nodulosis despite good control of the articular manifestations of the disease.

Digital infarcts and leukocytoclastic vasculitis are other features of RA-associated **small vessel vasculitis** and should prompt more aggressive treatment with disease-modifying antirheumatic drugs (DMARDs). A vasculitis of small and medium arteries, which is indistinguishable from polyarteritis nodosa, can be seen and requires aggressive systemic therapy. Finally, **pyoderma gangrenosum** occurs with increased frequency in patients with RA.

Patients with RA have significantly increased morbidity and mortality from **coronary artery disease.** The reasons for this have not been completely elucidated, but chronic inflammation with an elevated C-reactive protein, some of the medications used, and sedentary lifestyle may be significant risk factors.

Clinical manifestations of **cardiac involvement** directly related to RA are uncommon. Rarely, rheumatoid nodules develop in the conduction system and cause heart block. **Pericardial effusions** are common (detected in up to 50% of patients by echocardiography) but are usually asymptomatic. Uncommonly, long-standing pericardial disease results in a fibrinous pericarditis and **constrictive pericarditis.**

Pulmonary manifestations of RA include pleural effusions, rheumatoid nodules, and parenchymal lung disease. **Pleural effusions** occur more commonly in men and are usually small and asymptomatic. Of interest, pleural fluid in RA is characterized by low glucose and pH, and therefore may at times be confused with empyema. **Rheumatoid nodules** may occur in the lung, especially in men; they are usually solid but may calcify, cavitate, or become infected. Differentiating rheumatoid nodules from lung cancer may be difficult, particularly if they are solitary, and may require an excisional biopsy.

Diffuse interstitial fibrosis causes dyspnea and may progress to a honeycomb appearance on radiographs. Rarely, bronchiolitis obliterans, with or without organizing pneumonia, occurs and carries a poor prognosis.

Keratoconjunctivitis sicca (dry eyes) from secondary Sjögren syndrome is the most common ophthalmologic manifestation of RA. Patients often have associated xerostomia (dry mouth), parotid gland swelling, and occasionally lymphadenopathy.

Scleritis also occurs in RA and is usually painful. Severe involvement can lead to thinning of the sclera (seen as a bluish discoloration as the deep pigment shows through) and even to perforation of the orbit (scleromalacia perforans).

Neurologic manifestations include peripheral nerve entrapment syndromes, such as carpal tunnel syndrome (entrapment of the median nerve at the wrist) and tarsal tunnel syndrome (entrapment of the anterior tibial nerve at the ankle). Vasculitis can lead to **mononeuritis multiplex** and a host of neurologic problems. Subluxations at C1–C2 can produce myelopathy. Rheumatoid nodules in the central nervous system have been described but are rare and usually asymptomatic.

Felty syndrome is the triad of RA, splenomegaly, and neutropenia. Felty syndrome is seen in patients with severe seropositive disease and may be accompanied by hepatomegaly, thrombocytopenia, lymphadenopathy, and fevers. Most patients with Felty syndrome do not require specific therapy; rather, treatment should be focused on severe RA. Splenectomy may be indicated if severe neutropenia exists (< 500 cells/mm^3) and is accompanied by recurrent bacterial infections or by chronic nonhealing leg ulcers.

A few RA patients have white blood cell counts characterized by a dominance of large granular lymphocytes and a nearly complete absence of neutrophils. This condition, known as the "large granular lymphocyte syndrome," is thought to be a form of T-cell leukemia. When seen in the setting of RA, these patients have a good prognosis, with the neutropenia often responding dramatically to methotrexate therapy.

B. Laboratory Findings and Imaging

Anemia of chronic disease is seen in the majority of patients with RA, and the degree of anemia is proportional to the activity of the disease. Therapy that controls the disease results in normalization of the hemoglobin. Rarely, erythropoietin administration may be indicated. Thrombocytosis is common, with platelet counts returning to normal as the inflammation is controlled. Acute phase reactants, **erythrocyte sedimentation rate** and **C-reactive protein** levels, also parallel the activity of the disease, and their persistent elevation portends a poor prognosis, both in terms of joint destruction and mortality. White blood cell counts may be elevated, normal, or in the case of Felty syndrome, profoundly depressed.

The historically most characteristic laboratory abnormality in RA was the presence of **rheumatoid factor,** an autoantibody directed against the constant (Fc) region of IgG. Rheumatoid factor is positive in about 50% of cases at presentation and an additional 20–35% of cases become positive in the first 6 months after diagnosis. Rheumatoid factor has an unfortunate name because it is not unique to RA and occurs in many other diseases, particularly those characterized by chronic stimulation of the immune system (Table 15–2). In RA, the presence of rheumatoid factor is associated with more severe articular disease, and essentially all patients with the extra-articular features are seropositive for rheumatoid factor. Recently, it has been recognized that the autoantibodies most

Table 15–2. Differential of a Positive Rheumatoid Factor

- Rheumatic diseases
  - RA, Sjögren syndrome, SLE, others
- Infections
  - Viral: Hepatitis C, EBV, parvovirus, influenza, others
  - Bacterial: Endocarditis, osteomyelitis, others
- Chronic inflammatory conditions
- Liver disease, inflammatory bowel disease, others
- Aging

RA, rheumatoid arthritis; SLE, systemic lupus erythematosus; EBV, Epstein-Barr virus.

Table 15–3. American College of Rheumatology Criteria for Rheumatoid Arthritis

- Morning stiffness[a]
- Arthritis of three joint areas[a]
- Arthritis of the hands[a]
- Symmetric arthritis[a]
- Rheumatoid nodules
- Serum rheumatoid factor
- Radiographic changes

[a]These criteria must be present for more than 6 weeks.

specific for RA are directed against citrullinated proteins, the so-called **anticyclic citrullinated peptide (anti-CCP) antibodies.** Anti-CCP antibodies are present in 60–70% of patients with RA at diagnosis, are 90–98% specific for RA, are often present in the serum years before RA is diagnosed (similar to rheumatoid factor), and correlate strongly with erosive disease. RA is associated with multiple other autoantibodies, including **antinuclear antibodies** (seen in ~ 30% of patients) and antineutrophilic cytoplasmic antibodies, particularly of the perinuclear type (seen in ~ 30% of patients).

Synovial fluid in RA is inflammatory; white blood cell counts typically range from 5000–50,000 per microliter with approximately two-thirds of the cells being neutrophils. No synovial fluid findings are pathognomonic of RA.

Making the Diagnosis

Unfortunately, there is no one single finding on physical examination or laboratory testing that is diagnostic of RA. Instead, the diagnosis of RA is a clinical one, requiring a collection of historical and physical features, as well as an alert and informed clinician.

The American College of Rheumatology provides classification criteria which, although not designed specifically for the purpose, are widely used as an aid to diagnosis of RA (Table 15–3). The first five criteria are clinical; only the last two criteria require laboratory tests or radiographs. Of note the first four criteria need to be present for at least 6 weeks before a diagnosis of RA can be made. This time requirement was imposed because a number of conditions, most notably viral-related syndromes, can cause self-limited polyarthritis indistinguishable from RA, including, at times, the presence of rheumatoid factor (Table 15–4). These syndromes usually last 2–3 weeks, but unfortunately have caused some clinicians to be overly cautious and to delay the diagnosis of RA for months or longer. The recent recognition that anti-CCP antibodies are highly specific

for RA should help to expedite the diagnosis of RA. If a patient with symmetrical polyarthritis—even of only several weeks' duration—is found to be anti-CCP–positive, that patient should be promptly referred to a rheumatologist with the presumptive diagnosis of RA. The goal for the majority of RA patients should be to establish a diagnosis and to start DMARD therapy within the first 3 months of disease.

Although most patients with RA present with the onset of pain, stiffness, and swelling in multiple joints over the course of weeks to months, some may have a fulminant presentation and others may have an onset so insidious that the patient hardly notices. Alternatively, patients may have persistent monarthritis or oligoarthritis for prolonged periods before manifesting the more typical pattern of polyarticular involvement. Rarely, patients may present with extra-articular features of RA before the joint problems occur.

The distribution of involved joints is a critical clue to the underlying diagnosis (see Figure 15–1). The joints that are involved in patients with RA at presentation are also variable; the typical presentation has been described above. While the patient's history of joint symptoms (arthralgia) is important, the diagnosis of RA requires the presence of inflammation (swelling or warmth or both) on examination of the joints.

Table 15–4. Differential Diagnosis

- Viral syndromes, especially hepatitis B and C, Epstein-Barr virus, parvovirus, rubella
- Psoriatic arthritis, reactive arthritis
- Tophaceous gout
- Systemic lupus erythematosus
- Calcium pyrophosphate disease
- Polymyalgia rheumatica
- Paraneoplastic syndromes
- Osteoarthritis, especially hereditary osteoarthritis of the hand
- Sarcoidosis, Lyme disease, rheumatic fever, etc

Morning stiffness is a hallmark of inflammatory arthritis and is a prominent feature of RA. Patients with RA are characteristically at their worst upon arising in the morning or after prolonged periods of rest. This stiffness in and around joints will often last for hours and quantifying it is one way to measure improvement. Stiffness is relieved by warmth and activity, and reducing or eliminating it is a clear goal of therapy.

Differential Diagnosis

The early and accurate diagnosis of RA, while at times challenging, is critical if patients are to receive maximal benefit from therapeutic intervention. Once disease has been present and active for a number of years and the characteristic deformities on physical examination (see Figure 15–2B) and radiographs (see Figures 15–3 and 15–4A) have occurred, the diagnosis in most cases is all too obvious. RA rarely if ever burns out and its inflammatory component will respond to therapy at any time. Unfortunately, once deformities are present, their mechanical component will not respond to medical therapy.

Many diseases can mimic RA early in its course (see Table 15–4). **Acute viral syndromes,** especially hepatitis B and C, parvovirus, rubella (infection or vaccination), and Epstein-Barr virus can produce a polyarthritis that mimics RA initially but is self-limited, usually resolving over 2–4 weeks. **Systemic lupus erythematosus, psoriatic arthritis,** and **reactive arthritis** may present diagnostic challenges. With these three mimics, a targeted history and examination to elucidate their associated clinical features (such as rashes, oral ulcers, nail changes, dactylitis, and urethritis) and renal, pulmonary, gastrointestinal or ophthalmologic problems is critical. Hypothyroidism, which causes a collection of rheumatic manifestations and also occurs commonly in conjunction with RA, should be kept in mind. In the elderly patient with fulminant-onset RA, remitting seronegative symmetric synovitis with pitting edema or paraneoplastic syndromes should be considered. Chronic tophaceous gout may mimic severe nodular RA. Finally, osteoarthritis with severe deformities of the hands from bony proliferation of the DIP and PIP joints (Heberden and Bouchard nodes) may confuse some inexperienced clinicians; the keys here are DIP joint involvement and the bony, instead of soft tissue, joint abnormalities.

Comorbidity

Increasingly, cardiovascular disease is being recognized as the major cause of the excess mortality in RA. Chronic inflammation, which is strongly associated with the development of cardiovascular disease, is likely the most significant factor. Therapies that control RA earlier and better can be expected to decrease cardiovascular morbidity and mortality. A recent study indicates that methotrexate reduces cardiovascular mortality by 70% in patients with RA. Clinicians should consider RA a risk factor for cardiovascular disease and should aggressively address other cardiovascular risk factors in these patients.

Osteoporosis is ubiquitous in patients with RA, and early therapy directed at this problem will result in long-term benefits. Patients with RA are at an increased risk for infections, and this risk is further increased by some therapies. Patients should be cautioned to seek medical attention early for even minor symptoms suggestive of infection, especially if receiving anti–tumor necrosis factor therapy. All patients with RA should receive pneumococcal and yearly influenza vaccinations. Finally, patients with RA have an increased risk of lymphomas. Occasionally, B-cell lymphomas may be associated with immunosuppression and regress after immunosuppression is discontinued. Interestingly, RA patients have a significantly decreased risk (odds ratio 0.2) of developing colon cancer. This is thought to be secondary to chronic inhibition of cyclooxygenase by the nonsteroidal anti-inflammatory agents commonly used in this group of patients.

Complications

RA is a lifelong, progressive disease that can produce significant morbidity and premature mortality. Long-term studies have found that 50% of RA patients have had to stop working after 10 years (approximately 10 times the average rate). Patients who have anti-CCP antibodies, who are rheumatoid factor positive, or who have HLA-DR alleles expressing the shared epitope have a worse prognosis with more erosions and more extra-articular disease. Once deformities are found on examination or erosions on radiography, the damage is largely irreversible. Erosions develop in the majority of patients in the first 1 or 2 years of disease, and it has now been clearly shown that the rate of radiographic damage can be affected by early therapy. Therefore, early DMARD therapy is critical. Although long-term data are not yet available, short-term data strongly suggest that current patients have the opportunity to benefit greatly if the newer principles of therapy are practiced (Table 15–5).

Table 15–5. Keys to Optimize Outcome

- Early diagnosis
- DMARD therapy as early as possible
- Strive for remissions in all patients
- Recognize and treat comorbid conditions
- Cooperation and communication between primary care physician and rheumatologist

DMARD. disease-modifying antirheumatic drug.

Prognosis

Because he duration of disease prior to DMARD therapy may be one of the strongest predictors of outcome, making the correct diagnosis quickly is of critical importance. All current treatment paradigms for RA stress the early aggressive use of DMARDs.

Treatment

Please see Chapter 16.

REFERENCES

Gabriel SE. The epidemiology of rheumatoid arthritis. *Rheum Dis Clin North Am.* 2001;27:269. [PMID: 11396092] (This is an excellent article on the epidemiology of rheumatoid arthritis.)

Goldbach-Mansky R, Lee J, McCoy A, et al. Rheumatoid arthritis associated autoantibodies in patients with synovitis of recent onset. *Arthritis Res.* 2000;2:236. [PMID: 11056669] (This study of patients with early rheumatoid arthritis is a terrific summary of what is known about early antibody markers of rheumatoid arthritis.)

Crowson CS, Nicola PJ, Kremers HM, et al. How much of the increased incidence of heart failure in rheumatoid arthritis is attributable to traditional cardiovascular risk factors and ischemic heart disease? *Arthritis Rheum.* 2005;52:3039. [PMID: 16200583] (An excellent discussion on this, the most significant comorbidity for patients with RA.)

Maradit-Kremers H, Crowson CS, Nicola PJ, et al. Increased unrecognized coronary heart disease and sudden deaths in rheumatoid arthritis: a population-based cohort study. *Arthritis Rheum.* 2005;52:402. [PMID: 15693010] (A great original article on heart disease in RA.)

Mikuls TR, Saag KG. Comorbidity in rheumatoid arthritis. *Rheum Dis Clin North Am.* 2001;27:283. [PMID: 11396093] (This article summarizes the importance of comorbidity in rheumatoid arthritis and discusses strategies to address these comorbid conditions.)

van Gaalen FA, et al. Autoantibodies to cyclic citrullinated peptides predict progression to rheumatoid arthritis in patients with undifferentiated arthritis: a prospective cohort study. *Arthritis Rheum.* 2004;50:709. [PMID: 16237041] (The best discussion of the usefulness of anti-CCP antibodies in early arthritis.)

Relevant World Wide Web Site

[American College of Rheumatology]
http://www.rheumatology.org

Treatment of Rheumatoid Arthritis   16

James R. O'Dell, MD

There is no cure for rheumatoid arthritis (RA), which is a lifelong disease process requiring lifelong treatment. Currently available therapies are effective, but therapeutic regimens are often complex. Moreover, although multiple treatment options exist, comparative trials are relatively few, placing a premium on clinical experience. For these reasons, and because of the rapid pace of the introduction of new medications, a rheumatologist should monitor the care of all patients with RA. The optimal care for patients with RA requires effective interactions between primary care physicians and rheumatologists. Often, once the diagnosis is established and effective therapeutic programs are in place, follow-up may be primarily with primary care physicians, with rheumatologists involved two to four times per year. In most cases, patients also should consult with physical and occupational therapists to learn about range-of-motion exercises, joint protection, and assistive devices.

The goal of therapy for RA is to put the disease in remission and to maintain this remission by continuing therapy. If RA is treated early using currently available therapies, remission is possible in 20–40% of patients. Unfortunately, remissions require the ongoing use of medications and even then are not always durable. Four broad categories of medical therapies are used for the treatment of RA: nonsteroidal anti-inflammatory drugs (NSAIDs), glucocorticoids, conventional disease-modifying antirheumatic drugs (DMARDs), and biological DMARDs. Almost all patients require use of more than one type of medication, and with rare exceptions, all patients should receive DMARD therapy (Figure 16–1). Indeed, optimal control of disease activity often requires combinations of different conventional DMARDs or combinations of conventional and biological DMARDs (Figure 16–1). Therapy must be escalated rapidly to assure maximal suppression of disease while making efforts to minimize toxicity and expense. The effectiveness of therapy is usually assessed by monitoring symptoms (eg, pain and the duration of morning stiffness) and signs of synovitis, as well as acute phase reactants (the erythrocyte sedimentation rate or C-reactive protein). Recent data suggest that setting specific therapeutic goals using formally determined disease activity scores may achieve better results than this "clinical gestalt," but this approach is not in widespread use.

NSAIDs are important for symptomatic relief but play only a minor role, if any, in altering the underlying disease process. **Therefore, NSAIDs should rarely, if ever, be used to treat RA without the concomitant use of DMARDs.** Many clinicians still waste valuable time switching from one NSAID to another before starting DMARD therapy; this is unfortunate, as early DMARD therapy is associated with better long-term outcomes.

The gastrointestinal toxicity of NSAIDs is a major issue for RA patients, who often have multiple risk factors for gastrointestinal toxicity. The use of proton pump inhibitors reduces the incidence of clinically significant gastrointestinal side effects. Selective inhibitors of cyclooxygenase-2 had been particularly popular in this group of patients until increased cardiovascular morbidity and mortality was associated with some of these agents, especially when used at higher doses. This finding is of particular concern for RA patients, who already are at significantly increased risk of cardiovascular problems as a consequence of their underlying disease.

Glucocorticoids can be dramatically and rapidly effective in patients with RA. Glucocorticoids are not only useful for symptomatic improvement, but significantly decrease the radiographic progression of RA. Unfortunately, the toxicities of long-term glucocorticoid therapy are legendary. Therefore the optimal use of these drugs requires an understanding of the principles of glucocorticoid use in RA (Table 16–1).

Glucocorticoids are among the most potent anti-inflammatory treatments available; because of this and their rapid onset of action, they are ideally suited to help control synovial inflammation while introducing the much slower-acting conventional DMARDs. Thus the paradigm ("bridge therapy") is to shut off inflammation rapidly with glucocorticoids, and then to taper these as the slower-acting DMARD begin to work. Prednisone, the most commonly used glucocorticoid, should rarely be used in doses higher than 10 mg daily to treat articular disease (extra-articular manifestations of RA, such as vasculitis and scleritis, may require higher doses). This dose should be slowly tapered to the lowest effective dose, and the concomitant DMARD therapy should be adjusted to make this possible. Glucocorticoids should rarely, if ever, be used to treat RA without concomitant DMARD therapy. In all patients receiving glucocorticoids, strong

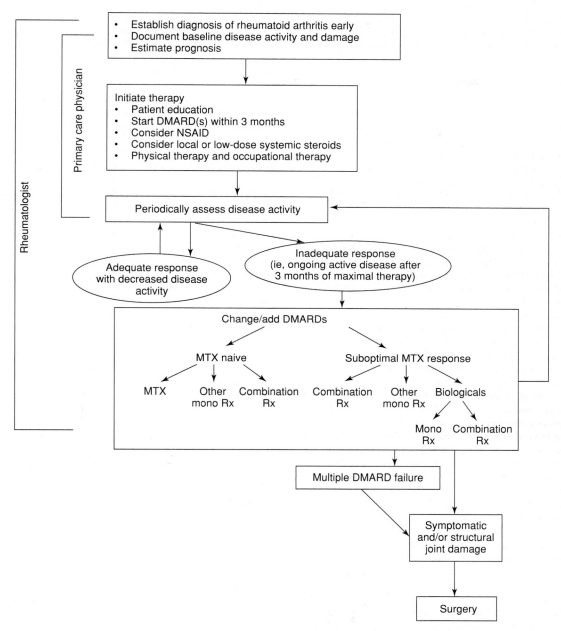

Figure 16–1. Guidelines for the management of rheumatoid arthritis. MTX, methotrexate; DMARD, disease-modifying antirheumatic drug; NSAID, nonsteroidal anti-inflammatory drug. (From the American College of Rheumatology 2002 Guidelines for the Management of Rheumatoid Arthritis. With permission.)

Table 16–1. Guidelines for the Use of Glucocorticoids in the Treatment of Rheumatoid Arthritis

---

- Prednisone > 10 mg daily is rarely indicated for articular disease
- Avoid using glucocorticoids without DMARDs
- Use glucocorticoids as a "bridge" to effective DMARD therapy
- Minimize duration and dose by slowly tapering to the lowest dose that controls arthritis
- Always consider prophylaxis to minimize osteoporosis

DMARDs, disease-modifying antirheumatic drugs.

consideration should be given to the prevention of osteoporosis, and bisphosphonates have been shown to be particularly effective in this regard.

DMARDs, both conventional and biological, are a group of medications that have the ability to modify or change the course of RA. Drugs included in this class have, in most cases, met the gold standard of halting or slowing the radiographic progression of RA.

Conventional (synthetic) DMARDs: Included in the conventional DMARD group of medications are methotrexate, sulfasalazine, gold, antimalarials, leflunomide, azathioprine, penicillamine, and minocycline. It is critically important that clinicians and patients alike understand that these medications take 2–6 months to reach maximal effect. Therefore other measures, such as glucocorticoid therapy, may be needed to control the disease while these medications are starting to work.

All of the above-mentioned DMARDs have been shown to be effective in treating both early and more advanced RA. The choice of which DMARD to use first depends on the activity of the disease, comorbid conditions, concerns about toxicity, and monitoring issues. Until additional research elucidates factors that allow clinicians to select the best initial therapy for each patient, there are many reasonable choices. The critical factor is not which DMARD to choose first, but the fact that DMARD therapy should be started early in the disease process.

Methotrexate is the preferred DMARD of most rheumatologists, largely because many patients have a durable response and serious toxicities are rare with careful monitoring. It is dramatically effective in slowing the radiographic progression of RA. Methotrexate also is the anchor drug in most successful combinations of DMARDs in RA. Specifically, a decade ago, methotrexate in combination with sulfasalazine and hydroxychloroquine was shown to be more effective than methotrexate alone and ushered in the current paradigm of combination DMARD therapy for all RA patients who are not controlled on DMARD monotherapy. Importantly, all of the biologicals have been shown to be more effective when combined with methotrexate.

Methotrexate is usually given orally in doses ranging from 5–25 mg as a single dose once a week. **This once-a-week administration is worthy of emphasis.** Prior experience with daily therapy in psoriasis has taught us that toxicity, particularly liver toxicity, is substantially greater when the same amount of drug is administered on a daily basis rather than as a weekly pulse. Oral absorption of methotrexate is variable; therefore, subcutaneous methotrexate may be effective when oral therapy is not and should be tried before discontinuing the drug for lack of efficacy. Side effects include oral ulcers, nausea, hepatotoxicity, bone marrow suppression, and pneumonitis. With the exception of pneumonitis (which is a hypersensitivity reaction), these toxicities respond to dose adjustments and are reduced by the concomitant use of folic acid (1–4 mg PO daily). Monitoring of blood cell counts and liver blood tests (albumin and alanine transaminase or aspartate transaminase) should be done every 4–8 weeks for the duration of methotrexate therapy, with dosage adjustments as needed. Renal function is critical for clearance of methotrexate and its active metabolites; previously stable patients may experience severe toxicities when renal function deteriorates. Pneumonitis, while rare, is less predictable and may be fatal, particularly if the methotrexate is not stopped or is restarted.

Hydroxychloroquine is frequently used for the treatment of RA, usually in combination with other DMARDs, particularly methotrexate. Hydroxychloroquine, which is given orally at a dose of 200–400 mg daily, has the least toxicity of any of the DMARDs but also is probably the least effective as monotherapy. Regular monitoring (every 6 months to a year) by an ophthalmologist is recommended to detect any signs of retinal toxicity.

Sulfasalazine is the most commonly used DMARD in Europe. It is an effective treatment when given in doses of 1–3 g daily. Monitoring blood cell counts, particularly white blood cell counts, in the first 6 months is recommended. In the United States, sulfasalazine is usually combined with methotrexate, hydroxychloroquine, or both.

Minocycline, 100 mg twice daily, is an effective treatment for RA, particularly when used in early seropositive disease. The mechanism of action in RA is uncertain but probably is independent of its antibacterial effects. Long-term therapy (more than 2 years) may lead to cutaneous hyperpigmentation.

Leflunomide, a pyrimidine antagonist, is the newest conventional DMARD approved for use in RA. It has a very long half-life and is given daily in a dose of 10–20 mg. When leflunomide was first introduced, a loading dose of 100 mg daily for 3 days was routinely used because of the long half-life, but most experts no longer use a loading dose because of increased side effects. The most common toxicity with leflunomide is diarrhea, which may respond to dose reduction. Leflunomide is teratogenic. Because of its exceptionally long half-life, women who have previously received leflunomide (even if therapy was years ago) should have blood levels drawn if they wish to become pregnant. If toxicity occurs or if pregnancy is being considered, cholestyramine can rapidly eliminate leflunomide.

Intramuscular gold, the oldest DMARD, remains an extremely effective therapy for a small percentage of patients. It is uncommonly used now because of its slow onset of action, the need for intramuscular administration, the requirement for frequent monitoring (complete blood cell count and urinalysis), and its frequent toxicities, which include skin rashes, bone marrow suppression, and proteinuria. A recent study in patients with active disease despite methotrexate has once again confirmed the efficacy of this drug.

Biological DMARDs: Biological therapies have had a significant impact on the treatment of patients with RA. It is now clear that proinflammatory cytokines, most notably tumor necrosis factor-α (TNF-α) and interleukin-1, play a central role in the pathophysiology of RA. This insight led to the development and clinical use of biological agents directed against TNF-α (etanercept, infliximab, and adalimumab) and interleukin-1 (anakinra). More recent studies have shown promise for therapies that block T-cell co-stimulation (abatacept) and that target B-cells (rituximab).

Etanercept, a recombinant TNF receptor fusion protein, is administered subcutaneously in a dose of 25 mg twice weekly. **Infliximab** is a mouse/human chimeric monoclonal antibody against TNF-α that is given intravenously (3–10 mg/kg) every 4–8 weeks. **Adalimumab** is a recombinant human IgG1 monoclonal antibody directed against TNF-α and is administered subcutaneously in a dose of 40 mg every other week. All three anti-TNF agents have been shown to reduce the signs and symptoms of synovitis—even in patients who have active disease despite treatment with methotrexate—and to substantially diminish radiographic progression of RA. A rapid onset of action (days to weeks) is apparent with all of these agents and is a significant advantage that these treatments have over conventional DMARDs. The major disadvantages are cost and concerns about long-term toxicities, notably infections (especially cellulitis, septic joints, tuberculosis, histoplasmosis, coccidioidomycosis, and *Listeria*) and demyelinating syndromes. Unfortunately, there is a paucity of data comparing anti-TNF agents with conventional DMARD therapy, especially for patients who have active disease despite methotrexate.

Anakinra, a recombinant human interleukin-1 receptor antagonist, is given subcutaneously in a dose of 100 mg daily. It has been shown to be effective for signs and symptoms of RA, as well as radiographic progression. Its onset of action is somewhat slower and less dramatic than that of the TNF inhibitors, and anakinra currently is used far less than the anti-TNF agents. Toxicities include injection-site reactions and pneumonia (especially in patients with asthma).

Abatacept is a recombinant fusion protein of the extracellular domain of human CTLA4 and a fragment of the Fc domain of human IgG1. It is the first of a new class of selective T-cell modulators and blocks the co-stimulatory signal, necessary for the full activation of T cells, that is delivered by the interaction of the T-cell molecule CD28 with its ligands (CD80 and CD86) on antigen-presenting cells. Abatacept reduces signs and symptoms of RA in patients with active disease despite methotrexate, and also in the subset of RA patients who have active disease refractory to the TNF inhibitors. The effect of abatacept on radiographic progression remains to be determined. It is administered by intravenous infusion every 4 weeks in a dose of approximately 10 mg/kg; its onset of action is slower than that of the anti-TNF agents.

Rituximab is a genetically engineered chimeric murine/human monoclonal antibody directed against the CD20 molecule found on the surface of B cells. Rituximab is approved for the treatment of CD20+ B-cell lymphomas, and RA. Initial studies indicate that rituximab has substantial efficacy when combined with methotrexate for the treatment of patients with refractory RA. It is given intravenously as two infusions 2 weeks apart, with retreatment if necessary. This treatment protocol leads to prolonged depletion of peripheral blood B cells. Total serum immunoglobulin levels do not drop significantly, probably because these are maintained by long-lived plasma cells that do not express CD20. The mechanism by which B-cell depletion leads to clinical improvement in RA is not certain, but speculation focuses on the loss of B cells either as antigen-presenting cells or as the precursors for short-lived producers of critical autoantibodies.

Comorbidity

Optimal care of patients with RA requires recognition of the comorbid conditions that are associated with RA. These include increased risk of cardiovascular death, osteoporosis, infections (especially pneumonia), and certain cancers.

Cardiovascular disease is now recognized as the cause of much of the excess mortality in RA. Clinicians should consider RA a risk factor for cardiovascular disease and should aggressively seek and treat known cardiovascular risk factors in these patients. A number of factors probably contribute to the increased cardiovascular disease, but the recent appreciation of the strong association between chronic inflammation and cardiovascular disease points to the inflammatory nature of RA as the most significant factor. Accordingly, therapies that control RA earlier and better would be expected to decrease cardiovascular morbidity and mortality. Indeed, a recent study indicates that methotrexate decreases cardiovascular mortality by 70% in patients with RA.

Osteoporosis is ubiquitous in patients with RA, and early therapy directed at this problem will result in long-term benefits. Glucocorticoids, even at the low doses generally used for the treatment of RA, markedly exacerbate this problem.

Patients with RA are at an **increased risk for infections,** and this risk is further increased by some therapies. Patients should be cautioned to seek medical attention early for even minor symptoms suggestive of infection, especially if receiving anti-TNF therapy. All patients with RA should receive pneumococcal and yearly influenza vaccinations.

Finally, patients with RA have an increased risk of **lymphomas.** Occasionally, B-cell lymphomas may be associated with immunosuppression and regress after immunosuppression is discontinued. Interestingly, RA patients have a significantly decreased risk (odds ratio 0.2) of developing colon cancer. This is thought to be secondary to chronic inhibition of cyclooxygenase by NSAIDs in this group of patients.

Prognosis

The duration of disease prior to DMARD therapy may be one of the strongest predictors of outcome; therefore making the correct diagnosis quickly and instituting effective treatment are of critical importance. All current treatment paradigms for RA stress the early aggressive use of DMARDs.

REFERENCES

American College of Rheumatology Subcommittee on Rheumatoid Arthritis Guidelines. 2002 Update: guidelines for the management of rheumatoid arthritis. *Arthritis Rheum.* 2002;46:328. [PMID: 11840435] (State of the art guidelines for the treatment of rheumatoid arthritis as formulated by the American College of Rheumatology in 2002.)

Bathon JM, Martin RW, Fleischmann RM, et al. A comparison of etanercept and methotrexate in patients with early rheumatoid arthritis. *N Engl J Med.* 2000;343:1586. [PMID: 11096165] (An important article focusing on the use of biologicals in the treatment of early rheumatoid arthritis.)

Lipsky PE, van der Heijde DM, St Clair EW, et al. Infliximab and methotrexate in the treatment of rheumatoid arthritis. Anti-Tumor Necrosis Factor Trial in Rheumatoid Arthritis with Concomitant Therapy Study Group. *N Engl J Med.* 2000;343:1594. [PMID: 11096166] (An important article that focuses on the use of biologicals in the treatment of advanced rheumatoid arthritis.)

Moreland LW, O'Dell JR. Glucocorticoids and rheumatoid arthritis: back to the future? *Arthritis Rheum.* 2002;46:2553. [PMID: 12384910] (This article reviews the use of glucocorticoids in the treatment of rheumatoid arthritis from their initial use in 1949 to the current use. It also reviews toxicities and measures to help prevent these toxicities.)

O'Dell JR. Drug therapy: Therapeutic strategies for rheumatoid arthritis. *N Engl J Med.* 2004;350:2591. [PMID: 15201416] (The most recent review of therapy of RA.)

O'Dell JR, Haire CE, Erikson N, et al. Treatment of rheumatoid arthritis with methotrexate alone, sulfasalazine, and hydroxychloroquine, or a combination of all three medications. *N Engl J Med.* 1996;334:1287. [PMID: 8609945] (This is the classic initial paper that showed that combinations of DMARDs are superior to what had previously been the gold standard, methotrexate, in the treatment of patients with rheumatoid arthritis.)

O'Dell JR. Treating rheumatoid arthritis early: a window of opportunity. *Arthritis Rheum.* 2002;46:283. [PMID: 11840429] (This editorial summarizes the rationale for treating patients with rheumatoid arthritis early in their course of disease and discusses different approaches.)

Olsen NJ, Stein CM. New drugs for rheumatoid arthritis. N Engl J Med 2004;350:2167. [PMID: 15152062] (A great review of some of the newest drugs.)

Relevant World Wide Web Site

[American College of Rheumatology]
http://www.rheumatology.org

Ankylosing Spondylitis and the Arthritis of Inflammatory Bowel Disease

17

Jennifer D. Gorman, MD, MPH, & John B. Imboden, MD

THE SPONDYLOARTHROPATHIES

Ankylosing spondylitis is the prototype of the spondyloarthropathies, a group of inflammatory diseases that also includes reactive arthritis, psoriatic arthritis, and the arthritis associated with inflammatory bowel disease. In aggregate the spondyloarthropathies have a prevalence estimated between 0.5% and 1.9%. Their shared clinical features include arthritis of the axial skeleton (sacroiliac joints and spine), an oligoarticular arthritis of peripheral joints, and enthesitis (inflammation at sites where tendons, ligaments, and joint capsule insert onto bone). Inheritance of human leukocyte antigen (HLA)-B27 increases the relative risk of developing spondyloarthropathy, particularly when there is involvement of the axial skeleton. These diseases are not associated with rheumatoid factor and thus are often referred to as the "seronegative" spondyloarthropathies.

Although the spondyloarthropathies share a number of features, each one has distinct epidemiologic and clinical features that distinguish it from the others (Table 17–1) (see Chapters 18 and 19). Some patients, particularly those early in the disease course, cannot be clearly placed in one of these disease categories and are referred to as having "undifferentiated spondyloarthropathy." Many patients with an undifferentiated spondyloarthropathy eventually evolve into ankylosing spondylitis.

Enthesitis is a characteristic feature of spondyloarthropathy and is observed in only a few other inflammatory arthropathies (primarily gout, disseminated gonococcal infection, and sarcoidosis). Enthesitis is the hallmark of spondyloarthropathy in children (juvenile spondyloarthropathy; see Chapters 5 and 21), and in many cases the disease is limited to this manifestation. Dactylitis, the distinctive sausagelike swelling of a finger or toe, has increased specificity for psoriatic arthritis and reactive arthritis. The characteristic clinical appearance of dactylitis is caused by inflammation of the tendons, and in some cases, the adjacent synovium.

ANKYLOSING SPONDYLITIS

 ESSENTIALS OF DIAGNOSIS

- *Inflammatory back pain in young adults.*
- *Radiographic demonstration of sacroiliitis.*
- *Reductions in spinal mobility, particularly lumbar flexion.*
- *Association with anterior uveitis.*
- *Increased relative risk conferred by inheritance of HLA-B27.*
- *Positive family history.*

General Considerations

Axial skeletal involvement predominates in ankylosing spondylitis, which invariably involves the sacroiliac joints and typically presents with the insidious onset of inflammatory low back pain during late adolescence or early adulthood. Onset of symptoms after the age of 40 is uncommon.

Although environmental factors are important in the development of ankylosing spondylitis, the environmental triggers appear to be ubiquitous, and genetic background is the major determinant of susceptibility to ankylosing spondylitis. The only known susceptibility gene, HLA-B27, confers a relative risk of close to 100 but probably accounts for only 10–50% of the overall genetic risk for ankylosing spondylitis.

The disease course varies considerably, ranging from mild disease with little impact on functional status to severe disease that produces substantial disability. The extent of spinal involvement is a major determinant of the

Table 17–1. Clinical and Epidemiologic Features of the Spondyloarthropathies

	Ankylosing Spondylitis	Psoriatic Arthritis	Reactive Arthritis	Enteropathic Arthritis
Prevalence[a]	0.1%	0.1%	>0.05%	>0.05%
Male:female ratio	3:1	1:1	9:1	1:1
Axial arthritis 　Frequency 　Radiographic features 　　Sacroiliitis 　　Syndesmophytes	100% Bilateral Symmetric Marginal	20% Unilateral Asymmetric Bulky	20% Unilateral Asymmetric Bulky	15% Bilateral Symmetric Marginal
Peripheral arthritis 　Frequency 　Typical distribution 　Typical affected joints	25% Monarticular, 　oligoarticular Hip, knee, ankle	60–95% Oligoarticular, 　polyarticular Knee, ankle, DIPs	90% Monarticular, 　oligoarticular Knee, ankle	20% Monarticular, 　oligoarticular Knee, ankle
Uveitis frequency	30%	15%	15–20%	~ 5%
Dactylitis frequency	Uncommon	~ 25%	~ 30–50%	Uncommon
Cutaneous findings	None specific	Psoriasis Onycholysis Nail pitting	Oral ulcerations Keratoderma blennorrhagica	Erythema nodosum Pyoderma gangrenosa
HLA-B27 positivity[a] 　All cases 　With axial disease	 90% 90%	 40% 50%	 50–80% 90%	 30% 50%

[a]Disease prevalence and HLA-B27 positivity greatly vary according to geographic and race/ethnicity. DIPs, distal interphalangeal joints.

impact of the disease on functional status. Unfortunately, there are no reliable predictors of long-term functional outcome early in the disease course.

On average, 9 years elapse between the onset of symptoms and the diagnosis of ankylosing spondylitis. Several factors contribute to this delay: (1) The onset of low back symptoms is insidious, and patients may delay seeking medical attention. (2) Mechanical low back pain is prevalent, and patients with ankylosing spondylitis are often misdiagnosed as having that disorder. (3) It can be difficult to diagnose ankylosing spondylitis in its early stages. Radiographic evidence of bilateral sacroiliitis, which is the most definitive finding, usually takes several years to develop. (4) There are no diagnostic criteria for the disease. The widely used modified New York Criteria for the classification of ankylosing spondylitis require unequivocal radiographic evidence of sacroiliitis and have limited sensitivity for early disease.

Clinical Findings

A. SYMPTOMS AND SIGNS

1. Axial spine—The typical presenting symptom in ankylosing spondylitis is the insidious onset of inflammatory low back pain due to sacroiliitis. The pain is dull and located in the lower lumbar regions, although some describe a deep alternating buttock pain. The characteristic inflammatory nature of the pain differentiates it from mechanical back pain; most notably, the pain worsens with rest, improves with activity, and is accompanied by morning stiffness that lasts 30 minutes or longer. Patients often describe awakening from sleep and pacing in order to relieve nocturnal pain—a rare complaint in patients with mechanical back pain.

There may be few objective findings in patients with early disease, making diagnosis a challenge. Palpation and specific maneuvers can elicit pain in the sacroiliac joints, but these tests are relatively insensitive and nonspecific due to the number of other anatomic structures that overlap within the same area.

Involvement of the spine (spondylitis) is the major source of morbidity. Unlike rheumatoid arthritis, which only affects the cervical spine, ankylosing spondylitis can involve the lumbar, thoracic, and cervical spine. Over time the accumulation of pathologic changes can lead to loss of spinal mobility, particularly of the lumbar spine. The **Schober test** is the standard examination to assess impaired lumbar flexion. Two marks are made on the patient's back: one at the level of the sacral dimples (approximately at the fifth lumbar spinous process) and the other 10 cm above. The patient then bends forward as far as possible (ie, attempts to touch toes with knees extended), and the distance between the two marks is again measured. In normal individuals, the overlying skin will stretch to 15 cm; values less than this can be indicative of reduced lumbar mobility. Some physicians prefer the **modified Schober test** in which marks are made 5 cm below and 10 cm above the sacral dimples; the distance between these marks should increase from 15 cm to at least 20 cm with lumbar flexion. Reductions in lumbar lateral bending and rotation are also commonly observed. Spinal fusion results in irreversible impairments, but reductions in mobility also can be induced by pain or muscle spasm, and therefore vary somewhat with time and treatment. With advancing disease, a characteristic posture often develops as the spine fuses in flexion, leading to loss of lumbar lordosis, exaggeration of thoracic kyphosis, an inability to extend the neck, and compensatory hip flexion deformities (Figure 17–1A, 17–1B, and 17–1C). The extent of spondylitis varies greatly, from minimal to complete fusion of the cervical, thoracic, and lumbar spine.

Involvement of the costovertebral and costochondral joints commonly leads to impaired chest expansion (<5 cm difference between full inspiration and full expiration when measured at the fourth intercostal space) and occasionally produces pain with deep breathing, coughing, or sneezing. Restriction in chest wall motion commonly produces reliance on diaphragmatic breathing and mild impairment of pulmonary function; characteristic spirometry findings include a slight reduction of vital and total lung capacity and normal diffusion capacity. Most patients, however, are asymptomatic, and clinically significant pulmonary disease is uncommon.

2. Peripheral joint manifestations—Peripheral arthritis, typically monarticular or asymmetric oligoarticular, develops in approximately one-third of patients with ankylosing spondylitis and most often affects large joints of the lower extremities. Hip disease develops in approximately 50% of patients and is a major source of morbidity.

3. Enthesitis—Involvement of insertion sites around the pelvis (the ischial tuberosities, iliac crests, and greater trochanters) is common and appears on radiographs as bony "whiskering" at these sites of attachment. Achilles tendinitis and enthesitis at the site of the insertion of the plantar fascia onto the calcaneus can cause unilateral or bilateral heel pain, although not as often as in reactive arthritis.

4. Ocular—The most common extra-articular manifestation of ankylosing spondylitis is acute anterior uveitis, and one-third of patients experience at least 1 episode. It is heralded by the acute or subacute onset of unilateral eye pain, photophobia, blurred vision, and increased lacrimation. Ciliary flush (an increased conjunctival injection at the rim of the iris) is a characteristic finding. The presence of cells and flare in the anterior uveal chamber detected by slitlamp examination establishes the diagnosis. The need for specialized equipment and expertise necessitates prompt ophthalmologic consultation when this diagnosis is suspected. Anterior uveitis can precede the onset of ankylosing spondylitis by several years, and a history of anterior uveitis is a helpful diagnostic clue in a patient with inflammatory back pain or other symptoms of ankylosing spondylitis. Anterior uveitis is strongly associated with HLA-B27.

5. Osteoporosis—Spinal immobility and persistent inflammation are believed to contribute to the increased prevalence of osteoporosis in ankylosing spondylitis and other spondyloarthropathies. However, the formation of syndesmophytes in these diseases creates a unique problem in evaluation of bone mineral density. For example, in an ankylosed spine with paravertebral calcification, anteroposterior measurement of bone density by dual energy x-ray absorptiometry can lead to spuriously increased values for bone mineral density of the spine.

6. Other organs—The majority of patients with ankylosing spondylitis have histologic evidence of inflammation on biopsy specimens of the small or large bowel. These changes are asymptomatic but may be of pathogenetic importance in view of the link between clinically overt inflammatory bowel disease and spondyloarthropathy and the apparent importance of colitis in the transgenic rat model of HLA-B27–associated disease.

Cardiac involvement in the form of ascending aortitis, aortic regurgitation, conduction abnormalities, and myocardial disease occurs in approximately 10% of patients with ankylosing spondylitis, and like uveitis and axial disease, is strongly associated with HLA-B27. The prevalence of aortic regurgitation, which is the most common

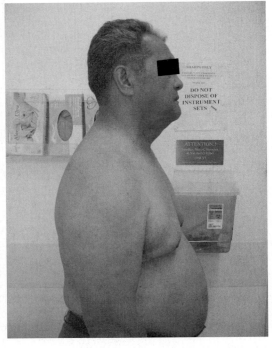

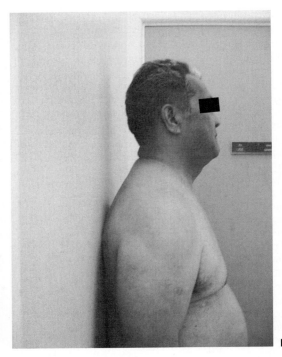

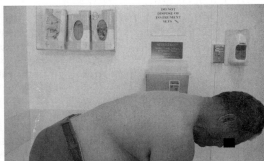

Figure 17–1. Long-standing ankylosing spondylitis. Despite extensive spinal involvement the patient has maintained an upright posture with only a slightly exaggerated thoracic kyphosis (A). The occiput-to-wall test, however, reveals marked reduction of cervical extension (B). Fusion of the lumbar spine causes straightening of the lower back and an inability to reverse the lumbar lordosis when the patient attempts to touch his toes with knees extended (C). (Courtesy of Dr. Lianne S. Wener, University of California, San Francisco.)

cardiac problem, increases with the duration of disease but remains <10% even after 30 years of disease.

A rare pulmonary finding in ankylosing spondylitis is the development of apical fibrobullous disease that radiographically resembles reactivation of tuberculosis and that can become a site for bacterial or fungal infections.

Of the neurologic consequences of spondyloarthritis, the most important is spinal fracture, which often goes unrecognized and leads to neurologic compromise in about one-third of cases (see the following section on Complications). Cauda equina syndrome can develop in long-standing ankylosing spondylitis and is associated with large subarachnoid diverticula on magnetic resonance imaging.

Rare manifestations of the spondyloarthropathies include the late development of secondary amyloidosis. An association of ankylosing spondylitis with retroperitoneal fibrosis has been suggested.

B. LABORATORY FINDINGS

1. Routine studies—No laboratory test is diagnostic of ankylosing spondylitis or the other spondyloarthropathies. Routine laboratory investigations often reveal a mild, normocytic, normochromic anemia, reflective of chronic disease. Only about half of patients with active disease will have elevations of the erythrocyte sedimentation rate or C-reactive protein. These inflammatory markers appear to correlate more with peripheral arthritis than the activity of axial skeleton disease. There is no association with rheumatoid factor, antibodies to cyclic citrullinated peptides, or antinuclear antibodies.

2. Testing for HLA-B27—Inheritance of HLA-B27 is strongly associated with ankylosing spondylitis. Under certain conditions, testing for HLA-B27 can be useful in clinical practice. For example, testing for HLA-B27 may be helpful early in the disease course prior to the development of definite sacroiliitis on radiographs. In general, HLA-B27 testing should be ordered when the diagnosis is suggested by the presence of inflammatory back pain but remains uncertain after appropriate clinical evaluation and radiographs. When used in these circumstances, the test results can substantially increase or reduce the probability of disease (but do not definitively establish or exclude the diagnosis).

Several facts should inform the use and the interpretation of the HLA-B27 test. First, inheritance of HLA-B27 is not sufficient to produce ankylosing spondylitis. The great majority of HLA-B27–positive persons (95% in some studies) do not have ankylosing spondylitis (or any other spondyloarthropathy); indiscriminant testing for HLA-B27 will produce many more false-positive tests than true-positives. Second, inheritance of HLA-B27 is not absolutely essential for the development of ankylosing spondylitis. Third, although HLA-B27 confers an increased relative risk of ankylosing spondylitis in most ethnic groups studied, ethnicity influences the prevalence of HLA-B27 in disease populations. For example, HLA-B27 is present in 8% of the general white population, and 90% of whites with ankylosing spondylitis are HLA-B27–positive. In contrast, HLA-B27 is present in 2% of the African American population and only 50% of African Americans with ankylosing spondylitis are HLA-B27–positive. Therefore, in a patient with symptoms suggestive of ankylosing spondylitis, the absence of HLA-B27 substantially decreases the probability of disease if the patient is white, but not if the patient is African American.

C. IMAGING STUDIES

The inflammatory disease of the axial spine results in characteristic pathologic changes; however, it may take years before these become evident by plain radiographic techniques.

1. Sacroiliac joints—The most distinctive finding is inflammation of both sacroiliac joints. A standard anteroposterior radiograph of the pelvis is commonly used to evaluate these S-shaped joints, although some believe a superior image is achieved with the Ferguson view, in which the radiograph is taken at a 15-degree angle to the prone pelvis.

The first radiographic finding is the appearance of iliac erosions, described as resembling postage stamp serra-

tions, in the lower one-third of the sacroiliac joint. With time, the erosions become more prominent and produce "pseudowidening" of the sacroiliac joint. Progressive inflammation leads to fusion, and the end result can be complete obliteration of the sacroiliac joint by bone and fibrous tissue. The pattern of sacroiliac joint involvement is bilaterally symmetric in ankylosing spondylitis and enteropathic arthritis, in contrast to the unilateral changes observed in early psoriatic and reactive arthritis. In the latter diseases, the progressive joint changes can become bilateral with time but usually remain asymmetrical.

The superior technique for diagnosing early axial inflammation is by magnetic resonance imaging with gadolinium-DPTA or fat suppression. This method is the most sensitive and specific for the diagnosis of sacroiliitis and also avoids exposure to pelvic radiation (substantial with computed tomography of the sacroiliac joints), making it particularly advantageous in the assessment of women of childbearing age and children. Magnetic resonance imaging allows for visualization of acute sacroiliitis, spondylitis, and spondylodiscitis, and can also detect acute inflammation of the entheses, bone, and synovium. The ability to detect early inflammation and accurately visualize cartilaginous and enthesal lesions makes magnetic resonance imaging a useful assessment tool in the spondyloarthropathies.

In clinical practice, a reasonable initial evaluation of patients with symptoms of inflammatory back pain is to obtain a plain radiograph of the pelvis. If this study fails to demonstrate sacroiliitis, then magnetic resonance imaging should be considered, particularly if the patient is HLA-B27–positive.

2. Spine—A subtle radiographic change observed relatively early in the course of spondylitis is the appearance of vertebral "shiny corners." Also referred to as Romanus lesions, these are a reaction to inflammation at the site where the annulus fibrosus of the disks inserts onto the vertebral bodies. With progressive erosions and formation of new periosteal bone, the lumbar vertebral bodies become "squared off" in the lateral view.

The most characteristic finding is the formation of syndesmophytes—bony bridges between vertebral bodies due to gradual ossification of the edges of the annulus fibrosus. The vertical orientation of syndesmophytes and preservation of the disk space distinguish these from osteophytes associated with degenerative disease of the spine. The morphology and symmetry of syndesmophytes can help distinguish among the spondyloarthropathies. Ankylosing spondylitis and enteropathic arthritis exhibit symmetric delicate-appearing syndesmophytes that are marginal, meaning that they are almost completely vertical in their alignment and arise from the margins of the vertebral body. In contrast, psoriatic arthritis and reactive arthritis typically have more bulky, asymmetric bony growths that tend to initially protrude laterally before progressing vertically (nonmarginal syndesmophytes).

3. Peripheral joints—Radiographic changes in the peripheral joints mainly result from disease of the synovium or entheses. Hip involvement can produce symmetric narrowing of the joint space. Enthesitis can result in a faint periosteal reaction at bony prominences, such as the greater trochanters, calcaneus, and malleoli.

Differential Diagnosis

The diagnosis of ankylosing spondylitis usually rests on the combination of inflammatory back pain and radiographic evidence of bilateral sacroiliitis. The bilateral nature of the sacroiliitis, the prominence of axial skeleton involvement, and the absence of mucocutaneous disease help distinguish ankylosing spondylitis from reactive arthritis and psoriatic arthritis. The presence of bowel symptoms in a patient with "ankylosing spondylitis" should prompt a search for inflammatory bowel disease. The sacroiliitis and spondylitis of inflammatory bowel disease are radiographically indistinguishable from ankylosing spondylitis.

Inflammatory sacroiliac joint disease is not limited to the spondyloarthropathies, and a number of disease processes can cause radiographic sacroiliac changes (Table 17–2). Degenerative disease of the sacroiliac joints does occur, although its radiographic appearance is distinct from the inflammatory changes of the spondyloarthritides. Osteitis condensans ilii is a condition seen in multiparous women and radiographically manifests as a characteristic triangle of ilial sclerosis adjacent to the sacroiliac joint. The sacroiliac joint itself is normal, and patients are usually asymptomatic.

Sacroiliac erosions from prolonged hyperparathyroidism, such as that induced by chronic renal failure, can mimic ankylosing spondylitis. Other causes of sacroiliac erosions include familial Mediterranean fever, Whipple and Paget disease, and rarely, paraplegia. Whether Behçet disease is associated with sacroiliitis is still debated. Infections with a particular tropism for the sacroiliac joints include tuberculosis and brucellosis. However, infection with more typical organisms is also described, such as *Staphylococcus aureus,* particularly in injecting drug users. In rare instances, the sacroiliac joint and surrounding structures are the site for primary malignancies or metastatic lesions.

The flowing ligamentous calcifications of diffuse idiopathic skeletal hyperostosis can mimic syndesmophytes and can be a source of diagnostic confusion. In diffuse idiopathic skeletal hyperostosis, however, the sacroiliac joints should appear normal. Symptomatically, the dis-

Table 17–2. Differential Diagnosis of the Spondyloarthropathies

Sacroiliac abnormalities	
Sacroiliitis	Hyperparathyroidism
	Familial Mediterranean fever
	Whipple disease
	Paget disease
	Paraplegia
	Behçet disease
	Tuberculosis
	Brucellosis
	Pyogenic sacroiliitis
	Malignancy
	Retinoid treatment
	SAPHO syndrome
Other changes	Degenerative joint disease
	Osteitis condensans ilii
	Chondrocalcinosis
	Gout
Vertebral hyperostosis	DISH
	Ochronosis
	SAPHO syndrome
	Retinoid treatment
Enthesopathy	Gout
	Disseminated gonococcal infection
	SAPHO syndrome
	Retinoid treatment
	BCG-induced

SAPHO, synovitis-acne-pustulosis-hyperostosis-osteitis; DISH, diffuse idiopathic skeletal hyperostosis; BCG, bacillus Calmette-Guérin.

eases are easily differentiated because diffuse idiopathic skeletal hyperostosis patients lack inflammatory back pain.

Ochronosis can cause calcification of vertebral disk spaces and bony bridging that can mimic marginal syndesmophytes. In some cases, sacroiliac involvement is also observed, complicating diagnosis. The SAPHO (synovitis-acne-pustulosis-hyperostosis-osteitis) syndrome has sometimes been considered a spondyloarthropathy due to the frequency of sacroiliitis, enthesopathies, and oligoarticular peripheral arthritis. In addition, bony hyperostosis can be induced by retinoid treatment.

Treatment

The goals of therapy are to reduce inflammation and pain and to improve function, mobility, and strength. Best results are achieved by a multidisciplinary treatment approach, with physical therapy being an essential adjunct to pharmacologic methods. In general, patients should be advised to be aware of their posture and to avoid maintaining a flexed spine. For example, the height of work surfaces should be adjusted to avoid prolonged leaning over or slouching.

A. NONSTEROIDAL ANTI-INFLAMMATORY DRUGS

Nonsteroidal anti-inflammatory drugs (NSAIDs) reduce pain and stiffness for most patients. Although many patients require additional pharmacologic agents, NSAIDs remain the cornerstone of initial therapy. As in other rheumatic diseases, there can be a wide individual variation in response to a given NSAID, and it is reasonable to try several NSAIDs sequentially if the response is suboptimal.

Because of the considerable toxicity of chronic NSAID use and because these agents were not considered to be disease-modifying, most physicians used NSAIDs intermittently for symptom relief. A recent randomized control trial, however, demonstrated that continuous treatment with NSAIDs for 2 years significantly reduces radiographic progression.

B. ANTI–TUMOR NECROSIS FACTOR AGENTS

The anti–tumor necrosis factor (TNF) agents, etanercept and infliximab, are the most potent of the currently available therapies. Prospective controlled trials have established that these produce impressive improvements in symptoms, function, and markers of inflammation, and the FDA has approved both for use in ankylosing spondylitis. Responses generally occur within weeks and are durable, but disease activity usually recurs when the anti-TNF agent is discontinued. Preliminary results with relatively small numbers of patients suggest that anti-TNF agents may slow radiographic progression of the spinal disease.

Current treatment guidelines, based solely on expert opinion, recommend anti-TNF agents for patients who have a definite diagnosis of ankylosing spondylitis, have active disease, and have failed adequate therapeutic trials with at least two NSAIDs.

C. DISEASE-MODIFYING ANTIRHEUMATIC DRUGS

Despite their effectiveness for rheumatoid arthritis, disease-modifying antirheumatic drugs have limited usefulness in the treatment of ankylosing spondylitis.

Sulfasalazine has modest efficacy in treating the peripheral arthritis of ankylosing spondylitis. It does not appear to be effective for chronic disease of the axial skeleton, but may be of benefit if used early in the course of axial disease. The typical therapeutic dose is 2–3 g daily in divided doses.

Methotrexate is sometimes used, but the rationale for this stems from its efficacy in rheumatoid arthritis, not on evidence of effectiveness in ankylosing spondylitis.

A recent controlled study found no benefit of low-dose methotrexate (7.5 mg weekly) relative to placebo.

D. PAMIDRONATE

A single double-blind study indicated that pamidronate, administered as a monthly 60-mg intravenous dose for 6 months, reduces disease activity. There was no significant effect on the erythrocyte sedimentation rate or the level of C-reactive protein. Acute arthralgia, myalgia, and fever after the first infusion are not uncommon, but reactions are generally mild and usually decrease with continued treatment.

E. OTHER PHARMACOLOGIC THERAPIES

Systemic glucocorticoids are not commonly used and can worsen osteopenia. In certain cases, intra-articular glucocorticoid injection into the sacroiliac joint can provide short-term symptomatic relief. However, the anatomy of the joint is extremely complicated, and radiographic guidance for this procedure is required.

F. SURGICAL THERAPY

The deformities that result from extensive disease of the spine can lead to disabling decreases in the field of vision and ambulation. Corrective surgeries of spinal alignment, however, are major procedures and have limited indications. Typically, osteotomy with fixation is performed, with corrections of the lumbar spine being most common. The risks of neurologic complications and perioperative mortality are not insignificant with these procedures.

Hip involvement requires artificial replacement in approximately 5% of patients with ankylosing spondylitis. The outcome of total hip arthroplasty is good, with long-term joint survival of 60% at 20 years. The occurrence of postoperative heterotopic bone formation is increased in those undergoing repeat hip surgery and those with more spinal ankylosis.

Complications

A. SPINAL FRACTURES

The fused, osteopenic spine of ankylosing spondylitis is at great risk for fracture, which can be precipitated by such minor trauma as insignificant falls, sneezing, or manual manipulation of the spine. The most common sites of fracture are the thoracolumbar and cervicothoracic junctions. Although cervical fractures may result immediately in quadriplegia or death, the symptoms of spinal fracture are often subtle and include new, localized back or neck pain, and in some cases, the description of recently increased spinal mobility. Many fractures are not acutely identified, in part because of the absence of preceding significant trauma and the failure to recognize a change in the characteristics of the back pain. Plain radiographs are relatively insensitive and fail to identify many spinal fractures, especially in the acute setting. Magnetic resonance imaging is the preferred technique when plain radiographs are unrevealing. Depending on the fracture site, the degree of instability, and the neurologic status, treatment may require early surgical stabilization.

B. INTUBATION RISK

Because of the ability to manually fracture the ankylosed spine, particularly in patients with altered mental status, preoperative assessment for patients with significant axial disease is essential before surgical procedures requiring general anesthesia. Specifically, since damage to the spine and spinal cord can result from endotracheal intubation, the need for awake fiberoptic intubation should be considered in appropriate situations.

C. ANTERIOR UVEITIS

Most uveitis associated with the ankylosing spondylitis can be effectively treated with topical glucocorticoids and mydriatics. However, the diagnosis requires specialized evaluation, and prompt referral to an ophthalmologist is required. In addition, some cases require more aggressive therapy, such as direct injection of glucocorticoid agents into the affected area, requiring professional expertise.

D. RISKS OF PRIOR RADIATION THERAPY

Spinal irradiation for the treatment of ankylosing spondylitis was widely performed from the early 1920s until the last few decades, but is no longer used because of the unacceptable long-term morbidity and mortality. Patients previously treated with spinal irradiation have an increase in cancer, specifically myeloid leukemias and other hematologic malignancies. Questions regarding previous therapeutic radiation should be included in a complete past medical history of patients with longstanding ankylosing spondylitis.

ENTEROPATHIC ARTHRITIS

Enteropathic arthritis, which develops in approximately 20% of patients with either Crohn disease or ulcerative colitis, has two forms: (1) a peripheral arthritis whose activity generally correlates with the activity of the inflammatory bowel disease, and (2) arthritis of the axial skeleton whose activity is independent of the bowel disease. The peripheral arthritis can take the form of either migratory arthralgias or an asymmetric oligoarthritis of the lower extremities. Erythema nodosum and pyoderma gangrenosa sometimes occur coincident with peripheral arthritis. Involvement of the axial skeleton is clinically and radiographically indistinguishable from that of ankylosing spondylitis.

Treatment of the underlying inflammatory bowel disease can ameliorate peripheral arthritis. Sulfasalazine appears to be effective for peripheral arthritis. There is some evidence that NSAIDs can induce gastrointestinal flares of inflammatory bowel disease; therefore their use in treating enteropathic arthritis should be considered on a case-by-case basis. Small uncontrolled studies report that infliximab, which is approved for use in the treatment of Crohn disease, is beneficial for both peripheral arthritis and arthritis of the axial skeleton.

REFERENCES

Braun J, Pham T, Sieper J, et al. International ASAS consensus statement for the use of anti-tumour necrosis factor agents in patients with ankylosing spondylitis. *Ann Rheum Dis.* 2003;62:817. [PMID: 12922952]

Rudwaleit M, van der Heijde D, Khan MA, Braun J, Sieper J. How to diagnose axial spondyloarthritis early. *Ann Rheum Dis.* 2004;63:535. [PMID: 15082484]

van der Heijde D, Dijkmans B, Geusens P, et al. Efficacy and safety of infliximab in patients with ankylosing spondylitis: results of a randomized, placebo-controlled trial (ASSERT). *Arthritis Rheum.* 2005;52:582. [PMID: 15692973]

Wanders A, Heijde D, Landewe R, et al. Nonsteroidal antiinflammatory drugs reduce radiographic progression in patients with ankylosing spondylitis: a randomized clinical trial. *Arthritis Rheum.* 2005 52:1756. [PMID: 15934081]

Relevant World Wide Web Sites

[The Spondylitis Association of America]
  http://www.spondylitis.org

[National Ankylosing Spondylitis Society]
  http://www.nass.co.uk

[British Society for Rheumatology guidelines for prescribing TNF blockers in ankylosing spondylitis]
  http://www.rheumatology.org.uk/guidelines/clinicalguidelines

Reactive Arthritis

Gordon K. Lam, MD, & Clifton O. Bingham III, MD

ESSENTIALS OF DIAGNOSIS

- *Inflammatory arthritis triggered by antecedent gastrointestinal or genitourinary infections.*
- *Asymmetric oligoarthritis most commonly affecting the lower extremities.*
- *Enthesitis and dactylitis.*
- *Association with extra-articular manifestations such as conjunctivitis, anterior uveitis, urethritis, circinate balanitis, oral ulcers, and keratoderma blennorrhagicum.*

General Considerations

Reactive arthritis is a systemic inflammatory condition that is triggered by bacterial infections of the gastrointestinal or genitourinary tracts. Despite the link with infection, cultures of synovial fluid are sterile, and there is no established role for antibiotics. Reactive arthritis is one of the spondyloarthropathies, a group of diseases that also includes psoriatic arthritis, ankylosing spondylitis, and enteropathic arthritis associated with inflammatory bowel disease. Inflammatory oligoarthritis of peripheral joints, arthritis of the axial skeleton (spine and sacroiliac joints), and enthesitis (inflammation of the insertion sites of tendons, ligaments, and fascia to bone) are shared characteristics of the spondyloarthropathies.

"Reactive arthritis" should replace the term "Reiter syndrome," which refers to the triad of reactive arthritis, conjunctivitis, and urethritis. "Reiter syndrome" is confusing because many patients with reactive arthritis do not have all components of the triad. Recent revelations concerning Reiter's involvement in war crimes during World War II provide an additional reason to avoid this eponym.

Reactive arthritis typically develops 1–4 weeks after a bout of gastroenteritis caused by *Shigella, Salmonella, Campylobacter,* or *Yersinia,* or after a genitourinary tract infection with *Chlamydia trachomatis.* Recent reports indicate that enteric infections with *Clostridium difficile* also can trigger reactive arthritis. Most cases are sporadic, but reactive arthritis also can occur in clusters following outbreaks of gastroenteritis. Sometimes there is no antecedent history of infection, suggesting that reactive arthritis can follow subclinical infections or that other environmental triggers are at play. Reactive arthritis usually develops in young adults between 20 and 40 years of age. *Chlamydia*-induced disease is more common in men; men and women are at equal risk to develop postenteric disease. The annual incidence of reactive arthritis is estimated to be approximately 30–40 per 100,000.

Genetic factors have a role in susceptibility to reactive arthritis. Human leukocyte antigen (HLA)-B27 is linked to reactive arthritis, but the strength of the association is not as robust as that seen between HLA-B27 and ankylosing spondylitis. The prevalence of HLA-B27 in series of reactive arthritis ranges from 50–80%, with the higher figures generally seen in cohorts with persistent disease. The incidence of reactive arthritis tends to reflect the prevalence of HLA-B27 in populations; in the United States, therefore, reactive arthritis is more common in Caucasians (8% of whom have HLA-B27) than in African Americans, who have a far lower frequency of HLA-B27. A notable exception to the link between reactive arthritis and HLA-B27 is in sub-Saharan Africa, where an aggressive form of reactive arthritis occurs in HLA-B27–negative individuals who are infected with human immunodeficiency virus.

The course of reactive arthritis varies considerably. Mild conjunctivitis and urethritis, which can be due either to infection with *Chlamydia* or to mucosal inflammation in cases induced by enteric infection, may precede the onset of arthritis. The arthritis is often low grade but can be severe and accompanied by significant weight loss, fever, and other constitutional symptoms. Enthesitis is often a prominent manifestation. Reactive arthritis can consist of a single attack that runs its course within a matter of months. Alternatively, patients may experience self-limited attacks, lasting weeks to months, that recur for years after the onset of initial symptoms. A chronic, destructive, and disabling arthritis evolves in a minority of patients. Unfortunately, there are no reliable predictors of long-term outcomes. Reactive arthritis generally has less long-term morbidity and mortality than rheumatoid arthritis.

Clinical Findings

A. SIGNS AND SYMPTOMS

1. Articular manifestations—The dominant manifestation of reactive arthritis is a peripheral arthritis that usually develops in an asymmetric and oligoarticular fashion. The affected joints are usually swollen, warm, and tender to palpation; range of motion movement often causes discomfort. The joints of the lower extremities (eg, knees, ankles, and feet) are more commonly affected than the joints of the upper extremities. The sternoclavicular and temporomandibular joints are sometimes involved.

Axial skeleton disease most commonly manifests as inflammatory low back pain, which occurs in up to half of patients with reactive arthritis. Approximately 20–25% of patients develop radiographic evidence of sacroiliitis, which is often unilateral, and if bilateral, is asymmetric and thus distinct from the bilateral, symmetric sacroiliitis of ankylosing spondylitis. A minority of those with sacroiliitis have spondylitis as well; extensive fusion of the spine resembling severe ankylosing spondylitis can develop but is uncommon. The prevalence of axial skeleton disease is greater among those with chronic disease and those with HLA-B27 (90% of patients with radiographic evidence of sacroiliitis are HLA-B27–positive).

2. Enthesitis—Inflammation of the sites where fascia, tendons, and ligaments attach to bone, or enthesitis, is usually a prominent feature of reactive arthritis. The most common manifestation is heel pain due to inflammation where the Achilles tendon inserts onto the calcaneus. In addition, some symptoms of low back pain may be due to enthesitis involving the pelvic girdle. Findings of enthesitis include swelling of the involved tendon or ligament with overlying warmth and tenderness to palpation.

3. Dactylitis—The combination of synovitis and enthesitis in a toe or finger can cause the entire digit to become diffusely swollen, producing dactylitis or "sausage digit." Dactylitis is a feature of the spondyloarthropathies, particularly reactive arthritis and psoriatic arthritis, but not of rheumatoid arthritis. Dactylitis involves the toes more commonly than the fingers.

4. Mucocutaneous lesions—Circinate balanitis is an inflammatory lesion on the glans or shaft of the penis, and it is one of the characteristic lesions associated with reactive arthritis. If the male is circumcised, these lesions can appear as multiple, serpiginous, shallow ulcers with raised borders. In uncircumcised males, the lesions can appear as dry, hyperkeratotic plaques that are reminiscent of psoriasis.

Urethritis can be a consequence of infection with *Chlamydia* but also can be a manifestation of mucosal inflammation in cases of reactive arthritis triggered by enteric infection. Prostatitis is common.

Another cutaneous lesion associated with reactive arthritis is keratoderma blennorrhagicum, a skin rash that typically affects the palms and soles and is best described as papular, waxy lesions which can evolve into scaly, hyperkeratotic lesions resembling psoriasis. These lesions can coalesce to cover large areas of skin, extending proximally beyond the palms and soles of the feet. Keratoderma blennorrhagicum cannot be distinguished histologically from pustular psoriasis.

Aphthous ulcerations can form in patients with reactive arthritis. These lesions are often painless and develop along the oral or genital mucosa.

As occurs in psoriatic arthritis, nails can become thickened and develop subungual debris and onychodystrophy. Pitting, however, does not occur. The clinical appearance is similar to onychomycosis, and often the two are confused.

5. Ocular inflammation—Conjunctivitis is common, particularly early in disease, and is usually mild and self-limited. Uveitis occurs in up to one-fourth of cases and mainly affects the iris and ciliary body (anterior uveitis) (see Chapter 61). Uveitis causes photophobia and ocular pain and can lead to visual impairment if not recognized and treated appropriately. Scleral injection is often, but not always, present. Diagnosis requires slitlamp examination, which reveals the presence of inflammatory cells and protein exudate in the anterior chamber. Attacks of uveitis are usually monocular, last weeks to months, and tend to recur (in either eye). Virtually all patients with reactive arthritis and uveitis are HLA-B27–positive.

6. Cardiovascular involvement—Inflammation of the interventricular septum can affect the atrioventricular node, resulting in varying degrees of heart block. Aortitis is an uncommon manifestation of long-standing reactive arthritis. Inflammation of the aortic root and aortic valve can lead to aortic valve regurgitation.

B. LABORATORY FINDINGS

A mild normocytic normochromic anemia, modest leukocytosis, thrombocytosis, and polyclonal elevations of serum immunoglobulins can accompany active disease. Acute phase reactants such as C-reactive protein and erythrocyte sedimentation rate are often elevated during attacks.

There are no serologic tests diagnostic for reactive arthritis. Rheumatoid factor, antibodies to cyclic citrullinated peptides, and antinuclear antibodies are typically negative.

Arthrocentesis reveals inflammatory synovial fluid with cell counts usually in the range of 2000–50,000 white blood cells per cubic millimeter and a predominance of neutrophils. Cultures of the synovial fluid are sterile, and no organisms are seen on Gram stain.

The inciting organism can be detected in approximately 50% of patients with suspected *Chlamydia*-induced reactive arthritis; ligase reactions on the first-voided urine are probably the single best test. In contrast, stool cultures are usually negative when cases of post-enteric reactive arthritis present. Serologic tests for antibodies against *Salmonella, Yersinia,* and *Campylobacter* may be helpful, but these are not well-standardized and are not universally available. There are no reliable serologic tests for infection with *Shigella.*

Testing for HLA-B27 can provide supportive evidence for the diagnosis under certain circumstances but is generally of limited value. The sensitivity and specificity of the test are not well-established, particularly for early disease when a test is most likely to be of value, and are influenced by the differential expression of HLA-B27 in ethnic groups.

C. IMAGING STUDIES

The hallmark radiographic finding is bony reaction at sites of inflammation. Fluffy periostitis develops where there is enthesitis, such as the insertions of the plantar fascia and the Achilles tendon onto the calcaneus. Reactive arthritis can produce articular erosions associated with periosteal reactions ("proliferative erosions"). Periostitis can be seen along the shafts of the small bones of the hands and feet. Osteolytic destruction and bony fusion of joints may also occur, although these changes are more characteristic of psoriatic arthritis (see Figure 19–2). Radiographic evidence of sacroiliitis can be seen in patients who have axial skeleton disease. The sacroiliitis of reactive arthritis is usually unilateral, and if bilateral, is asymmetric—in contrast to the bilateral, symmetric sacroiliitis seen in ankylosing spondylitis. Syndesmophytes (abnormal bony bridges between vertebrae) may develop. The syndesmophytes of reactive arthritis are bulky, asymmetric, and tend to protrude laterally before progressing vertically, whereas the syndesmophytes of ankylosing spondylitis are symmetric, delicate, and vertical.

Differential Diagnosis

The diagnosis of reactive arthritis is based on the clinical presentation and the exclusion of alternative explanations for an inflammatory oligoarthritis.

With early disease it is critical to exclude infectious causes of arthritis. Disseminated gonococcal infection (DGI) can be difficult to differentiate from acute-onset reactive arthritis because oligoarthritis, tenosynovitis, and fever can occur in both diseases. The synovial fluid white blood cell count in DGI is usually within the range seen in reactive arthritis. Synovial fluid cultures, moreover, are sterile in >50% of cases of DGI, and therefore do not distinguish reactive arthritis from DGI.

Urethral, pharyngeal, cervical, and rectal swabs for gonococci, however, have a combined sensitivity of 70–90% in DGI. Occasionally a therapeutic trial of antibiotics is necessary to make this diagnostic distinction; a prompt response to appropriate antibiotic therapy points to a diagnosis of DGI.

Nongonococcal septic arthritis can be oligoarticular and occasionally mimics reactive arthritis; synovial fluid cultures are usually positive, underscoring the importance of diagnostic arthrocentesis in cases of unexplained acute oligoarthritis. Bacterial endocarditis can produce an oligoarthritis due to either direct infection (with positive synovial fluid cultures) or immune complexes (with sterile synovial cultures); back pain is common, especially with acute endocarditis. Acute viral infections, such as parvovirus B19, usually cause an acute polyarthritis, but occasionally the arthritis involves only a few joints. An antecedent sore throat suggests poststreptococcal arthritis, which in adults usually is additive and is not associated with the extra-articular manifestations of acute rheumatic fever.

Occasionally rheumatoid arthritis begins as an oligoarthritis and causes some diagnostic confusion with reactive arthritis. The presence of antibodies to cyclic citrullinated peptides predicts evolution to rheumatoid arthritis, but testing for these antibodies has only about 50% sensitivity for early rheumatoid arthritis. Inflammatory low back pain and dactylitis are not features of rheumatoid arthritis. Dactylitis can be a helpful clue to the presence of a spondyloarthropathy (particularly reactive arthritis or psoriatic arthritis) but also can be seen in gout and sarcoidosis. Gout and pseudogout can cause an acute oligoarthritis; examination of synovial fluid is usually diagnostic.

Reactive arthritis, psoriatic arthritis, ankylosing spondylitis, and the arthritis associated with inflammatory bowel disease share many clinical features, and it may not be possible to distinguish among these, particularly in the early phases, leading to a diagnosis of undifferentiated spondyloarthropathy.

Treatment

A. NONSTEROIDAL ANTI-INFLAMMATORY DRUGS AND GLUCOCORTICOIDS

Nonsteroidal anti-inflammatory drugs form the cornerstone of treatment for reactive arthritis. Often prescription-strength doses (eg, ibuprofen 600–800 mg PO every 8 hours) are needed for appropriate anti-inflammatory and analgesic effects. Intra-articular injections of glucocorticoids can be effective for symptoms of inflammatory arthritis. There have been no systematic studies of oral glucocorticoids in reactive arthritis, but some rheumatologists advocate short courses of oral glucocorticoids in moderate doses (eg, prednisone 30–40 mg daily).

B. ANTIBIOTICS

Appropriate antibiotic therapy should be administered if there is active chlamydial infection (active enteric infection is uncommon). There is little evidence that the antibiotic itself curbs the symptoms of reactive arthritis, and the long-term use of antibiotics is probably not of value.

C. DISEASE-MODIFYING ANTIRHEUMATIC DRUGS

Sulfasalazine may be of modest benefit for peripheral arthritis. There are no clinical trials on the use of disease-modifying antirheumatic drugs like methotrexate or azathioprine, but these agents are sometimes used for patients with chronic disease refractory to nonsteroidal anti-inflammatory drugs. Inhibitors of tumor necrosis factor are effective in ankylosing spondylitis and psoriatic arthritis, but their efficacy in reactive arthritis has not been determined.

Prognosis

The prognosis of reactive arthritis is generally good. Even patients who experience severe disease at onset may have complete recovery, although recurrences are frequent and can occur for years after the initial episode.

REFERENCES

Flores D, Marquez J, Garza M, Espinoza LR. Reactive arthritis: newer developments. *Rheum Dis Clin North Am.* 2003;29:37.

Leirisalo-Repo M. Reactive arthritis. *Scand J Rheumatol.* 2005; 34:251.

Toivanen A, Toivanen P. Reactive arthritis. *Best Pract Res Clin Rheumatol.* 2004;18:689.

Psoriatic Arthritis

19

Gordon K. Lam, MD, & Clifton O. Bingham III, MD

ESSENTIALS OF DIAGNOSIS

- *Inflammatory arthritis associated with psoriasis.*
- *Often an asymmetric, peripheral oligoarthritis but monarthritis, polyarthritis, and spondylitis occur as well.*
- *Frequent involvement of the distal interphalangeal joints.*
- *Association with dactylitis, enthesitis, and characteristic nail changes.*
- *Absence of rheumatoid factor (seronegative).*
- *Radiographic findings of erosions or osteolytic destruction of the interphalangeal joints, often with concomitant proliferative changes.*

General Considerations

Psoriatic arthritis is an inflammatory arthritis that occurs in association with the skin disease psoriasis. It is one of the spondyloarthropathies, a group of inflammatory arthritides characterized by enthesitis (inflammation at the insertion sites of tendons to bone), arthritis of the axial skeleton (ie, the sacroiliac joints and spine), an asymmetric oligoarthritis of peripheral joints, and the absence of rheumatoid factor. Psoriatic arthritis has a predilection for the distal interphalangeal (DIP) joints.

Arthritis develops in approximately 10% of patients with psoriasis. The overall prevalence of psoriatic arthritis has been estimated to be 0.04–0.1% of the general population, but this may be an underestimate. In the United States, the incidence of psoriatic arthritis has been reported to be approximately 6–7 per 100,000 per annum. The mean age of disease onset ranges from 30–55 years, with men and women affected equally.

The etiology of psoriatic arthritis is unknown. There are confirmed associations with major histocompatibility alleles human leukocyte antigen-B27, -B7, -B13, -B17, and -Cw6. As in the pathogenesis of many other autoimmune disorders, an infectious trigger has been suspected. Group A streptococcal infections have been implicated

in guttate psoriasis, and ribosomal RNA from this species has been detected in blood and synovial fluid of psoriatic arthritis patients. In addition, the human immunodeficiency virus is strongly associated with the development of psoriasis and psoriatic arthritis; the incidence and prevalence of both psoriasis and psoriatic arthritis are substantially higher in individuals infected with human immunodeficiency virus than in the general population.

Psoriatic arthritis typically develops after or coincident with the onset of psoriasis. In 15–20% of cases, however, arthritis precedes the onset of psoriasis by as much as 2 years. An asymmetric oligoarticular arthritis is the classic description of psoriatic arthritis, but articular manifestations range from an isolated monarthritis to polyarthritis to widespread destructive arthritis (arthritis mutilans). The course of psoriatic arthritis varies considerably. Unfortunately, no reliable markers for diagnosis or predictors of long-term outcomes are available. There may be a direct correlation between the severity of arthritis at the time of presentation and the subsequent clinical course. As seen in rheumatoid arthritis, psoriatic arthritis can significantly impact quality of life and physical function. Articular damage often develops, and destruction of single joints can occur rapidly.

Clinical Findings

A. SIGNS AND SYMPTOMS

1. Articular involvement—The majority of patients with psoriatic arthritis present with an oligo- or monarthritis. Often the DIP joints become stiff, swollen, and tender in an asymmetric fashion. When present, involvement of the DIPs helps to distinguish psoriatic arthritis from rheumatoid arthritis, but sometimes results in confusion with osteoarthritis. In a smaller proportion of patients, symptoms begin in a symmetric fashion and involve the hands and feet in a pattern resembling that of rheumatoid arthritis. Other joints that are affected by psoriatic arthritis include the knees, hips, and sternoclavicular joints.

Regardless of the number of symptomatic joints at the onset, most patients will progress to additional joint involvement in the absence of effective treatment. There is ongoing destruction of joints, as evidenced clinically by the appearance of joint deformities and radiographically

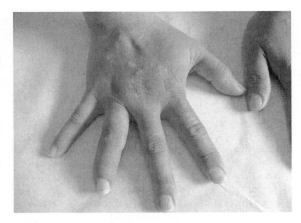

Figure 19–1. Dactylitis of the ring finger of a patient with psoriatic arthritis. (Courtesy of Dr. J. Graf, University of California, San Francisco.)

by the development of juxta-articular erosions, joint space narrowing, and in some cases, bony ankylosis. Arthritis mutilans describes the end stage of the destructive process, where loss of bony architecture allows complete subluxation and telescoping of the involved digit ("doigt en lorgnette" or opera-glass finger). This phenomenon is uncommon and is associated with long-standing disease.

2. Dactylitis—Dactylitis, or "sausage digit," is the complete swelling of a single digit in the hand or foot (Figure 19–1). It is a distinctive feature of the spondyloarthropathies, and it is common in psoriatic arthritis, occurring in one-third to one-half of patients at some point in their disease. Toes are more frequently involved than fingers.

3. Enthesitis—Enthesitis is an inflammatory process at the site of the insertion of tendons into bone. This is a feature common to other spondyloarthropathies and occurs in up to 40% of psoriatic arthritis patients. On physical examination, there is soft tissue swelling usually accompanied by tenderness to palpation and sometimes by overlying erythema and warmth as well. A common site for enthesitis is the insertion of the Achilles tendon into the calcaneus. Entheseal inflammation may evolve to destruction of the adjacent bone and joints.

4. Skin and nail changes—All forms of psoriasis are associated with arthritis, although classic psoriasis vulgaris is seen most frequently. Typical psoriatic lesions are erythematous plaques that produce scaling with scratching. Interestingly, many patients with psoriatic arthritis have only mild to moderate skin disease, and there has been no consistent correlation between the degree of psoriasis and the extent of joint involvement. The psoriasis may be subtle. Therefore careful examination of the entire skin surface must be performed when psoriatic arthritis is suspected, with particular attention to the hairline, scalp, external auditory canal, periumbilical area, and gluteal cleft.

As with uncomplicated psoriasis, nail involvement is common in psoriatic arthritis (Figure 19–2). Psoriatic nail changes include ridging, pitting, onycholysis, and hyperkeratosis, and may represent the only manifestation of psoriasis before the presence of more characteristic skin lesions. Nail changes on the affected finger virtually always occur when psoriatic arthritis affects a DIP joint.

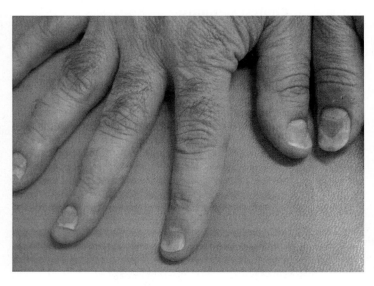

Figure 19–2. Psoriatic nail changes with onycholysis and subungual debris. (Courtesy of Dr. J. Graf, University of California, San Francisco.)

5. Spondyloarthropathy—Symptomatic involvement of the sacroiliac joints and axial skeleton is less common than peripheral arthritis. Inflammation of the sacroiliac joints (sacroiliitis) in psoriatic arthritis is usually unilateral and presents with pain and stiffness in the lower back or buttock. Tenderness often can be elicited by direct palpation of the joints by applying firm pressure with the thumbs when the examiner places his or her palms over the patient's iliac crest—the thumbs will tend to fall directly over the joint. Another maneuver that may detect sacroiliitis is the Gaenslen test, in which the patient hyperextends the leg over the examination table. This applies stress to the ipsilateral sacroiliac joint and is considered positive if pain is elicited with this maneuver. However, the reliability of physical examination findings for detection of sacroiliitis is poor, and noninflammatory processes may elicit positive findings. Plain radiography of the pelvis and Ferguson views that focus on the sacroiliac joints may aid in the detection of inflammatory disease of this joint.

A common site of skeletal involvement in psoriatic arthritis is the cervical spine. Here, as in rheumatoid arthritis, extensive inflammation and erosion can lead to atlantoaxial (C1–C2) instability, which can produce cervical myelopathy as the odontoid process erodes. This process is often clinically silent and painless. Involvement of other levels of the spine is also seen in psoriatic arthritis with syndesmophytes which often arise from the midpoint of a vertebral body, bridge adjacent vertebrae, and restrict motion of the spine. In contrast to the continuous ascending spinal involvement in ankylosing spondylitis, psoriatic spinal involvement is usually discontinuous, affecting noncontiguous vertebrae or areas (Figure 19–3).

6. Extra-articular manifestations—Ocular inflammation (conjunctivitis, iritis, scleritis, and episcleritis), oral ulcerations, and urethritis occur in psoriatic arthritis, but less frequently than in the other spondyloarthropathies.

B. LABORATORY FINDINGS

There are no laboratory tests diagnostic for psoriatic arthritis. Up to 20% of patients have hyperuricemia. Because of the systemic, inflammatory nature of the disease, acute phase reactants such as the C-reactive protein

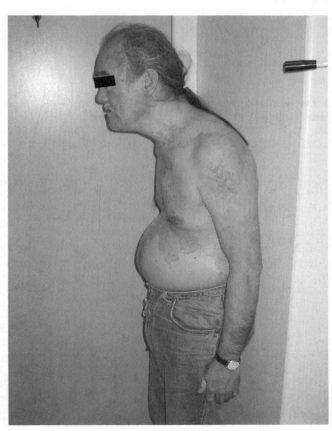

Figure 19–3. Psoriatic spondylitis. Extensive spinal involvement has led to exaggerated thoracic kyphosis and loss of cervical extension. As a result the patient is unable to touch the occiput to the wall when standing against the wall ("occiput-to-wall" test). There is limited chest expansion leading to a protuberant abdomen and to diaphragmatic breathing. (Courtesy of Dr. J. Graf, University of California, San Francisco.)

and the erythrocyte sedimentation rate may be elevated, though typically not as high as those seen in other inflammatory arthritides such as rheumatoid arthritis. In some patients, elevations of acute phase reactants correlate with disease activity, more commonly in patients with a higher number of affected joints.

Synovial fluid analysis reveals inflammatory fluid, with white blood cell counts usually in the 5000–50,000/mm^3 range.

Patients with psoriatic arthritis usually do not have rheumatoid factor, but up to 10% of patients with psoriatic arthritis will test positive. A positive rheumatoid factor is not an exclusion criterion for the diagnosis of psoriatic arthritis. Antibodies to cyclic citrullinated peptides are extremely sensitive and specific for rheumatoid arthritis. These antibodies have only rarely been reported in patients with psoriatic arthritis, and in most cases to date have been seen in patients with polyarticular symmetrical presentations that suggest the co-occurrence of psoriasis with rheumatoid arthritis. Antinuclear antibodies are detected in 10–20% of patients, which is comparable to the prevalence of antinuclear antibody positivity in healthy control populations.

C. IMAGING STUDIES

The most common radiographic findings in psoriatic arthritis are joint space narrowing and erosions involving the distal interphalangeal and proximal interphalangeal joints. Typically, these findings are asymmetric, paralleling the pattern of the clinical arthritis. The metacarpophalangeal joints and wrists are usually spared, in contrast to rheumatoid arthritis. In addition, periarticular osteopenia (decreased density of the bone adjacent to the joints) is usually absent in psoriatic arthritis, another feature that helps distinguish psoriatic arthritis from rheumatoid arthritis.

Severe destructive changes of the joints may occur with long-standing disease, but may also develop rapidly in a single joint, resulting in a whittling phenomenon of the bone. When a phalanx is involved, it becomes "penciled," thus giving rise to the classic "pencil-in-cup" deformity when it abuts the base of an adjacent phalanx (Figure 19–4). Marked osteolysis results in widening of the spaces between joints and eventual complete disorganization of the joint architecture, described as arthritis mutilans. Subluxations can occur, which give the clinical manifestation of telescoping digits.

In contrast to rheumatoid arthritis, psoriatic arthritis can produce proliferative bony changes adjacent to erosive and osteolytic changes in the same bone. This new bone formation often occurs along the shaft of the metacarpal and metatarsal bones and is seen as a fluffy periostitis. Rheumatologists and radiologists may use the term "whiskering" to describe these proliferative changes.

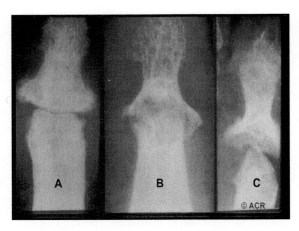

Figure 19–4. Radiographic changes from psoriatic arthritis of the distal interphalangeal joint. **A:** Subtle periosteal erosions at the margins of the joint space are an initial appearance. **B:** Progressive erosive and proliferative changes occur over time and can be greatly destructive. **C:** Distinctive "pencil-in-cup" appearance with severe disease. (©1972–1999, American College of Rheumatology Clinical Slide Collection. Used with permission.)

Differential Diagnosis

The diagnosis of psoriatic arthritis may be difficult when the skin manifestations are subtle or the arthritis antedates the onset of skin lesions. The wide range of clinical manifestations of psoriatic arthritis, the lack of defined diagnostic criteria, and the possibility of overlap syndromes with other rheumatic diseases also add to the complexity of diagnosis.

The differential diagnosis for psoriatic arthritis includes other forms of inflammatory arthritis, most notably rheumatoid arthritis and the other seronegative spondyloarthropathies (reactive arthritis, ankylosing spondylitis, and enteropathic arthritis). When acute in onset, the monarticular and oligoarticular forms of psoriatic arthritis can cause confusion with the crystal arthropathies (gout and pseudogout) and septic arthritis, necessitating the analysis of synovial fluid to exclude these alternative diagnoses. When performing an arthrocentesis in a patient with psoriasis it is critical to avoid passing the aspirating needle through psoriatic plaques, which are heavily contaminated with bacteria.

Treatment

A. NONSTEROIDAL ANTI-INFLAMMATORY DRUGS

Nonsteroidal anti-inflammatory drugs (NSAIDs) are the first-line therapy for psoriatic arthritis, and most patients derive some clinical benefit from them. Often, higher doses of nonselective NSAIDs may be required, and hence, vigilance must be maintained for gastrointestinal adverse effects. Administration of misoprostol or a proton pump inhibitor may be necessary for prophylaxis. The cyclooxygenase-2–selective inhibitor celecoxib is also an option, but recent concerns regarding increased risk of cardiovascular events temper the use of the coxibs.

B. DISEASE-MODIFYING ANTIRHEUMATIC DRUGS

Many disease-modifying antirheumatic drugs have been used in the treatment of psoriatic arthritis, including methotrexate, sulfasalazine, azathioprine, antimalarials (specifically hydroxychloroquine), and cyclosporine. Methotrexate is generally considered to be the agent of choice for patients who are refractory to NSAIDs and has the advantage of having efficacy for the skin manifestations of psoriasis as well as the arthritis. The typical starting dose is 7.5–15 mg either orally or subcutaneously once weekly, with titration to 25 mg once weekly as dictated by clinical response or by adverse events. Methotrexate is typically given as a single dose once weekly, as with rheumatoid arthritis, for the management of joint disease, in contrast to its administration sometimes in divided doses for skin psoriasis. The most common and significant side effects are nausea and vomiting, hair loss, hepatotoxicity, bone marrow suppression, immunosuppression, and teratogenicity. Hence, careful follow-up, laboratory monitoring, and counseling for family planning are required. Because of the hepatotoxicity of methotrexate, patients are strongly advised to limit alcohol intake to one drink per week, and methotrexate use is relatively contraindicated in patients with preexisting liver disease or hepatitis B or C infection. Folic acid supplementation (1 mg/d) should be given concomitantly to all patients, as this decreases the frequency and severity of side effects.

Sulfasalazine has also been shown to have a good clinical effect in psoriatic arthritis. In studies done in patients from the Department of Veterans Affairs who were unresponsive to NSAIDs, sulfasalazine at 2 g per day decreased the joint pain/tenderness scores and swelling scores over 36 weeks. However, these findings did not reach statistical significance. Subsequent studies indicated that peripheral articular manifestations of psoriatic arthritis responded to sulfasalazine, whereas axial disease did not. Hence, axial and peripheral involvement of psoriatic arthritis may represent two distinct subgroups with regard to treatment response to sulfasalazine. While sulfasalazine was well tolerated in these studies, gastrointestinal intolerance is a commonly reported adverse event, which may be decreased with the use of enteric-coated formulations. Up to 40% of patients may discontinue this medication at higher doses secondary to gastrointestinal distress. As a result, when prescribed, it should be started at a low dose (500 mg twice daily) and slowly increased over weeks to a maximum dose of 2–3 g daily. Like methotrexate, sulfasalazine is metabolized by the liver. Hence, liver function tests should be monitored periodically. Sulfasalazine may cause allergic reactions and rash, which could be severe. It should be avoided in sulfa-allergic patients and in individuals with aspirin sensitivity. Screening for glucose-6-phosphate dehydrogenase deficiency should also be considered, as patients are at increased risk for hemolysis. Because of anemia and other potential complications of sulfasalazine, blood counts should also be periodically followed.

C. BIOLOGICAL THERAPIES

Tumor necrosis factor-α (TNF-α) is a proinflammatory cytokine that plays a central role in the pathogenesis of inflammatory arthritis and is detected in psoriatic plaques, synovium, and at entheses. Recently, three biological inhibitors of TNF-α, etanercept, infliximab, and adalimumab, have been approved for treating psoriasis and psoriatic arthritis. In clinical trials, all three agents had significant and early efficacy in decreasing the signs and symptoms of arthritis, as well as in the severity of psoriatic skin lesions in many patients. TNF antagonists have also been shown to slow the rate of radiographic progression of psoriatic arthritis. Two of these biological agents (etanercept and adalimumab) are given as subcutaneous injections, while infliximab is given as an intravenous infusion. The main adverse effects include injection site and infusion reactions and immunosuppression. Reactivation of latent tuberculosis has been seen with all agents, and it is a mechanism-based side effect; thus each patient should be screened for latent tuberculosis with a purified protein derivative test and a chest radiograph prior to the initiation of a TNF-α inhibitor.

A second class of biological agents is currently being studied for the treatment of psoriatic arthritis. Alefacept is a recombinant fusion protein of soluble lymphocyte function antigen with Fc fragments of IgG1 that is presently approved for the treatment of moderate to severe psoriasis. Its mechanism of action is not completely understood, but it is thought to induce apoptosis of memory T cells, inhibit co-stimulation of T cells, and decrease inflammatory cell infiltration, thus leading to an anti-inflammatory effect. Recently, a randomized, double-blind, placebo-controlled study of alefacept in combination with methotrexate showed that alefacept-methotrexate–treated patients had a greater decrease in signs and symptoms of psoriatic arthritis, compared to the placebo-methotrexate group. There were no serious adverse reactions. Hence, alefacept in combination with methotrexate appeared to be safe and effective for psoriatic arthritis in a short-term study. Further studies of longer duration are in progress. Because of its effects on peripheral T cells, CD4 counts should be monitored in all patients on alefacept.

D. GLUCOCORTICOIDS

Intra-articular injections of glucocorticoids are an effective treatment when only one or two joints dominate a patient's symptoms. Psoriatic plaques are heavily contaminated with bacteria, and considerable care should be taken to avoid introducing an infection by passing the injecting needle through a psoriatic plaque into the joint.

Systemic glucocorticoids should be used with caution if at all. Some rheumatologists use oral prednisone at doses of 10–20 mg daily with a subsequent taper to quell an acute attack of psoriatic arthritis. Many dermatologists, however, avoid systemic glucocorticoids because of the risk that the glucocorticoid taper can precipitate a severe flare of pustular psoriasis. Regardless, baseline therapy in the form of NSAIDs, and in most cases disease-modifying antirheumatic drugs or biologicals, should be on board for maintenance immunomodulatory control.

E. SURGERY

Long-standing erosive and destructive disease can lead to extensive joint deformities. If severe destructive disease is present, orthopedic surgery consultation may be considered for joint replacement or stabilization.

REFERENCES

Gladman DD, Antoni C, Mease P, Clegg DO, Nash P. Psoriatic arthritis: epidemiology, clinical features, course, and outcome. *Ann Rheum Dis.* 2005;64(Suppl 2):ii14.

Helliwell PS, Taylor WJ. Classification and diagnostic criteria for psoriatic arthritis. *Ann Rheum Dis.* 2005;64(Suppl 2):ii3.

Mease PJ, Antoni CE. Psoriatic arthritis treatment: biological response modifiers. *Ann Rheum Dis.* 2005;64(Suppl 2):ii78.

Mease PJ. Psoriatic arthritis therapy advances. *Curr Opin Rheumatol.* 2005;17:426.

Reddy SM, Bingham III CO. Outcome measures in psoriatic arthritis clinical trials. *Curr Rheumatol Rep.* 2005;7:299.

Adult Still Disease

Peggy Schlesinger, MD

ESSENTIALS OF DIAGNOSIS

- *Fever that spikes in "rabbit ears" pattern with daily return to normal.*
- *Salmon-colored macular rash only occurring with fever.*
- *Arthritis, splenomegaly, pleuritis, pericarditis, and marked leukocytosis common.*
- *Pharyngitis often the initial symptom.*

General Considerations

Adult-onset Still disease (AOSD) is a multisystem inflammatory disease that typically begins with a sore throat. Nonsuppurative pharyngitis may develop days to weeks before the typical quotidian fever, evanescent rash, and joint pains begin. Other constitutional symptoms soon follow, including profound fatigue, weight loss, and anorexia. Malignancy and infectious causes of these symptoms must be excluded because AOSD is diagnosed mainly on clinical grounds.

The cause of AOSD has yet to be identified. The presence of daily spiking fevers has focused research efforts on the possibility that the cause of AOSD is infection-related. To date, however, there has not been any infectious agent or genetic predisposition identified in patients with this disease.

Fortunately, AOSD is rare. One series reported an incidence of 0.16 cases per 100,000 population. Women and men are equally affected. The peak onset is between ages 20 and 45, although cases have been reported in all age groups. Pediatric patients with systemic-onset juvenile idiopathic arthritis can have a recurrence of active Still disease at any age into adulthood.

Clinical Findings

There is no definitive lab test for AOSD, but a high serum ferritin and marked leukocytosis with fever, rash, and arthritis in the absence of other possible causes is highly suggestive of this diagnosis.

A. SYMPTOMS AND SIGNS

The fever of AOSD is relentless, often lasting weeks at a time before the diagnosis can be established. Temperature spikes occur daily in these patients, often in the afternoon or evening. These elevations in temperature can be associated with shaking chills and sweating. The daily return to baseline or normal temperature is a distinguishing feature that separates patients with AOSD from those with chronic infection. Typically, in patients with chronic infection the temperature remains elevated between fever spikes.

The rash of AOSD is salmon-colored, macular, and can occur anywhere on the trunk and extremities. It is evanescent, and manifests during the febrile episodes but clears completely when the temperature returns to normal. It may be mildly pruritic and extend to areas that are scratched (Koebner phenomenon). Biopsy of involved skin, even with immunofluorescence, is usually not diagnostic. The presence of this particular rash in association with a daily fever is diagnostic of AOSD, even though the rash itself is nondescript, and can easily be mistaken for a drug reaction or viral exanthem. In some patients, the rash may reappear in the identical location during subsequent flares of active disease. Usually the face, palms, and soles are spared.

Joint pain is a common feature of AOSD, but true arthritis may be slow to develop. Initially, patients often have significant joint and muscle pain without true synovitis. Marked arthralgias and myalgias may be present initially and can develop into frank arthritis over time. Arthritis develops in large joints such as the hip, knee, ankle, shoulder and wrist more often than the small joints of the hands and feet. Persistent synovitis and restricted range of motion in affected joints can occur even after the fever has resolved. Destructive arthritis occurs in 20% of patients with AOSD. Carpal and cervical ankylosis can occur as a result of arthritis in both the adult and childhood-onset forms of the disease. Avascular necrosis is a significant risk for those patients with AOSD who require glucocorticoids for control of their systemic symptoms or persistent arthritis or both. Hip involvement and

Table 20–1. Clinical Manifestations of Adult-Onset Still Disease

Fever
Acute pharyngitis
Arthritis/arthralgia
Severe myalgias
Lymphadenopathy
Splenomegaly
Hepatic dysfunction
Pleuritis
Pericarditis

Table 20–2. Common Laboratory Test Abnormalities in Adult-Onset Still Disease

Elevated erythrocyte sedimentation rate
Elevated white blood cell count[a]
Elevated platelet count
Anemia
Elevated liver enzymes
Elevated ferritin
Negative antinuclear antibodies
Negative rheumatoid factor

[a] White blood cell count $>15,000/\mu$L with $>80\%$ polymorphonuclear leukocytes.

persistent synovitis are poor prognostic signs and justify an aggressive treatment approach.

Pleuritis, pericarditis, lymphadenopathy, hepatomegaly, and splenomegaly are common in AOSD (Table 20–1). Biopsy specimens of lymph nodes show reactive changes due to polyclonal B-cell hyperplasia.

B. Laboratory

There is no definitive lab test for AOSD; however, marked leukocytosis ($>15,000/\mu$L) with a predominance of neutrophils ($>80\%$) and a markedly elevated erythrocyte sedimentation rate (>90 mm/h) is seen in almost all patients with this disorder. The lab findings in AOSD suggest both acute and chronic inflammation with a low serum albumin, anemia of chronic disease, elevated C-reactive protein, and elevated complement levels. Marked elevation of the serum ferritin (above 3000 mg/mL) is seen in over 70% of AOSD patients. A high ferritin can be seen in hematologic malignancies but does not occur in other rheumatic disease syndromes. There is a low percentage ($<20\%$) of serum ferritin that is glycosylated in patients with AOSD which may be even more specific for this disease. However, this test is not routinely clinically available. Recent studies have documented elevated levels of interleukin-18 that correlate with clinical activity of AOSD. This may help to explain the unusual pattern of inflammatory markers specific to this disease.

The antinuclear antibody test and rheumatoid factor are negative in almost all cases (Table 20–2). Mild elevation of liver function tests are a frequent but nonspecific finding. There is no threat to renal function associated with AOSD, and the creatinine and urinalysis typically remain normal.

Differential Diagnosis

Diagnostic criteria have been proposed by several authors to help identify patients with AOSD using major and minor criteria taken from the list of clinical and laboratory findings listed in Tables 20–1 and 20–2. These proposed classification systems rely on different combinations of major and minor criteria once infection, malignancy, and other rheumatic disorders have been excluded.

When patients present with sore throat, daily fever, rash, arthritis, and muscle pain, infection tops the list of possible causes. The most common causes of rash, fever, and arthritis are infectious, including viral infections (such as rubella, parvovirus, Epstein-Barr virus, cytomegalovirus, hepatitis B and C, and HIV) and bacterial infections (*Borrelia burgdorferi* [Lyme disease], *Borrelia hermsii* [relapsing fever], streptococcal-associated arthritis and rheumatic fever recurrence, and subacute bacterial endocarditis, among others). It is vitally important to exclude infection before beginning treatment for AOSD.

Malignancy can cause fever, rash, arthralgias, and also many of the nonspecific lab abnormalities seen in AOSD. Patients with hematologic malignancies often have enlarged lymph nodes, elevated ferritin levels, splenomegaly, abnormal liver function, and fever that can be difficult to distinguish from AOSD.

Other rheumatic disease syndromes can also mimic the signs and symptoms of AOSD. Sarcoidosis, polyarteritis nodosa, antineutrophilic cytoplasmic anti-body–associated vasculitis, inflammatory bowel disease, and recurrent fever syndromes such as familial Mediterranean fever, autoimmune neutropenia, hemophagocytic syndromes, and systemic lupus erythematosus must all be ruled out to establish a diagnosis of AOSD.

Treatment

Treatment of this condition can be challenging. Early in the disease course, treatment with nonsteroidal anti-inflammatory drugs can help reduce fever, joint pain, and muscle aches, but can lead to markedly elevated liver function tests. Aspirin was previously considered to be the mainstay of therapy, but frequently caused significant hepatitis. Nonsteroidal anti-inflammatory drugs are less likely to cause similar problems but the potential remains. Systemic glucocorticoids are indicated to control persistent synovitis and to treat life-threatening manifestations and constitutional symptoms that interfere with the activities of daily living. If arthritis persists, treatment with a disease-modifying agent, such as methotrexate or cyclosporine, or an anti-cytokine agent, such as anakinra (an interleukin-1 inhibitor) or etanercept (a tumor necrosis factor inhibitor), can induce remission and minimize glucocorticoid exposure. There are remarkable responses to anakinra reported in the literature. Newer biological agents that target interleukin-6 may be even more effective in treating this disease.

Therapy should be continued until laboratory parameters show no signs of inflammation and clinical examination indicates no active disease is present. Medication can then be tapered slowly with the hope of maintaining a remission on the lowest effective dose. Disease-modifying agents should be continued for a 1-year disease-free interval before being discontinued altogether.

The clinical course of AOSD is variable. One-third of patients remit after one extended symptomatic period that can last up to 1 year. One-third of patients with AOSD relapse with a polycyclic course. In these patients, remission can occur between flares. Another third of patients with AOSD will have a persistent active clinical course with chronic active arthritis the main ongoing symptom. Relapse in this disorder can occur years after the initial diagnostic episode.

REFERENCES

Chen DY, Lan JL, Lin FJ, Hsieh TY, Wen MC. Predominance of Th1 cytokine in peripheral blood and pathological tissues of patients with active untreated adult onset Still's disease. *Arthritis Rheum Dis.* 2004;63:1300.

Cush J. Adult-onset Still's disease. *Bull Rheum Dis.* 2002;49:1.

Fautrel B, Zing E, Golmard JL, et al. Proposal for new set of classification criteria for adult-onset still disease. *Medicine (Baltimore).* 2002;81:194.

Fitzgerald AA, Leclercq SA, Yan A, Homik JE, Dinarello CA. Rapid responses to anakinra in patients with refractory adult-onset Still's disease. *Arthritis Rheum.* 2005;52:1794.

Magadur-Joly G, Billaud E, Barrier JH, et al. Epidemiology of adult Still's disease: estimate of the incidence by a retrospective study in west France. *Ann Rheum Dis.* 1995;54:587.

Mandl LA, Esdaile JM. Adult Still's disease. *UpToDate Online* [serial online]. April 2005; UpToDate Online 13.2.

Mert A, Ozaras R, Tabak F, et al. Fever of unknown origin: a review of 20 patients with adult-onset Still's disease. *Clin Rheumatol.* 2003;22:89.

Juvenile Idiopathic Arthritis 21

Peggy Schlesinger, MD

 ESSENTIAL FEATURES

- *Juvenile idiopathic arthritis (JIA) causes chronic arthritis in children.*
- *There are seven subgroups of JIA: systemic onset (Still disease); enthesitis-related arthritis; juvenile psoriatic arthritis; oligoarticular, polyarticular seronegative, and polyarticular seropositive arthritis; and "other."*
- *The type of JIA subgroup is determined by the age of the child; the number and type of joints involved; the presence of associated symptoms such as rash, fever, and iritis; and the course of the illness during the first 6 months after the diagnosis is confirmed.*

General Considerations

Juvenile idiopathic arthritis (JIA) refers to the group of disorders that cause chronic arthritis in children. The diagnosis of JIA is made clinically when chronic synovitis is present in any one joint for more than 6 weeks in a child less than 16 years of age. Synovitis is defined as inflammation of the synovial lining that manifests clinically as swelling and limited motion of a joint, often with warmth, pain, and stiffness. The chronicity of the joint involvement in JIA distinguishes this group of disorders from the many short-term causes of joint pain and swelling that can occur in childhood.

JIA is more common than is often appreciated, with an incidence of 1–22 children per 100,000, and a prevalence of anywhere from 8–150 per 100,000. It is the most common chronic rheumatic disease of childhood, and can be a significant cause of both short-term and long-term disability.

The subtypes of JIA (Table 21–1) are identified and classified based on several factors: age at onset, number of joints involved initially and as the disease progresses, associated clinical features, and lab test results (rheumatoid factor positive or negative). Identification of the correct subtype leads to appropriate therapy and can give prog-

nostic information. The classification system for juvenile arthritis has undergone important changes in the last 30 years in an attempt to define more fully the scope and prognosis of this group of disorders.

The International League of Associations for Rheumatology classification of 1997 will be used in this chapter. This system identifies seven different types of JIA based on the pattern of joint involvement at onset of the illness. These seven types are: systemic onset JIA (SOJIA), oligoarticular (previously known as pauciarticular) JIA, polyarticular rheumatoid factor positive JIA, polyarticular rheumatoid factor negative JIA, juvenile psoriatic arthritis, enthesitis-related arthritis, and "other." The subtypes are listed in the table (see Table 21–1) from left to right in order of frequency with their distinguishing clinical features. The signs and symptoms of each subtype will be discussed individually.

Oligoarticular JIA occurs in very young children with symptoms beginning any time between the ages they begin walking until they are school age. An asymmetric pattern of joint involvement is common and fewer than five joints total can be affected. Morning stiffness is a prominent finding, and although the affected joint is often swollen and quite large, the child frequently has less pain than one would anticipate. Knees are the most commonly involved joints; there may also be diffuse swelling of a toe or finger. The neck at the atlantoaxial (C1–C2) joint and the temporomandibular joint are relatively hidden sites where joint inflammation can also occur.

Children with oligoarticular JIA, especially very young girls with a positive antinuclear antibody test, are at increased risk of developing iritis. This chronic, anterior, nongranulomatous uveitis or iridocyclitis is usually painless and occurs early in the course of the illness. One out of five patients with oligoarticular JIA will have asymptomatic iritis, usually girls. Seventy-five percent of these young girls with oligoarticular JIA and iritis will have a positive antinuclear antibody test. The iritis of oligoarticular JIA is treatable when the diagnosis is made early. Treatment options include steroid drops, sub-tenon injections of long-acting steroid preparations, and mydriatics, used as needed to control the inflammation in the anterior chamber of the affected eye. Systemic therapy with methotrexate and/or biological agents is sometimes necessary to quiet completely the inflammatory response

Table 21–1. Subgroups of Juvenile Idiopathic Arthritis (JIA)

JIA Subgroup	Oligoarticular	Polyarticular Negative	Polyarticular Positive	Systemic Onset	Juvenile Psoriatic	Enthesitis-Related (ERA)
Percentage of all JIA	40%	20%	15%	10–20%	≤ 10%	≤ 10%
Age at onset and gender	<8 years g > b	8–12 years g = b	Teen years g > b	Any age	Any age	8–12 years b > g
No. of joints involved	<5	Many	Many	Varies	Varies	Varies
Pattern	Asymmetric	Varies	Symmetric	Asymmetric	Asymmetric	Lower extremity joints
Hips involved	Rarely	No	No	Occasionally	Sometimes	Yes
Back pain	No	No	No	Myalgic	Sometimes	Yes
Clinical features	Painless iridocyclitis Requires regular slitlamp exam	Poor weight gain	Aggressive course Nodules Poor weight gain	Fever Evanescent rash Serositis Lymphadenopathy Hepatosplenomegaly MAS Complications can be fatal	DIP joints Nail pitting Psoriatic rash or positive family history Dactylitis Can look like polyarticular JIA or ERA	Enthesitis Heel pain Sausage digits Abnormal Schober test Sacroiliitis Oral ulcers
Distinguishing lab abnormalities	Antinuclear antibody positive	Rheumatoid factor positive	Rheumatoid factor negative	Increased ESR, WBC, CRP, ferritin, platelets Anemia Abnormal LFTs	None	HLA-B27 positive

g, girls; b, boys; CRP, C-reactive protein; ESR, erythrocyte sedimentation rate; HLA, human leukocyte antigen; WBC, white blood cell count; LFTs, liver function tests; DIP, distal interphalangeal; MAS, macrophage activation syndrome.

Table 21–2. Recommended Ophthalmologic Screening for Children with Juvenile Idiopathic Arthritis[a]

JIA Subgroup	Iritis Risk		
	High (Screen Every 3 Months)	**Moderate (Screen Every 6 Months)**	**Low (Screen Annually)**
Oligoarticular dx at <7 years old; positive ANA	Years 1–3 after dx	Years 4–6 after dx	After year 7 after dx
Extended oligoarticular or oligo- to polyarticular	Years 1–3 after dx	Years 4–6 after dx	After year 7 after dx
Polyarticular dx at <7 years old; positive ANA	Years 1–3 after dx	Years 4–6 after dx	After year 7 after dx
Polyarticular dx at >7 years old; negative ANA		Year 1–6 after dx	After year 7 after dx
Psoriatic arthritis			Low risk: annual screen
Systemic onset			Low risk: annual screen
Enthesitis-related			Low risk: annual screen

[a]Screening should include a slitlamp exam to evaluate the anterior chamber for cells and flare *even in the absence of eye symptoms.*

in the eye. Serious complications such as blindness, glaucoma, cataracts, and band keratopathy can result from untreated eye disease. Prevention and early treatment is preferable to the disappointing results seen in the later-stage cases. All children with oligoarticular JIA should have regular slitlamp exams done until they reach 18 years of age, *even in the absence of a red eye or joint symptoms* (Table 21–2). Untreated iritis can cause more long-term morbidity in these children than their arthritis, which often resolves by the time they reach school age and usually does not lead to permanent joint damage.

In some children, arthritis may begin in a few joints but later progress to involve more than five joints. These patients have crossed out of the oligoarticular subgroup and into the polyarticular subgroup of JIA, which can persist into adulthood and can cause joint destruction over time. Patients who are "oligo to poly" retain the same increased risk of iridocyclitis as children with the persistent oligoarticular type and continue to require periodic eye exams.

Polyarticular JIA defines a group of children whose arthritis begins in five or more joints at onset. In this heterogeneous group of patients the rheumatoid factor test is a useful prognosticator. Rheumatoid factor positive patients are usually teenage girls with symmetric small-joint arthritis involving hands and feet. These girls may have rheumatoid nodules, with aggressive erosive joint disease. This is the only one of the JIA group that clinically resembles the adult form of classic rheumatoid factor positive, rheumatoid arthritis, with similar HLA-DR4 associations. Iritis or uveitis is uncommon in this subgroup.

Polyarticular rheumatoid factor negative JIA affects younger children, more girls than boys. The arthritis may or may not be symmetric but usually affects large joints predominantly. There are no associated extra-articular features and uveitis is rare. These children can have active arthritis for many years without erosive change on x-ray. The course is variable, and transition to the rheumatoid factor positive group can occur. Patients with a psoriatic rash or a family history of psoriasis are excluded from this group.

The child with high daily spiking fever, an evanescent rash present during febrile episodes that disappears when the temperature is back to normal, severe myalgias, and polyserositis likely has Still disease (see Chapter 20) or **systemic onset JIA** (SOJIA). This disease affects children and adults at any age, without preference for girls or boys. The onset can be devastating with such significant fever and pain that the child fails to thrive and malignancy is suspected. True arthritis may manifest months after the onset of fever, which can make early diagnosis difficult. The hallmarks of this disorder are the daily spiking fever in a "rabbit ears" pattern in association with an evanescent, salmon-colored, macular rash on the trunk and extremities. Marked leukocytosis,

Table 21–3. Nonsteroidal Anti-Inflammatory Drugs Used in Pediatric Juvenile Idiopathic Arthritis (JIA) Patients[a]

Drug	Dose	Formulation
Naproxen	20 mg/kg/d; 10 mg/kg/dose bid up to 1000 mg/d	Liquid: 125 mg/5 mL Tablet: 220 mg, available over the counter Twice-daily dosing is convenient
Ibuprofen	40 mg/kg/d; 10 mg/kg/dose qid up to 2400 mg/d	Liquid: 100 mg/5 mL Tablet: 200 mg, available over the counter
Tolmetin	30 mg/kg/d; 10 mg/kg/dose tid up to 1800 mg/d	Tablets: 200, 400, and 600 mg
Indomethacin	1–3 mg/kg/d tid or qid up to 200 mg/d	Liquid: 25 mg/5 mL Approved for patients younger than 14 years Used in younger patients with systemic onset JIA or spondylitis
Meloxicam	0.125 mg/kg/d up to 7.5 mg/d	Liquid: 7.5 mg/mL Tablet: 7.5 and 15 mg Once-a-day dosing is convenient

[a]As of this writing, other NSAIDs have not been approved by the Food and Drug Administration for use in the pediatric age group.

very high sedimentation rates, and elevated ferritin levels are the rule in this disease. Complications, including the macrophage activation syndrome and hemodynamically significant pleuropericarditis, can be life-threatening. Recurrent episodes of active SOJIA can occur into adulthood after an extended disease-free interval.

The **psoriatic arthritis** subgroup of JIA includes patients with any of the following signs and symptoms: sacroiliitis, distal interphalangeal joint synovitis, dactylitis, "sausage" digit, nail pitting, psoriatic rash, or a positive family history of psoriasis. A history of psoriasis in a first-degree relative can be enough to raise the suspicion that psoriasis will develop in time and thus confirm the diagnosis. In some patients, it may take years from the onset of arthritis until the typical skin lesions appear.

The **enthesitis-related JIA** group includes patients with juvenile onset spondylitis, reactive arthritis, and the arthritis associated with inflammatory bowel disease. Boys from 8 years of age onward are most often affected, with pain, stiffness, and loss of flexibility in the spine, in addition to synovitis of peripheral joints, predominantly in lower extremities. Heel pain, rash including pyoderma gangrenosum or ulcers, and acute, painful uveitis can occur. Enthesitis refers to inflammation at the tendon/bone insertion site that can lead to point tenderness at that site. The HLA-B27 gene can be found in many patients in this category, but is not diagnostic.

The last category, "**other,**" includes patients whose arthritis either does not fit into any of the six categories, or patients whose arthritis symptoms fit into more than one of these categories.

Laboratory

Children suspected of having JIA should have a complete blood cell count, erythrocyte sedimentation rate, C-reactive protein quantitation, and assessment of liver and renal function, in addition to an antinuclear antibody test and rheumatoid factor assay. The anti–cyclic citrullinated peptide antibody is currently being evaluated in this age group to identify its diagnostic potential in JIA. Serum ferritin is useful in the work-up of SOJIA and an HLA-B27 test can at times be helpful in the evaluation of enthesitis-related JIA. As there is no single laboratory test that is diagnostic of JIA, these tests and others are needed to exclude other possible causes of arthritis symptoms.

Imaging

Plain radiographs of affected joints are helpful in the initial evaluation of joint pain in children, and serial exams done at 6- to 12-month intervals in selected patients with aggressive disease can document the presence of erosive disease and growth restriction. At times a bone scan can help identify other sites of inflammation in patients in whom the diagnosis of arthritis is in question, or in patients whose symptoms are difficult to evaluate. MRI is useful in identifying joint erosions at an early stage.

Special Tests

Regular ophthalmologic screening with periodic slitlamp exams is necessary in all oligoarticular JIA patients every

Table 21–4. Disease-Modifying Antirheumatic Drugs (DMARDs) Used to Treat Juvenile Idiopathic Arthritis (JIA) in Pediatric Patients[a]

Drug	Dose	Form	Special Considerations
Hydroxychloroquine	6 mg/kg/d qd or bid daily	200-mg pills	• Periodic eye exams; retinal toxicity rare at these doses
Sulfasalazine	30–50 mg/kg/d tid or bid daily	500-mg tablets	• Contraindicated in sulfa-allergic or aspirin-sensitive patients • Useful in polyarticular or spondylitis subgroups • *Not* for use in systemic onset JIA • Enteric-coated formulation is often better tolerated
Methotrexate	15 mg/m^2 per dose or 0.5–1.0 mg/kg per dose PO, IM, or SC once a week	Pills: 2.5 mg Liquid: 25 mg/mL 2.5 mg = 0.1 mL	• Higher doses well tolerated in children • Poor absorption can cause decreased clinical response; try same dose SC • Avoid concomitant sulfa, tetracycline • Liquid can be taken PO or SC • This is the least expensive DMARD
Cyclosporine	3 mg/kg/d bid	Neoral pills: 25- and 100-mg capsules Liquid: 100 mg/mL	• Neoral has increased bioavailability • Grapefruit juice increases absorption • Most effective in systemic onset JIA • Monitor kidney function and BP frequently • Many drug interactions
Leflunomide	100-mg loading dose + 10 mg PO qod if < 20 kg 100 mg/2 days then 10 mg PO qd if 20–40 kg 100 mg/3 days then 20 mg/d if >40 kg	10- and 20-mg pills	• Hair thinning in ⅛ of patients • Loose stools respond to dose adjustment, loperamide • Avoid pregnancy while on treatment until cholestyramine washout completed
Etanercept	0.4 mg/kg/dose SC 2 times/week	Powder to reconstitute with water in prefilled syringe; *refrigerate*	• Avoid live virus immunization during etanercept therapy • Approved and indicated for polyarticular JIA • Combination with methotrexate prolongs effect • Serious infection can occur
Anakinra	1–2 mg/kg/d SC	Prefilled syringe 100 mg; *refrigerate*	• Very effective in systemic onset JIA • Injection-site reaction is common • Infection risk
Infliximab	3–5 mg/kg per infusion given IV at 0, 2, and 6 weeks, then every 8 weeks	IV infusion requires premedication with diphenhydramine and acetaminophen	• Infection risk is high • Chimeric molecule requires concomitant treatment with methotrexate • Avoid live virus immunization • Useful in psoriatic arthritis, inflammatory bowel disease, and spondyloarthropathy
Adalimumab	24 mg/m^2 SC every other week	Prefilled syringe 40 mg; *refrigerate*	• Currently under study for JIA • Early clinical response and ease of administration • Infection risk

[a]Leflunomide, anakinra, infliximab, and adalimumab are currently under investigation regarding their usefulness in the pediatric age group.

3–6 months for the first 5 years of their disease (see Table 21–2). JIA patients in other subgroups are at lower risk for iridocyclitis but should still have slitlamp exams done yearly through their 18th birthday.

Differential Diagnosis

See Chapter 5, Approach to the Adolescent with Arthritis, for a more complete discussion of the differential diagnosis.

Complications

Serious complications including mandibular asymmetry, generalized growth retardation, leg length inequality, osteopenia/osteoporosis, gait abnormalities, muscle atrophy, difficult orthodontic problems, loss of vision, glaucoma, and cataracts, can occur in the child with JIA who is inadequately treated. In treated patients, complications of therapy such as infection, delayed immunizations, steroid complications, and dyspepsia from nonsteroidal anti-inflammatory drugs can occur.

Treatment

The goals of the treatment of JIA are to reduce pain and restore the child to normal function. Once joint pain, stiffness, and swelling are reduced, then gait patterns and patterns of use will return to normal, and muscle atrophy will reverse, making joint contracture less likely. Other sequelae such as specific growth impairment of the mandible, leg length, and generalized growth restriction do not develop when active arthritis is well controlled. Uveitis is less likely to persist when arthritis is in remission.

Nonsteroidal anti-inflammatory drugs and corticosteroids, either oral or intra-articular, are the mainstays of therapy for the majority of children with JIA (Table 21–3). Ibuprofen, naproxen, tolmetin, and indomethacin have been FDA-approved for use in the pediatric age group. Meloxicam has recently been approved for use in children with JIA and the once-daily dosing is convenient. Rofecoxib enjoyed a similar indication for use in JIA for 1 month before being removed from the market in fall 2004.

Most children in the oligoarticular, polyarticular rheumatoid factor negative, and enthesitis-related subgroups will not need disease-modifying antirheumatic drugs to control their arthritis symptoms. Patients with rheumatoid factor positive polyarticular disease should be treated aggressively with disease-modifying antirheumatic drugs (Table 21–4) early to avoid joint erosions and deformities. SOJIA patients may require corticosteroids initially to get control of their symptoms, and biologic therapy with an interleukin-1 inhibitor (anakinra) or other disease-modifying antirheumatic drugs to maintain remission.

The availability of etanercept in 1999 was a significant step forward in the treatment of JIA, producing remission in polyarticular disease early in the course, prior to the development of complications such as erosions, deformity, and growth abnormalities. Other biological therapies (see Table 21–4) are currently in clinical trials to clarify the safety and efficacy of these agents in the pediatric age group.

The treatment team involved in the care of a child with JIA can include the primary care provider, pediatric rheumatologist, social worker, clinic nurse, and pharmacist. Others, such as a psychologist or school counselor, nutritionist, and parent advocate may also be needed. Physical and occupational therapy may be needed in some cases to strengthen muscles, provide adaptive equipment when needed, and prevent contractures while improving range of motion.

Recognizing the needs of the child with JIA in her surroundings, at school and as well as at home, is vital to successful management of the disease. Attention to school issues and peer acceptance or lack thereof can lead to helpful involvement of a social worker for assistance with the management of these issues. It is vitally important that the child with JIA be encouraged to remain active and participate fully in both school and extracurricular activities. Participation in physical education and competitive sports can help a child with arthritis build strength and endurance as well as boost self-esteem.

There are several treatment options available for children with JIA that are very effective at producing remission. Early treatment should be made available to all children with JIA to minimize disability from this disease. Consultation with a pediatric rheumatologist can ensure that the child with JIA is receiving optimal therapy and thus reduce overall morbidity from this disease.

REFERENCES

Burgos-Vargas R. The juvenile-onset spondyloarthritides. *Rheum Dis Clin North Am.* 2002;28:531.

Cassidy JT. *Textbook of Pediatric Rheumatology.* 4th ed. WB Saunders, 2001. (An excellent text.)

Emery H. Juvenile rheumatoid arthritis and the spondyloarthropathies. *Adolesc Med.* 1998;9:45.

Milojevic DS, Ilowite NT. Treatment of rheumatoid diseases in children. *Rheum Dis Clin North Am.* 2002;28:461.

Rabinovich CE. Bone metabolism in childhood rheumatic disease. *Rheum Dis Clin North Am.* 2002;28:655.

Schneider R, Passo MH. Juvenile rheumatoid arthritis. *Rheum Dis Clin North Am.* 2002;28:503.

Weiss, JE, Ilowite NT. Juvenile idiopathic arthritis. *Pediatr Clin North Am.* 2005;52:413. (The entire volume is devoted to childhood rheumatic disease.)

Rheumatic Disease Clinics of North America, 2002, Volume 28 gives the best overall update of pediatric rheumatology.

SECTION III

Lupus & Related Autoimmune Disorders

Systemic Lupus Erythematosus | 22

Michelle Petri, MD, MPH

 ESSENTIALS OF DIAGNOSIS

- *Onset after puberty in young women.*
- *More common in African Americans.*
- *Common presentations are photosensitive rashes, polyarthritis, or nephritis.*
- *Characterized by autoantibody formation (specific autoantibodies include anti-dsDNA and anti-Sm) and often low complement levels (C3, C4, and CH50).*

GENERAL CONSIDERATIONS

Systemic lupus erythematosus (SLE) is usually a multi-organ, multisystem autoimmune disease. It must be distinguished from chronic cutaneous lupus (in which only discoid lupus occurs and progression to a systemic disease occurs in only 5%), and from drug-induced lupus erythematosus (associated with isoniazid, procainamide, hydralazine, minocycline, anti–tumor necrosis factor biologicals, and some other drugs, presenting as arthritis and serositis, but resolving after cessation of the culprit drug).

"Mixed connective tissue disease" is a term proposed for patients with high-titer anti-ribonucleoprotein anti-bodies and a syndrome of Raynaud phenomenon, polyarthritis, and myositis. Long-term follow-up has suggested that the diagnosis is often not appropriate because true systemic lupus erythematosus or scleroderma develops in many patients. In addition, the term is often misused to designate patients with an undefined autoimmune disease. A better diagnostic code for such patients is "undifferentiated connective tissue disease."

SLE predominantly occurs in women, with a gender ratio of 9:1. Onset is usually after puberty, typically in the 20s and 30s. It is more common in African Americans than in whites. The incidence in white females is 3.9 per 100,000 and in white males is 0.4 per 100,000. The prevalence in white females is 130 per 100,000. The incidence of SLE may have tripled since the 1970s.

Multiple predisposing factors have been identified. The genetic predisposition is complex, likely involving more than 100 genes. HLA-DR and DQ alleles are associated not just with the risk of developing lupus, but with the kinds of autoantibodies produced. Genes that control programmed cell death (apoptosis) are important in murine lupus models and likely in human lupus as well. The proteins to which the lupus patient mounts an autoantibody response are exposed on nuclear blebs during programmed cell death. Genes involved in immune complex clearance (Fc-γ receptor alleles) may predispose patients to lupus nephritis. Gene expression studies have identified an "interferon signature"—a group of genes regulated by interferon-α—in the majority of

SLE patients. The genetic predisposition to SLE is not overwhelming. Only 10% of patients have a first-degree relative with SLE, and SLE develops in only 2% of children who have an afflicted parent.

Environmental factors play a role not only in the onset of SLE but also in triggering the "flares" (relapses). The most recognized environmental trigger is ultraviolet light exposure. Ultraviolet light, both ultraviolet-B and ultraviolet-A, can trigger photosensitive rashes, and more rarely, systemic flares. SLE patients are more likely than controls to have drug allergies, especially to sulfonamide antibiotics. The common cold remedy echinacea has precipitated SLE flares in several patients. In several case-control studies, smoking has been found to be a risk factor for SLE. Once SLE is diagnosed, patients who continue to smoke are at greater risk for discoid lupus. Infection with Epstein-Barr virus has been strongly associated with SLE in a multicase family registry. Silica and mercury exposure are increased in SLE patients.

Hormonal factors are obviously important, given the female predominance of SLE and the usual onset of SLE after puberty. In the Nurses' Cohort study, use of oral contraceptives or estrogen replacement therapy was a risk factor for later SLE. In clinical trials, hormone replacement therapy increased mild-to-moderate flares in SLE, but oral contraceptives did not. Pregnancy is associated with SLE flares in some, but not all, studies. Elevation of prolactin may be associated with activity of SLE.

The activity of SLE follows several patterns. The classic pattern, the flare pattern, is characterized by a relapsing-remitting course. However, an equal number of SLE patients have a pattern of continuously active disease. Only a minority of patients are lucky enough to have long periods of disease quiescence. The antimalarial drug hydroxychloroquine, which is widely used for cutaneous lupus and lupus arthritis, reduces future flares if patients continue to take it. Dehydroepiandrosterone, which is not approved by the Food and Drug Administration, has also been shown to reduce flares.

Over half of SLE patients have acquired permanent damage in one or more organ systems. Although damage, such as renal failure and interstitial pulmonary fibrosis, can occur from SLE itself, glucocorticoid therapy accounts for a large proportion as well. For example, long-term prednisone therapy may cause osteoporotic fractures, osteonecrosis of bone, and cataracts and glaucoma.

Survival of SLE patients peaked at about 80% at 10 years after diagnosis in the 1980s. The Centers for Disease Control and Prevention reported in 2002 that mortality in young women had actually increased. The major cause of death in SLE is accelerated atherosclerosis. Although SLE itself can damage the endothelial surface of the coronary arteries, part of the atherosclerotic process results from elevated levels of traditional cardiovascular risk factors, including hypertension, hyperlipidemia, obesity, and homocysteine levels. Prednisone increases the patient's weight, blood pressure, glucose, and lipid levels. SLE nephritis can lead to hypertension and hyperlipidemia. Renal insufficiency can increase homocysteine levels.

Clinical Findings

A. SYMPTOMS AND SIGNS

The American College of Rheumatology has established criteria for the classification (not diagnosis) of SLE. Four of the eleven criteria must be present for the classification of SLE (Table 22–1). The criteria are heavily weighted toward mucocutaneous findings but do serve to emphasize the multisystem nature of the disease. However, a patient with a classic finding, such as lupus nephritis, has SLE even if she or he does not have 4 of the 11 classification criteria.

Early signs and symptoms of SLE may not be specific; a delay in diagnosis is commonplace. Early signs and symptoms include fatigue, mild hair loss, anemia, arthralgias, nausea, and weight loss.

Table 22–1. Systemic Lupus Erythematosus Classification Criteria

Systemic lupus erythematosus may be classified if 4 or more of the following 11 disorders are present:
Malar rash
Discoid rash
Photosensitivity
Oral ulcers
Arthritis
Serositis
Renal disorder
a. > 0.5 g/d proteinuria, or
b. ≥ 3+ dipstick proteinuria, or
c. Cellular casts
Neurologic disorder
a. Seizures, or
b. Psychosis (without other cause)
Hematologic disorder
a. Hemolytic anemia, or
b. Leukopenia ($<4000/\mu$L), or
c. Lymphopenia ($<1500/\mu$L), or
d. Thrombocytopenia ($<100,000\ \mu$L)
Immunologic disorder
a. Antibody to native DNA, or
b. Antibody to Sm, or
c. Positive test for antiphospholipid antibodies, including:
(1) abnormal IgG or IgM anticardiolipin
(2) lupus anticoagulant
(3) false-positive serologic test for syphilis
Positive antinuclear antibodies

Table 22–2. Organ Involvement in Systemic Lupus Erythematosus

Involved Organ or System	Typical	Unusual
Head, ears, eyes, nose, and throat	Alopecia Discoid lupus of scalp, ears Oral/nasal ulcers Keratoconjunctivitis sicca Dry mouth Episcleritis, scleritis	Angioedema Polychondritis Retinitis Optic neuritis Uveitis
Cutaneous	Malar rash Discoid rash Maculopapular rash Subacute cutaneous lupus Nailfold capillary changes Livedo reticularis	Bullous lupus Cutaneous vasculitis
Cardiopulmonary	Pleurisy/pleural effusion Pericarditis/pericardial effusion Interstitial pneumonitis (acute or chronic) Pulmonary hypertension	Myocarditis Libman-Sacks endocarditis Pulmonary hemorrhage Coronary arteritis/aneurysm
Gastrointestinal	Esophageal dysmotility Hepatomegaly Splenomegaly Elevated liver function tests	Mesenteric vasculitis (with or without infarcts) Colitis Protein-losing enteropathy Primary biliary cirrhosis Budd-Chiari syndrome Ascites
Neurologic	Cognitive impairment Seizures Psychosis Stroke (or transient ischemic attack) Mononeuritis multiplex Peripheral neuropathy	Cranial neuropathy Chorea Pseudotumor cerebri Transverse myelitis Encephalopathy/coma
Constitutional	Fever Weight loss Fatigue Lymphadenopathy	
Musculoskeletal	Polyarthralgias/arthritis Myalgias	Myositis

1. Head, ears, eyes, nose, and throat—Alopecia can occur as a diffuse alopecia or as an alopecia that is especially marked around the face (Table 22–2). Discoid lupus can cause a scarring alopecia. Ear involvement is sometimes seen in discoid lupus. Rarely, polychondritis may develop in a patient with lupus. Secondary Sjögren syndrome occurs in some patients with SLE, leading to keratoconjunctivitis sicca (dry eyes and mouth). Additional ocular involvement includes episcleritis, scleritis, uveitis, retinitis, and optic neuropathy. Both the nose and mouth (palate and buccal mucosa) may have aphthous ulcers (both painful and painless). Discoid lupus can also occur in the mouth.

2. Cutaneous—SLE rashes are most often, but not always, photosensitive. The malar rash occurs in sun-exposed areas, such as nose and cheeks, and spares the nasolabial folds and below the nares. Maculopapular lupus eruptions can occur on the face, the V of the neck, forearms, and elsewhere. Discoid lupus lesions occur in these areas and also in the ears and scalp. Discoid lesions often heal with hypo- or hyperpigmentation. Subacute cutaneous lupus, which may be mistaken for a fungal rash, occurs as a psoriaform type or an annular type. It may develop idiopathically or in a response to a drug, including hydrochlorothiazide, angiotensin-converting enzyme inhibitors, and calcium channel blockers. About half of patients with subcutaneous lupus have systemic lupus erythematosus. Livedo reticularis occurs with or without antiphospholipid antibodies. Nailfold capillary changes can be seen. A rare lupus rash, bullous lupus, presents as blistering lesions. Lupus panniculitis (also called "lupus profundus") can heal with a cavitating appearance because of fat necrosis.

3. Cardiopulmonary—Pleuritic pain (sometimes with pleural effusions) and pericardial pain (with or without effusion) occur in SLE. Pleurisy is more common than pericarditis, but they can occur together. Rare cardiac manifestations include Libman-Sacks endocarditis with valvular vegetations, myocarditis, and coronary arteritis. Pulmonary hypertension can be primary or secondary to pulmonary emboli. Pulmonary hypertension in lupus is usually mild, but it can progress. Interstitial pneumonitis, both acute and chronic, may occur. Life-threatening pulmonary hemorrhage is an unusual finding.

4. Gastrointestinal—Esophageal dysmotility occurs in SLE, but is usually mild. Hepatomegaly and splenomegaly may occur, especially in children. Pancreatitis is a rare manifestation. Mesenteric vasculitis can lead to postprandial pain, abdominal pain, infarcts, and bowel perforation. Colitis and protein-losing enteropathy are extremely rare. A few SLE patients will have overlap with primary biliary cirrhosis or autoimmune hepatitis. About one-third of SLE patients have a mild elevation of liver function tests.

5. Neurologic—SLE can present with or include psychosis, seizures, encephalopathy (organic brain syndrome), coma, stroke, pseudotumor cerebri, meningitis, transverse myelitis, mononeuritis multiplex, and peripheral neuropathy. The diversity of neurologic manifestations is not represented by the classification criteria, which include only seizures and psychosis. For this reason, the American College of Rheumatology devised, by consensus, definitions of the neurologic symptoms and manifestations seen in SLE.

The most common form of neurologic involvement is cognitive impairment, occurring in 80% of SLE patients 10 years after diagnosis. This likely represents permanent damage in most patients. It is more likely to progress in patients who are persistently positive for antiphospholipid antibodies.

Psychosis in lupus is rare. If it occurs in a patient on glucocorticoids, the differential diagnosis would include glucocorticoid psychosis. Glucocorticoid psychosis is rare if the prednisone dose is less than 20 mg daily.

Seizures can represent active lupus, or represent an epileptic focus from a past stroke. Antiphospholipid antibodies increase the risk of stroke. Seizures can also be secondary to metabolic or toxic factors. Hydroxychloroquine reduces the seizure threshold, and should not be introduced unless seizures are well controlled.

Encephalopathy, formerly called organic brain syndrome, is very rare. Patients present with a change in mentation and consciousness, sometimes progressing to frank coma. The EEG will be abnormal, usually with diffuse slowing. The lumbar puncture will often show an elevated protein level, or will show an elevated IgG index or oligoclonal bands. The differential diagnosis includes metabolic or toxic factors.

Pseudotumor cerebri presents as headache. The differential diagnosis includes lupus, glucocorticoids, antiphospholipid antibodies leading to a dural sinus thrombosis, and idiopathic.

Lupus can cause meningitis, presenting as headache, often with fever and meningeal signs. The cerebrospinal fluid will be sterile, but often the protein level is increased, the white blood cell count is increased, or there are oligoclonal bands or an increased IgG index. Nonsteroidal anti-inflammatory drugs, including ibuprofen and naproxen, have rarely caused meningitis in lupus patients.

Transverse myelitis is rare in lupus. It can be seen from lupus itself, or secondary to thrombosis from antiphospholipid antibodies. Patients may first present with sensory symptoms. The physical examination will show the spinal cord level.

Mononeuritis multiplex is a vasculitis of the vaso nervorum. It presents with sensory symptoms followed by motor weakness such as foot drop, most often in the distal lower extremities. Peripheral neuropathy, including sensory neuropathies, also occur in lupus. Cranial neuropathies, such as ptosis, are rare.

Strokes can occur from active lupus. However, most strokes in SLE patients are from comorbid conditions such as hypertension, atherosclerosis, or antiphospholipid syndrome.

6. Constitutional—Many SLE patients have low-grade fever (a few with temperatures higher than 39°C). Weight loss can occur, especially at presentation, but is rare. Lymphadenopathy can be found, usually small and symmetric. An acute fatigue can occur with lupus flares. Chronic fatigue is common, often as part of fibromyalgia, which occurs in as many as 30% of SLE patients.

7. Musculoskeletal—Polyarthralgias and polyarthritis eventually occur in 90% of SLE patients. The arthritis is usually nonerosive, involving the small joints of the hands (proximal interphalangeal and metacarpophalangeal joints, but not distal interphalangeal joints) and wrists initially. If deformities occur, they are usually reversible ("Jaccoud arthropathy"), because they are due to tendon and ligament laxity, not to bone erosions. Myositis, or an overlap with dermatomyositis, is rarely found. As many as 30% of SLE patients have coexisting fibromyalgia, which is a noninflammatory chronic

Table 22–3. Laboratory Findings in Systemic Lupus Erythematosus

Test	Typical	Unusual
Hematologic	Anemia of chronic disease Hemolytic anemia with elevated reticulocyte count Leukopenia Thrombocytopenia Elevated erythrocyte sedimentation rate or C-reactive protein Prolonged partial thromboplastin time, dR VVT, or other test for lupus anticoagulant	Neutropenia
Comprehensive metabolic panel	Elevated blood urea nitrogen or creatinine	Elevated liver function tests
Other chemistry	Elevated creatine kinase or aldolase Elevated homocysteine Elevated cholesterol	
Urinalysis	Proteinuria Red blood cells or red blood cell casts	

dR VVT, dilute Russel viper venom time.

pain syndrome, presenting with symmetric tender points above and below the waist.

8. Lupus nephritis—Lupus nephritis occurs in 50% of Caucasian patients, and as many as 75% of African-American patients. Patients are usually asymptomatic, with the urinalysis or serum creatinine leading to the initial evaluation. The International Society of Nephrology has updated the previous World Health Organization classification of lupus nephritis. A renal biopsy is necessary to correctly classify the patient. Even in the lupus patient with proteinuria or hematuria, it should not be assumed that the underlying pathology is lupus nephritis. The renal biopsy may identify other lesions, including comorbidity from diabetes mellitus and hypertension, interstitial nephritis from drugs, renal vasculitis from hepatitis C (cryoglobulinemia), or microangiopathic changes (often due to antiphospholipid antibodies).

The most severe form of lupus nephritis is diffuse proliferative glomerulonephritis. There are subendothelial immune complex deposits. This disorder can rapidly lead to renal failure. Usually, the urinalysis shows proteinuria, hematuria, and if a first morning urine is obtained, red blood cell casts (Table 22–3). Focal lupus nephritis (class III) is less severe, but occasional patients do progress to renal failure. Membranous lupus nephritis can occur as a pure form, or along with diffuse proliferative glomerulonephritis or focal lupus nephritis. There are subepithelial immune complex deposits with concomitant mesangial deposits. Patients usually have nephrotic syndrome. Its course is more indolent, but there is eventual progression to renal insufficiency and failure. Nephrotic syndrome is not to be considered benign, because it causes hyperlipidemia and hypercoagulability. The mildest form of lupus nephritis is mesangial lupus nephritis (class I).

B. LABORATORY FINDINGS

1. Hematologic—Anemia is very common in SLE but is multifactorial. The classic anemia, a hemolytic anemia with increased reticulocyte count, direct Coombs test, and low haptoglobin, is not the most common. Anemia of chronic disease is the most common finding. Anemia may also be due to iron deficiency, renal insufficiency or failure, or to sickle cell (or trait) and thalassemia.

Leukopenia is common but usually mild. It is rare for the white blood cell count to be below $1000/\mu L$. Lymphopenia is frequent (glucocorticoids also cause lymphopenia). Neutropenia can occur but is rare.

Mild or profound thrombocytopenia can occur. Antiphospholipid antibodies are also associated with thrombocytopenia.

The partial thromboplastin time may be prolonged due to a lupus anticoagulant.

The erythrocyte sedimentation rate or C-reactive protein level may be elevated. The erythrocyte sedimentation rate and C-reactive protein do not correlate with or predict clinical disease activity.

2. Chemistries—The blood urea nitrogen and creatinine may be elevated due to renal insufficiency or failure. Cholesterol may be elevated secondary to nephrotic syndrome or to high-dose prednisone.

The transaminases may be elevated (usually mildly) due to SLE. An elevated alkaline phosphatase may indicate renal osteodystrophy or primary biliary cirrhosis.

Creatine kinase may be elevated secondary to myositis. Homocysteine, a risk factor for atherosclerosis and thrombosis, is elevated in up to 30%, especially if there is renal insufficiency.

3. Urinalysis—Lupus nephritis may present as proteinuria alone or proteinuria with an active urine sediment (red blood cells or red blood cell casts). Pyuria may occur as well. Nephrotic syndrome is common with membranous lupus nephritis. Isolated hematuria is unlikely to be due to lupus nephritis, and would prompt a search for other pathologies, such as menstrual contamination, trauma, bladder pathology such as hemorrhagic cystitis, polyp or tumor, and renal calculi.

C. IMAGING STUDIES

Magnetic resonance imaging of the brain is preferred over computed tomography in the evaluation of central nervous system lupus. The most common finding is small white matter lesions, which may represent immune complex deposition. Cerebral atrophy can also occur. A true vasculitis is almost never seen on cerebral arteriogram.

Magnetic resonance imaging of the hip is the best way to find osteonecrosis at an early stage, when it may be ameliorated by core decompression. Bone scan can detect subclinical involvement of other sites.

D. SPECIAL TESTS

1. Autoantibodies—Most (96% or more) SLE patients have a positive antinuclear antibody (ANA) test result. Because up to 20% of healthy young women also have a positive ANA, the presence of an ANA alone is not given much weight. Titers of 1:640 or higher are more indicative of a connective tissue disease of some sort.

Some autoantibodies are very specific for lupus, such as anti-dsDNA (which occurs in about 30%) or anti-Sm (this is an abbreviation for Smith, not smooth muscle). Other autoantibodies, such as anti-Ro/SS-A, anti-La/SS-B, and anti-ribonucleoprotein, occur in SLE but also in rheumatoid arthritis and in Sjögren syndrome.

Antiphospholipid antibodies (lupus anticoagulant, anticardiolipin, and anti-β_2 glycoprotein-1) are found in about 50% of SLE patients during the course of disease. They are associated with an increased risk of thrombosis and pregnancy loss.

A recently identified autoantibody, anti-SR, has received Food and Drug Administration approval for testing in SLE.

2. Complement—Reduction in the complement components C3 and C4 or in total hemolytic complement occurs frequently, but is not specific for lupus.

E. SPECIAL EXAMINATION

A skin biopsy with immunofluorescence is helpful in the diagnosis of SLE cutaneous lesions.

In patients with nephritis, a renal biopsy can determine the ISN subtype (mesangial, focal proliferative, diffuse proliferative, or membranous) and give information on both activity and chronicity (damage).

In patients with neuropathy, a nerve conduction study and biopsy may be necessary to document vasculitis. An electromyelogram and muscle biopsy may be needed in the evaluation of myositis.

Differential Diagnosis

SLE is diagnosed in some patients based on a positive ANA, which is inappropriate. Patients with a positive ANA and fatigue or chronic pain are likely to have fibromyalgia rather than lupus.

SLE may be confused with other connective tissue diseases, especially rheumatoid arthritis. SLE patients may have positive rheumatoid factor. The usual presentation of lupus arthritis is identical to that of rheumatoid arthritis, but SLE arthritis is rarely erosive. SLE and dermatomyositis may be hard to differentiate, or they may overlap.

Drug-induced lupus must be excluded. In young women, minocycline can cause a drug-induced lupus, often with autoimmune hepatitis and perinuclear-antineutrophilic cytoplasmic autoantibodies. Anti–tumor necrosis factor biological agents used for rheumatoid arthritis can induce lupus.

Some viral infections may mimic lupus. Parvovirus can cause a polyarthritis and positive ANA. HIV can cause thrombocytopenia and positive direct Coombs test. Hepatitis B can cause vasculitis, and hepatitis C can cause cryoglobulinemia (with renal and neurologic manifestations) that can be confused with lupus.

A malignancy can cause anemia, elevated erythrocyte sedimentation rate, positive ANA, vasculitis, and other autoimmune phenomena. Anemia and an elevated erythrocyte sedimentation rate should also bring to mind multiple myeloma.

Complications

A. SLE COMPLICATIONS

The major cause of death in patients with SLE is accelerated atherosclerosis. This is a multifactorial process, with lupus playing a role along with traditional cardiovascular risk factors (many of which are aggravated by glucocorticoid therapy). Attention to weight, hypertension, hyperlipidemia, smoking, diabetes, and homocysteinemia is crucial.

Renal failure occurs in lupus nephritis in spite of aggressive treatment with intravenous cyclophosphamide

Table 22–4. Antiphospholipid Antibody Syndrome Classification Criteria

Vascular thrombosis
Arterial, venous, or small vessel
Pregnancy morbidity
One or more fetal deaths
One or more premature births due to severe preeclampsia or placental insufficiency
Three or more first trimester losses
PLUS lupus anticoagulant
Anticardiolipin IgG or IgM (medium to high titer)
Anti-β_2 glycoprotein-1 IgG or IgM on two occasions 3 months (or more) apart

Ig, immunoglobulin.

and other regimens. Hypertension is a major comorbidity and should be aggressively managed with angiotensin-converting enzyme inhibitors, which may have a renal protective effect.

Strokes can occur from active central nervous system lupus, but also from antiphospholipid antibody syndrome, hypertension, atherosclerosis, and infection. Antiphospholipid antibody syndrome (see Chapter 24) is a major source of morbidity in SLE and contributes to mortality (Table 22–4).

B. GLUCOCORTICOID COMPLICATIONS

Glucocorticoid use contributes to cataracts; osteoporotic fractures; osteonecrosis; diabetes mellitus; multiple cardiovascular risk factors; infections; and quality-of-life issues with cushingoid habitus, weight gain, acne, and emotional lability or frank depression.

Recognition of glucocorticoid toxicity has led to a steroid-sparing approach, with prednisone taper; if taper is unsuccessful, then other immunosuppressive drugs are added to control disease activity.

C. OPPORTUNISTIC INFECTIONS

Until proved otherwise, consider infection in a patient with SLE who is febrile. Opportunistic infections are often missed until a postmortem examination. Prophylaxis against *Pneumocystis carinii* pneumonia can be given to neutropenic SLE patients using 100 mg of dapsone three times a week. Also, use of sulfonamide antibiotics should be avoided, as they can sometimes precipitate lupus flares.

D. MALIGNANCY

Recent studies have suggested an increased risk of malignancy in SLE, even without cyclophosphamide exposure. SLE patients who received oral cyclophosphamide at the National Institutes of Health had an increase in skin cancer, and later lymphoproliferative disease. Women with SLE are more likely to have cervical dysplasia and carcinoma. Pap smears should be done yearly.

E. ASSOCIATED AUTOIMMUNE DISEASES

Hypothyroidism develops in about 10% of SLE patients. Secondary Sjögren syndrome can occur in SLE patients, with or without the Sjögren antibodies anti-Ro and anti-La.

If anti-Ro (especially with anti-La) is present, there is a risk of neonatal lupus in the fetus, presenting as congenital heart block or neonatal lupus rash (the latter being transient).

When to Refer to a Specialist

A rheumatologist is usually needed to make a firm diagnosis of SLE. Often the need for procedures, such as skin, nerve/muscle, or renal biopsy, will lead to the involvement of dermatologists, neurologists, and nephrologists, as appropriate.

SLE patients receiving glucocorticoids or other immunosuppressive drugs require follow-up by a rheumatologist. Bone density scans should be done routinely to monitor for glucocorticoid-induced osteoporosis and to assess the adequacy of treatment.

Often, comorbid conditions, such as depression or fibromyalgia, lead to complaints that appear to mimic lupus. Recognition before the patient is unnecessarily exposed to glucocorticoids is essential.

Communication between the patient, primary care provider, and rheumatologist is crucial in laboratory monitoring and identifying which new events or complications are lupus-related.

Prognosis

The 10-year survival of lupus patients peaked at 80% in the 1980s. The improvement up to the 1980s reflected not just rheumatologic care but successful treatment of infections and supportive care for renal failure. Early deaths in lupus tend to reflect disease activity and infections, whereas late deaths are largely due to cardiovascular complications.

REFERENCES

American College of Rheumatology Ad Hoc Committee on Systemic Lupus Erythematosus Guidelines. Guidelines for referral and management of systemic lupus erythematosus in adults. *Arthritis Rheum.* 1999;42:1785. [PMID: 10513791] (The committee report reviews general guidelines in the care of SLE.)

Barr SG, Zonana-Nacach A, Magder LS, Petri M. Patterns of disease activity in systemic lupus erythematosus. *Arthritis Rheum.* 1999;42:2682. [PMID: 10616018] (Two patterns of activity characterize SLE: a relapsing-remitting pattern [flare] and a chronically active pattern. Long periods of disease quiescence are rare.)

Bernatsky S, Boivin JF, Joseph L, et al. An international cohort study of cancer in systemic lupus erythematosus. *Arthritis Rheum.* 2005;52:1481. [PMID: 15880596]

Brey RL, Holliday SL, Saklad AR, et al. Neuropsychiatric syndromes in lupus: prevalence using standardized definitions. *Neurology.* 2002;58:1214. [PMID: 11971089]

Esdaile JM, Abrahamowicz M, Grodzicky T, et al. Traditional Framingham risk factors fail to fully account for accelerated atherosclerosis in systemic lupus erythematosus. *Arthritis Rheum.* 2001;44:2331. [PMID: 11665973] (Atherosclerosis in SLE cannot be explained by traditional risk factors alone.)

Manzi S, Meilahn EN, Rairie JE, et al. Age-specific incidence rates of myocardial infarction and angina in women with systemic lupus erythematosus: comparison with the Framingham Study. *Am J Epidemiol.* 1997;145:408. [PMID: 9048514] (Atherosclerosis in SLE is much more frequent than in Framingham controls.)

Tan EM, Cohen AS, Fries JF, et al. The 1982 revised criteria for the classification of systemic lupus erythematosus. *Arthritis Rheum.* 1982;25:1271. [PMID: 7138600]

The American College of Rheumatology nomenclature and case definitions for neuropsychiatric lupus syndromes. *Arthritis Rheum.* 1999;42:599. [PMID: 10211873]

Uramoto KM, Michet CJ Jr, Thumboo J, et al. Trends in the incidence and mortality of systemic lupus erythematosus, 1950–1992. *Arthritis Rheum.* 1999;42:46. [PMID: 9920013] (This population-based study in Rochester, Minnesota, shows an apparent tripling in the incidence of SLE.)

Urowitz MB, Gladman DD. Late mortality in SLE—"the price we pay for control." *J Rheumatol.* 1980;7:412. [PMID: 7401073] (Mortality in SLE is bimodal, with later deaths largely due to atherosclerosis.)

Weening JJ, D'Agati VD, Schwartz MM, et al. The classification of glomerulonephritis in systemic lupus erythematosus revisited. *J Am Soc Nephrol.* 2004;15:241. [PMID: 14747370]

Zonana-Nacach A, Barr SG, Magder LS, Petri M. Damage in systemic lupus erythematosus and its association with corticosteroids. *Arthritis Rheum.* 2000;43:1801. [PMID: 10943870] (In this prospective study, both chronic use of prednisone and exposure to high doses led to later morbidity.)

Relevant World Wide Web Sites

[Lupus Foundation of America]

http://www.lupus.org

[The National Institute of Arthritis and Musculoskeletal and Skin Diseases (NIAMS)]

http://www.niams.nih.gov/

[Arthritis Foundation]

http://www.arthritis.org

Treatment of Systemic Lupus Erythematosus

Maria Dall'Era, MD, & David Wofsy, MD

Systemic lupus erythematosus (SLE) is a heterogeneous multisystem disease. Each lupus patient manifests her or his disease in a unique way, and treatment should be tailored to the type and severity of organ system involvement. Unfortunately, this is more easily said than done, because there are few large studies to guide decision making. The lack of large-scale, randomized controlled trials has resulted in therapeutic strategies that are largely empiric. Indeed, in the four decades since the U.S. Food and Drug Administration adopted its current approach to drug evaluation, no drug has been approved for the treatment of SLE. Despite these limitations, well-accepted community standards exist and are helpful in guiding treatment. In the end, the patient and his or her physician must weigh the potential risks and benefits of a particular therapy and agree upon a course of action.

As a foundation for any lupus treatment regimen, lifestyle modification including regular exercise, sufficient rest, a healthful diet, smoking cessation, and sun protection is critical. Lupus patients are at increased risk for accelerated atherosclerosis, and thus aggressive risk factor modification is also required. In particular, hypertension and hyperlipidemia should be appropriately treated. Each patient should receive a yearly influenza vaccine and a pneumococcal vaccine every 5 years. Attention to bone health and prevention of steroid-induced osteoporosis with calcium, vitamin D, and bisphosphonates is necessary. Because of this adverse effect as well as many others, it is important to minimize the use of chronic glucocorticoids if at all possible. Studies suggest that there may be an increased risk of malignancy in SLE patients and that SLE patients are less likely than the general population to undergo routine cancer screening. Thus age-appropriate cancer screening should be reinforced. Unlike the general population, women with SLE should undergo screening for cervical cancer on a yearly basis.

CONSTITUTIONAL SYMPTOMS

Fatigue is prevalent in SLE patients and can be a disabling symptom. Treatment depends on the underlying etiology of the fatigue, with reversible factors such as hypothyroidism, anemia, and diabetes being addressed first. Pain and depression are positive predictors of fatigue in SLE patients, while social support mitigates fatigue. Thus a multidisciplinary approach with attention to these issues can be helpful. Regular aerobic exercise followed by periods of rest should also be encouraged. In some patients, successful treatment of other manifestations of SLE (eg, with antimalarials) has a beneficial impact on fatigue as well.

CUTANEOUS MANIFESTATIONS

Sun Protection

Photosensitivity occurs in approximately 75% of SLE patients. Although sensitivity to ultraviolet-B light as found in sunlight and fluorescent lights occurs most commonly, some individuals are also sensitive to ultraviolet-A light and/or visible light. Photosensitive lesions include the malar rash, discoid lupus, and subacute cutaneous lupus. Prompt treatment of cutaneous lupus is necessary to prevent the development of scarring, dyspigmentation, and alopecia.

Sun protection forms the cornerstone of the management of cutaneous lupus. Patients should be educated about the use of sunscreens and the avoidance of intense sun exposure during peak daylight hours. Daily use of sunscreen with an SPF value of 30 is recommended. Patients are urged to apply the sunscreen 30–60 minutes prior to exposure and to reapply the sunscreen every 4–6 hours. Sun-protective clothing is also very important and is widely available. Smoking cessation is very important because smokers tend to have worse skin disease than nonsmokers.

Topical Therapies

Cutaneous lupus is often initially treated with topical glucocorticoids. The selection of a topical glucocorticoid is based on the location of the lesion as well as the type of lesion. In general, a low-potency glucocorticoid such as hydrocortisone is used first, with escalation to more potent, fluorinated preparations as needed. When treating facial lesions, the use of fluorinated glucocorticoids is limited to 2 weeks because of the well-recognized side effects of skin atrophy, striae, depigmentation, and telangiectasias. Medium-potency preparations such as triamcinolone acetonide or betamethasone valerate are often used for trunk and limb lesions, while high-potency preparations such as clobetasol are reserved for severe, hypertrophic lesions. It is thought that ointments are generally more effective than creams and that lotions are most useful for hairy areas such as the scalp. Intralesional injections of triamcinolone acetonide are often used to treat refractory lesions, such as discoid lupus occurring on the scalp. The injection is performed with a 30-gauge needle and is directed into the active, erythematous regions of the lesions. It is important to remember that adrenal suppression can occur with the use of high-potency topical glucocorticoids.

Topical tacrolimus and pimecrolimus, which are approved for the treatment of atopic dermatitis, are sometimes used as second-line agents for the treatment of acute lupus lesions, subacute cutaneous lupus, and discoid lupus. They are often used in an attempt to minimize exposure to chronic topical glucocorticoids. Enthusiasm for their use has been slightly tempered by an FDA advisory in May of 2005 warning physicians about the risk of lymphoma and nonmelanoma skin cancer with topical tacrolimus. This warning was based primarily on information from animal studies and case reports from small numbers of patients. Another class of topical therapies, retinoids, might be effective in patients with discoid lupus.

Systemic Therapies

Systemic therapies are necessary when cutaneous lupus cannot be controlled with the topical and/or intralesional methods described above. The antimalarial hydroxychloroquine is the initial treatment of choice. Its onset of action is approximately 1 month, and full benefit might not be seen for several months. Hydroxychloroquine is also useful in controlling mild arthritis and fatigue. In addition, it might prevent more serious disease flares. A 24-week randomized placebo-controlled trial examining the effect of discontinuing the use of hydroxychloroquine in 47 patients with SLE determined that the risk of major and minor flares was 2.5 times greater in the patients that discontinued the hydroxychloroquine. Lastly, the antithrombotic and lipid-lowering effects of hydroxychloroquine are beneficial for all SLE patients, especially those who have antiphospholipid antibodies.

Hydroxychloroquine is typically dosed at 200 or 400 mg per day and should not exceed 6.5 mg/kg/d. At these doses it is usually well tolerated. The most common side effects of hydroxychloroquine include gastrointestinal upset, headaches, and rashes. The most feared complication of the drug is retinal deposition leading to potentially irreversible retinopathy if it is not detected early. Thus a baseline ophthalmologic examination followed by yearly exams is recommended in all patients. This complication is exceedingly rare at the doses of hydroxychloroquine currently used.

The antimalarial agents chloroquine (200–500 mg/d) or quinacrine (100 mg/d) can be used in patients who do not fully respond to treatment with hydroxychloroquine. Because of the possibility of increased ocular toxicity, hydroxychloroquine should not be used in combination with chloroquine. Quinacrine does not cause retinal toxicity, and thus can be used in combination with either hydroxychloroquine or chloroquine. In practice, quinacrine is used infrequently because it causes a yellow skin discoloration with long-term use. It is only available through compounding pharmacists.

Patients with refractory cutaneous lupus may respond to treatment with a variety of other systemic agents. Dapsone (25–200 mg/d) is effective in some patients, particularly those with bullous LE. Open-label trials have shown efficacy for thalidomide, but significant toxicities including drowsiness, dizziness, neuropathy, and teratogenicity limit its utility for long-term use. Azathioprine, methotrexate, mycophenolate mofetil, intravenous immune globulin (IVIG), and cyclophosphamide may also be beneficial for severe cutaneous disease.

Callen JP. Update on the management of cutaneous lupus erythematosus. *Br J Dermatol.* 2004;151:731. [PMID: 15491411] (Concise evidence-based review of the treatment of lupus skin disease.)

The Canadian Hydroxychloroquine Study Group. A randomized study of the effect of withdrawing hydroxychloroquine sulfate in systemic lupus erythematosus. *N Engl J Med.* 1991;324:150. [PMID: 1984192] (Patients who discontinued hydroxychloroquine had a 2.5-times greater risk of major and minor flares than those who continued the drug.)

MUSCULOSKELETAL MANIFESTATIONS

Arthritis and arthralgias are extremely common in patients with SLE. First-line therapy usually consists of nonsteroidal anti-inflammatory drugs (NSAIDs) and/or acetaminophen. A proton pump inhibitor is necessary for those at risk of NSAID-induced gastropathy, especially for patients taking concomitant aspirin and/or glucocorticoids. Testing for and treating *Helicobacter pylori* infection is also prudent in this group of patients. Hydroxychloroquine is often added in patients who have had an incomplete response to NSAIDs. Short-term use of low doses of glucocorticoids (5–10 mg) might be necessary to obtain quick control over an inflammatory arthritis while waiting for the full effect of hydroxychloroquine. Methotrexate is frequently used as a steroid-sparing agent. Azathioprine and mycophenolate mofetil might be helpful in patients who have an incomplete response to, or are unable to tolerate, methotrexate.

SEROSITIS

Pleuritis and pericarditis often respond to treatment with NSAIDs and/or low-to-moderate doses of glucocorticoids. Hydroxychloroquine may be helpful in patients with persistent or recurrent symptoms. In patients with severe and/or refractory disease, moderate-to-high doses of glucocorticoids (0.5–1 mg/kg) can be used for short periods of time. In these patients, methotrexate, azathioprine, or mycophenolate mofetil can be helpful in tapering the prednisone.

RENAL DISEASE

Basic Principles

The treatment of lupus renal disease is divided into an induction of remission phase and a maintenance phase. The goal of this approach is to achieve a remission with cytotoxic agents given over several months, and then to maintain the remission by using less toxic medications. In addition to addressing the inflammatory etiology of the nephritis, it is also important to treat concomitant risk factors for the progression to chronic kidney disease. To this end, angiotensin-converting enzyme inhibitors and/or angiotensin II receptor blockers are used to treat proteinuria and hypertension. A combination of antihypertensive agents might be necessary to achieve the goal blood pressure of <130/80 mm Hg. Statins are often needed to lower serum low density lipoprotein cholesterol levels to the goal of <100 mg/dL.

Renal biopsy is recommended for most patients with suspected lupus nephritis. The pathologic type of nephritis as defined by the International Society of Nephrology/Renal Pathology Society classification system helps to guide the choice of the treatment regimen. For example, patients with proliferative disease and a high activity index usually receive cytotoxic medications and high-dose glucocorticoids. Conversely, patients with class I or class II disease can often be treated solely with angiotensin-converting enzyme inhibitors and/or angiotensin II receptor blockers. A renal biopsy is also useful in ruling out other etiologies for the nephropathy such as diabetes, hypertension, or focal segmental glomerulosclerosis, for which immunosuppressive medication would not be appropriate. Patients who fail to respond to therapy might require a second biopsy to determine if they still have active nephritis, or alternatively, if they have developed significant renal scarring that should not be treated with further immunosuppressives.

Mittal B, Rennke H, Singh AK. The role of kidney biopsy in the management of lupus nephritis. *Curr Opin Nephrol Hypertens.* 2005;14:1. [PMID: 15586009] (A recent review of the utility of renal biopsy in lupus nephritis, written by experts in the field.)

Weening JJ, D'Agati VD, Schwartz MM, et al. The classification of glomerulonephritis in systemic lupus erythematosus revisited. *Kidney Int.* 2004;65:521. [PMID: 14717922] (An informative review of the new International Society of Nephrology/Renal Pathology Society classification system for lupus nephritis including micrographs of various patterns of glomerular injury.)

Proliferative Lupus Nephritis

Several important trials conducted at the National Institutes of Health provided the rationale behind the current therapeutic regimens used to treat proliferative lupus nephritis. Key findings from these trials are as follows: (1) treatment with intravenous pulse cyclophosphamide (CYC) is superior to high-dose oral prednisone alone in preventing progression to end-stage renal disease, and (2) an extended course of CYC (six monthly pulses followed by quarterly pulses for 2 years) is more effective than pulse methylprednisolone and shorter courses of CYC in preserving renal function and preventing renal relapse. Thus the use of monthly intravenous pulse CYC (in conjunction with high-dose glucocorticoids) followed by quarterly pulse CYC became the standard of care in the community. CYC is initially dosed at 0.5–1 g/m^2, with the lower dose range administered to patients with renal dysfunction, obesity, or advanced age. The dose is then adjusted based on the leukocyte nadir 7–10 days after the infusion.

The use of CYC is associated with significant toxicities including infections (most commonly herpes zoster), cytopenias, hemorrhagic cystitis, malignancy, and premature ovarian failure. Adequate hydration and the use of mesna decrease the occurrence of bladder toxicity, and *Pneumocystis carinii* pneumonia prophylaxis is indicated for all patients on CYC. Ovarian toxicity deserves special mention because it has become a major reason why increasing numbers of patients are trying to avoid treatment with CYC. The risk of permanent ovarian failure is related to the cumulative CYC dose and the age of the patient. One sobering study revealed that in patients on the standard long course of pulse CYC, the rate of amenorrhea was 17% for patients ≤25 years old, 43% for patients between 26 and 30 years old, and 100% for patients ≥31 years old. Recent data suggest that the administration of 3.75 mg leuprolide intramuscularly 2 weeks prior to each CYC infusion might offer some protection against ovarian failure. Because of the potentially devastating toxicities described above, many physicians and their patients are opting to use shorter courses and/or lower doses of pulse CYC than originally described in the National Institutes of Health regimen. Most commonly, once a patient enters remission after 3–6 months of CYC, agents such as azathioprine or mycophenolate mofetil are used for maintenance. Not only are physicians increasingly attracted to less intensive CYC regimens, but some have challenged the primacy of CYC as an induction agent altogether. One recent trial suggests that mycophenolate mofetil may be comparable, or perhaps superior, to CYC in terms of both induction and maintenance of renal remission. A large multicenter trial of mycophenolate mofetil in lupus nephritis is currently underway in an effort to confirm these findings. Numerous other agents are also under investigation as possible therapies for lupus nephritis. Like mycophenolate mofetil, which is widely used to facilitate organ transplantation, some of these agents have already been approved for other indications (eg, rituximab for B-cell lymphoma) and therefore are currently available and are occasionally tried in refractory cases.

Austin HA, Klippel JH, Balow JE, et al. Therapy of lupus nephritis. Controlled trial of prednisone and cytotoxic drugs. *N Engl J Med.* 1986;314:614. [PMID: 3511372] (A classic study showing that pulse CYC is more effective than oral prednisone alone in preventing renal failure in patients with lupus nephritis.)

Boumpas DT, Austin HA, Vaughn EM, et al. Controlled trial of pulse methylprednisolone versus two regimens of pulse cyclophosphamide in severe lupus nephritis. *Lancet.* 1992;340:741. [PMID: 1356175] (A landmark trial showing that a prolonged course of pulse CYC is more effective than a shorter course of CYC or pulse methylprednisolone alone in the treatment of lupus nephritis.)

Contreras G, Pardo V, Leclercq B, et al. Sequential therapies for proliferative lupus nephritis. *N Engl J Med.* 2004;350:971. [PMID: 14999109] (Treatment with azathioprine or mycophenolate mofetil was safer and more efficacious than prolonged pulse CYC for maintenance of remission of lupus nephritis.)

Ginzler EM, Dooley MA, Aranow C, et al. Mycophenolate mofetil or intravenous cyclophosphamide for lupus nephritis. *N Engl J Med.* 2005;353:2219. [PMID: 16306519] (This 24-week, randomized, open-label trial demonstrated that mycophenolate mofetil was more effective than cyclophosphamide in inducing remission in lupus nephritis.)

Houssiau FA, Vasconcelos C, D'Cruz D, et al. Immunosuppressive therapy in lupus nephritis: the Euro-Lupus Nephritis Trial, a randomized trial of low-dose versus high-dose intravenous cyclophosphamide. *Arthritis Rheum.* 2002;46:2121. [PMID: 12209517] (In this European trial, treatment of lupus nephritis with a low-dose CYC regimen followed by azathioprine was as effective as a more traditional high-dose CYC regimen.)

Petri M. Cyclophosphamide: new approaches for systemic lupus erythematosus. *Lupus.* 2004;13:366. [PMID:15230294] (A well-written review describing traditional and new uses of CYC for the treatment of organ-threatening SLE.)

Somers EC, Marder W, Christman GM, et al. Use of a gonadotropin-releasing hormone analog for protection against premature ovarian failure during cyclophosphamide therapy in women with severe lupus. *Arthritis Rheum.* 2005;52:2761. [PMID: 16142702] (In 20 patients undergoing treatment with CYC for lupus nephritis, 5% of patients treated with leuprolide versus 20% of control patients had premature ovarian failure.)

Membranous Lupus Nephritis

The treatment of membranous nephritis is controversial. Although the renal prognosis of membranous nephropathy is better than that of proliferative nephritis, the morbid cardiovascular effects of the nephritic syndrome are well recognized. Thus, membranous nephritis is often aggressively treated to control the extrarenal aspects of the disease. Similarly to proliferative nephritis, immunosuppressives are used in conjunction with the renoprotective medications discussed previously. Angiotensin-converting enzyme antagonists are of paramount importance for the reduction of proteinuria. Therapeutic regimens might include glucocorticoids, cyclosporine, cyclophosphamide, or mycophenolate mofetil.

Austin HA, Illei GG. Membranous lupus nephritis. *Lupus.* 2005;14:65. [PMID: 15732291] (An up-to-date, evidence-based review of the clinical features and treatment of membranous lupus nephritis.)

NEUROPSYCHIATRIC SLE

Neuropsychiatric SLE encompasses a wide variety of abnormalities of the central, peripheral, and autonomic nervous systems. The specific abnormality as well as its severity dictates the appropriate treatment measures. To begin with, it is critical to determine if a particular neuropsychiatric finding is due to active SLE or to a secondary cause such as drug side effect, infection, uremia, or a concomitant systemic disease such as diabetes or hypertension.

If active SLE is determined to be the culprit, treatment will differ widely depending on the specific manifestation. Severe neuropsychiatric manifestations include stroke syndromes, demyelinating syndromes, seizures, transverse myelopathy, and organic brain syndrome (acute confusional state). Many of these severe manifestations require high-dose glucocorticoids. Several small studies have suggested an additional benefit with pulse IV cyclophosphamide. However, there are exceptions to this general approach. In particular, stroke syndromes and seizures are particularly challenging. Stroke syndromes in SLE can be caused by a variety of factors including antiphospholipid antibodies, cardiac vegetations, and atherosclerosis. Chronic anticoagulation with warfarin or aspirin is the treatment of choice for strokes associated with antiphospholipid antibodies. Unless there is a concomitant SLE flare, treatment with glucocorticoids is not needed. Similarly, glucocorticoids are not the first line of treatment for most lupus patients with seizures. Rather, seizures in SLE patients are usually treated with the same anticonvulsant medications that are used in non-SLE patients. However, it is sometimes difficult to determine if seizures represent an ongoing inflammatory process or are the result of a fixed scar. If ongoing inflammation is the cause, glucocorticoids and/or cytotoxic drugs may be necessary. Headaches are very common in SLE patients and are treated similarly to those occurring in non-SLE patients. Glucocorticoids are added if there are other manifestations of active SLE. Cognitive dysfunction is also present in many SLE patients. The use of glucocorticoids in these patients is controversial. If treatment is initiated, it is important to perform serial neuropsychiatric testing to demonstrate benefit. If no benefit is seen, glucocorticoids should be discontinued. Some studies have demonstrated an association between cognitive dysfunction and the presence of antiphospholipid antibodies, but it has yet to be determined whether aspirin or any other antithrombotic therapy might be helpful in this subgroup of patients.

HEMATOLOGIC MANIFESTATIONS

Leukopenia, anemia, and thrombocytopenia are frequently noted in SLE patients, and their etiology can be multifactorial. Side effects from medication should always be considered. Because hematologic abnormalities caused by SLE are often mild, treatment is not always necessary. In patients with leukopenia in association with recurrent infections, cautious use of prednisone to raise the white blood cell count might be indicated. Granulocyte colony-stimulating factor is usually avoided because there are data to suggest that it can precipitate SLE flares.

Severe SLE-related autoimmune thrombocytopenia is generally treated according to the guidelines established for idiopathic thrombocytopenic purpura. The overall treatment goal is to maintain a safe platelet count while minimizing the potential toxicity of therapy. Although data suggest that life-threatening bleeding does not occur until platelet counts are <10,000/mm^3, treatment is usually indicated for all patients with platelet counts of <20,000/mm^3 and for patients with platelet counts of <50,000/mm^3 with clinically important bleeding and/or a history of bleeding. Initial treatment consists of a course of high-dose glucocorticoids, often commencing with pulse methylprednisolone in extreme circumstances. After improvement in the platelet count (usually within 1 week), the glucocorticoids are tapered. In patients who do not respond to glucocorticoids or who relapse during tapering, IVIG is often tried. Because IVIG often produces a rapid platelet response, it should be used in conjunction with glucocorticoids from the outset in patients who are actively bleeding or in those requiring an invasive procedure. Although IVIG is often initially effective, relapse is common. Note that

IVIG is contraindicated in patients with IgA deficiency. Splenectomy is often considered as the next therapeutic modality in refractory patients. A recent systematic review estimated that 66% of patients with idiopathic thrombocytopenic purpura achieve a complete remission after splenectomy. Laparoscopic splenectomy appears to be safer than laparotomy. The majority of patients achieve a response within 2 weeks after the procedure. Vaccinations for *Streptococcus pneumoniae, Haemophilus influenzae* b, and *Neisseria meningitidis* are recommended 2 weeks prior to the splenectomy. A variety of other agents can be tried in patients with refractory disease. Other SLE disease manifestations will guide the choice of additional medications. Options include danazol, azathioprine, mycophenolate mofetil, cyclophosphamide, and rituximab (Table 23–1).

The treatment of severe autoimmune hemolytic anemia is similar to the treatment of autoimmune thrombocytopenia. High-dose prednisone or pulse methylprednisolone is used initially, and tapering begins once the hematocrit rises. In refractory patients, additional immunosuppressive agents may be necessary. Splenectomy is occasionally necessary after all other therapeutic options have been exhausted. SLE-related microangiopathic hemolytic anemia is treated with plasmapheresis, following the standard of care for the treatment of thrombotic thrombocytopenic purpura.

Kojouri K, Vesely SK, Terrell DR, et al. Splenectomy for adult patients with idiopathic thrombocytopenic purpura: a systematic review to assess long-term platelet count responses, prediction of response, and surgical complications. *Blood.* 2004;104:2623. [PMID: 15217831] (This systematic review of 135 case series of patients with idiopathic thrombocytopenic purpura revealed that 66% of patients achieved a remission after splenectomy.)

UNCOMMON COMPLICATIONS

Acute pneumonitis and diffuse alveolar hemorrhage are rare pulmonary manifestations of SLE. Both syndromes carry a poor prognosis, and treatment recommendations are based upon uncontrolled data and case reports. Because infection is usually part of the differential diagnosis, most patients are initially covered with broad-spectrum antibiotics. Acute pneumonitis is treated with high-dose glucocorticoids, and additional immunosuppressives can be added if necessary. Diffuse alveolar hemorrhage is typically treated with high-dose glucocorticoids in conjunction with pulse cyclophosphamide. In addition, plasmapheresis may be effective in some patients. Mesenteric vasculitis is another uncommon but life-threatening manifestation of SLE. Bowel perforation is the most feared complication. High-dose

Table 23-1. Commonly Used Medications in Systemic Lupus Erythematosus (SLE)

Agent	Typical Dose	Potential Toxicities	Follow-up	Comments
Glucocorticoids	Mild SLE: ≤10 mg/d Moderate to severe SLE: ≥10 mg/d	Hypertension, dyslipidemia, atherosclerosis, hyperglycemia, osteoporosis, avascular necrosis, infection, weight gain, adrenal insufficiency	Lipid profile yearly, urinalysis for glucose, bone densitometry, blood pressure	Regimen for organ/life-threatening disease-prednisone: 1 mg/kg/d or pulse intravenous methylprednisolone 1 g/d × 3 d
Hydroxychloroquine	≤400 mg/d, not to exceed 6.5 mg/kg/d	Ocular effects including inability to focus, corneal deposits, and retinopathy; rash, hyperpigmentation, myopathy, headache, nausea	Ophthalmologic exam with funduscopy and visual field testing yearly	Reduce dose in renal insufficiency; ophthalmologic exam every 3 months when using chloroquine
Methotrexate	7.5–15 mg/d	Myelosuppression, lymphoproliferative disorders, cirrhosis, pulmonary inflammation and fibrosis	Complete blood cell count (CBC), platelets, liver function tests, albumin, creatinine every 8 weeks or more frequently during dose changes	Do not use in patients with impaired renal function: use concomitant folic acid 1 mg/d or folinic acid 2.5 mg/wk
Azathioprine	Target dose of 2 mg/kg/d	Myelosuppression, hepatotoxicity, malignancy, nausea and vomiting, infection	CBC and platelets every 2 weeks with dosage change, and every 8 weeks thereafter	Consider testing for the thiopurine methyltransferase gene prior to drug initiation; reduce dose in renal insufficiency
Mycophenolate mofetil	Target dose of 2–3 g/d	Myelosuppression, nausea, diarrhea	CBC and platelets every 2 weeks with dosage change, and every 8 weeks thereafter	Reduce dose in renal insufficiency
Cyclophosphamide	IV dosing: 0.5–1.0 g/mm^2 monthly for 3–6 months for induction; every 3 months for maintenance Oral dosing: Target dose of 2 mg/kg/d	Myelosuppression, malignancy, hemorrhagic cystitis, bladder cancer, gonadal failure, infection	IV dosing: CBC with platelets 7–14 days after dose to determine leukocyte nadir, then every 1–3 months thereafter Oral dosing: CBC and platelets every 1–2 wk with dose change, every 1–3 months thereafter IV and oral: Urinalysis and urine cytology every month while on treatment, every 6–12 months lifelong	Reduce dose in renal insufficiency, obesity, and advanced age; use *Pneumocystis carinii* pneumonia prophylaxis; ensure adequate hydration during treatment; use antiemetics and mesna with IV dosing; consider use of leuprolide in women with IV dosing

glucocorticoids and pulse cyclophosphamide are the most commonly used therapies.

PEDIATRIC SLE

The treatment of children and adolescents with SLE generally follows the same guidelines as the treatment of adults with SLE. However, special attention must be paid to the unique circumstances of the pediatric population. In particular, consideration of issues related to physical growth, emotional well-being, and coping with a chronic and potentially appearance-changing illness are paramount to a successful treatment plan. Multidisciplinary care with education of the family is critical. In terms of pharmacologic therapies, the negative effects of systemic glucocorticoids on bone, physical growth, and appearance are well recognized. Thus every effort must be made to minimize the long-term use of these medications. Mild SLE is typically treated with NSAIDs and antimalarials. In patients with persistent disease, there is experience with the use of azathioprine, methotrexate, and mycophenolate mofetil as steroid-sparing agents. Organ-threatening disease is usually treated with intravenous pulse cyclophosphamide.

FUTURE DEVELOPMENTS

The prognosis of SLE has improved significantly over the past several decades with cohort studies after 1980 showing a 5-year survival rate of >90%, compared to a rate of <50% a few decades earlier. Better therapeutic options are probably one of several factors contributing to this observation. Despite this improvement in short-term mortality, however, it is well known that our current treatment armamentarium is associated with considerable toxicity and is not effective in every patient. Thus safer and more beneficial therapies are needed. To this end, our improved understanding of the immunopathogenesis of SLE has led to the development of multiple novel biologic agents that are currently being tested in clinical trials. Some of these agents specifically target T cells; others target B cells, cytokines, or complement components that appear to contribute to the development and/or perpetuation of SLE. The hope is that these targeted therapies might provide a better risk:benefit profile than the generalized immunosuppressives in current use and that they will broaden the therapeutic options for people with SLE.

Antiphospholipid Antibody Syndrome

24

Michelle Petri, MD, MPH

ESSENTIALS OF DIAGNOSIS

- *An acquired hypercoagulable state.*
- *Presentation with arterial or venous thrombosis, pregnancy loss, or thrombocytopenia.*
- *About 50% have systemic lupus erythematosus.*
- *Antiphospholipid antibodies include the lupus anticoagulant, anticardiolipin antibody, and anti-β_2 glycoprotein-1.*

General Considerations

About 5% of the general population, but 50% of patients with systemic lupus erythematosus, have an antiphospholipid antibody, such as the lupus anticoagulant, anticardiolipin antibody, or anti-β_2 glycoprotein-1. Because phospholipids are integral parts of the control of coagulation, these antibodies can lead to a hypercoagulable state, antiphospholipid antibody syndrome (APS). If no connective tissue disease is present, the term "primary" is used.

Classification criteria for APS are listed in Table 24–1. The two clinical criteria are (1) arterial or venous thrombosis or vasculopathy or (2) pregnancy loss (three first-trimester losses; one or more late fetal deaths) or morbidity from placental insufficiency, in the setting of a lupus anticoagulant or moderate to high immunoglobulin (Ig)G or IgM anticardiolipin, or anti-β_2 glycoprotein-1 IgG or IgM (confirmed twice over at least 12 weeks).

Venous thrombosis, usually a deep venous thrombosis with or without pulmonary emboli, is the most common thrombotic presentation. Arterial thrombosis is most commonly a transient ischemic attack or stroke. Some strokes in APS patients are embolic, from vegetations on the mitral or aortic valve.

Antiphospholipid antibodies are associated with pregnancy loss, both early spontaneous abortions and late intrauterine fetal death. The latter likely is due to placental vasculopathy rather than actual infarcts.

Some patients with antiphospholipid antibodies are thrombocytopenic. The reasons for thrombocytopenia are varied and include an autoimmune thrombocytopenia, platelet activation, or most worrisome, platelet consumption. Usually the thrombocytopenia is mild, but on occasion it can be profound, potentially putting the patient at risk for both bleeding and clotting.

The most dire presentation of APS is the catastrophic form, in which thrombosis is occurring in three or more organs over a short period of time. Such patients may initially be given an incorrect diagnosis such as thrombotic thrombocytopenic purpura or disseminated intravascular coagulation. Precipitants of the catastrophic form of APS include infections, surgery, discontinuation of anticoagulation therapy, and hormonal factors such as oral contraceptives and pregnancy.

Obviously, not all persons with antiphospholipid antibodies clot. In a patient with systemic lupus erythematosus and lupus anticoagulant, the risk of a venous thrombosis is 50% over 20 years. In general, patients with a lupus anticoagulant, higher-titer anticardiolipin, or anti-β_2 glycoprotein-1, and persistence of antibody over time are at greater risk for thrombosis. In addition, the presence of other risk factors for clotting, such as oral contraceptive pills, pregnancy, homocysteinemia, and so on, can increase the risk of thrombosis.

Clinical Findings

A. Symptoms and Signs

1. Cutaneous—Livedo reticularis is the classic cutaneous sign associated with antiphospholipid antibodies. It is not specific, because it can occur with lupus, vasculitis, cholesterol emboli, and cryoglobulinemia. Splinter hemorrhages, superficial thrombophlebitis, and leg ulcers are additional cutaneous manifestations.

2. Head, eyes, ears, nose, and throat—Optic neuropathy can occur as a thrombotic manifestation of APS.

Table 24–1. Antiphospholipid Antibody Syndrome Classification Criteria

Vascular thrombosis
  Arterial, venous, or small vessel
Pregnancy morbidity
  One or more fetal deaths
  One or more premature births due to severe preeclampsia
    or placental insufficiency
  Three or more first trimester losses
PLUS lupus anticoagulant
  Anticardiolipin IgG or IgM (medium to high titer)
  Anti-β_2 glycoprotein-1 IgG or IgM on two occasions 12 weeks
    (or more) apart

Ig, immunoglobulin.

3. Cardiopulmonary—Pulmonary emboli and pulmonary infarcts are thrombotic sequelae of APS. Rarely, pulmonary capillaritis is a presentation. Myocardial infarction, even without atherosclerosis, can occur. Libman-Sacks endocarditis—sterile valve vegetations—can occur from APS, typically on the mitral or aortic valve. Valvular involvement can be severe enough to require valve replacement.

4. Gastrointestinal—Hepatic or splenic infarcts can occur as part of APS. Budd-Chiari syndrome can occur as well.

5. Neurologic—Transient ischemic attacks or strokes are the most common neurologic manifestations. Dementia can occur without infarcts. Cognitive impairment may be associated with antiphospholipid antibodies. Two neurologic manifestations, chorea and transverse myelitis, may represent nonthrombotic consequences of APS.

6. Endocrinologic—Adrenal insufficiency can occur in APS, either due to an infarct that turns hemorrhagic or as a primary hemorrhage.

7. Reproductive—In addition to pregnancy losses, antiphospholipid antibodies may be associated with other pregnancy morbidity, including severe preeclampsia, HELLP (*h*emolysis, *e*levated *l*iver enzymes, and *l*ow *p*latelet count) syndrome, and intrauterine growth restriction.

B. Laboratory Findings

1. Antiphospholipid antibody tests

  a. False-positive test for syphilis—The FP-RPR is caused by an antiphospholipid antibody. However, it is not as strongly associated with thrombosis as those antiphospholipid antibodies directed against negatively charged phospholipids.

  b. Lupus anticoagulant (LA)—The name LA is unfortunate, because only 50% of patients with the LA have lupus and because it is a procoagulant, not anticoagulant,

in vivo. In vitro, though, the LA prolongs clotting times. The activated partial thromboplastin time is not a sensitive enough screening test. By international consensus, it is recommended that two sensitive screening tests should be done, such as a dilute Russell viper venom time and a sensitive partial thromboplastin time. The second step is to do a mix with normal plasma (1:1 and then 4:1 ratios) because there will be a lack of correction of the prolonged clotting time in the presence of an LA. The final confirming step is to add back phospholipids, such as with a platelet neutralization procedure.

  c. Anticardiolipin—Anticardiolipin is a solid-phase enzyme-linked immunosorbent assay. Usually all three isotypes (IgG, IgM, and IgA) are measured, although a polyclonal assay is also possible. International criteria for negative, low, medium, and high levels have been set, and standards are available for laboratory calibration.

  d. Anti-β_2 glycoprotein-1—Anti-β_2 glycoprotein-1 is the "co-factor" or target of anticardiolipin antibodies. Anti-β_2 glycoprotein-1 assay results, however, do not completely overlap with anticardiolipin results. There are no current international standards for anti-β_2 glycoprotein-1.

2. Complete blood cell count—Thrombocytopenia is a common finding in patients with APS.

3. Urinalysis—Proteinuria, secondary to renal vasculopathy from APS, can be found.

C. Imaging Studies

Imaging studies are frequently required in the evaluation of APS. Obviously, appropriate imaging studies will be done to diagnose a thrombotic event (duplex ultrasonogram or venogram for deep venous thrombosis, computed tomography or magnetic resonance imaging of the brain for stroke) or other APS manifestations (echocardiography for valve vegetations).

Arteriograms (coronary, mesenteric, and so on) may be necessary to ascertain the presence of thrombosis or vasculopathy in an organ.

Differential Diagnosis

Common genetic causes of hypercoagulability must be considered. The two most common are the factor V Leiden mutation (presenting predominantly as venous thrombosis) and the prothrombin mutation (usually venous, but some arterial thrombosis). Less common genetic hypercoagulable states include protein C, protein S, and antithrombin III deficiency, all of which are associated with venous thrombosis. Homocysteinemia, mediated by multiple genetic mutations, is a risk factor for both arterial thrombosis and atherosclerosis.

Acquired causes of hypercoagulability include pregnancy (especially the postpartum period), oral contraceptives, estrogen replacement therapy, bed rest, trauma, surgery, vasculitis, and malignancy.

The catastrophic form of APS may be confused with several entities. Thrombotic thrombocytopenia purpura—a disorder of von Willebrand monomers—often involves fever, and schistocytes will be seen on the peripheral blood smear. Disseminated intravascular coagulation will also be in the differential diagnosis.

Treatment

A. VENOUS AND ARTERIAL THROMBOSIS

The acute treatment of venous or arterial thrombosis does not change. Over the long term, two treatment caveats are important. First, because of the high risk of recurrence, long-term anticoagulation with warfarin is recommended. Second, although retrospective studies found high-intensity warfarin to be preferable, a recent clinical trial found usual-intensity (International Normalized Ratio 2.0–3.0) and high-intensity warfarin (International Normalized Ratio 3.1–4.0) to be equally efficacious.

B. PREGNANCY LOSS

A landmark clinical trial showed that 40 mg of prednisone and low-dose aspirin versus 10,000 U of subcutaneous heparin twice daily and low-dose aspirin were equally successful in terms of live births; however, there was much more maternal morbidity (ie, preeclampsia and diabetes) in the prednisone arm. Heparin and aspirin have been the preferred therapy since then. Low-molecular-weight heparin may be substituted for unfractionated heparin, but twice-daily dosing is preferred in pregnant women. However, unfractionated heparin should be substituted for low-molecular-weight heparin before delivery. Otherwise, the long duration of action of low-molecular-weight heparin might lead to a bleeding complication during delivery.

In two trials, heparin plus aspirin were better than aspirin alone. In a third trial, there was no difference in pregnancy outcomes.

In women who continue to miscarry while receiving heparin plus aspirin, intravenous immune globulin has been used, based on a strong scientific rationale that it binds antiphospholipid antibodies and may downregulate their production. However, no additional benefit was demonstrated in a small clinical trial.

C. THROMBOCYTOPENIA

Patients with APS and thrombosis cannot be given anticoagulant therapy safely if they are also profoundly thrombocytopenic (platelets $<50,000/\mu L$). Additional therapies (prednisone and intravenous immune globulin) should be added to keep the platelet count above $50,000/\mu L$. A few patients have required splenectomies, with variable success.

D. CHOREA AND TRANSVERSE MYELITIS

Chorea and transverse myelitis are often not thrombotic manifestations of APS. They may respond to intravenous methylprednisolone, which should always be given promptly. Such patients are at risk, though, for later APS-associated thrombosis.

E. CATASTROPHIC APS

The catastrophic form of APS has a high mortality rate of 50%. Essentials of treatment include heparin, intravenous methylprednisolone pulse therapy, and plasmapheresis or intravenous immune globulin to reduce the burden of circulating antiphospholipid antibodies.

F. PROPHYLACTIC TREATMENT

There is a strong case for using low-dose aspirin in patients with the lupus anticoagulant or medium- to high-titer anticardiolipin or anti-β_2 glycoprotein-1. A retrospective study suggested that this reduced the thrombosis rate. Prospective clinical trials are underway.

Hydroxychloroquine has also been shown to reduce the thrombosis rate in longitudinal studies in systemic lupus erythematosus and to prevent thrombosis in an animal model of a damaged femoral vein. Because 50% of patients with systemic lupus erythematosus make antiphospholipid antibodies, hydroxychloroquine may already be considered for its beneficial effect on disease activity.

Complications

An arterial or venous thrombotic event may lead to profound morbidity or even be fatal. APS patients have a high risk of recurrent thrombotic events if they do not receive long-term anticoagulant therapy.

Unfortunately, anticoagulation is not completely safe. Severe bleeding complications can occur. Monitoring the International Normalized Ratio every 2 weeks is recommended.

Prognosis

With careful management of anticoagulation, recurrent thrombotic events can usually be prevented. Classic lupus may develop in a few patients who have APS.

REFERENCES

Alarcon-Segovia D, Cabral AR. The anti-phospholipid antibody syndrome: clinical and serological aspects. *Baillieres Best Pract Res Clin Rheumatol.* 2000;14:139. [PMID: 10882219] (A review of APS manifestations in a large Mexican systemic lupus erythematosus cohort.)

Asherson RA, Cervera R, de Groot PG, et al. Catastrophic antiphospholipid syndrome: international consensus statement on classification criteria and treatment guidelines. *Lupus.* 2003;12:530. [PMID: 12892393] (Catastrophic antiphospholipid antibody syndrome carries a mortality of 50%.)

Cowchock FS, Reece EA, Balaban D, Branch DW, Plouffe L. Repeated fetal losses associated with antiphospholipid antibodies: a collaborative randomized trial comparing prednisone with low-dose heparin treatment. *Am J Obstet Gynecol.* 1992;166:1318. [PMID: 1595785]

Crowther MA, Ginsberg JS, Julian J, et al. A comparison of two intensities of warfarin for the prevention of recurrent thrombosis in patients with the antiphospholipid antibody syndrome. *N Engl J Med.* 2003;349:1133. [PMID: 13679527] (A clinical trial demonstrating that normal-intensity warfarin is equal to high-intensity warfarin in the prevention of future thrombotic events.)

Erkan D, Merrill JT, Yazici Y, et al. High thrombosis rate after fetal loss in antiphospholipid syndrome: effective prophylaxis with aspirin. *Arthritis Rheum.* 2001;44:1466. [PMID: 11407709] (A retrospective chart review study suggesting benefit of aspirin as prophylactic therapy.)

Exner T, Triplett DA, Taberner D, Machin SJ. Guidelines for testing and revised criteria for lupus anticoagulants. SSC Subcommittee for the Standardization of Lupus Anticoagulants. *Thromb Haemost.* 1991;65:320. [PMID: 1904657] (A review of lupus anticoagulant testing.)

Harris EN, et al. The anti-cardiolipin assay. In: Harris EN, Exner T, Hughes GRV, Asherson RA, eds. *Phospholipid-Binding Antibodies.* CRC Press, 1991:175–187. (A review of anticardiolipin standardization and testing.)

Miyakis S, et al. International consensus statement on an update of the preliminary classification criteria for antiphospholipid syndrome (APS). *J Thromb Haemost* 2006;4:295. (A recent update on the classification criteria for APS, which now includes the anti-β_2 glycoprotein-1 assay.)

Schulman S, et al and the Duration of Anticoagulation Study Group. Anticardiolipin antibodies predict early recurrence of thromboembolism and death among patients with venous thromboembolism following anticoagulant therapy. *Am J Med.* 1998;104:332. [PMID: 9576405] (A prospective study proving the high risk of recurrent thrombosis in APS.)

Raynaud Phenomenon

Sangeeta Dileep Sule, MD, & Fredrick M. Wigley, MD

ESSENTIALS OF DIAGNOSIS

- *An exaggerated response to cold temperatures that results in transient digital ischemia.*
- *Classified clinically into primary or secondary forms.*
- *Complications of digital tissue ischemia may occur in patients with secondary Raynaud phenomenon, leading to recurrent digital ulcerations, rapid deep tissue necrosis, and amputation.*
- *Avoidance of cold temperatures is crucial to the management of Raynaud phenomenon. The entire body must be kept comfortably warm.*
- *Medications are indicated if there are signs of critical tissue ischemia (eg, digital ulcers) or if the quality of life of the patient is so affected that normal function is restricted.*

General Considerations

When humans are exposed to cold temperatures, the body will sacrifice the viability of peripheral tissues by shifting blood flow from the skin and other organs to maintain a stable core body temperature. A unique circulatory system exists in the skin, especially in the hands, feet, and areas of the face that includes both thermoregulatory and nutritional blood vessels. In these areas of the body, local blood flow is regulated by a complex interaction of neural signals, cellular mediators, and circulating vasoactive molecules. Temperature responses are principally mediated through the sympathetic nervous system by rapidly altering blood flow through arteriovenous shunts in the skin. During hot weather, these shunts open (vasodilate), allowing heat to dissipate. In cool weather, the shunts constrict, shifting blood centrally and helping maintain a stable core body temperature.

Raynaud phenomenon (RP) is an exaggerated response to cold temperatures that results in transient digital ischemia. The vasoconstriction of digital arteries, precapillary arterioles, and cutaneous arteriovenous shunts leads to a sharp demarcation of skin pallor or cyanosis

of the digits (Figure 25–1). This ischemic phase is followed by recovery of blood flow that appears as cutaneous erythema, secondary to rapid reperfusion of the digits.

RP is classified clinically into primary or secondary forms. Primary RP occurs in the absence of any associated disease or definable cause. In fact, most experts think that the primary form is merely an exaggeration of normal physiologic responses to cold environmental temperatures or emotional stress or both, rather than a disease. Secondary RP is associated with an underlying pathologic condition or disease that alters regional blood flow by damaging blood vessels, interfering with neural control of the circulation, or changing either the physical properties of the blood or the levels of circulating mediators that regulate the digital and cutaneous circulation. Although there are a large number of suspected causes of secondary RP, the primary care physician will most commonly encounter RP associated with a rheumatic or connective tissue disease, such as scleroderma, systemic lupus erythematosus, Sjögren syndrome, or dermatomyositis.

Clinical Findings

A. SYMPTOMS AND SIGNS

RP results from an exaggerated vascular response to cold temperatures or stress. This vascular constriction leads to color changes visible on the skin. The fingers are most commonly affected, although attacks also occur in the toes and occasionally on areas of the face. A typical RP attack is characterized by the sudden onset of cold digits associated with a demarcation of skin pallor (white attack) or cyanosis (blue attack). After rewarming, the skin blushes from reperfusion, resulting in the erythema secondary to rebound of blood flow. Although many people in the general population (~30%) are "sensitive to the cold," a true RP attack is defined clinically by a history of both cold sensitivity and associated color changes of the skin (pallor or cyanosis or both) limited to the digits. RP attacks typically begin in a single finger and then spread to other digits of the same or both hands. The index, middle, and ring fingers are the most commonly involved digits. Primary RP occurs in the absence of a definable cause for the attacks. It is most common in otherwise healthy females with an age of onset between 15 and 30 years. A history that another first-degree family

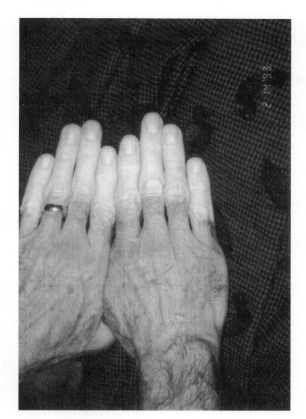

Figure 25–1. A typical Raynaud phenomenon attack characterized by a sharp demarcation of skin pallor.

Table 25–2. Secondary Causes of Raynaud Phenomenon

Rheumatologic	Hematologic disorders
Systemic sclerosis (scleroderma) Systemic lupus erythematosus Rheumatoid arthritis Sjögren syndrome Dermatomyositis Polymyositis Vasculitis	Cryoglobulinemia Paraproteinemia Polycythemia Cold agglutinins
Mechanical	**Endocrine disorders**
Vibration injury Frostbite Thoracic outlet syndrome Vascular embolus or occlusion	Hypothyroidism Carcinoid syndrome Pheochromocytoma
Vasospasm	**Drugs**
Migraine headaches	Sympathomimetic drugs (decongestants, diet pills) Serotonin agonists (sumatriptan) Chemotherapeutic agents (bleomycin, cisplatin, carboplatin, vinblastine) Ergotamine tartrate Caffeine Nicotine

member is affected with RP is reported in about 30% of cases. Criteria for the diagnosis of primary RP are shown in Table 25–1.

Underlying causes of RP—usually connective tissue diseases—eventually emerge in 10–15% of patients in whom primary RP was initially diagnosed. If a patient meets criteria for primary RP and no new symptoms

Table 25–1. Criteria for the Diagnosis of Primary Raynaud Phenomenon[a]

Symmetric intermittent RP attacks
No evidence of peripheral vascular disease
No evidence of tissue gangrene or digital pitting
No abnormal nailfold capillary microscopy
Negative antinuclear antibody test and normal erythrocyte sedimentation rate

[a]From LeRoy EC, Medsger TA Jr. Raynaud's phenomenon: a proposal for classification. *Clin Exp Rheumatol.* 1992;10:485, with permission.

develop over 2 years of follow-up, the development of secondary disease is unlikely. The presence of abnormal nailfold capillaries on microscopy (see below) is the best predictor of secondary RP.

The most common causes of secondary RP are scleroderma, systemic lupus erythematosus, and other connective tissue disorders (Table 25–2). Patients with secondary RP generally have more severe RP, often accompanied by pain, which may herald an episode of serious digital ischemia, fingertip ulceration, and tissue loss. Tissue ischemia and digital ulceration may result. The more severe nature of the RP in these cases is due to secondary processes causing direct vessel damage. The clinical features that help distinguish primary from secondary RP are outlined in Table 25–3.

All patients with a history of RP should be asked about symptoms suggestive of an autoimmune disease, such as arthritis, dry eyes or dry mouth, myalgias, fevers, skin rash, or cardiopulmonary abnormalities. Careful examination for signs of a secondary process should include examination of the pulses, auscultation over large arteries, examination for evidence of tissue ischemia or inflammatory skin lesions, and nailfold capillary microscopy. If

Table 25–3. Clinical Features of Secondary Raynaud Phenomenon

---

Male sex
Pain associated with attacks
Signs of tissue ischemia (digital ulcerations)
Age of onset >40 years
Asymmetry of digits affected
Signs or symptoms of other diseases (rheumatic endocrine, etc)
Abnormal laboratory tests (positive antinuclear antibodies, cryoglobulins)

---

the clinician suspects an underlying autoimmune disease, the patient should be evaluated for the presence of specific autoantibodies (see section on Laboratory Findings, below).

B. LABORATORY FINDINGS

Patients who are young when symptoms begin; who have a normal history and physical examination, including normal nailfold capillaries and larger vessel examination; and who have no history of digital ischemic lesions can be considered to have primary RP. These patients can be monitored clinically, and no further laboratory testing is needed.

However, if a secondary cause of RP is suspected, appropriate testing is recommended, including serum chemistries, complete blood cell count, thyroid function tests, serum and urine protein electrophoresis, and testing for cryoglobulins or cryofibrinogens. In addition, inflammatory markers such as erythrocyte sedimentation rate or C-reactive protein are often elevated in patients with secondary RP.

Antinuclear antibody assays are highly sensitive for the types of connective tissue disorders that are often associated with RP. However, positive antinuclear antibody tests are quite nonspecific and therefore should be followed by testing for autoantibodies with higher positive predictive values for such conditions. An anticentromere pattern detected on antinuclear antibody testing is associated strongly with limited scleroderma (eg, the CREST syndrome [*c*alcinosis, *R*aynaud phenomenon, *e*sophageal dysmotility, *s*clerodactyly, and *t*elangiectasias]; see Chapter 26). Antitopoisomerase antibodies may be observed in patients with RP secondary to scleroderma. Anti-dsDNA, anti-Ro/SS-A, anti-La/SS-B, anti-Sm, and anti-RNP antibodies are detected in many patients with systemic lupus erythematosus. Anti-Jo-1 antibodies are often associated with inflammatory myopathies.

C. SPECIAL TESTS

Nailfold capillary microscopy can be used to examine the nailfold capillary bed of patients with RP. This can provide a clue for the classification of RP (primary versus secondary); patients with secondary RP may have capillary loop changes, including enlargement and dropout caused by the underlying vascular disease process (Figure 25–2). To perform nailfold capillary microscopy, a drop of grade B immersion oil is placed on the patient's skin at the base of the fingernail. This area is then viewed using an ophthalmoscope set to 10–40 diopters or a stereoscopic microscope. Normal capillaries appear as symmetric, nondilated loops. In contrast, distorted,

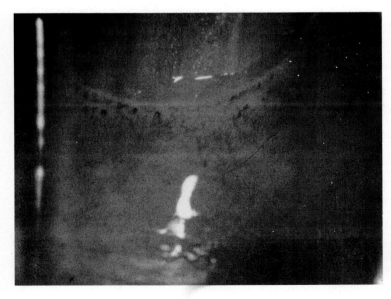

Figure 25–2. Nailfold capillary microscopy demonstrating nailfold capillary loop dilation and dropout.

dilated, or absent capillaries suggest a secondary disease process.

Differential Diagnosis

The diagnosis of RP is clinical, based on a patient's report of sudden, episodic color changes of the digits provoked by cold temperature or emotional stress. However, many people without RP report an increased sensitivity to the cold. Thus, true RP should be distinguished from the nondemarcated mottling seen in a normal response to cool temperatures. True RP must also be distinguished from acrocyanosis—a condition seen when the patient has cool hands and feet with persistently cyanotic skin. Although acrocyanosis is aggravated by cold temperatures, there are none of the episodic attacks or sharp demarcations of color changes observed in RP.

Repeated mechanical stress on the nerves or vessels in the hand or fingers may also cause sensitivity to the cold temperature. Use of tools that vibrate, carpal tunnel syndrome, or neuropathy should be considered in a patient who complains of color changes of the hands and numbness with or without sensitivity to the cold. Paraproteinemias and hyperviscosity syndromes should also be considered in the differential diagnosis. RP in these patients results from sluggish blood flow through cutaneous and digital vessels. Patients may also have cold-sensitive proteins; RP is common among patients with cryoglobulinemia. The use of certain drugs (eg, sympathomimetic agents) that induce vasoconstriction can aggravate or cause RP. In addition, patients with hypothyroidism often have cold hands, acrocyanosis, or RP.

Distinguishing primary from secondary RP is critical. The connective tissue diseases are the most common secondary disorders that the internist will encounter. Thus, a thorough review of systems focusing on symptoms of a connective tissue disease is essential. Patients should be asked about dry eyes or mouth (Sjögren syndrome); painful joints or morning stiffness (arthritis); rashes, photosensitivity, or cardiopulmonary abnormalities (systemic lupus erythematosus); and skin tightening, respiratory distress, or gastrointestinal disease (scleroderma).

Most patients with RP report symmetric involvement of the digits. Therefore, if a patient reports asymmetric RP, a mechanical occlusion of the large vessels, either from atherosclerosis, emboli, or arterial occlusion, should be considered. In such cases, noninvasive vascular flow studies are helpful and vascular imaging such as a magnetic resonance arteriogram or arteriography may be appropriate. Although systemic vasculitides such as polyarteritis nodosa, Wegener granulomatosis, and Buerger disease may cause critical digital ischemia and tissue necrosis, these patients do not have typical RP.

Treatment

A. PREVENTIVE STRATEGIES

Avoidance of cold temperatures is crucial to the management of RP. Although the importance of keeping the hands and feet warm is obvious, the whole body must be kept comfortably warm. Thus, wearing several layers of loose-fitting clothing, mittens, stockings, and headwear in cold temperatures is very important. Damp windy weather or rapid shifts in ambient temperature are more likely to precipitate RP attacks. Air conditioning during summer months can be a problem because of sudden shifts in temperature or uncontrolled drafts of cold air over the hands or body. Emotional stress can not only trigger an RP attack but also lower the threshold for cold-induced attacks. Therefore, stress control and relaxation techniques are helpful in preventing RP attacks.

Medications that have the potential to vasoconstrict the peripheral arteries should be avoided in patients with both primary and secondary RP. Sympathomimetic drugs (decongestants, diet pills, ephedra) and serotonin agonists such as sumatriptan should be avoided because they are vasoconstrictors and could aggravate RP. In addition, certain chemotherapeutic agents (bleomycin, cisplatin, carboplatin, and vinblastine) may cause vascular occlusion and trigger RP attacks. RP patients should avoid smoking because nicotine reduces cutaneous and digital blood flow. Nonselective β blockers were once thought to be contraindicated, but new studies refute this finding. Clonidine and narcotics also vasoconstrict the cutaneous circulation and should be used with caution. A recent warning has noted potential vasospasm with concomitant administration of ergotamine tartrate plus caffeine, a migraine medication, and cytochrome P450-3A4 inhibitors such as macrolide antibiotics and protease inhibitors.

B. VASODILATOR THERAPY

Medications are indicated in the treatment of RP if there are signs of critical tissue ischemia (eg, digital ulcers) or if the quality of life of the patient is affected to the degree that normal functions are restricted. If preventive strategies fail, vasodilator therapy is the next available option. Calcium channel blockers are the most widely used vasodilators; however, other agents are rapidly becoming available. In general, no medication has proved to be more effective or safer than the calcium channel blockers. Although combinations of vasodilators are often used, there are no studies that address this strategy.

1. Calcium channel blockers—Calcium channel blockers are the most popular pharmacologic treatment for RP. Short-acting nifedipine reduces the frequency and severity of attacks by about one-third. The benefit is more robust in the patients with primary RP than in those with secondary RP. Calcium channel blockers differ in their peripheral vasodilatory properties. Nifedipine, amlodipine, felodipine, nisoldipine, and isradipine appear more effective than diltiazem and verapamil in the treatment of RP. The most significant side effects from calcium channel blockers are headache, hypotension, tachycardia, and lower extremity edema. However, aggravation of gastroesophageal reflux disease, constipation, and hypertrophy of the gums can also occur. In one study of sustained-release nifedipine, approximately 15% of healthy patients with primary RP had to stop taking the drug because of headache and lower extremity edema.

Slow-release preparations are preferred because they are as effective and safer than the rapid-release medications. Slow-release nifedipine may be used in the treatment of RP at doses from 30–180 mg/d. Currently, oral amlodipine at doses of 5–20 mg/d is preferred over nifedipine because amlodipine exerts less negative inotropy on the heart. Individual responses and tolerance to calcium channel blockers vary among patients. If one calcium channel blocker is ineffective, another calcium channel blocker may be tried. There is no evidence that combinations of calcium channel blockers are better than a single drug.

2. Angiotensin-converting enzyme inhibitors—These drugs are used in the treatment of hypertension and scleroderma renal crisis. The role of angiotensin-converting enzyme inhibitors in RP is debated and not well defined, but there is evidence that they may improve digital blood flow by increasing kinins and causing vasodilation. A small clinical trial using losartan, an angiotensin II receptor blocker, found a decrease in the number and severity of RP attacks in both primary and secondary RP. Captopril, a traditional angiotensin-converting enzyme inhibitor, improved RP attacks in primary RP, but not RP secondary to scleroderma. Although the use of angiotensin-converting enzyme inhibitors in RP needs further investigation, the use of these drugs alone in complex or refractory cases or in combination with calcium channel blockers is reasonable.

3. Sympatholytic agents—Sympathetic adrenergic stimulation, particularly β_2-adrenergic receptors on the digital arteries, is thought to play an important role in control of digital blood flow. Therefore in severe RP, another option is to block sympathetic tone in the hope of inducing vasodilation of digital vessels. However, there are few controlled trials of sympatholytic agents in RP. The best studied is prazosin, an α_1-adrenergic receptor blocker. In two controlled trials, prazosin was more effective than placebo in primary and secondary RP. However, patients became resistant to prazosin after prolonged use. Thus, sympatholytic agents may be helpful in the treatment of RP, but the vasodilation lessens over time and side effects are often intolerable.

4. Nitrates and other topical therapy—Although not well studied in controlled trials, nitroglycerin ointment is frequently used in combination with a calcium channel blocker or alone in the treatment of both primary and secondary RP. There have been numerous anecdotal reports of improvement in RP with 0.25–0.5 inch of 2% nitroglycerin ointment applied daily to fingers, forearms, or wrists of affected hands. The medication is systemically absorbed; thus patients may still have such side effects as hypotension and headaches. Recently, topical application of prostaglandin E_1 was reported to reduce secondary RP attacks. The potential of topical prostaglandin therapy needs further investigation.

5. Prostaglandins/endothelin-receptor inhibitors—Prostacyclin and other prostaglandins are vasodilators and have been used in the treatment of RP in Europe. Iloprost, a stable prostacyclin analog, has been shown to be beneficial in the treatment of RP secondary to scleroderma. Therapy with iloprost (0.5–2 ng/kg/min intravenous infusion) can provide relief for several weeks following treatment. However, the drug is not currently available in the United States. Orally administered prostaglandins (oral iloprost, cicaprost, and beraprost) are not beneficial in RP, probably because of poor oral bioavailability.

Endothelin is a potent vasoconstrictor produced by a variety of cells including endothelial cells, smooth muscle cells, leukocytes, macrophages, and mesangial cells. Endothelin receptor antagonist drugs (ie, bosentan) have been developed to prevent this potent vasoconstriction. Currently, bosentan is used for the treatment of pulmonary hypertension. Anecdotal reports suggest an improvement in RP among patients with scleroderma. A recent study involving patients with scleroderma demonstrated that patients treated with bosentan had fewer new digital ulcers than those treated with placebo. Liver toxicity, availability, and the expense of bosentan limit its use, but future studies may define its place in the treatment of difficult cases.

6. Phosphodiesterase inhibitors—Case reports suggest that phosphodiesterase type 5 inhibitors (eg, sildenafil, tadalafil, and vardenafil) may reduce the severity and frequency of RP and improve healing of digital ulcers. An initial clinical trial found that sildenafil reduced the number and severity of RP attacks compared to placebo. More studies are needed but in complex cases with digital ischemia not responding to a calcium channel blocker, the use of a phosphodiesterase inhibitor is reasonable. Phosphodiesterase type 5 inhibitors should not be combined with the use of nitroglycerin. Other phosphodiesterase inhibitors tested in RP include cilostazol and pentoxifylline, but these appear to be less potent.

7. Selective serotonin reuptake inhibitors—Recent experience has demonstrated that fluoxetine improves

RP, suggesting that inhibition of serotonin uptake prevents the vasoconstriction caused by circulating serotonin. While the evidence is still preliminary, the use of fluoxetine or another selective serotonin reuptake inhibitor can be considered in complex cases, particularly if their baseline blood pressure is low.

8. Sympathectomy—Surgical sympathectomy is used to ligate the sympathetic nerves that cause vasoconstriction. Both proximal (cervical) and localized (digital) sympathectomy can be used in the treatment of RP. Cervical sympathectomy is reported to be helpful in primary but not in secondary RP. However, a proximal sympathectomy may not be fully effective and this procedure is associated with significant risks including neuralgia, Horner syndrome, and decreased localized sweating. Therefore a localized digital sympathectomy is the preferred procedure. Nevertheless, the procedure is limited to patients with severe RP, especially those who are in an active ischemic crisis and are not responding to medical management. Most of the available evidence shows that RP attacks recur several weeks to months following either proximal or digital sympathectomy.

9. Anticoagulation—Anticoagulation therapy with aspirin (81 mg/d) is recommended in selected patients with severe secondary RP who are at risk for digital ulceration or larger-artery thrombotic events. Heparin may be used acutely during an ischemic crisis to prevent further digital vessel thrombosis, but long-term anticoagulation with heparin or warfarin is not recommended unless there is evidence of a hypercoagulable disorder (eg, antiphospholipid syndrome or malignancy).

Complications

RP can be a mild nuisance to patients or it can alter their quality of life and prevent them from living in even cool temperatures. The primary form of RP is not associated with critical ischemia or tissue ulcerations, but cold sensitivity, digital numbness, and discomfort can alter hand function. Emotional problems can occur from the social stigma of cold hands with unsightly skin color changes.

Complications of digital tissue ischemia may occur in patients with secondary RP, leading to recurrent digital ulcerations, rapid deep tissue necrosis, and amputation. These patients, unlike patients with primary RP, have structurally abnormal digital vessels as the underlying problem.

A persistently demarcated ischemic digit with accompanying numbness and pain in the digit, hand, or arm characterizes critical digital ischemia. Pain is so severe that the patient seeks medical attention or is positioning the hand downward to improve blood flow, indicating that the tissue is ischemic and vulnerable to ulceration. Severe RP and signs or symptoms of critical tissue ischemia should be considered a medical emergency, and patients should be considered for hospitalization. They should be kept warm and at rest. Vasodilator therapy with a short-acting calcium channel blocker (eg, nifedipine 10–20 mg orally every 8 hours) should be started in combination with aspirin. If ischemia continues, a combination of vasodilators (eg, a calcium channel blocker plus a nitrate [topical nitroglycerin], a sympatholytic agent [prazosin], or an intravenous vasodilator such as prostaglandin infusion [eg, epoprostenol]) may be added. A temporary chemical digital sympathectomy (eg, xylocaine) may reverse vasospasm. Surgical digital sympathectomy may be considered if ischemia persists despite vasodilator therapy. Early intervention with hospitalization and vasodilator therapy is the key to preventing irreversible vessel occlusion and breaking the cycle of vasospasm and digital ischemia.

Digital ulcers from tissue ischemia often develop in patients with secondary RP. In order to avoid infection, it is important to keep these ulcers clean by washing with soap and water twice daily, followed by an appropriate protective dressing. Topical or systemic antibiotics are used if an infection develops.

REFERENCES

LeRoy EC, Medsger TA Jr. Raynaud's phenomenon: a proposal for classification. *Clin Exp Rheumatol.* 1992;10:485. [PMID: 1458701]

Thompson AE, Shea B, Welch V, Fenlon D, Pope JE. Calcium-channel blockers for Raynaud's phenomenon in systemic sclerosis. *Arthritis Rheum.* 2001;44:1841. [PMID: 11508437]

Spencer-Green G. Outcomes in primary Raynaud phenomenon: a meta-analysis of the frequency, rates, and predictors of transition to secondary diseases. *Arch Intern Med.* 1998;158:595. [PMID: 9521223]

Wigley FM. Clinical practice. Raynaud's phenomenon. *N Engl J Med.* 2002;347:1001. [PMID: 12324557]

Relevant World Wide Web Sites

[Arthritis Foundation]
http://www.arthritis.org
[Scleroderma Foundation]
http://www.scleroderma.org
[Scleroderma Research Foundation]
http://www.srfcure.org

Scleroderma

Laura K. Hummers, MD, & Fredrick M. Wigley, MD

ESSENTIALS OF DIAGNOSIS

- The most frequent symptoms are (in descending order) Raynaud phenomenon, gastroesophageal reflux with or without dysmotility, skin changes, swollen fingers, and arthralgias.
- Patients with Raynaud phenomenon and features atypical for primary Raynaud phenomenon should be evaluated for the possibility of scleroderma or another connective tissue disease.
- A negative antinuclear antibody test makes the diagnosis of scleroderma very unlikely.
- The degree of skin involvement is highly variable. Many patients with limited scleroderma have only subtle cutaneous findings (eg, mild sclerodactyly).
- The available diagnostic criteria do not include many patients with milder forms of scleroderma.
- Some patients may have overlapping clinical features with other systemic autoimmune rheumatic disorders such as polymyositis/dermatomyositis, Sjögren syndrome, systemic lupus erythematosus, and rheumatoid arthritis.

General Considerations

Systemic sclerosis (scleroderma) is a chronic multisystem disease that belongs to the family of systemic autoimmune disorders. The word scleroderma literally means "hard skin" and describes the most dramatic clinical feature of the disease—namely, skin fibrosis. Scleroderma affects approximately 20 new patients per million per year and has an estimated prevalence of approximately 250 patients per million in the United States. As with many other autoimmune disorders, scleroderma is approximately 4–5 times more common in women than men. The average age at the time of diagnosis is approximately 50 years.

The prevalence and manifestations of scleroderma vary among racial and ethnic groups. For example, the disease is approximately 100 times more common among the Choctaw Native Americans in Oklahoma, in whom the disease is characterized by diffuse skin disease and pulmonary fibrosis. Milder, limited disease is more common among white women, and African-American patients are more likely to have severe lung disease. The finding of various subtypes of scleroderma among different ethnic or racial groups, the presence of familial clustering, and the appearance of specific autoantibodies that are associated with specific human leukocyte antigen types define genetic influences on disease expression. Certain environmental factors are also thought to play etiologic roles. For example, characteristic antibodies and scleroderma disease manifestations can develop in coal miners exposed to high levels of silica.

Clinical Findings

Scleroderma is a rare disorder but is characterized by symptoms that occur frequently in the general population, such as Raynaud phenomenon, gastroesophageal reflux, fatigue, and musculoskeletal pain. Therefore it is important for primary care practitioners to be aware of scleroderma because early intervention can reduce morbidity and detect treatable, life-threatening complications.

The American College of Rheumatology diagnostic criteria for scleroderma include either thickened (sclerodermatous) skin changes proximal to the metacarpophalangeal joints or at least two of the following:

- Sclerodactyly.
- Digital pitting (residual loss of tissue on the finger pads due to ischemia).
- Bibasilar pulmonary fibrosis.

A diagnosis of scleroderma can also be made if the patient has three of the five features of the CREST syndrome (*c*alcinosis, *R*aynaud phenomenon, *e*sophageal dysmotility, *s*clerodactyly, and *t*elangiectasias). Patients with definite Raynaud phenomenon who have abnormal nailfold capillary loops and the presence of autoantibodies known to be associated with scleroderma (see section on Laboratory Findings and Table 26–2) may be considered to have early scleroderma or a mild expression of the disease.

Table 26–1. Classic Presentations of Patients with Limited and Diffuse Scleroderma

Limited scleroderma
   Long history of Raynaud phenomenon
   Gastroesophageal reflux and dysphagia
   Swelling or skin thickening of the fingers
   Infrequent systemic symptoms such as arthralgias, weight
      loss, and dyspnea
Diffuse scleroderma
   New onset of Raynaud phenomenon
   Rapid change in skin texture with new onset of edema,
      pruritus, and pain
   Significant systemic symptoms with severe arthralgias,
      weight loss, and tendon friction rubs
   Early evidence of internal organ involvement such as dyspnea
      or hypertension

Although skin changes are usually the major diagnostic clue, scleroderma is a systemic disease that most commonly targets the peripheral circulation, muscles, joints, gastrointestinal tract, lung, heart, and kidney. Symptoms encountered in the early presentation of scleroderma include musculoskeletal discomfort, fatigue, weight loss, and heartburn associated with gastroesophageal reflux disease. When these symptoms are accompanied by the new onset of cold sensitivity or Raynaud phenomenon, then scleroderma should be considered and further diagnostic investigation is warranted.

A. Symptoms and Signs

1. Skin—Thickening of the skin is the most easily recognizable manifestation of scleroderma but is not prominent in all patients. Patients with scleroderma are typically classified based on the amount and location of skin involvement. Patients with limited disease have skin changes on the face and distal to the knees and elbows. One form of limited scleroderma, the CREST syndrome, typically only involves the skin of the fingers (sclerodactyly) distal to the metacarpophalangeal joints (Table 26–1). In contrast, diffuse scleroderma refers to the group of patients with proximal extremity or truncal skin thickening (Figure 26–1). The amount of skin thickening can be quantified by performing a "skin score," in which the skin is pinched between the examiner's thumbs in 17 specified areas of the patient's body, scoring the thickness of the skin from 0 (normal) to 3 (very thick). The skin score provides a systematic approach to longitudinal disease evaluations and is commonly used in clinical trials to assess treatment efficacy. Moreover, epidemiologic studies indicate that higher skin scores correlate with greater degrees of internal organ involvement and worse overall prognosis.

Early in the course of diffuse scleroderma, the skin appears edematous and inflamed with erythema and pigmentary changes. Hyperpigmented areas alternating with vitiligolike areas of depigmentation impart to the skin a "salt and pepper" appearance. The early inflammatory phase is associated with pruritus and discomfort that usually lasts for weeks to months. In vitro studies show that dermal fibroblasts derived from patients with scleroderma overproduce extracellular matrix that leads to increased tissue collagen deposition in the skin. Collagen cross-linking then causes progressive skin tightening. In the later stages of the disease, the involved skin becomes atrophic, dry, and scaly because of the loss of its natural oils (sebaceous gland damage). These dry thickened areas of skin are often intensely pruritic, causing the patient to excoriate the skin, which leads to more damage and thickening (lichenification).

Patients often have other prominent skin changes, including marked telangiectasias (dilated capillaries) that occur on the skin of the face, the palmar surface of the hands (Figure 26–2), and the mucous membranes which tend to be more prominent in the subset of patients with CREST syndrome. A smaller proportion of patients have subcutaneous calcinosis, primarily on the fingers and along the extensor surfaces of the forearms.

2. Vascular disease—Involvement of the vasculature is ubiquitous among patients with scleroderma. A diffuse vasculopathy of peripheral arteries is manifested pathologically by intimal proliferation, activation of the arterial smooth muscle and endothelium, and narrowing or occlusion of the vessel lumen. Critical ischemia occurs in the tissues when vasoconstriction occludes these diseased vessels. Evidence suggests that this vascular disease is fundamental to organ damage and subsequent malfunction of the heart (cardiomyopathy), lung (pulmonary hypertension), kidney (scleroderma renal crisis [SRC]), and other organs in scleroderma (see below).

Raynaud phenomenon is the first manifestation of the disease in almost every patient. It tends to develop concurrently with other symptoms in those with diffuse disease and typically precedes other symptoms by years in those with limited disease. Stress and cold temperatures induce an exaggerated vasoconstriction of the small arteries, arterioles, and arteriovenous shunts of the skin of the digits. This is manifested clinically as pallor and cyanosis of the digits, followed by a reactive hyperemia after rewarming. Unlike episodes of uncomplicated primary Raynaud phenomenon, attacks of Raynaud phenomenon in patients with scleroderma are often painful and frequently lead to digital ulcerations, gangrene, or amputation.

Clinical features found to be predictive of an autoimmune rheumatic disease among patients with Raynaud phenomenon include the presence of antinuclear

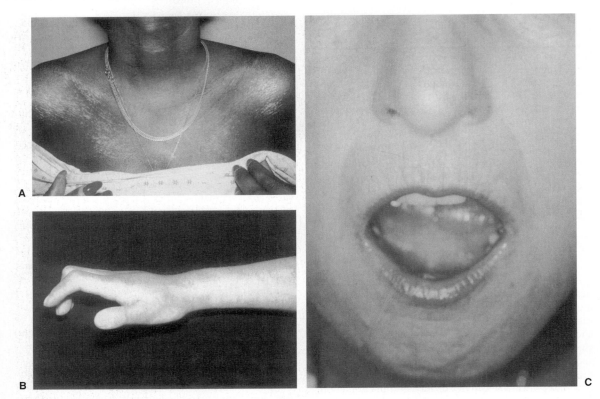

Figure 26–1. (**A**) Skin thickening of the chest in a patient with diffuse scleroderma. (**B**) Marked skin thickening of the forearm, hands, and fingers with joint contractures in a patient with diffuse scleroderma. (**C**) Typical skin changes of the face with reduced oral aperture and furrowing around the lips.

antibodies (ANAs) and abnormal nailfold capillaries (see section on Special Examinations, below). Patients over the age of 30 who develop new-onset Raynaud phenomenon should be screened with an ANA test and nailfold capillary examination, particularly if they have severe, painful episodes, signs of digital ischemia, or any other systemic symptoms. Although patients with scleroderma almost always have a positive ANA, it is important to remember that the presence of a positive ANA does not by itself make the diagnosis of a connective tissue disorder (see section on Laboratory Findings, below).

3. Lung involvement—Two main forms of lung disease occur in patients with scleroderma: inflammatory alveolitis leading to interstitial fibrosis and pulmonary arterial hypertension. These two processes can occur independently or concomitantly. Active interstitial lung disease occurs typically in patients with early diffuse scleroderma in the first 4 years of illness, whereas pulmonary hypertension more commonly affects those with long-standing limited disease. Lung involvement (both types) usually

presents as dyspnea on exertion, but can be asymptomatic early in the course of the lung disease. Therefore routine screening tests for lung disease (complete pulmonary function testing and echocardiograms) are important because early intervention may prevent progression. In the case of interstitial fibrosis, physical examination reveals fine crackles at the lung bases. This finding, however, is not present in early disease and its presence may indicate stable fibrosis and not active disease. Pulmonary function testing (PFT) or high-resolution computed tomography scanning can detect very mild and early disease and are better indicators of disease activity (ie, change in forced vital capacity over a short interval and ground glass opacities on computed tomography). Approximately 80% of patients with scleroderma have restrictive ventilatory defects on PFTs, consistent with interstitial lung disease. However, only about 10–20% of these patients suffer from progressive interstitial lung disease.

Pulmonary vascular disease with or without fibrosis can lead to pulmonary arterial hypertension and ultimately right heart failure. Estimates of the prevalence

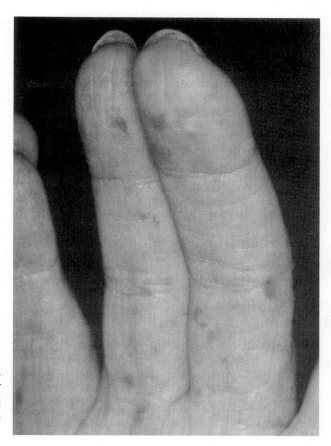

Figure 26–2. Raynaud phenomenon and telangiectasias of the skin in a patient with the CREST (*calcinosis*, *Raynaud* phenomenon, *esophageal* dysmotility, *sclerodactyly*, and *telangiectasias*) syndrome.

of pulmonary arterial hypertension among patients with scleroderma vary, but may be as high as 25%, although severe disease is only seen in roughly 10–15%. Typically, patients with isolated pulmonary arterial hypertension seek medical care complaining of dyspnea on exertion; however, signs of progressive, life-threatening right heart failure develop rapidly in later stages. Physical examination in these patients reveals systolic murmurs (from tricuspid regurgitation), a prominent P_2 component of S_2, right ventricular heaves, hepatomegaly, and lower extremity edema.

4. Gastrointestinal involvement—Gastrointestinal disease in scleroderma usually involves both the upper and lower gastrointestinal tract but is highly variable in its clinical expression. Patients with measurable gastrointestinal involvement can be relatively asymptomatic (eg, mild constipation). Alternatively, they may have profound gastrointestinal tract dysfunction, with malnutrition and significant morbidity. The majority of patients with scleroderma have symptomatic gastroesophageal reflux disease with dysphagia. Complaints include a sensation of food getting stuck in the mid-esophagus, atypical chest pain, or cough. Patients often complain that they must drink liquids to swallow solid food, particularly dry food such as meat or bread. Reflux and dysphagia occur because of dysmotility of the esophagus and stomach (gastroparesis). This type of organ dysfunction results from atrophy of the gastrointestinal tract wall smooth muscle that occurs in the absence of significant tissue fibrosis or vascular insult. If left untreated, the upper gastrointestinal disease can cause esophagitis, esophageal ulceration with bleeding, esophageal stricture, or Barrett esophagus.

The small and large intestines can also be affected by smooth muscle atrophy of the bowel wall causing abnormal motility of the gut. The most common symptom is the combination of constipation alternating with diarrhea and patients frequently give a history compatible with irritable bowel syndrome. Severe disease causes recurrent bouts of pseudo-obstruction, bowel distention with leakage of air into the bowel wall (pneumatosis coli intestinalis), and even bowel rupture. Lower bowel dysmotility slows the movement of bowel contents severely, allowing bacterial overgrowth, diarrhea, and malabsorption. Fecal incontinence develops in a small subset of patients.

5. Renal involvement—Clinically significant kidney disease occurs in only a minority of patients, but when it develops, renal disease poses a major threat to life. Scleroderma renal crisis (SRC) develops in approximately 10% of patients. It is characterized by the sudden onset of malignant hypertension that, if untreated, can lead rapidly to renal failure and death. Prior to the discovery that angiotensin-converting enzyme inhibitors (ACEIs) can control hypertensive crises in scleroderma effectively, SRC was the leading cause of death. Patients in the early stages of diffuse scleroderma, particularly those treated with glucocorticoids, are at the greatest risk for SRC. Patients in whom SRC develops may have symptoms associated with the acute onset of severe hypertension, including headache, visual changes, or seizures. Some, however, are asymptomatic and have undetected hypertension and an abrupt rise in creatinine; therefore, patients at high risk (those with early, active diffuse skin involvement) must have their blood pressure monitored frequently. Renal biopsy specimens reveal changes similar to those of malignant hypertension, thrombotic thrombocytopenic purpura/hemolytic uremic syndrome, and eclampsia. There is intimal hyperplasia and vasospasm of cortical arteries. This leads to activation of the renin-angiotensin system and accelerated hypertension, proteinuria, microscopic hematuria, and microvascular hemolysis (schistocytes on peripheral blood smear).

6. Cardiac involvement—Cardiac involvement in scleroderma can frequently be demonstrated by objective testing (eg, echocardiography, thallium scan, or electrocardiogram), but is usually subclinical. Cardiovascular morbidity is seen primarily in the late stages of diffuse scleroderma. Ischemia-reperfusion injury secondary to small arterial disease of the myocardium leads to contraction band necrosis and tissue fibrosis. This process can result in arrhythmias, a cardiomyopathy with diastolic dysfunction, or overt symptoms of heart failure. Although pericardial effusions are frequently detected by echocardiography, they are usually clinically silent. Large pericardial effusions are associated with pulmonary arterial hypertension and confer a poor prognosis. Symptoms from scleroderma cardiac disease include chest pain from pericarditis, palpitations from arrhythmias, or dyspnea on exertion from heart failure.

7. Musculoskeletal involvement—Musculoskeletal symptoms range from mild arthralgias to frank nonerosive arthritis with synovitis resembling rheumatoid arthritis. The sclerosis of the skin of the fingers or limbs is often associated with contractures of the joints. Deeper tissue fibrosis can also involve the fascia and underlying muscle. If areas around the tendons are involved, active and passive range of motion of the joints are limited and painful. The physician can appreciate this on examination by feeling a tendon friction rub when placing the hand over the tendons as the patient flexes and extends the joint. Tendon friction rubs are found most commonly around the ankles, wrists, or knees in those patients with early diffuse scleroderma.

Muscle weakness is a common complaint with a variety of causes including pain, prolonged muscle disuse, malnutrition, and a slowly progressive fibrosis of striated muscle. A true inflammatory myopathy is seen in a small subset of patients. Patients with "overlap" phenotypes who have scleroderma features (eg, Raynaud phenomenon, interstitial lung disease, and sclerodactyly) and a true inflammatory polyarthritis or polymyositis may be categorized as having mixed connective tissue disease. Patients with mixed connective tissue disease have high-titer anti-U1-ribonuclearprotein antibodies.

8. Other symptoms—Sicca complex (dry eyes and dry mouth) are common in patients with scleroderma but are usually not as severe as in patients with primary Sjögren syndrome (see Chapter 27).

Pain is very common and usually is associated with digital ulcers, fibrosis of tendons, joint contractures, or musculoskeletal disease. Rarely, neuropathic pain is present secondary to carpal tunnel syndrome or trigeminal neuralgia.

Depression is frequent among patients with scleroderma but does not correlate directly with disease severity. Depression more likely reflects other factors such as degree of pain, personality traits, and lack of good social support systems.

Erectile dysfunction is very common among men with scleroderma and is often not detected or properly managed. Fortunately, erectile dysfunction in scleroderma patients can respond to conventional therapy such as phosphodiesterase 5 inhibitors. Sexual dysfunction among women is also common; symptoms include vaginal dryness and dyspareunia secondary to a narrowed, fibrotic introitus.

B. LABORATORY FINDINGS

There is no single laboratory study or test that confirms the diagnosis of scleroderma. The diagnosis is made by obtaining a careful history and performing a physical examination. However, autoantibodies are found in nearly every patient with scleroderma (sensitivity >95%). ANAs are the most frequently detected, but they are not specific for scleroderma. ANAs can be detected in other connective tissue diseases, other diseases associated with autoimmunity (eg, Hashimoto thyroiditis), chronic infections (such as hepatitis C), and up to 10% of healthy individuals (at low titers). Anticentromere antibodies are detected in approximately

Table 26–2. Autoantibodies Associated with Scleroderma

Autoantibody	Prevalence	Associated Clinical Features
Antinuclear antibody	>95%	—
Anti-Scl-70 (anti-topoisomerase I)	20–40%	Lung disease, diffuse skin involvement. African Americans, worse prognosis
Anti-centromere	20–40%	CREST syndrome, digital ulcerations/digital loss
Anti-RNA polymerases	4–20%	Diffuse skin involvement, scleroderma renal crisis, cardiac disease, worse prognosis
Anti-B23	10%	Pulmonary hypertension
Anti-Pm-Scl	2–10%	Limited cutaneous involvement, myositis
Anti-U3-RNP (anti-fibrillarin)	8%	Lung disease, diffuse skin involvement, African-American males
Anti-U1-RNP	5%	Mixed connective tissue disease
Anti-Th/To	1–5%	Limited cutaneous involvement, pulmonary disease

CREST, calcinosis. *R*aynaud phenomenon, *e*sophageal dysmotility, *s*clerodactyly, and *t*elangiectasias; RNP, ribonucleoprotein.

20–40% of patients with scleroderma and are associated specifically with the CREST syndrome and severe digital ischemia with digital loss and pulmonary arterial hypertension. Anticentromere antibodies can also be found in patients with primary biliary cirrhosis and Sjögren syndrome. Antitopoisomerase I (anti-Scl-70) antibodies are also found in 20–40% of patients with scleroderma. Patients with antitopoisomerase I antibodies typically have diffuse skin changes, interstitial lung disease, and an overall worse prognosis. Antitopoisomerase I antibodies are highly specific for scleroderma. Antibodies to RNA polymerases (anti-RNAP I, II, and III) are also associated with diffuse skin changes, cardiac and renal involvement, and increased mortality. Antibodies to other nucleolar proteins are found in a small percentage of scleroderma patients, but assays for these are generally not commercially available (Th/To, Nor-90, Fibrillarin, Pm-Scl, and B23). The scleroderma-associated autoantibodies are outlined in Table 26–2.

C. IMAGING STUDIES

Chest films are an insensitive method to diagnose scleroderma lung disease. High-resolution computed tomography scans of the chest have an increased sensitivity and may provide some insight into disease activity (eg, ground glass opacities). Radiographic testing for evaluation of upper gastrointestinal disease is not often required unless patients have atypical symptoms or do not respond to standard treatments. A cine esophagram, however, will typically show a dilated esophagus, lower esophageal dysmotility, and gastroesophageal reflux.

D. SPECIAL TESTS

The use of specialized diagnostic testing depends on the organ system to be investigated. Every patient with scleroderma should be screened routinely at baseline and monitored for the development of pulmonary and cardiac disease. Patients should have PFTs (spirometry, lung volumes, and diffusing capacity) performed at baseline and then every 4–12 months depending on symptoms. PFTs provide the most sensitive measure for the development of interstitial lung disease, typically revealing a restrictive pattern with or without a reduction in diffusing capacity. PFTs can also suggest the presence of pulmonary arterial hypertension by the finding of an isolated reduction in diffusing capacity or a reduction out of proportion to the degree of the decline in forced vital capacity. The degree of pulmonary arterial hypertension can be estimated on a two-dimensional echocardiogram by measuring the right ventricular systolic pressure. Follow-up echocardiograph studies are recommended each year. Additional specialized studies such as bronchoalveolar lavage or right heart catheterization may be performed to determine degree of activity or severity of disease in those patients with abnormal screening studies and cardiopulmonary symptoms.

Studies of the upper gastrointestinal tract are often unnecessary in a patient with scleroderma who has symptomatic gastroesophageal reflux alone. Patients with atypical symptoms, poor responses to proton pump inhibitors, or long-standing untreated symptoms warrant further studies such as a barium swallow or upper gastrointestinal endoscopy. The barium swallow is relatively insensitive to measure motility problems but is useful for the exclusion of other potentially treatable causes of dysphagia such as a stricture. Any patient with long-standing reflux should be referred for endoscopy to evaluate for the complications of gastroesophageal reflux disease, including Barrett esophagus.

E. SPECIAL EXAMINATIONS

The capillaries of the skin can be visualized at the nailfold by using simple tools available in a typical examination room, thus giving insight into a patient's microvasculature status. Nailfold capillary dropout and dilated capillary loops are seen in nearly every patient with scleroderma but are not specific for scleroderma because nailfold changes can also be seen in other connective tissue diseases (such as dermatomyositis and mixed connective tissue disease). To examine the nailfold capillaries, a drop of either microscope oil or lubricant jelly is placed on the nail bed. An ophthalmoscope, set at minus 20–40 diopters (40 green) is used as a microscope to visualize the capillaries. Normally, the nailfold capillaries should be thin, linear, and uniform. In patients with scleroderma, these capillaries become dilated and areas of vessel dropout are apparent.

Differential Diagnosis

Given the multisystem nature of systemic sclerosis, the differential diagnosis is broad. Scleroderma is a rare disease but a protean one. Often the diagnosis only becomes obvious after several evaluations over time.

Patients with symptoms compatible with early scleroderma are encountered frequently in the primary care office. For this reason, primary care providers should be aware of this potentially life-threatening disease and be able to distinguish it from other disorders with similar features so that appropriate referrals can be made. The differential diagnosis includes other disorders that are associated with Raynaud phenomenon, those with similar skin changes, and those with other components of systemic autoimmune rheumatic diseases, such as arthralgias and positive autoantibodies. This differential diagnosis is detailed in Table 26–3.

Treatment

A. GENERAL PRINCIPLES

No single drug has been found to treat all of the manifestations of scleroderma, so no effective disease-specific therapy exists. Management, therefore, is based on the symptoms and disease manifestations of each individual patient and is often *organ-specific*. Recent therapeutic advances and improved screening tests have decreased the morbidity and mortality in scleroderma. For example, since the routine use of ACEIs in the management of SRC, the incidence of end-stage renal disease and mortality from this once-fatal complication has declined significantly.

Some important principles to keep in mind when treating patients with scleroderma follow:

- Each patient with scleroderma is unique with regard to disease features and prognosis (see below).
- No *proven* disease-modifying medication exists.

Table 26–3. Differential Diagnosis of Scleroderma

Clinical Feature	Differential Diagnosis

Raynaud phenomenon	Primary Raynaud phenomenon
	Systemic lupus erythematosus
	Vibration-hand syndrome
	Medication-induced
	    Chemotherapy (eg, cisplatin
	      or bleomycin)
	    Sympathomimetics
	Thoracic outlet syndrome
	Cryoglobulinemia/cryofibrino
	    genemia/cold agglutinins
	Systemic vasculitis
	Chilblains

Skin thickening	Scleredema Scleromyxedema POEMS syndrome Eosinophilic fasciitis Graft-versus-host disease Eosinophilia-myalgia syndrome Morphea Nephrogenic fibrosing dermopathy Diabetic cheiroarthropathy
Overlapping clinical features	Systemic lupus erythematosus Sjögren syndrome Inflammatory myopathies Rheumatoid arthritis

POEMS, *polyneuropathy, organomegaly, endocrinopathy, monoclonal gammopathy, and skin changes.*

- Scleroderma skin disease tends to reach peak involvement over the first 18–24 months, but then gradually improves with or without therapy.
- Routine screening and early intervention for internal organ manifestations may significantly reduce morbidity and mortality.

B. FIBROSIS

Although the pathogenesis of fibrosis is now better understood, this understanding has yet to translate into medications that treat cutaneous fibrosis effectively. Although some early, uncontrolled observations suggested that D-penicillamine may be beneficial, a controlled trial of low-dose versus high-dose D-penicillamine has cast doubt on the benefit of this drug (patients in the low-dose group had better outcomes). Most experts feel that until new antifibrotic drugs are available, the inflammatory process that triggers or causes the tissue injury and fibrosis needs to be controlled rapidly. Therefore, various immunosuppressive agents are used early in the disease course of those with diffuse skin involvement in an attempt to modify the course of skin fibrosis. Unfortunately, no convincing controlled trial using these agents is available to provide complete guidelines for their use. Agents that are currently used include glucocorticoids, methotrexate, mycophenolate mofetil, cyclophosphamide, antithymocyte globulin, and intravenous immune globulin. Each drug has unique toxicities and risks. Great care and expert guidance should be sought when prescribing these medications.

C. Vascular Disease

While the vascular insult is common to all patients with scleroderma, the clinical expression varies widely. Many patients have only mildly symptomatic Raynaud phenomenon, whereas others can have recurrent digital ulcerations that can progress to gangrene and digital loss. In addition, the scleroderma vasculopathy (intimal proliferation of arteries) is often a contributing factor in the internal organ involvement that is the major cause of morbidity and mortality. Episodes of critical ischemia are multifactorial and are a culmination of severe vasospasm (with ischemia-reperfusion injury), progressive vascular intimal proliferation with narrowing of the vessel lumen, and microvascular thrombosis. A combined therapeutic approach that addresses each of these processes is often used. The management of Raynaud phenomenon is discussed in detail in Chapter 25.

D. Inflammation

In early diffuse scleroderma, biopsy specimens of the skin reveal inflammatory infiltrates, and patients often complain of pain and swelling and stiffness of skin, joints, and periarticular structures. Inflammation can also be demonstrated in the lungs of some patients with interstitial lung disease (see below). It is postulated, therefore, that an early inflammatory insult leads to the downstream processes of fibrosis, atrophy, and loss of function. Because of this, a variety of immunosuppressive agents have been tried in the treatment of scleroderma, including methotrexate, mycophenolate mofetil, cyclophosphamide, antithymocyte globulin, and intravenous immune globulin. Unfortunately, data from rigorous clinical trials assessing the efficacy of these agents in scleroderma are limited. Regimens of intense immunosuppression are also currently being studied (bone marrow transplantation and immunoablation with high-dose cyclophosphamide) in patients with severe, early disease. These interventions carry the risk of significant adverse events, and their use should be limited to patients at high risk for significant morbidity and mortality. Patients with early, potentially modifiable disease but features associated with poor prognoses are the ideal candidates for these yet unproven aggressive therapies.

E. Organ-Specific Therapy

1. Scleroderma renal crisis (SRC)—Scleroderma patients considered to be at high risk for the development of renal crisis (those with early diffuse skin changes and prednisone use) should have their blood pressure monitored several times a week. A physician should promptly evaluate any unexplained rise in blood pressure, and renal function should be checked (urinalysis and creatinine). If there is persistently elevated blood pressure or signs of renal insufficiency, SRC should be suspected. In this setting, further diagnostic work-up (such as a renal biopsy) may be unnecessary. Prompt institution of ACEI therapy is needed to control blood pressure, with a target blood pressure of 130/80 mm Hg or lower. ACEIs should be titrated upward to gain control of blood pressure as quickly as possible. If blood pressure remains high, patients may require hospitalization for the management of medications and close monitoring of blood pressure and renal function. Some data suggest that angiotensin II receptor blockers are as beneficial as ACEIs in SRC. Despite the current availability of effective therapy and aggressive management, approximately 40% of patients with SRC have poor outcomes (death within 6 months or permanent dialysis), likely due to underrecognition of early symptoms and signs.

2. Interstitial lung disease—All patients with scleroderma should be monitored for the development of lung disease. Patients with a restrictive pattern on PFTs or interstitial fibrosis on high-resolution computed tomography scanning should be treated with immunosuppression if there is evidence of progression. Bronchoalveolar lavage should be performed to define the level of active disease in cases with suspected active alveolitis. There are now data from a multicenter, randomized, placebo-controlled trial that suggest that daily oral cyclophosphamide is beneficial in those patients with evidence of an active alveolitis (increased neutrophils or eosinophils on bronchoalveolar lavage or ground glass opacities on computed tomography scan). Monthly intravenous cyclophosphamide also showed benefit in another trial and is an alternative mode of therapy. Younger patients (under 60 years of age) with severe interstitial lung disease who do not respond to therapy should be considered for lung transplantation.

3. Pulmonary arterial hypertension—Unlike the other significant organ involvement in scleroderma, isolated pulmonary arterial hypertension is more commonly seen in those patients with limited scleroderma. All patients with scleroderma, however, should be evaluated with echocardiograms to screen for elevated pulmonary pressures. Patients with isolated pulmonary hypertension may also have a reduction in the diffusing capacity on PFTs.

In the past several years, new medications have been developed to treat patients with pulmonary hypertension. Currently approved therapies include endothelin-1 antagonists, prostaglandins, and phosphodiesterase inhibitors. The oral endothelin-1 dual receptor antagonist bosentan has proved effective in randomized trials to improve symptoms and exercise tolerance in scleroderma patients with pulmonary arterial hypertension. Sildenafil has also recently been approved for therapy of pulmonary arterial hypertension, but its use in scleroderma patients has not been fully investigated. Prostaglandin therapy (delivered by continuous intravenous or subcutaneous infusion or intermittent inhalation) is currently used for the management of severe or refractory pulmonary hypertension. In the United States, the only available formulations are intravenous epoprostenol, and the other prostacyclin analogs treprostinil and iloprost. Iloprost is approved in the United States for delivery by inhalation. Recent data suggest that aggressive management of severe pulmonary arterial hypertension with these agents may improve survival in scleroderma. However, more experience is necessary with these agents to define their long-term benefit in the management of scleroderma. Patients with severe pulmonary arterial hypertension should also be considered candidates for lung transplantation (occasionally performed simultaneously with heart transplantation).

4. Gastrointestinal disease—The gastrointestinal involvement in scleroderma is usually fairly easy to manage in the majority of patients. The most frequent symptoms, gastroesophageal reflux and esophageal dysmotility, may be treated effectively with proton pump inhibitors (ie, omeprazole 20–40 mg once or twice daily). All patients with upper gastrointestinal symptoms should also be instructed in simple behavioral measures that can reduce symptoms:

- Eat small, frequent meals.
- Do not eat meals within 2–3 hours of bedtime.
- Keep the head of the bed elevated.
- Avoid aggravating factors (eg, tobacco, alcohol, and caffeine).

Those with persistent symptoms may require the use of promotility agents such as metoclopramide. Any patient with severe dysphagia or symptoms unresponsive to the above measures should be referred to a gastroenterologist for an upper gastrointestinal endoscopy.

Lower gastrointestinal symptoms are less frequent but often more difficult to manage. Over-the-counter preparations such as loperamide or fiber supplements are used to treat mild symptoms. Persistent, frequent diarrhea may be a sign of bacterial overgrowth that requires treatment with antibiotics (eg, metronidazole). Promotility agents may also improve lower gastrointestinal symptoms (eg, erythromycin, tegaserod, metoclopramide, or octreotide). Severe dysmotility that is refractory to medical therapy and associated with either recurrent bouts of pseudo-obstruction or progressive weight loss and malnutrition is best treated with bowel rest and total parenteral nutrition.

Prognosis

The prognosis in scleroderma is highly dependent on the extent of major organ disease. This can be predicted to some extent by the degree of skin involvement. Patients with limited scleroderma have a normal life expectancy with approximately a 90% 5-year survival rate. Patients with diffuse skin disease have only about a 70–80% 5-year survival rate. Clinical features that predict poor outcomes include high skin scores, progressive lung disease, tendon friction rubs, evidence of heart disease, the presence of pulmonary arterial hypertension, anemia, and SRC. Aggressive management early in the course of the disease can improve quality of life and reduce morbidity. In the future, new therapies and better methods of recognizing disease complications early will improve the prognosis of patients with scleroderma. In the meantime, primary care physicians are encouraged to refer scleroderma patients to a rheumatologist or specialty scleroderma treatment center.

REFERENCES

Highland KB, Silver RM. New developments in scleroderma interstitial lung disease. *Curr Opin Rheumatol.* 2005;17:737. [PMID: 16224252]

Kahaleh MB. Raynaud phenomenon and the vascular disease in scleroderma. *Curr Opin Rheumatol.* 2004;16:718. [PMID: 15577610]

Mayes MD. Scleroderma epidemiology. *Rheum Dis Clin North Am.* 2003;29:239. [PMID: 12841293]

Ramirez A, Varga J. Pulmonary arterial hypertension in systemic sclerosis: clinical manifestations, pathophysiology, evaluation and management. *Treat Respir Med.* 2004;3:339. [PMID: 15658881]

Relevant World Wide Web Sites

[American College of Rheumatology]
http://www.rheumatology.org
[Scleroderma Clinical Trials Consortium]
http://www.sctc-online.org
[Scleroderma Foundation]
http://www.scleroderma.org
[Scleroderma Research Foundation]
http://www.srfcure.org

Primary Sjögren Syndrome

27

Manuel Ramos-Casals, MD, PhD, & Josep Font, MD, PhD

ESSENTIALS OF DIAGNOSIS

- *Sjögren syndrome (SS) is a systemic autoimmune disease that presents with sicca symptomatology of mucosal surfaces.*

- *The main sicca features (xerophthalmia and xerostomia) are determined by specific ocular (rose bengal staining and Schirmer test) and oral (salivary flow measurement and parotid scintigraphy) tests.*

- *The histologic hallmark is a focal lymphocytic infiltration of the exocrine glands, determined by a biopsy of the minor labial salivary glands.*

- *The spectrum of the disease includes systemic features (extraglandular manifestations) in some patients, and may be complicated by the development of lymphoma.*

- *Patients with SS present a broad spectrum of analytic features (cytopenias, hypergammaglobulinemia, and high erythrocyte sedimentation rate) and autoantibodies, of which antinuclear antibodies are the most frequently detected, anti-Ro/SS-A the most specific, and cryoglobulins and hypocomplementemia the main prognostic markers.*

General Considerations

Sjögren syndrome (SS) is a systemic autoimmune disease that mainly affects the exocrine glands and usually presents as persistent dryness of the mouth and eyes due to functional impairment of the salivary and lacrimal glands. An estimated 2–4 million persons in the United States have SS, of whom approximately 1 million have established diagnoses. The prevalence in European countries ranges between 0.60% and 3.3%. The incidence of SS has been calculated as 4 cases per 100,000. SS primarily affects white perimenopausal women, with a female:male ratio ranging from 14:1 to 24:1 in the largest reported series. The disease may occur at all ages but typically has its onset in the fourth to sixth decades of life. When sicca symptoms appear in a previously healthy person, the syndrome is classified as primary SS. When sicca features are found in association with another systemic autoimmune disease, most commonly rheumatoid arthritis, systemic sclerosis, or systemic lupus erythematosus, it is classified as secondary SS. Recent studies have found a prevalence of secondary SS of between 11% and 19% in systemic lupus erythematosus patients, and 7% in a large rheumatoid arthritis registry.

Major clinical manifestations are summarized in Table 27–1. Although most patients present with sicca symptoms, there are various clinical and analytic features that may indicate undiagnosed SS Table 27–2. The variability in the presentation of SS may partially explain delays in diagnosis of up to 9 years from the onset of symptoms. SS is a disease that can be expressed in many guises depending on the specific epidemiologic, clinical, or immunologic features. The therapeutic management of SS is mainly centered on the control of sicca features, using substitutive and oral muscarinic agents, while glucocorticoids and immunosuppressive agents play a key role in the treatment of extraglandular features.

Clinical Findings

A. Signs and Symptoms

1. Sicca features—Xerostomia, the subjective feeling of oral dryness, is the key feature in the diagnosis of primary SS, occurring in more than 95% of patients. Other oral symptoms may include soreness, adherence of food to the mucosa, and dysphagia. Reduced salivary volume interferes with basic functions such as speaking or eating. The lack of salivary antimicrobial functions may accelerate local infection (eg, candidiasis), tooth decay, periodontal disease, and angular cheilitis. Xerostomia can lead to difficulty with dentures and the need for expensive dental restoration, particularly in elderly patients. Various oral signs may be observed in SS patients. In the early stages, the mouth may appear moist, but as the disease progresses, the usual pooling of saliva in the floor of the mouth disappears. Typically the surface of the tongue becomes red and lobulated, with partial or complete depapillation (Figure 27–1). In advanced disease, the oral mucosa appears dry and glazed and tends to form fine wrinkles.

Table 27–1. Major Clinical Manifestations of Sjögren Syndrome

Organ	Manifestations
Mouth	Oral dryness (xerostomia), soreness, caries, periodontal disease, oral candidiasis, parotid swelling
Eyes	Ocular dryness (xerophthalmia), corneal ulcers, conjunctivitis
Nose and throat	Nasal dryness, chronic cough
Skin	Cutaneous dryness, palpable purpura, Ro-associated polycyclic lesions, urticarial lesions
Joints	Arthalgias, non-erosive symmetric arthritis
Lungs	Obstructive chronic pneumopathy, interstitial pneumopathy
Cardiovascular	Raynaud phenomenon, pericarditis, autonomic disturbances
Liver	Associated hepatitis C virus infection, primary biliary cirrhosis, type 1 autoimmune hepatitis
Kidneys	Renal tubular acidosis, glomerulonephritis
Peripheral nerve	Mixed polyneuropathy, pure sensitive neuropathy, mononeuritis multiplex
Central nervous system	White matter lesions, cranial nerve involvement (V, VIII, and VII), myelopathy
Ears	Sensorineural hearing loss
Thyroid	Autoimmune thyroiditis
General symptoms	Low-grade fever, generalized pain, myalgias, fatigue, weakness, fibromyalgia, polyadenopathies

Table 27–2. Non-Sicca Manifestations Suggestive of Sjögren Sydrome

Clinical features
 Chronic fatigue
 Fever of unknown origin
 Leukocytoclastic vasculitis
 Parotid or submandibular gland swelling
 Raynaud phenomenon
 Peripheral neuropathy
 Pulmonary fibrosis
 Mother of a baby born with congenital heart block
Analytic features
 Elevated erythrocyte sedimentation rate
 Hypergammaglobulinemia
 Leukopenia and thrombocytopenia
 Serum and/or urine monoclonal band
 Positive antinuclear antibodies or rheumatoid factor in an asymptomatic patient

epithelium (keratoconjunctivitis sicca). In severe cases, slitlamp examination may reveal filamentary keratitis, marked by mucus filaments that adhere to damaged areas of the corneal surface (Figure 27–2). Tears also have inherent antimicrobial activity and SS patients are more susceptible to ocular infections such as blepharitis, bacterial keratitis, and conjunctivitis. Severe ocular complications may include corneal ulceration, vascularization, and opacification.

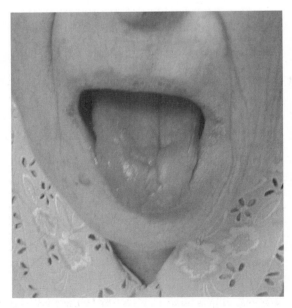

Figure 27–1. Dry mouth in a patient with primary SS: red tongue with depapillation.

Xerophthalmia, the subjective feeling of ocular dryness, produces sensations of itching, grittiness, soreness, and dryness, although the eyes have a normal appearance. Other ocular complaints include photosensitivity, erythema, eye fatigue, or decreased visual acuity. Environmental irritants such as smoke, wind, air conditioning, and low humidity may exacerbate ocular symptoms. Diminished tear secretion may lead to chronic irritation and destruction of corneal and bulbar conjunctival

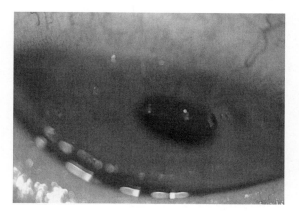

Figure 27–2. Dry eye with filamentary keratitis.

Chronic or episodic swelling of the major salivary glands (parotid and submandibular glands) is reported in 10–20% of patients and may commence unilaterally, but often becomes bilateral (Figure 27–3). Reduction or absence of respiratory tract glandular secretions can lead to dryness of the nose, throat, and trachea resulting in persistent hoarseness and chronic, nonproductive cough. Likewise, involvement of the exocrine glands of the skin leads to cutaneous dryness. In female patients with SS, dryness of the vagina and vulva may result in dyspareunia and pruritus, affecting their quality of life.

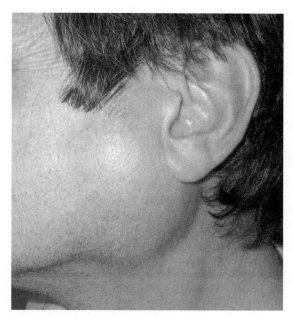

Figure 27–3. Parotid enlargement.

2. Extraglandular manifestations

a. General symptomatology—Patients with primary SS often present with general symptomatology, including fever, generalized pain, fatigue, weakness, sleep disturbances, anxiety, and depression, which may have a much greater impact on the quality of life of patients than sicca features. Low-grade fevers may occur in SS, usually in young patients with positive immunologic markers. Fatigue, generalized pain, and weakness are among the most debilitating clinical features of primary SS. The coexistence of primary SS with a defined fibromyalgia is reported often.

b. Joint and muscular involvement—Joint involvement, primarily generalized arthralgias, is seen in 25–75% of patients. Less frequently, joint disease presents as an intermittent symmetric arthritis primarily affecting small joints. Joint deformity and mild erosions are rare, except for those cases associated with rheumatoid arthritis. Clinical myopathy is rare but myalgias are frequently observed, and a recent study reported that subclinical muscular inflammation is often observed.

c. Skin—Although the main cutaneous manifestation of patients with primary SS is skin dryness, a wide spectrum of cutaneous lesions may be observed, the most frequent of which is a small-vessel vasculitis. The vasculitis may be characterized by either a lymphocytic vasculitis or leukocytoclastic vasculitis. The skin findings include palpable purpura (Figure 27–4), urticaria, and erythematous macules or papules, and are associated with cryoglobulins in 30% of patients. Life-threatening vasculitis is also closely related to cryoglobulinemia.

Primary SS patients may also present with nonvasculitic cutaneous lesions. Some patients with anti-Ro/SS-A antibodies may present with polycyclic, photosensitive cutaneous lesions (Figure 27–5), clinically identical to the so-called annular erythema described in Asian SS patients and subacute cutaneous lupus.

d. Lungs—Two types of pulmonary involvement are predominant in primary SS: bronchial/bronchiolar involvement and interstitial disease. The results of pulmonary function tests often correlate with the computed tomographic scan pattern, with predominantly obstructive profiles being found in bronchial/bronchiolar disease and restrictive patterns in interstitial disease. Subsequent diagnostic procedures, including bronchoscopy with bronchoalveolar lavage and transbronchial biopsy, may be required to exclude other disorders. Lung disease in primary SS has been reported to occur early following clinical presentation of the disease. Anti-Ro antibody positivity is believed to be a risk factor for pulmonary disease in SS. Most patients do not develop progressive pulmonary disease after 10-year follow-up.

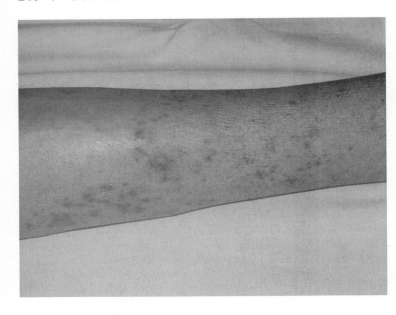

Figure 27–4. Cutaneous purpura in the legs in a patient with SS and cryoglobulinemia.

e. Cardiovascular features—Raynaud phenomenon, with a prevalence of 13%, is probably the most common vascular feature observed in primary SS. The clinical course of Raynaud phenomenon in primary SS is milder than in other systemic autoimmune diseases such as systemic sclerosis. Vascular complications (eg, digital loss, digital pulp pitting, or fingertip infarctions)

are uncommon, and pharmacologic interventions are required in only 40% of cases. Cardiac involvement is rarely observed, with pericardial effusions (usually mild and asymptomatic) being the most frequent feature. Recent studies have described autonomic cardiovascular disturbances.

f. Gut—Gastrointestinal involvement may include altered esophageal motility, chronic gastritis, and less frequently, malabsorption. *Helicobacter pylori* infection should be excluded in patients with gastritis, due to the close association with gastric mucosa-associated lymphoid tissue lymphoma. Pancreatic involvement, usually asymptomatic, is demonstrated by altered pancreatic function tests. Some patients may present with chronic pancreatitis. Liver function tests may be elevated in 10–20% of patients with primary SS. After exclusion of potentially hepatotoxic drugs, the main causes are chronic hepatitis C viral infection (especially in geographic areas with a high prevalence) and primary biliary cirrhosis. Less frequently, SS patients may present with type 1 autoimmune hepatitis, and even more rarely, autoimmune or sclerosing cholangitis.

g. Nephro-urologic involvement—Many SS patients have renal dysfunction, including mild proteinuria in 28%, reduced creatinine clearance in 16%, and distal renal tubular acidosis in 13%. However, overt renal involvement was only found in 5% of the nearly 1000 patients included in the two largest reported series. The main types of renal involvement described are interstitial renal disease, characterized by hyposthenuria and type I (distal) tubular acidosis, and glomerulonephritis. Finally,

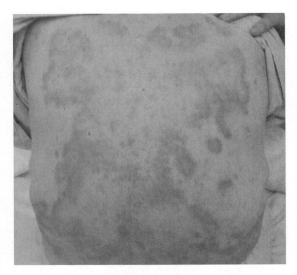

Figure 27–5. Polycyclic, photosensitive cutaneous lesions in a 67-year-old woman with primary SS and anti-Ro/SS-A antibodies.

interstitial cystitis, sometimes with severe symptoms, has recently been identified as a frequent extraglandular SS feature.

h. Neurologic involvement—Peripheral neuropathy is the most common neurologic involvement. A joint analysis of 1025 patients with primary SS showed peripheral neuropathy in 18%. The most frequent types of neuropathy were mixed polyneuropathy, pure sensory neuropathy, and mononeuritis multiplex. Of these, pure sensory neuropathy is recognized as a characteristic neurologic complication of primary SS, caused by damage to the sensory neurons of the dorsal root and gasserian ganglia. In contrast, mixed polyneuropathy and multiplex mononeuritis are usually associated with vasculitis and often with concomitant cryoglobulinemia. SS patients may present cranial nerve involvement, mainly of the trigeminal (V), vestibulocochlear (VIII), and facial (VII) cranial pairs.

Although earlier studies described central nervous system involvement as a frequent extraglandular manifestation of primary SS, clinically significant central nervous system involvement is actually very rare (3). The most frequently detected central nervous system feature in primary SS is probably asymptomatic white matter lesions in magnetic resonance examinations. These are considered as having a nonspecific etiopathogenic role, although isolated cases of SS patients presenting with a multiple sclerosis–like disease have been reported. Some patients may present with an associated myelopathy.

i. Other organs—Nearly one-third of patients with primary SS have thyroid disease. Subclinical hypothyroidism is the most frequent finding, especially in patients with antithyroid autoantibodies (suggesting previous Hashimoto thyroiditis). Although ear, nose, and throat involvement has been little studied in patients with primary SS, recent studies have described sensorineural hearing loss in nearly 25% of SS patients. Psychiatric disorders, including depression and anxiety, have been described in many patients with SS.

B. LABORATORY FINDINGS

The results of routine laboratory tests and immunologic markers in primary SS are summarized in Table 27–3. The most frequent analytic features are cytopenia (33%), elevated erythrocyte sedimentation rate (22%), and hypergammaglobulinemia (22%). The most frequent cytopenias detected are normocytic anemia (20%), leukopenia (16%), and thrombocytopenia (13%), all of which are found more commonly in patients with positive immunologic markers. Cytopenias are usually asymptomatic, but may be clinically overt in some cases. Erythrocyte sedimentation rate levels correlate closely with the percentage of circulating gamma globulins

Table 27–3. The Laboratory Evaluation in Sjögren Syndrome

Test	Typical Result
Complete blood cell count	• Normochromic, normocytic anemia. Isolated cases of hemolytic anemia • Mild leukopenia ($3–4 \times 10^9$/L) • Mild thrombocytopenia ($80–150 \times 10^9$/L)
Erythrocyte sedimentation rate (ESR) and C-reactive protein (CRP)	• Raised ESR (>50 mm/h) in 20–30% of cases, especially in patients with hypergammaglobulinemia • Normal values of CRP
Serum protein	• Hypergammaglobulinemia • Monoclonal band
Liver function tests	• Raised transaminases (associated with hepatitis C virus or autoimmune hepatitis) • Raised alkaline phosphatase and/or bilirubin (associated with primary biliary cirrhosis)
Electrolytes and urinalysis	• Proteinuria (glomerulonephritis) • Hyposthenuria, low plasma bicarbonate and low blood pH (renal tubular acidosis)
Antinuclear antibody test	• Positive in more than 80%
Rheumatoid factor	• Positive in 40–50% of patients, often leading to diagnostic confusion with rheumatoid arthritis
Anti-extractable nuclear antigens antibodies	• Positive anti-Ro/SS-A (30–60%) and anti-La/SS-B (15–40%)
Complement (C3, C4, and CH50) Cryoglobulins Other autoantibodies	• Complement levels are decreased in 10–20% of patients • Present in 10–20% of patients • Antimitochondrial antibodies (associated with primary biliary cirrhosis) • Antithyroid antibodies (associated with thyroiditis) • Anti-dsDNA (associated with systemic lupus erythematosus) • Anticentromere (associated with a limited form of systemic sclerosis)

(hypergammaglobulinemia), while serum C-reactive protein levels are usually normal. Biochemical evaluation of patients with SS should routinely include renal and liver analysis. Finally, circulating monoclonal immunoglobulins may be detected in nearly 20% of patients with primary SS, with monoclonal IgG being detected most frequently.

C. SPECIAL TESTS

1. Salivary gland biopsy—Minor salivary gland biopsy remains a highly specific test for the diagnosis of SS, although it is an invasive technique that, when not correctly performed, may be accompanied by local side effects. Focal lymphocytic sialadenitis, defined as multiple, dense aggregates of 50 or more lymphocytes in perivascular or periductal areas in the majority of sampled glands, is the characteristic histopathologic feature of SS. The key requirements for a correct histological evaluation are an adequate number of informative lobules (at least four) and the determination of an average focus score (a focus is a cluster of at least 50 lymphocytes). However, nonspecific sialadenitis is quite common in biopsy samples of minor salivary glands in healthy control populations. Although sialoadenitis is the key histopathologic feature of SS, this finding in the absence of symptoms and markers suggestive of SS should be interpreted with caution.

2. Assessment of oral involvement—Several methods to assess oral involvement have been proposed, such as measurement of the salivary flow rate, sialochemistry, sialography, or scintigraphy. Measurement of the salivary flow, with or without stimulation, is the simplest method in evaluating xerostomia, and is acceptable to patients and needs no special equipment. The other tests, though useful for the purposes of research, rarely have clinical applications.

3. Assessment of ocular involvement—The main ocular tests are the Schirmer test and rose bengal staining. The Schirmer test for the eye quantitatively measures tear formation via placement of filter paper in the lower conjunctival sac. The test can be performed with or without the instillation of anesthetic drops to prevent reflex tearing. The test result is positive when less than 5 mm of paper is wetted after 5 minutes. Rose bengal scoring involves the placement of 25 mL of rose bengal solution in the inferior fornix of each eye and having the patient blink twice. Slitlamp examination detects destroyed conjunctival epithelium due to desiccation.

4. Immunologic tests—The main immunologic markers found in primary SS are antinuclear antibodies, anti-Ro/SS-A or anti-La/SS-B antibodies, rheumatoid factor, hypocomplementemia, and cryoglobulins (see Table 27–3). Antinuclear antibodies are the most frequently detected antibodies in primary SS (in more than 80% of cases), and titers $\geq 1:80$ play a central role in differentiating SS from non-autoimmune causes of sicca syndrome. Anti-Ro/SS-A and La/SS-B antibodies, detected in 30–60% of patients, are closely associated with most extraglandular features, especially with cutaneous lesions, neurologic features, congenital heart block, and cytopenias. In nearly 50% of cases, patients with primary SS also present with positive rheumatoid factor.

Hypocomplementemia and cryoglobulinemia (see Chapter 37 on mixed cryoglulinemia) are two closely-related immunologic markers that have been linked with more severe SS. Recent studies have associated low complement levels with chronic hepatitis C viral infection, lymphoma development, and mortality. Similarly, cryoglobulins (usually type II, which are found in 10–20% of patients) have been associated with extraglandular manifestations, hepatitis C viral infection, and prospectively with the development of lymphoma. The detection of these markers (which is usually simultaneous) identifies patients at high risk of developing severe disease, including a high prevalence of extraglandular features and the development of lymphoma.

Differential Diagnosis

The proven diagnosis of SS requires not only documentation of sicca symptoms, but also objective evidence of dry eyes and mouth and analytic evidence of autoimmunity, as sicca syndrome has many causes. The most frequent cause of sicca features is the chronic use of dry drugs (mainly antihypertensive, antihistamine, and antidepressant agents), especially in the elderly. After this cause is excluded, there are three main causes of sicca syndrome. First, some processes may mimic the clinical picture of SS through nonlymphocytic infiltration of the exocrine glands by granulomas (sarcoidosis and tuberculosis), amyloid proteins (amyloidosis), or malignant cells (hematologic neoplasia). Second, extrinsic factors, mainly chronic viral infections such as hepatitis C virus or HIV, may induce a lymphocytic infiltration of exocrine glands. Third, patients may have primary SS or secondary SS (Table 27–4).

Diagnosis

Sicca features are symptoms that usually receive little attention and may be considered trivial by both doctor and patient. Although often elusive, an early, accurate diagnosis of SS can help prevent, or ensure timely treatment of, many of the complications associated with the disease. For example, early restoration of salivary function can relieve symptoms of dry mouth and may prevent or slow the progress of the oral complications of SS, including dental caries, oral candidiasis, and periodontal disease. Untreated severe dry eye can result in corneal ulcers and further perforation, which may eventually lead to loss of

Table 27–4. Classification of Sjögren Syndrome (SS): Primary, Secondary, Mimicked, and Associated SS

---

1. **Primary SS**
2. **Secondary SS**
   Chronic HCV infection (Mediterranean countries)
   HTLV-I infection (Asian countries)
   HIV infection
3. **Mimicked SS**
   Other diseases infiltrating exocrine glands
      Granulomatous diseases (sarcoidosis and tuberculosis)
      Amyloidosis
      Neoplasias (lymphoma)
      Type V hyperlipidemia
   Other processes
      Graft-versus-host disease
      Eosinophilia-myalgia syndrome
      Radiation injury
      Medication-related dryness
4. **Associated SS**
   Systemic autoimmune diseases
      Systemic lupus erythematosus
      Systemic sclerosis
      Rheumatoid arthritis
      Still disease
      Sarcoidosis
      Inflammatory myopathies
   Organ-specific autoimmune diseases
      Primary biliary cirrhosis
      Autoimmune thyroiditis
      Multiple sclerosis
      Diabetes mellitus

HCV, hepatitis C virus; HIV, human immune deficiency virus; HTLV, human T-cell lymphoma virus.

the eye. An early diagnosis is also mandatory for the main extraglandular features, in order to prevent chronic organ damage by prompt recognition and treatment. Two sets of criteria for the diagnosis of SS have been established (Table 27–5).

Complications

Primary SS usually progresses very slowly, with no rapid deterioration in salivary function or dramatic changes in sicca symptoms. The main exceptions to this benign course are the development of extraglandular manifestations and the high incidence of lymphoma.

With respect to extraglandular involvement, SS patients may be divided into two groups with different prognoses. A more stable, chronic SS course is usually found in patients with predominantly peri-epithelial lesions (such as interstitial nephritis or liver or lung disease), while those with predominantly extraepithelial

Table 27–5. Classification Criteria for Sjögren Syndrome

I. Ocular symptoms: a positive response to at least one of the following questions:
   a) Have you had daily, persistent, troublesome dry eyes for more than 3 months?
   b) Do you have a recurrent sensation of sand or gravel in the eyes?
   c) Do you use tear substitutes more than three times a day?
II. Oral symptoms: a positive response to at leasst one of the following questions:
   a) Have you had a daily feeling of dry mouth for more than 3 months?
   b) Have you had recurrently or persistently swollen salivary glands as an adult?
   c) Do you frequently drink liquids to aid in swallowing dry food?
III. Ocular signs: objective evidence of ocular involvement defined as a positive result for at least one of the following two tests:
   a) Schirmer test, performed without anesthesia (5 mm in 5 minutes)
   b) Rose bengal score or other ocular dye score (4 according to the van Bijsterveld scoring system)
IV. Histopathology: In minor salivary glands (obtained through normal-appearing mucosa) focal lymphocytic sialoadenitis, evaluated by an expert histopathologist, with a focus score of 1, defined as a number of lymphocytic foci (which are adjacent to normal-appearing mucous acini and contain more than 50 lymphocytes) per 4 mm^2 of glandular tisue.
V. Salivary gland involvement: objective evidence of salivary gland involvement defined by a positive result for at least one of the following diagnostic tests:
   a) Unstimulated whole salivary flow (1.5 mL in 15 minutes)
   b) Parotid sialography showing the presence of diffuse sialectasias (punctate, cavitary, or destructive patttern), without evidence of obstruction in the major ducts
   c) Salivary scintigraphy showing delayed uptake, reduced concentration, and/or delayed excretion of tracer
VI. Autoantibodies: presence in the serum of the following autoantibodies:
   a) Antinuclear antibodies
   b) Rheumatoid factor
   c) Antibodies to Ro/SS-A or La/SS-B antigens, or both

Patients are classified as having primary SS when they fulfill four or more of the six classification criteria (1993 European Classification Criteria).

According to the recently proposed 2002 American-European Classification Criteria, either criterion IV (salivary gland biopsy) or criterion VIc (anti-Ro/La antibodies) are mandatory.

expression (glomerulonephritis, polyneuropathy, and vasculitis) suffer higher morbidity and mortality. Cryoglobulinemia probably plays a central etiopathogenic role in this latter group of patients, contributing to the development of the main extraepithelial manifestations.

Lymphoma is traditionally considered as the main complication in the natural history of SS, although cross-sectional studies have reported that lymphoma develops in 5% or less of patients with primary SS. Lymphadenopathy, skin vasculitis, peripheral neuropathy, fever, anemia, and lymphopenia are observed significantly more frequently among patients who develop lymphoma compared with the general SS population.

The few studies that have analyzed the causes and rates of mortality in these patients compared to the general population found that the overall mortality of patients with primary SS increased only in patients with adverse predictors. The presence of cutaneous vasculitis and low C4 levels, for example, help differentiate patients at higher risk for adverse outcomes from those likely to have uncomplicated disease courses.

Treatment

At present, there is no treatment capable of modifying the evolution of SS. The therapeutic approach is based on symptomatic replacement or stimulation of glandular secretions. Extraglandular involvement requires organ-specific therapy, sometimes with glucocorticoids and immunosuppressive agents, as appropriate to the level of severity.

Treatment of sicca manifestations is mainly symptomatic and is typically intended to limit the damage resulting from chronic involvement. Moisture replacement products can be effective for patients with mild or moderate symptoms. Some severe symptoms can occur as a result of oral candidiasis, which should be treated with nystatin. Use of anticholinergic medications, alcohol, and smoking, should be avoided whenever possible.

Frequent use of tear substitutes will help replace moisture, and preservative-free formulations help avoid the irritation that can occur with frequent use, while lubricating ointments and methylcellulose inserts are usually reserved for nocturnal use. In moderate-to-severe xerophthalmia, frequent use of preservative-free artificial tears in dosing intervals as often as hourly is highly recommended. Glucocorticoid-containing ophthalmic solutions should be avoided because they may induce corneal lesions or promote infection. In severe cases, temporary occlusion of the puncta through the insertion of plugs (collagen or silicone) or permanent occlusion by electrocautery can be used to block tear drainage and thus retain existing tears. Ocular infection, which may present with sudden aggravation of symptoms and/or excessive mucus production, should be treated promptly.

For patients with SS who have residual salivary gland function, stimulation of saliva flow with a secretagogue is the treatment of choice and at present is the most efficacious means to prevent long-term oral complications. Two muscarinic agonists (pilocarpine and cevimeline) have recently been approved for the treatment of sicca symptoms in SS. These agents stimulate the M_1 and M_3 receptors present on salivary glands, leading to increased secretory function. Clinical studies with pilocarpine (Salagen) tablets in the United States have demonstrated significant subjective and objective benefit for xerostomia and related oral symptoms at doses of 15–20 mg/d. The other muscarinic agonist is cevimeline hydrochloride, which is given at a dose of 30 mg three times daily. Further controlled studies of these muscarinic agonists at different dosages are needed in patients with SS, including evaluation of elderly patients or those with comorbid processes, such as chronic cardiovascular, pulmonary, or hepatic diseases.

As a rule, the management of extraglandular features should be organ-specific, with glucocorticoids and immunosuppresive agents limited to potentially severe scenarios. Nonsteroidal anti-inflammatory drugs usually provide relief from the minor musculoskeletal symptoms of SS, as well as from painful parotid swelling. Hydroxychloroquine may be used in patients with fatigue, arthralgias, and myalgias. For patients with moderate extraglandular involvement (mainly arthritis, extensive cutaneous purpura, and non-severe peripheral neuropathy), 0.5 mg/kg/d of prednisone may suffice. For patients with internal organ involvement (pulmonary alveolitis, glomerulonephritis, or severe neurologic features), a combination of prednisone and immunosuppressive agents (cyclophosphamide, azathioprine, or mycophenolate mofetil) is suggested.

With regard to biological agents, recent studies have demonstrated the lack of efficacy of tumor necrosis factor inhibitors in primary SS. In contrast, a promising treatment is rituximab (anti-CD20), a monoclonal agent approved for the treatment of B-cell lymphoma. Rituximab has been used to treat patients with systemic lupus erythematosus, rheumatoid arthritis, mixed cryoglulinemia, and recently, SS patients with lymphoma. The specific target of rituximab (B cells) suggests that this agent may play a role in modifying the etiopathogenic events of patients with primary SS, a disease characterized by B-cell hyperactivity.

REFERENCES

Fox RI. Sjogren's syndrome. *Lancet.* 2005;366:321.

Garcia-Carrasco M, Ramos-Casals M, Rosas J, et al. Primary Sjogren syndrome: clinical and immunologic disease patterns in a cohort of 400 patients. *Medicine (Baltimore).* 2002;81: 270.

Ioannidis JP, Vassiliou VA, Moutsopoulos HM. Long-term risk of mortality and lymphoproliferative disease and predictive classification of primary Sjogren's syndrome. *Arthritis Rheum.* 2002;46:741.

Kassan SS, Moutsopoulos HM. Clinical manifestations and early diagnosis of Sjogren syndrome. *Arch Intern Med.* 2004;164:1275.

Ramos-Casals M, Anaya JM, García-Carrasco M, et al. Cutaneous vasculitis in primary Sjögren syndrome. Classification and clinical significance of 52 patients. *Medicine (Baltimore).* 2004;83:96.

Ramos-Casals M, Cervera R, Yague J, et al. Cryoglobulinemia in primary Sjögren's syndrome: prevalence and clinical characteristics in a series of 115 patients. *Semin Arthritis Rheum.* 1998;28:200.

Ramos-Casals M, Loustaud-Ratti V, De Vita S, et al, and the SS-HCV Study Group. Sjogren syndrome associated with hepatitis C virus: a multicenter analysis of 137 cases. *Medicine (Baltimore).* 2005;84:81.

Theander E, Manthorpe R, Jacobsson LT. Mortality and causes of death in primary Sjögren's syndrome: a prospective cohort study. *Arthritis Rheum.* 2004;50:1262.

Relevant World Wide Web Sites

[The Sjögren's Syndrome Foundation]

www.sjogrens.org

(Information about the foundation and its membership as well as explanation of this disease, links, and news and events.)

[Dry.Org—Internet resources for Sjogren's syndrome]

www.dry.org

(Internet resources for dryness and other symptoms of Sjogren's syndrome.)

[eMedicine—Sjogren syndrome: Article by Darren Phelan, MD]

www.emedicine.com/emerg/topic537.htm

[Sjogren's Syndrome Support: Sjogren's World]

www.sjsworld.org

(Sjögren's syndrome support through live chat, message boards, forums, instant messaging, E-pals (internet pen pals), articles, and links.)

[Sjögren's syndrome]

www.clevelandclinic.org/health/health-info/docs/0200/0220.asp?index=4929

[Arthritis Research Campaign: Sjögren's syndrome]

www.arc.org.uk/about_arth/booklets/6041/6041.htm

[Sjogren syndrome: Guide to Sjogren's syndrome—Part 1 of 10

arthritis.about.com/od/sjogrens/ss/sjogrens.htm

[Sjögren, syndrome: sites et documents francophones]

www.chu-rouen.fr/ssf/pathol/sjogrensyndrome.html

[Sjogren syndrome—Swedish Medical Center, Seattle, Washington]

www.swedish.org/14541.cfm

[Spanish Association of Sjögren's syndrome: Information in Spanish]

www.aesjogren.org/publico/na_consejo.asp

Polymyositis & Dermatomyositis

Alan N. Baer, MD, & Robert L. Wortmann, MD

ESSENTIALS OF DIAGNOSIS

- *Proximal muscle weakness, elevated serum levels of enzymes derived from skeletal muscle, myopathic changes demonstrated by electromyography, and muscle biopsy evidence of inflammation are diagnostic criteria for polymyositis and other idiopathic inflammatory myopathies.*

- *Dermatomyositis is defined by the additional presence of a characteristic skin rash.*

- *These manifestations can occur in a variety of combinations or patterns, and no single feature is specific or diagnostic.*

- *The diagnosis is made by fulfilling these criteria in combination and excluding other potential causes for these abnormalities.*

- *Inclusion body myositis is an inflammatory myopathy that must be distinguished from polymyositis, especially in patients 50 years or older. Distinctive features of this disease include an asymmetric pattern of muscle weakness that includes distal muscle groups and characteristic histopathologic features.*

General Considerations

Inflammatory myopathies are rare diseases. Estimates of incidence range from 2.2–7.7 cases per million. The incidence appears to be increasing, although this may simply reflect increased awareness and more accurate diagnosis. Six types of myositis are currently classified as "idiopathic inflammatory myopathies" (Table 28–1).

These diseases are seen in all age groups, but overall the age at onset has a bimodal distribution with peaks observed between ages 10 and 15 years in children and between 45 and 60 years in adults. However, the mean ages for specific types of myositis differ. Both myositis associated with malignancy and inclusion body myositis are more common after age 50 years. The age at onset for myositis occurring with an established connective tissue disease is similar to that for the associated condition.

Women are affected twice as commonly as men, with the exception of inclusion body myositis, in which men are affected more often.

Clinical Features

A. SYMPTOMS AND SIGNS

Proximal and symmetric muscle weakness is the cardinal clinical feature of the inflammatory myopathies. Muscle pain and tenderness are infrequent. Weakness of the proximal muscles of the legs is usually noted first and results in difficulty arising from a chair or climbing stairs. Weakness of the proximal arm muscles may limit the ability to lift heavy items, to brush one's hair, or to reach up to shelves. Neck and axial muscles are also commonly involved. The detection of muscle weakness on physical examination typically relies on manual muscle strength testing and is usually rated on a scale of 0 to 5. However, this testing may miss subtle degrees of weakness and not be sufficiently sensitive or objective to detect changes in muscle strength with therapy. Accordingly, functional measurements of muscle strength are often helpful. These include determining how long it takes the patient to arise ten times from a chair without use of the arms or to walk 10 meters. The patient's ability to rise from a squat or stand on his or her toes and heels can also be assessed.

Polymyositis usually has an insidious onset over 3–6 months with no identifiable precipitating event. Pelvic and shoulder girdle musculature are affected most, but weakness of neck muscles, particularly the flexors, is also common. Ocular and facial muscles are virtually never involved. Dysphagia may develop secondary to esophageal dysfunction or cricopharyngeal obstruction. Pharyngeal muscle weakness may cause dysphonia and difficulty swallowing. Myalgias and arthralgias may occur, but severe muscle tenderness and frank synovitis are unusual. Raynaud phenomenon is sometimes present.

Pulmonary and cardiac manifestations may precede the onset of muscle weakness or develop at any time during the course of disease. Velcrolike crackles may be heard on chest auscultation of patients with interstitial fibrosis or interstitial pneumonitis. Cardiac involvement is usually limited to asymptomatic electrocardiographic abnormalities. However, supraventricular arrhythmia, cardiomyopathy, and congestive heart failure can occur.

Table 28–1. Clinical Classification of the Idiopathic Inflammatory Myopathies[a]

Polymyositis
Dermatomyositis
Juvenile dermatomyositis
Myositis associated with neoplasia
Myositis associated with connective tissue disease
Inclusion body myositis

[a]In the past, the terms "idiopathic inflammatory myopathy" and "polymyositis" have been used interchangeably. Today, idiopathic inflammatory myopathy is used to represent the spectrum of these conditions; polymyositis represents one of these diseases.

The clinical features of dermatomyositis include all those described for polymyositis plus a variety of cutaneous manifestations. The clinical onset of dermatomyositis is generally more rapid than that of polymyositis, developing over several weeks and occasionally over a matter of days. Skin involvement varies widely from patient to patient. The rash can antedate the onset of muscle weakness or follow its development by more than a year. Furthermore, the characteristics of the rash may change over time. Two cutaneous manifestations are considered pathognomonic. These include Gottron papules (symmetric lacy pink or violaceous raised lesions typically found on the dorsal and lateral aspects of the interphalangeal and metacarpophalangeal joints) and Gottron sign (symmetric macular violaceous erythema overlying the dorsal aspects of the interphalangeal and metacarpophalangeal joints, olecranon processes, patellae, and medial malleoli) (Figure 28–1). Other highly characteristic cutaneous findings include heliotrope (violaceous) discoloration of the eyelids, often with associated periorbital edema (Figure 28–2); macular erythema of the posterior shoulders and neck (shawl sign), anterior neck and upper chest (V sign), malar region, or forehead; dystrophic cuticles; and periungual telangiectases and nailfold capillary changes. The latter are similar to those observed in patients with scleroderma or systemic lupus erythematosus. "Mechanic's hands" refers to darkened or dirty-appearing horizontal lines and fissures that are seen across the lateral and palmar aspects of the fingers. This skin lesion can be seen in both dermatomyositis and the anti-synthetase syndrome subset of polymyositis (see below). In contrast to lupus erythematosus, the erythematous rash of dermatomyositis may be intensely pruritic.

The inflammatory myopathy that affects children tends to have a highly characteristic pattern, although a disease similar to adult polymyositis does occur. In juvenile dermatomyositis, the skin lesions and weakness are almost always coincidental, but the severity and progression of each varies greatly from patient to patient. In some patients, remission is complete with little or no therapy. The juvenile variant differs from the adult form because of the coexistence of vasculitis, ectopic calcification, and lipodystrophy. Unfortunately, the progression of dermatomyositis accompanied by vasculitis may be devastating despite therapy. Gastrointestinal ulcerations resulting from vasculitis can cause hemorrhage or perforation of a viscus. Ectopic calcification may occur in the subcutaneous tissues or in the muscles.

Some patients with biopsy-confirmed, classic cutaneous findings of dermatomyositis have normal muscle strength, muscle enzymes, electromyograms (EMGs), and muscle histology. The terms "amyopathic dermatomyositis" and "dermatomyositis sine myositis" have been

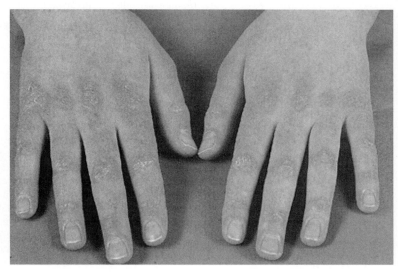

Figure 28–1. Dermatomyositis. Gottron papules on the dorsa of the hands and fingers, especially over the metacarpophalangeal and interphalangeal joints. (From Wolff K, Johnson RA, Suurmond D. *Fitzpatrick's Color Atlas and Synopsis of Clinical Dermatology.* 5th ed. McGraw-Hill, 2005:375. With permission.)

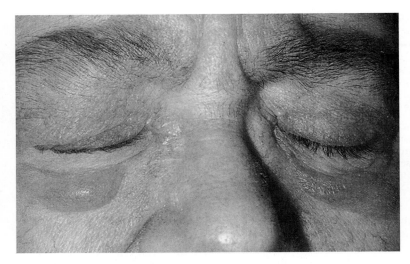

Figure 28–2. Dermatomyositis. Heliotrope erythema of upper eyelids and edema of the lower lids. (From Wolff K, Johnson RA, Suurmond D. *Fitzpatrick's Color Atlas and Synopsis of Clinical Dermatology.* 5th ed. McGraw-Hill, 2005:373. With permission.)

used to describe these patients. Although there is no evidence of myopathy, fatigue may be a dominant complaint. Some patients with this presentation continue to have skin disease only, whereas others progress over time, becoming weak and developing typical dermatomyositis. In some patients, magnetic resonance imaging (MRI) may show muscle abnormalities, suggesting the presence of clinically silent myositis. There may be an increased prevalence of neoplasia associated with this presentation.

Muscle weakness is a common finding in patients with connective tissue diseases. The features of inflammatory myopathy may dominate the clinical picture in some patients with scleroderma, systemic lupus erythematosus, mixed connective tissue disease, and Sjögren syndrome, but the classic picture of polymyositis is less common in rheumatoid arthritis, Wegener granulomatosis, polyarteritis nodosa, and adult Still disease. Weakness in these latter conditions is more commonly the result of vasculitis.

Muscle weakness associated with an underlying malignancy develops in a subset of patients with inflammatory myopathies. The true incidence of this relationship is not clear. Although malignancy may precede, or develop after, the onset of muscle weakness, usually the two are diagnosed within a 1-year period. The association occurs in patients of all ages but is rare in childhood. Although an associated malignancy is more common with dermatomyositis, cancer can be found in association with each type of myositis. The sites or types of malignancy that occur in association with myositis are those that are expected for the age and gender of the patient. A probable exception is ovarian cancer, which appears to be overrepresented in women with dermatomyositis.

Inclusion body myositis mainly affects persons over the age of 50 years and is the most common form of inflammatory myopathy in this age group. It affects men twice as often as women. The symptoms begin insidiously and progress slowly. Symptoms are often present for 5–8 years before the diagnosis is made. Predominant weakness of the quadriceps, long finger flexors, and anterior calf muscles is characteristic. Patients thus present with frequent falls due to buckling of the knees, a weak hand grip, and foot drop or tripping. The clinical picture in some patients is identical to that of typical polymyositis. Dysphagia is common in this disease. As the muscle weakness becomes severe, it can be accompanied by atrophy and diminished deep tendon reflexes. In some patients, inclusion body myositis follows a slow, steadily progressing course. In others the weakness seems to plateau, resulting in fixed weakness and atrophy of the involved musculature.

B. Laboratory Findings

An abnormal creatine kinase (CK) level is possibly the most sensitive indicator of skeletal muscle damage. The serum level of this enzyme is elevated at some time during the course of an inflammatory myopathy, and in most instances the serum CK level correlates with disease activity. Normal levels of CK may be found very early in the course of polymyositis or dermatomyositis, in advanced cases with significant muscle atrophy, or in myositis associated with a malignancy. CK levels are normal or only mildly elevated in inclusion body myositis. Other enzymes derived from diseased skeletal muscle include aldolase, aspartate aminotransferase, alanine aminotransferase, and lactate dehydrogenase. Accordingly, these enzymes may also be elevated in the course of the disease.

Tests of acute phase reactants, the erythrocyte sedimentation rate and C-reactive protein levels, are abnormal in only some patients with myositis. The erythrocyte sedimentation rate is normal in about half of patients with polymyositis and is elevated above 50 mm/h (Westergren method) in only 20%.

Antinuclear antibodies (ANAs) may be found in the serum of over 50% of patients with inflammatory muscle disease. The presence of a high-titer antinuclear antibody test may indicate the presence of an associated connective tissue disease (for example, anti-Sm or anti-dsDNA in systemic lupus erythematosus, anti-RNP in mixed connective tissue disease, or anti-Scl-70 antibodies in scleroderma). In the other forms of myositis, antinuclear antibodies tend to be present in low titer and are nonspecific in nature.

Certain autoantibodies are found almost exclusively in patients with idiopathic inflammatory myopathies, and therefore are termed myositis-specific autoantibodies (Table 28–2). With extremely rare exceptions, an individual patient will have only one myositis-specific autoantibody, and the particular autoantibody present appears to identify relatively homogeneous groups of patients with regard to clinical manifestations and prognosis.

Most myositis-specific autoantibodies are directed against amino acyl-tRNA synthetase activities. The most common of these is anti-histidyl-tRNA synthetase (Jo-1), present in approximately 20% of patients with polymyositis. Patients with these autoantibodies typically manifest myositis (polymyositis more commonly than dermatomyositis) plus several extramuscular features including interstitial lung disease, arthritis, mechanic's hands, and Raynaud phenomenon. The combination of these features and an inflammatory myopathy has been termed "antisynthetase syndrome." Patients with this syndrome have a variable response to therapy and often are difficult to treat because they tend not to sustain complete remission. Anti-Mi-2 antibodies are directed against helicase activities. These autoantibodies are found almost exclusively in patients with dermatomyositis who typically respond very well to treatment. In contrast, but with some exceptions, polymyositis of sudden onset develops in patients with antibodies to signal recognition particle; these patients are relatively resistant to treatment. Cardiomyopathy and distal muscle weak-

Table 28–2. Myositis-Specific Autoantibodies

Autoantibody	Clinical Features	Treatment Response
Antisynthetase[a]	Polymyositis or dermatomyositis with interstitial lung disease Fever Arthritis Raynaud phenomenon	Moderate with disease persistence
Anti-SRP	Polymyositis with very acute onset Onset often in fall Severe weakness Palpitations	Typically poor
Anti-Mi-2	Dermatomyositis with V and shawl signs Cuticular overgrowth	Good in most cases

[a] Anti-Jo-1 is the most common myositis-specific antibody. Other antisynthetase antibodies are anti-PL-7, anti-PL-12, anti-EJ, and anti-OJ.
SRP, signal recognition particle.

ness are also associated with the presence of anti–signal recognition particle antibodies.

C. IMAGING STUDIES

Although neither conventional radiography nor radionuclide imaging have proved particularly useful in patients with muscle diseases, computer-based image analysis using ultrasonography, computed tomography, and MRI can be helpful. Of these, MRI with T2-weighted images and fat suppression or short tau inversion recovery (STIR) technique offers the best imaging of soft tissue and muscle (Figure 28–3). MRI can detect early or subtle disease changes as well as patchy muscle involvement. Because of these capacities and the fact that it is noninvasive, MRI may prove superior to EMG in determining the

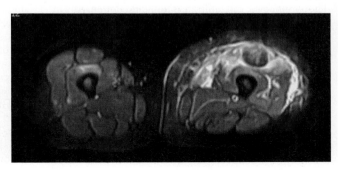

Figure 28–3. Axial STIR magnetic resonance image through the midsection of the thighs of a patient with dermatomyositis. There is marked enhancement of the fascia and the quadriceps muscles in the left thigh. Spotty enhancement of the quadriceps muscles is evident in the right thigh.

site for muscle biopsy. Furthermore, MRI can be used to semiquantitatively grade muscle involvement, and therefore can be used to monitor the response to therapy. This may be particularly useful when trying to differentiate between active myositis and glucocorticoid myopathy. In such situations the presence of edema in the muscle tissue, indicative of an inflammatory process, would be an argument for active myositis rather than for glucocorticoid myopathy.

D. SPECIAL TESTS

EMG is a valuable technique for determining the classification, distribution, and severity of diseases affecting skeletal muscle. Although the changes identified with this technique are not specific, EMG is quite effective for (1) differentiating between myopathic and neuropathic conditions, and (2) localizing a neurologic lesion to the central nervous system, spinal cord anterior horn cell, peripheral nerves, or neuromuscular junction. In addition, knowledge of the distribution and severity of abnormalities can guide selection of the most appropriate site to biopsy if MRI is not available.

In polymyositis and dermatomyositis, EMG classically reveals the following triad: (1) increased insertional activity, fibrillations, and positive sharp waves; (2) spontaneous, bizarre high-frequency discharges; and (3) polyphasic motor unit potentials of low amplitude and short duration. This triad is characteristic but not diagnostic. The complete triad is seen in approximately 40% of patients, whereas 10–15% of patients will have completely normal EMGs. In a small number of patients, abnormalities are limited to the paraspinal muscles. In patients with inclusion body myositis, EMG may also reveal neurogenic or mixed neurogenic and myopathic changes, especially in those with distal or asymmetric muscle weakness.

Muscle histology is useful for making the diagnosis of an inflammatory myopathy and for determining the specific type of disease, because there are characteristic changes seen in polymyositis, dermatomyositis, and inclusion body myositis. In classic polymyositis, muscle biopsies reflect a T-cell mediated autoimmune process. The lymphocytic cell infiltrate is found predominantly in endomysial locations. T lymphocytes, especially CD8+ cytotoxic T cells, can be seen surrounding and invading non-necrotic fibers expressing class I major histocompatibility antigen. Muscle fibers are in varying stages of necrosis and regeneration. In other cases, however, changes are minimal with fiber atrophy or degeneration observed in the absence of inflammatory cells. With disease progression, muscle fibers are replaced by fibrous connective tissue and fat. However, in some cases no fiber necrosis is observed, and the only recognized change is that of type 2 fiber atrophy.

The histopathology of muscle biopsies of classic adult or juvenile dermatomyositis reflects a humorally mediated autoimmune disorder characterized by a microangiopathy. Biopsies show a perivascular infiltration of inflammatory cells composed largely of B lymphocytes and CD4+ T-helper lymphocytes, with destruction of capillaries and perifascicular atrophy.

The muscle biopsy in inclusion body myositis closely resembles that of polymyositis, with endomysial inflammatory infiltrates and CD8+ T-cell invasion of non-necrotic muscle fibers. However, a characteristic feature of inclusion body myositis is the presence of intracellular vacuoles. The vacuoles contain basophilic (red on Gomori trichrome stain) granules in their center or along their walls, leading to their "red-rimmed" appearance. These vacuoles can be overlooked early in the disease but increase in number with disease progression. Amyloid proteins may be detected within vacuolated fibers with Congo red staining. The type of amyloid is identical to that present in the brains of patients with Alzheimer disease, suggesting that inclusion body myositis is a degenerative disease. Electron microscopy reveals either intracytoplasmic or intranuclear tubular or filamentous inclusions. These structures are straight and rigid-appearing with periodic transverse and longitudinal striations. Myelin figures (also called myeloid bodies) and membranous whorls are also common. Neither the red-rimmed vacuoles or changes seen with electron microscopy are specific for inclusion body myositis, but they may prove diagnostic in the appropriate clinical setting.

Differential Diagnosis

Polymyositis and dermatomyositis are relatively rare, and the list of diseases that can cause similar clinical manifestations is long (Table 28–3). When encountering a patient with proximal muscle weakness, a series of evaluations will help establish the correct diagnosis (Table 28–4). An initial step is to determine whether the process is myopathic or neuropathic in origin. Neurologic diseases can generally be identified by the additional presence of distal or asymmetric weakness or abnormalities on other components of the neurologic examination (eg, altered sensorium, cranial nerve deficits, and abnormal deep tendon reflexes). Typically, the weakness in myopathy is limited to proximal muscles, and the remainder of the physical examination of the nervous system is normal. Exceptions include inclusion body myositis, myositis with circulating anti–signal recognition particle antibodies, and myositis with neoplastic disease.

The two most common causes for an insidious onset of proximal muscle weakness in adult patients, apart from the idiopathic inflammatory myopathies, are thyroid disease and drug-induced myotoxicity. Both should be sought early in the evaluation, since they are readily

Table 28–3. Differential Diagnosis of Muscle Weakness[a]

Neuropathic diseases	Cytomegalovirus
Muscular dystrophies	Echovirus
Denervating conditions	Epstein-Barr virus
Neuromuscular junction disorders	Human immune deficiency virus
Proximal neuropathies	Influenza viruses
Myotonic disorders	Rubella virus
Neoplasm	Spirochetal
Paraneoplastic syndromes	*Borrelia burgdorferi* (Lyme disease)
Eaton-Lambert syndrome	Fungal
Drug-related conditions	*Cryptococcus*
Alcohol	Prasitic
Cocaine	*Toxoplasma gondii*
Colchicine	Helminthic
Cyclosporine	*Trichinella*
Fibrates	Inborn errors of metabolism
Gemfibrozil	Muscle glycogenoses
Glucocorticoids	Lipid storage disorders
Heroin	Mitochondrial myopathies
Hydroxychloroquine	Endocrine disorders
Ketoconazole	Acromegaly
Nicotinic acid	Cushing syndrome
D-penicillamine	Hypothyroidism
Phenytoin	Hyperthyroidism
Statins	Hyperparamyroidism
Valproic acid	Miscellaneous causes
Zidovndine	Sarcoidosis
Infections	Atherosclerotic emboli
Viral	Behçet disease
Adenovirus	Fibromyalgia
Coxsackievirus	Psychosomatic

[a]Does not include inflammatory diseases described in the text.

treatable. Hypothyroidism is commonly associated with proximal muscle weakness and elevation of the CK. Muscle weakness is also common in hyperthyroidism, but the CK level is usually normal. Numerous drugs can cause myopathic changes by a variety of mechanisms. Some, such as alcohol, may have direct toxic effects. Other drugs may cause metabolic or electrolyte abnormalities. For example, thiazide diuretics induce hypokalemia, which can cause weakness, myalgias, and cramps; clofibrate, lovastatin, gemfibrozil, and other lipid-lowering agents probably alter muscle fiber energetics; and zidovudine can induce a mitochondrial myopathy. D-Penicillamine can trigger polymyositis in addition to other autoimmune syndromes.

Neoplasia should also be considered in the evaluation of patients with myopathic symptoms. Although generalized weakness and fatigue can occur in these diseases from the systemic effects of cytokines released by tumor cells or as a result of immune response to the malignancy, prominent neuromuscular changes can also develop as features of paraneoplastic syndromes.

Numerous infections can cause a myopathy, with viruses being the most common. Children with influenza infections can experience severe myalgias associated with very high CK levels. Weakness is a common finding in patients suffering from AIDS and may be due to cachexia, central or peripheral nervous system diseases, polymyositis emerging as a consequence of altered immune function, zidovudine toxicity, or opportunistic infections (eg, cytomegalovirus, *Mycobacterium avium-intracellulare, Cryptococcus, Trichinella,* or *Toxoplasma*).

Metabolic myopathies are diseases caused by abnormalities in muscle energy metabolism that result in skeletal muscle dysfunction. These diseases, which can be inherited or acquired, are more prevalent than previously appreciated. Metabolic myopathies may also be a secondary manifestation of various endocrine disorders such as thyroid or adrenal diseases, electrolyte abnormalities, or drugs. Patients with a variety of these diseases can fulfill the criteria for the diagnosis of polymyositis.

The glycogen storage diseases, such as myophosphorylase deficiency (McArdle disease), share an underlying

Table 28–4. Initial Evaluation of Symmetrical, Proximal Muscle Weakness in Adults

Initial clinical evaluation
Exclude other neuromuscular cause for muscle weakness, although these rarely present with only symmetric, proximal muscle weakness
  Fatigability (myasthenia gravis, Eaton-Lambert syndrome, or mitochondrial myopathies)
  Marked muscle atrophy (anterior horn cell disorders, peripheral neuropathies, or some muscular dystrophies)
  Absent deep tendon reflexes (anterior horn cell disorder, peripheral neuropathy)
  Cranial nerve deficits
  Increased tone
  Abnormal sensation (peripheral neuropathy)
Determine age of onset of muscle weakness
  Teenage years: Becker muscular dystrophy, myophosphorylase deficiency (McArdle disease), or acid maltase deficiency (childhood form)
  Late teens: dysferlinopathy (limb girdle muscular dystrophy type 2B)
  Over age 18 but before the age of 50: polymyositis, dermatomyositis, or acid maltase deficiency (adult form)
  Over the age of 50: inclusion body myositis or myositis associated with malignancy
Determine temporal onset of muscle weakness
  Slow onset over months to years: inclusion body myositis or muscular dystrophy
  Subacute onset over weeks to months: polymyositis, dermatomyositis, or certain drug-induced myopathies
  Acute onset over days to weeks: infectious myositis, dermatomyositis (rarely), or drug-induced rhabdomyolysis
  Episodic: periodic paralyses
Determine range of muscle symptoms, in addition to weakness
  Muscle pain at rest (childhood dermatomyositis, myopathy associated with metabolic bone disease, infectious myopathies, or drug-induced myopathies)
  Exercise intolerance (metabolic myopathies)
  Myoglobinuria (metabolic myopathies or drug-induced necrotizing myopathies)
  Cramps (dystrophinopathies or metabolic myopathies)
Determine presence of extramuscular disease
  Cutaneous (rash of dermatomyositis, systemic lupus erythematosus, or scleroderma)
  Rheumatic disease (eg, polyarthritis, Raynaud phenomenon, sicca symptoms, or interstitial lung disease)
  Endocrine disorder (delayed tendon relaxation times or exophthalmos)
  Mitochondrial disorder (eg, external ophthalmoplegia, strokelike episodes, seizures, pigmentary retinopathy, sensorineural hearing loss, peripheral neuropathy, or cardiac conduction defect)
Determine family history of muscle disease
  Muscular dystrophies: X-linked, autosomal recessive or dominant
  Glycogenoses: most are autosomal recessive
  Mitochondrial disorders: maternal inheritance with threshold effect due to heteroplasmy
Determine medication use and toxin exposure
Evaluate for acute or chronic infection
Initial laboratory evaluation
  Serum electrolytes, calcium
  Thyroid function tests
  Creatine phosphokinase and other muscle enzymes (see Table 28–5)
Subsequent diagnostic testing
  Electromyography and nerve conduction testing
  Muscle biopsy
  Genetic testing where appropriate

defect that blocks the ability of tissues to use carbohydrate to produce energy. Abnormal accumulation of glycogen in skeletal muscle often results. The clinical manifestations of a glycogen storage disease include exercise intolerance that is attributed to pain, fatigue, stiffness, weakness, or intense cramping; severe rhabdomyolysis with myoglobinuria; or progressive proximal muscle weakness. In adults, the latter presentation can be difficult to distinguish from polymyositis because it is accompanied by an elevated CK level and myopathic changes on EMG. The diagnosis of glycogen storage diseases may be suggested by finding increased glycogen deposition on muscle histochemistry and is established by enzyme analyses in muscle tissue.

Table 28–5. Creatine Kinase Levels in Various Myopathies

	CK Level		
Disease	**Normal**	**Mildly Elevated (up to 10 × ULN)**	**Markedly Elevated (10 × ULN or Higher)**
Polymyositis		X	X
Dermatomyositis		X	X
Amyopathic dermatomyositis	X		
Inclusion body myositis	X	X	
Hypothyroidism		X	X (rare)
Hyperthyroidism	X		
Dystrophinopathy			X
Limb girdle muscular dystrophy	X	X	X
Facioscapulohumeral muscular dystrophy		X	
Acid maltase deficiency		X	
Myophosphorylase deficiency		X	X
Mitochondrial myopathy	X		
Carnitine palmitoyltransferase II deficiency	X (at rest)		X (following exercise)
Critical illness myopathy	X	X	
Drugs: chronic glucocorticoids, chloroquine	X		
Drugs: lipid-lowering agents, cocaine, colchicine, penicillamine		X	X
Zidovudine myopathy	X	X	
Toxins: snake venoms, alcohol	X (in some patients with chronic alcoholic myopathy)	X	X
Hypokalemic myopathy			X

The recognized disorders of lipid metabolism that cause myopathic problems are due to abnormalities in the transport and processing of fatty acids for energy in mitochondria. Patients with muscle carnitine deficiency present with chronic muscle weakness in late childhood, adolescence, or early adulthood. Muscle carnitine deficiency can also be confused with polymyositis because serum CK levels are elevated in more than half the patients, and EMG often reveals myopathic changes. Patients with other lipid storage disorders or mitochondrial defects also can have presentations that mimic inflammatory muscle disease.

Finally, the finding of an elevated CK level is not specific for an inflammatory myopathy (Table 28–5). Elevated CK levels can result from any disease or factor that causes muscle necrosis or membrane damage. Trauma is a well-recognized cause of high CK levels, as are unaccustomed exercise and activities that involve eccentric muscle contractions (such as downhill running or forearm curls) in which both muscle lengthening and contractile process shortening occur. Occasionally, elevated CK levels are observed in asymptomatic persons. Racial differences in normal CK levels must be considered in this context; healthy black men have higher CK levels than whites or Hispanics, with the majority of values appearing abnormal by usual laboratory values. Some asymptomatic persons with high CK levels are carriers for disease, such as one of the glycogen storage diseases, malignant hyperthermia, or muscular dystrophy. Over time, symptomatic myopathy may develop in some patients, but others remain asymptomatic for years. This latter condition has been termed "benign hyper-CK-emia."

Treatment

Before initiating medications, it is recommended that the patient's clinical status be evaluated as objectively as possible. Assessing the strength of individual muscle groups provides valuable information because these measures can be compared with those obtained after therapy is initiated. In addition to manual muscle testing, measurement of functional capacity by quantitative (eg, the time required to arise 10 times from a chair without use of the arms) and qualitative (responses to standardized questionnaires) is also helpful. Chest radiography, pulmonary function studies, and swallowing studies may be indicated. Muscle enzymes, including CK, aldolase, aspartate aminotransferase, alanine aminotransferase, and lactate dehydrogenase, should be measured in addition to other laboratory values that might be affected by therapy. The tests chosen to screen for cancer are those indicated by the patient's age and gender, as well as those that would address any areas of concern identified through the review of systems or physical examination. Women with dermatomyositis should have pelvic imaging to rule out ovarian cancer.

Physical therapy has an important role. Bed rest may be required during intervals of severe inflammation. Passive range-of-motion exercise is encouraged during these intervals to maintain movement and prevent contractures. With improvement, therapy should include active-assisted and then active exercises. The head of the bed should be elevated in patients with dysphagia or dysphonia in an attempt to reduce the risk of aspiration.

The choice of medications used to treat polymyositis and dermatomyositis is determined empirically because randomized trials are few and have evaluated only small numbers of patients. Glucocorticoids are the standard first-line medication for any idiopathic inflammatory myopathy. Initially, prednisone is usually given in a single dose of 1 mg/kg/d, but in severe cases, the daily dose can be divided or intravenous methylprednisolone can be used. Clinical improvement may be noted in the first weeks or gradually over 3–6 months. In general, the earlier in the course of disease that prednisone is started,

the faster and more effectively it works. As many as 90% of patients attain some response with glucocorticoid therapy and 50–75% of those achieve complete remission.

If a patient does not respond to glucocorticoid therapy, another agent is added, usually either azathioprine or methotrexate. Methotrexate is generally given on a weekly schedule at doses of 10–20 mg orally or 15–50 mg subcutaneously or intravenously. The typical dose of azathioprine is 2–3 mg/kg/d. Intravenous immune globulin is often beneficial in the treatment of dermatomyositis and polymyositis, but its effect is short-lived and repeat infusions are generally necessary every 6–8 weeks. Other immunosuppressive agents or therapeutic modalities have been used in treatment-resistant patients, including cyclophosphamide, cyclosporine, tacrolimus, rituximab, etanercept, infliximab, mycophenolate mofetil, plasmapheresis, and total-body (or total-nodal) irradiation. Oral hydroxychloroquine and topical glucocorticoids can be used to treat the cutaneous lesions of dermatomyositis, although they have no recognized effect on the myositis.

The pharmacologic treatment of inclusion body myositis is generally unsatisfactory. Nevertheless, occasional patients demonstrate a response to immunosuppressive therapy and a 6-month trial of such therapy is often recommended. Intravenous immune globulin has been shown to reduce the dysphagia associated with this form of myositis.

Complications

Progression of the underlying disease process produces the major complications that develop in patients with inflammatory muscle diseases. These are more likely to be seen in patients in whom the diagnosis was delayed or in patients with refractory disease. Persistent or progressive muscle weakness can result in the patient becoming wheelchair-dependent. Severe disease may be associated with loss of deep tendon reflexes, muscle atrophy, and especially in children, joint contractures. Patients with dysphagia or dysphonia are at great risk for aspiration pneumonia. Those with interstitial lung disease may progress to respiratory failure, and acute respiratory distress syndrome has been described. Cardiomyopathy with congestive heart failure can develop in the few patients with cardiac involvement.

Complications also result from therapy. Of major concern are the side effects and toxicities of glucocorticoid use. Although patients treated with these agents can manifest all of the features of iatrogenic Cushing syndrome, two of the more troubling complications are opportunistic infections and glucocorticoid-induced proximal muscle weakness. Opportunistic pulmonary infections such as *Pneumocystis carinii* pneumonia can be rapidly fatal. Glucocorticoid myopathy can be particularly frustrating because it can complicate the course of a patient who is getting stronger in response to therapy. Clinically, this is often observed in patients who show improvement with glucocorticoid therapy and then suddenly plateau or deteriorate. In this setting, it is difficult to determine whether the decrease in muscle strength is due to a disease flare or glucocorticoid toxicity. One method of distinguishing between these two possibilities is a provocative test of significantly increasing or decreasing the glucocorticoid dosage and assessing the response.

REFERENCES

Bohan A, Peter JB. Polymyositis and dermatomyositis: first of two parts. *N Engl J Med.* 1975;292:344. [PMID: 1090839] (This remains the classic description of diagnostic criteria used for the diagnosis and established the foundation for our current understanding of the idiopathic inflammatory myopathies.)

Buchbinder R, Hill CL. Malignancy in patients with inflammatory myopathy. *Curr Rheumatol Rep.* 2002;4:415. [PMID: 12217247] (Extensive review of the current information on the relation between these diseases with annotated bibliography.)

Callen JP. Dermatomyositis. *Lancet.* 2000;355:53. [PMID: 10615903] (Authoritative review of this disease from a dermatologist's perspective.)

Dalakas MC, Hohlfeld R. Polymyositis and dermatomyositis. *Lancet.* 2003;362:971. [PMID: 14511932] (A comprehensive review of the inflammatory myopathies which includes new diagnostic criteria based primarily on immunohistopathologic features.)

Dion E, Cherin P, Payan C, et al. Magnetic resonance imaging criteria for distinguishing between inclusion body myositis and polymyositis. *J Rheumatol.* 2002;29:1897. [PMID: 12233884] (Describes the findings in the various forms of myositis using the most recently developed evaluative tool, one that is becoming more and more important in the evaluation of patients with these diseases.)

Mastaglia FL, Garlepp MJ, Phillips BA, et al. Inflammatory myopathies: Clinical, diagnostic and therapeutic aspects. *Muscle Nerve.* 2003;27:407. [PMID: 12661042] (An authoritative review of the topic, with over 250 references.)

Mastaglia FL, Phillips BA. Idiopathic inflammatory myopathies: Epidemiology, classification, and diagnostic criteria. *Rheum Dis Clin North Am.* 2002;28:723. [PMID: 12510664] (An extensive analysis of the epidemiology and classification of the idiopathic inflammatory myopathies.)

Relevant World Wide Web Sites

[International Myositis Assessment and Clinical Studies Group]
https://dir-apps.niehs.nih.gov/imacs/index.cfm
[The Myositis Association]
http://www.myositis.org
[Washington University Neuromuscular Disease Center]
http://www.neuro.wustl.edu/neuromuscular/index.html

Relapsing Polychondritis

29

John H. Stone, MD, MPH

General Considerations

Relapsing polychondritis (RP) is an immune-mediated condition associated with inflammation in cartilaginous structures and other connective tissues throughout the body, including the ears, nose, joints, respiratory tract, and others. The incidence of RP is estimated to be approximately 3.5 cases per million people. Thirty percent of RP cases occur in association with another disease, usually some form of systemic vasculitis (particularly Wegener granulomatosis), connective tissue disorder (eg, rheumatoid arthritis or systemic lupus erythematosus), or a myelodysplastic syndrome. RP is often assumed to be "autoimmune" in nature, but the evidence for a true autoimmune pathogenesis is relatively weak. Some patients have been reported to have antibodies to type 2 collagen, but these assays are not widely available and their poor sensitivities and specificities make them inappropriate for general clinical use. In general, a cartilage biopsy is not required to make the diagnosis. Rather, the identification of cartilaginous inflammation in typical areas (auricular cartilage, nasal bridge, and costochondral joints) and the exclusion of other possible causes is usually sufficient.

Relapsing polychondritis is associated with a broad range of clinical courses. The spectrum extends from intermittent bouts of auricular cartilage inflammation (which respond quickly to treatment) at one end to widespread, aggressive lesions of cartilage that may have very serious complications at the other.

Clinical Findings

Table 29–1 lists the major clinical manifestations of RP.

A. SYMPTOMS AND SIGNS

1. Ears—Unilateral or bilateral auricular chondritis is often the first symptom of the disease. Onset of the inflammation is usually quite abrupt and not subtle. The inflammation may be confused with cellulitis of the ear, but a major clue to the diagnosis of RP is confinement of the inflammation to the auricular part of the ear, with sparing of the earlobe (Figure 29–1). The ears are erythematous and tender to touch. Swelling of the external ear canal may cause conductive hearing loss. RP may also be associated with sensorineural hearing loss, the mechanism of which remains obscure (vasculitis is often implicated, without proof).

2. Nose—Inflammation of the nasal cartilage leads to tenderness of the nasal bridge and often to epistaxis. In severe cases, saddle-nose deformities develop through collapse of the nasal bridge. This is usually preceded by the development of a nasal septal perforation.

3. Trachea—Subglottic stenosis results from tracheal inflammation and scarring inferior to the vocal cords. Early subglottic involvement often has minimal symptoms and may be manifest as only subtle changes in voice. With time, however, substantial airway scarring may occur, leading to potentially life-threatening tracheal narrowing. In addition to the subglottic region, other parts of the tracheal wall may be softened by cartilaginous inflammation, leading to a tendency of the airway to collapse. Tracheal inflammation may be associated with tenderness to palpation of the anterior cervical trachea, the thyroid cartilage, and larynx.

4. Bronchi and airways—Cartilaginous inflammation may extend to the lower respiratory tract, with bronchial involvement. This manifestation, unlike the tracheal disease, may have a lengthy subclinical period, but is usually detectable by investigations such as pulmonary function testing. RP may mimic bronchial asthma. Lower airway disease and its associated mucociliary dysfunction may heighten patients' susceptibility to infections.

5. Eyes—Nearly any part of the eye may be involved in RP. Scleritis causes photophobia and painful, often

Table 29–1. Major Clinical Manifestations of Relapsing Polychondritis

Feature	Data
Mean age at diagnosis	47 years
Auricular chondritis	90%
Reduced hearing	37%
Nasal chondritis	60%
Saddle-nose deformities	25%
Laryngotracheal involvement	52%
Ocular inflammation	54%
Arthritis	69%
Skin involvement	25%
Aortic or mitral regurgitation	8%
Vasculitis	12%

(Adapted from Molina JF, Espinoza LR. Relapsing polychondritis. *Baillieres Best Pract Res Clin Rheumatol.* 2000;14:97. With permission.)

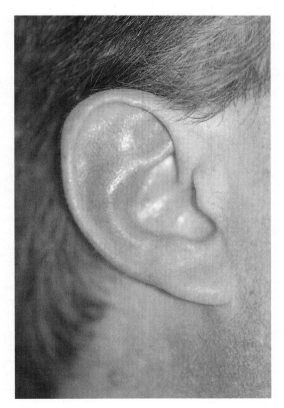

Figure 29–1. Auricular chondritis in a patient with relapsing polychondritis. Note the duskiness (erythema) of the skin overlying the cartilaginous part of the ear, and the relative sparing of the earlobe, which has no cartilage.

raised, scleral erythema. If unchecked, necrotizing scleritis may lead to scleral thinning, scleromalacia perforans, and visual loss. Peripheral keratitis may cause ulcerations on the margin of the cornea and lead to the syndrome of "corneal melt." Episcleritis and conjunctivitis are very common in RP. Extraocular involvement may include periorbital edema, chemosis, and proptosis.

6. Heart—Cartilaginous inflammation within the heart valve rings may lead to valvular dysfunction. The usual lesions are aortic and mitral regurgitation; aortic valve disease is more common. The proximity of the conduction system to some areas of valve ring inflammation may lead to cardiac conduction abnormalities. Pericarditis and rare cases of coronary arteritis have also been described in RP.

7. Joints—Articular lesions are often the first non-specific manifestation of RP. The pattern of joint involvement at presentation is typically an intermittent, migratory oligoarthritis, but symmetric polyarticular presentations are also seen. In general, the arthritis associated with RP is nondestructive, unless there is underlying rheumatoid arthritis. Joint symptoms tend to correlate very well with activity of disease at other sites.

8. Skin—Patients with RP may demonstrate a panoply of cutaneous lesions, none of which is specific for the disorder. Cutaneous findings are particularly common in cases of RP that are associated with myelodysplasia but occur frequently in other cases as well. Among patients with primary RP, the most common skin findings are aphthous ulcers, nodules (erythema nodosum–like lesions), purpura, papules, and sterile pustules. The cutaneous lesions of RP may resemble those of Behçet disease. An overlap condition of these two disorders—known as the MAGIC syndrome (*m*outh *a*nd *g*enital ulcers with *i*nflamed *c*artilage)—has been described.

9. Kidneys—Renal lesions in RP range from pauci-immune glomerulonephritis to mild mesangial expansion and cellular proliferation. Distinguishing RP from Wegener granulomatosis is difficult in the setting of pauci-immune glomerulonephritis.

B. LABORATORY FINDINGS

There are no specific laboratory findings in RP. Mild normochromic, normocytic anemias and mild degrees of thrombocytosis may be observed. Major cytopenias should trigger suspicion of myelodysplasia. Mild to moderate elevations of acute phase reactants are expected. Antinuclear antibodies and rheumatoid factor are usually negative, and complement levels are normal. In the setting of antineutrophil cytoplasmic antibody positivity, underlying Wegener granulomatosis should be suspected, particularly if the antibody specificity is to proteinase-3, or less commonly to myeloperoxidase.

C. IMAGING STUDIES

Advances in computed tomography make these studies increasingly useful in the evaluation of airway disease. Computed tomography findings include edema, wall thickening, granulation tissue, and fibrosis. Thin-cut computed tomography scans of the trachea are sensitive means of evaluating subglottic stenosis (in some cases of subglottic narrowing, however, direct visualization with fiberoptic laryngoscopy is required to make the diagnosis).

D. SPECIAL TESTS

1. Biopsy—Given the proper constellation of clinical symptoms and signs, tissue biopsy is rarely required to establish the diagnosis of RP. (Biopsy may be more important, however, in the exclusion of RP mimickers.) In contrast to Wegener granulomatosis, RP is not associated with granulomatous inflammation. Biopsy of the trachea or larynx should be performed only with great caution because acute airway narrowing may result from additional damage to already compromised tissues.

2. Pulmonary function tests—Full sets of pulmonary function tests, including inspiratory and expiratory flow-volume loops, are useful in RP. Patterns consistent with either extra- or intrathoracic obstruction (or both) may occur in RP. Pulmonary function tests (flow-volume loops) provide a useful noninvasive means of quantifying and following the degree of extrathoracic airway obstruction.

Differential Diagnosis

Aural chondritis is often confused initially with infectious processes, particularly cellulitis of the ear. Other infections in the differential diagnosis include tuberculous laryngitis, now rare in developed countries. The differential diagnosis of nasal inflammation (often accompanied by saddle-nose deformity) is quite short, including Wegener granulomatosis, Crohn disease, syphilis, leprosy, lymphoma, and leishmaniasis.

"Pure" RP must be distinguished from RP associated with an underlying condition because the complications of the underlying disorder may greatly affect the patient's prognosis. The major underlying disorders of concern are systemic vasculitides (particularly Wegener granulomatosis), connective tissue diseases (such as rheumatoid arthritis and systemic lupus erythematosus), and myelodysplastic syndromes.

Treatment

Glucocorticoids are the treatment of choice for reducing major inflammation in cartilaginous areas. In order to limit glucocorticoid exposure, dapsone, colchicine, and nonsteroidal anti-inflammatory drugs have all been used empirically. For patients with sustained disease, however, methotrexate is the most commonly used glucocorticoid-sparing agent. Cyclophosphamide is required for glomerulonephritis and other disease manifestations that are refractory to glucocorticoid alone. In the case of airway disease, it is essential to distinguish dysfunction secondary to active cartilaginous inflammation from that caused by damage from previously active disease.

The management of upper airway problems in RP requires collaboration with an experienced otolaryngologist or pulmonologist or both. Some upper airway disease manifestations (eg, subglottic stenosis) respond better to mechanical interventions and glucocorticoid injections than to systemic therapies. Stenting may also be required for cases in which the tracheal or bronchial walls have lost their integrity, provided that the regions of tracheomalacia or bronchomalacia are not too long. Continuous positive airway pressure may help some patients during sleep.

Complications

Prolonged or repeated bouts of aural chondritis may lead to deformation of the ear cartilage and "cauliflower ear." Similarly, nasal chondritis may cause nasal septal perforation and saddle-nose deformities.

Tracheomalacia may lead to extrathoracic airway obstruction and sometimes requires tracheostomy. Collapsible airways may be associated with postobstructive infections. Cardiac valvular regurgitation in RP may lead to valve replacement.

REFERENCES

Frances C, el Rassi R, Laporte JL, et al. Dermatologic manifestations of relapsing polychondritis. A study of 200 cases at a single center. *Medicine (Baltimore)*. 2001;80:173. [PMID: 11388093] (Examines both the skin lesions associated with primary RP and those potentially associated with underlying conditions. Aphthous ulcers, skin nodules, and purpura were the most common cutaneous lesions in primary RP.)

Tillie-Leblond I, Wallaert B, Leblond D, et al. Respiratory involvement in relapsing polychondritis. Clinical, functional, endoscopic, and radiographic evaluations. *Medicine (Baltimore)*. 1998;77:168. [PMID: 9653428]

SECTION IV

Vasculitis

Introduction to Vasculitis: Classification & Clinical Clues

30

David B. Hellmann, MD

General Considerations

Vasculitis refers to a heterogeneous group of disorders that is characterized by inflammatory destruction of blood vessels. Inflamed blood vessels are liable to occlude or rupture or develop a thrombus, and thereby lose the ability to deliver oxygen and other nutrients to tissues and organs. Depending on the size, distribution, and severity of the affected vessels, vasculitis can result in clinical syndromes that vary in severity from a minor self-limited rash to a life-threatening multisystem disorder.

Because it often begins with nonspecific symptoms and signs and unfolds slowly over weeks or months, vasculitis is one of the great diagnostic challenges in all of medicine. Yet, physicians who know the general and specific clinical clues for vasculitis can often learn to suspect when vasculitis is present at the bedside. Establishing the diagnosis of vasculitis requires confirmation by laboratory tests, usually a biopsy of an involved artery but sometimes an angiogram or a serologic test.

Treating vasculitis has become as rewarding as establishing the diagnosis. In the absence of treatment, most patients with systemic vasculitis will suffer and die. With treatment, the vast majority of patients will improve, many will achieve remission, and a few will be cured.

Classification

Because the causes of most forms of vasculitis are not known, the vasculitides are classified according to their clinicopathologic features. Although no schema has been accepted universally, one frequently used classification system separates the vasculitides based first on whether the process is primary (ie, of unknown cause) or secondary to some other condition (eg, a connective tissue disease or infection). The vasculitides can then be further separated by the size of vessels usually affected—large-sized, medium-sized, or small-sized arteries (Table 30–1). Finer distinctions among forms of vasculitis affecting the same size vessel can be made by other clinicopathologic characteristics. For example, Takayasu arteritis and giant cell arteritis are grouped together because they both can affect the aorta and other large arteries. However, they are distinguished from each other by their clinical differences, such as the age of onset. Takayasu arteritis is chiefly a disease of young women, while giant cell arteritis almost never occurs before age 50. To take another example, both Wegener granulomatosis and Churg-Strauss syndrome affect small-sized vessels and are associated with antineutrophil cytoplasmic antibodies. But only Churg-Strauss syndrome is associated with asthma and striking levels of eosinophilia.

Although classification systems are useful in highlighting differences among the vasculitides, the arbitrary categories suggest neater lines of demarcation than nature always recognizes. Despite being classified as a form of primary, medium-vessel vasculitis, polyarteritis nodosa results from chronic hepatitis B or C infection in about 20% of cases and can affect small vessels. Until the causes

Table 30–1. Classification of the Primary Vasculitides: Major Examples

Large-artery vasculitis
  Giant cell arteritis
  Takayasu arteritis
  Cogan syndrome
Medium-vessel vasculitis
  Polyarteritis nodosa
  Primary central nervous system disease
  Buerger disease
Small-vessel vasculitis
  ANCA-associated small-vessel vasculitis
  • Wegener granulomatosis
  • Microscopic polyangiitis
  • Churg-Strauss syndrome
  • Drug-induced ANCA-associated vasculitis
  Behçet disease
  Hypersensitivity vasculitis
  Urticarial vasculitis

ANCA, antineutrophil cytoplasmic antibody.

of all forms of vasculitis are known, exceptions in the classification schema will be common.

Epidemiology

The epidemiology of individual forms of vasculitis is covered in the relevant chapters. In general, the vasculitides are relatively uncommon but not rare in Western countries: about 1 out of 2000 adults has some form of vasculitis, and each year vasculitis develops in approximately 1 in 7000 adults. In the United States, the most common forms of primary systemic vasculitis are giant cell arteritis, Wegener granulomatosis, and microscopic polyangiitis (Table 30–2).

Clinical Findings

Although the presenting manifestations of vasculitis are protean, they can be grouped into five categories of clinical clues (Table 30–3). The first general clue is that

Table 30–2. Average Annual Incidence Rates of Different Forms of Vasculitis

Form of Vasculitis	Incidence Per Million
Giant cell arteritis	170[a]
Wegener granulomatosis	4–15
Polyarteritis nodosa	9
Microscopic polyangiitis	1–24
Takayasu arteritis	2

[a] Population 50 years of age or older.

Table 30–3. General Clinical Clues Suggesting the Presence of Systemic Vasculitis

1. Constitutional symptoms prominent
2. Subacute onset
3. Symptoms and signs of inflammation common
4. Pain common
5. Multisystem disease evident

most forms of systemic vasculitis begin with constitutional symptoms (such as malaise, fever, sweats, fatigue, decreased appetite, and weight loss). These nonspecific symptoms, in the absence of more specific signs, usually effectively camouflage the vasculitic nature of the patient's illness. A second clue is that most forms of vasculitis unfold subacutely over weeks or months. In contrast to many patients with acute infections, patients with vasculitis usually cannot pinpoint the hour or the day that their illness began. More typically, patients with vasculitis will struggle to define the month or the season in which their nonspecific symptoms accumulated sufficiently to become memorable. A corollary of the subacute course typical of vasculitis is that the initial diagnosis of vasculitis is rarely made (correctly) in the intensive care unit. Although pulmonary hemorrhage, bowel infarction, or other devastating complications of vasculitis frequently result in a patient being admitted to the intensive care unit, these catastrophic events usually develop late, weeks or months after other clinical clues have suggested or established the patient's diagnosis.

The tendency of most forms of vasculitis to produce striking signs of inflammation constitutes a third general clue. Manifestations of inflammation can include fever, arthritis, rash, pericarditis, anemia of chronic disease, or a markedly elevated erythrocyte sedimentation rate. Pain is a fourth common feature of the vasculitides and can originate from many different sources, such as arthritis; myalgia; or infarction of a digit, nerve, bowel, or testicle. The fifth general clinical clue is that vasculitis tends to cause multisystem disease. The skin, joints, nervous system, kidneys, lung, and gastrointestinal tract are especially favorite targets of many different forms of vasculitis. Although specific forms of vasculitis can defy generalization, most vasculitides start with constitutional symptoms that evolve over weeks and months to a painful disorder marked by signs of inflammation and multiorgan injury.

A. SYMPTOMS AND SIGNS

The signs and symptoms of specific forms of vasculitis are detailed in the individual chapters. The signs and symptoms common to many forms of systemic vasculitis are found in Table 30–4.

Table 30–4. Organ- or Tissue-Specific Manifestations of Vasculitis

Organ or Tissue	Manifestation
Skin	Livedo reticularis, palpable purpura, nodules, ulcers, gangrene
Peripheral nervous system	Mononeuritis multiplex, polyneuropathy
Central nervous system	Stroke, seizure, encephalopathy
Kidney	Hypertension, proteinuria, hematuria, renal failure
Heart	Myocardial infarction, cardiomyopathy, pericarditis, arrhythmia
Lung	Cough, chest pain, hemoptysis, breathlessness
Eyes	Blindness, scleritis
Gastrointestinal tract	Pain, bleeding, perforation
Genitals	Testicular infarction, ovarian mass

In general, the skin and the peripheral nervous system signs are especially useful because they often develop early in the course of the disease and because they can be detected at the bedside. The onset of small-vessel vasculitis (eg, hepatitis C–associated vasculitis) is often heralded by palpable purpura, usually on the lower extremities, whereas medium-vessel diseases (eg, polyarteritis nodosa) more commonly produce nodules, ulcers, or digital gangrene.

The most characteristic nervous system manifestation of vasculitis is mononeuritis multiplex, which is defined as a distinctive peripheral neuropathy in which named peripheral nerves are infarcted one at a time. The nerve infarctions result from vasculitis of the vessels of the vasa nervorum, causing ischemia of a nerve. Clinically, the two features that characterize this neuropathy are the **asynchrony** and **asymmetry** of the symptoms and findings. These features are best illustrated by comparing mononeuritis multiplex with other peripheral neuropathies. With most forms of nonspecific neuropathy the patient experiences numbness and tingling in a symmetric, stocking or glove distribution, which develop so slowly that the patient cannot accurately date the onset of the neuropathy. Examination of these patients usually fails to identify the involvement of large, named nerves. In sharp contrast, the onset of mononeuritis multiplex is strikingly memorable: The patient will often recall the day that his foot drop or wrist drop began. The patient

will also often vividly recall how the neuropathy progressed asynchronously so that each month or so a new area of the body (usually an extremity) became involved. On examination, the damage from mononeuritis multiplex can be mapped to individual, named nerves (eg, the peroneal, tibial, ulnar, radial, or median nerves). Almost all will have sensory abnormalities and about half will have weakness as well. Although mononeuritis multiplex is often bilateral, the lesions are usually asymmetric: The right hand may demonstrate a median nerve infarct while the left hand has an ulnar nerve lesion.

Mononeuritis multiplex produces such a characteristic clinical picture that usually it can be diagnosed at the bedside. Occasionally, identifying mononeuritis multiplex becomes difficult late in the course when the infarctions of so many nerves can coalesce to produce an unusually symmetric pattern of deficits. In most cases, the early history of sequential peripheral nerve lesions supports the diagnosis of vasculitic neuropathy. In some cases, proof of mononeuritis multiplex will require electrodiagnostic studies.

Mononeuritis multiplex is one of the physical findings in medicine of great differential diagnostic value. In the absence of diabetes or multiple compression injuries, mononeuritis multiplex usually means the patient has some form of vasculitis. Polyarteritis nodosa, microscopic polyangiitis, Churg-Strauss syndrome, and Wegener granulomatosis are the forms of vasculitis most likely to cause mononeuritis multiplex.

B. LABORATORY FINDINGS

Laboratory abnormalities accompany virtually every form of vasculitis (Table 30–5). Some abnormalities, such as anemia and an elevated erythrocyte sedimentation rate, are very nonspecific and can be seen with many other diseases. Other findings, such as red blood cell casts in the urine (indicating vasculitis of the glomeruli) or antineutrophil cytoplasmic antibodies (associated with Wegener granulomatosis), have much greater specificity.

C. IMAGING TESTS

The role of imaging tests depends greatly on the form of vasculitis suspected. Plain radiographs rarely provide important clues except in Wegener granulomatosis, where views of the sinuses and chest may yield findings (albeit usually not specific ones). Computed tomography scans of the chest are more sensitive in Wegener granulomatosis. Angiograms are especially helpful in supporting or establishing the diagnosis of Takayasu arteritis, polyarteritis nodosa, and primary central nervous system vasculitis.

D. SPECIAL TESTS

Biopsy of involved tissues is the most common method for establishing definitively the diagnosis of vasculitis.

Table 30–5. Common Laboratory Tests in Vasculitis

Test Result	Disease Association
Hematocrit	Low in many forms
Erythrocyte sedimentation rate	Usually high, especially in giant cell arteritis
Creatinine	Elevated by renal forms of vasculitis
Urinalysis	Often abnormal, red blood cell casts caused by vasculitis of the glomeruli
Liver function tests	Abnormal in hepatitis B- or C-associated polyarteritis
Serum cryoglobulins	Present in cryoglobulinemia
Complement levels	Low in SLE, cryoglobulinemia
Immunoelectrophoresis	Monoclonal gammopathies common in hepatitis C-related vasculitis
Antineutrophil cytoplasmic antibodies	Positive in WG, MPA, Churg-Strauss syndrome

SLE, systemic lupus erythematosus; WG, Wegener granulomatosis; MPA, microscopic polyangiitis.

Skin, peripheral nerves, airways, arteries, kidney, and gut are the most commonly sampled tissues. In general, biopsies of symptomatic areas have a yield of about 66%, whereas biopsy of sites with no symptoms or findings have low yield. Special stains are sometimes required to reveal the degree of damage to particular arterial layers (such as the internal elastic lamina) or the extent of immune complex deposition.

Differential Diagnosis

Specific diagnostic criteria have been established for most forms of vasculitis and are detailed in subsequent chapters. In general, the diagnosis of vasculitis requires a compatible clinical picture and a laboratory test—usually a biopsy but sometimes an angiogram or a specific sero-logic test (such as antineutrophil cytoplasmic antibodies for Wegener granulomatosis). It is also important to consider, and to exclude where appropriate, other diseases that can mimic primary systemic vasculitis. Cholesterol emboli, drug reactions, Whipple disease, syphilis, HIV, endocarditis, antiphospholipid antibody syndrome, and atrial myxoma are particularly common mimickers of primary vasculitis. Indeed, endocarditis and syphilis can cause vasculitis. In the appropriate setting, these conditions may need to be considered.

Treatment

An important general principle in the treatment of vasculitis is to make sure that the intensity of treatment fits the severity of vasculitis. Although most forms of vasculitis require aggressive treatment to prevent morbidity and mortality, some do not. Minor vasculitis limited to the skin and caused by drug reactions requires no therapy other than stopping the offending drug. In contrast, rapid and intensive therapy is required to prevent blindness from developing in giant cell arteritis or renal failure from complicating Wegener granulomatosis.

Another important principle of treatment is to limit the toxicity of therapy. When long-term prednisone is required, for example, appropriate measures to prevent osteoporosis should be initiated. If immunosuppression will result (as occurs with high-dose prednisone or immunosuppressive drugs), then prophylaxis against *Pneumocystis carinii* pneumonia should be started. Other potential toxicities of therapies must be monitored closely.

REFERENCES

González-Gay MA, García-Porrúa C. Epidemiology of the vasculitides. In: Stone JH, Hellmann DB, eds. *Rheumatic Disease Clinics of North America.* WB Saunders, 2001:729–749.

Hellmann DB, Stone J. Small and medium vessel primary vasculitis. In: Rich RR, et al, eds. *Clinical Immunology.* 2nd ed. Mosby, 2001:67.1–67.24.

Seo P, Stone JH. Large-vessel vasculitis. *Arthritis Rheum.* 2004;51:128. [PMID: 14872466]

Relevant World Wide Web Sites

[Johns Hopkins Vasculitis Center]
http://vasculitis.med.jhu.edu

Giant Cell Arteritis & Polymyalgia Rheumatica

31

David B. Hellmann, MD

Giant cell arteritis (GCA)—also known as temporal arteritis—is the most common form of systemic vasculitis in adults. GCA is a panarteritis that occurs almost exclusively in older people and preferentially affects the extracranial branches of the carotid artery. The most feared complication of GCA is blindness, which usually can be prevented by early diagnosis and treatment with glucocorticoids. Polymyalgia rheumatica (PMR) is an aching and stiffness of the shoulders, neck, and hip-girdle area that can occur with GCA, or more commonly, by itself.

ESSENTIALS OF DIAGNOSIS

- *For GCA, headache; for PMR, jaw claudication, and visual symptoms.*
- *The gold standard for diagnosing GCA is temporal artery biopsy.*
- *For PMR, stiffness and aching of the shoulders, neck, and hip region.*
- *PMR is a clinical diagnosis. The only common laboratory abnormality is an elevated erythrocyte sedimentation rate (ESR).*

General Considerations

Although the causes of PMR and GCA are unknown, the disorders share many risk factors and probably mechanisms of pathogenesis. Age is the greatest risk factor for developing either condition. Almost all patients who have GCA are older than 50 years (the average age of onset is 72). The incidence of GCA rises from 1.54 cases per 100,000 people in the sixth decade to 20.7 per 100,000 in the eighth decade.

PMR is 2–4 times more common than GCA, and its incidence also rises with age. Women are twice as likely as men to have GCA or PMR. Both conditions develop most often in Scandinavians and in Americans of Scandinavian origin. GCA rarely develops in black men.

GCA and PMR are associated with the same human leukocyte antigen genes as those seen in patients with rheumatoid arthritis (ie, human leukocyte antigen-DR4 variants *0401 and *0404). The pathogenesis of GCA appears to be initiated by T cells in the adventitia responding to an unknown antigen, which prompts other T cells and macrophages to infiltrate all layers of the affected artery and to elaborate cytokines that mediate both local damage to the vessel and systemic effects. The differential expression of inflammatory cytokines may explain the clinical subsets seen in GCA. Patients with the highest levels of interlukin-6, for example, are more likely to have fever and less likely to experience blindness. Magnetic resonance imaging and ultrasonography show that PMR is caused by inflammation of the synovial lining of the bursa and joints around the neck, shoulders, and hips.

Although GCA may develop later in some patients with PMR, patients who have only PMR are not at risk of losing their vision and usually require small doses of prednisone (ie, <20 mg/d). In contrast, patients with GCA are at risk for losing their vision and require higher doses of prednisone ($\geq$40 mg/d) to prevent blindness. Because patients who have GCA and PMR require treatment with glucocorticoids for months or years, it is important to minimize the likelihood of adverse effects from therapy (eg, osteoporosis, hypertension, and cataracts).

Clinical Findings

A. SYMPTOMS AND SIGNS

The classic symptoms of GCA include headache, jaw claudication, PMR, visual symptoms, and malaise (Table 31–1). The onset may be gradual or sudden. Three of the following five criteria must be met to diagnose GCA: (1) age >50 years, (2) new headaches, (3) abnormal temporal artery, (4) ESR $\geq$50 mm/h, and (5) positive temporal artery biopsy results for vasculitis (Figure 31–1).

Table 31–1. Classic Presenting Manifestations of Giant Cell Arteritis

Symptoms	Percentage of Cases
Headache	70
Jaw claudication	50
Constitutional symptoms	50
Polymyalgia rheumatica	40
Visual loss	20
Abnormal temporal artery	50
Anemia	80
Erythrocyte sedimentation rate >50 mm/h	90
Arthritis	15

The most frequent finding during a physical examination is an abnormal temporal artery, which develops in only 50% of patients; thus a normal temporal artery does not exclude the diagnosis of GCA. The temporal artery may be enlarged, difficult to compress, nodular, or pulseless. About 15–20% of patients will have axillary or subclavian disease, which manifests as diminished pulses, unequal arm blood pressures, or bruits heard above or be-low the clavicle or along the upper arm. Tongue ulcers, mass lesions of the breast and ovaries, and aortic regurgitation are other signs of GCA.

1. Headache—The intensity and location of the headache, the most common symptom, varies greatly from patient to patient. The headache is typically described as a dull, aching pain of moderate severity, localized over the temporal area, but variations in location, quality, and severity occur often. The most striking feature of the headache is that the patient notices that it is new or different. Even if the patient has had migraine or other headache problems in the past, features of the new headache are different. Patients frequently describe tenderness of the scalp, especially when they comb or brush their hair. Some patients will localize the tenderness to the temporal arteries, which may be enlarged or nodular in only a minority of cases.

2. Jaw claudication—Jaw claudication, defined as pain in the masseter muscles associated with protracted chewing, develops when the oxygen demand of the masseter muscles exceeds the supply provided by narrowed and inflamed arteries. Typically, patients with jaw claudication notice pain when eating foods that require vigorous chewing, such as meats, and little or no pain when chewing soft foods. Of all the possible symptoms of GCA, jaw claudication is the most specific for this disease. Many patients do not provide such a classic description of jaw claudication, and instead report a vague sense of discomfort along the jaw or face, with or without protracted chewing. Atypical manifestations of jaw claudication include discomfort over the ear or around the nose.

3. PMR and joints—PMR is defined as pain and stiffness in the neck, shoulders, and hip-girdle area that are usually much worse in the morning. All of the following criteria must be met to diagnose PMR: (1) age >50 years; (2) aching and stiffness for at least 1 month, affecting at least two of the three above-mentioned areas (ie, shoulders, neck, and pelvic girdle); (3) morning stiffness lasting at least 1 hour; (4) ESR >40 mm/h; (5) exclusion of other diseases except GCA; and (6) rapid response to prednisone (≤20 mg/d).

The shoulders are more commonly involved (70–95%) than the hips (50–70%). Shoulder pain in PMR may begin unilaterally but quickly becomes bilateral. Patients with PMR may report great difficulty getting out of bed, arising from the toilet, or brushing their teeth. People in whom GCA develops frequently describe feeling "old" for the first time at the onset of the disease. The stiffness is especially severe in the morning but may improve, usually a little but sometimes markedly, during the day. When asked to localize the pain, patients often say the pain is "in the flesh" rather than in the joints. Examination of the shoulders and hips is usually unremarkable except for decreased active and passive range of

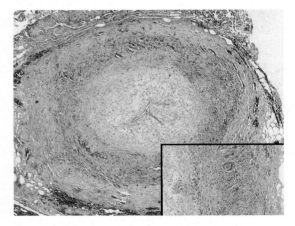

Figure 31–1. Giant cell arteritis. Temporal artery biopsy showing endothelial proliferation, fragmentation of internal elastic lamina, and infiltration of the adventitia and media by inflammatory cells. Giant cells are especially well seen in the inset. (From Hellmann DB. Vasculitis. In: Stobo J, et al, eds. *Principles and Practice of Medicine.* Appleton & Lange, 1996. With permission.)

motion. Swelling, erythema, and heat are usually absent. However, some patients with PMR or GCA experience arthralgia or arthritis of the sternoclavicular joint, wrists, fingers, knees, or ankles. Rarely, pitting edema develops in the patient's hands or feet.

4. Visual symptoms—About one-third of patients present with visual symptoms, chiefly diplopia or visual loss. Visual hallucinations occur rarely. The visual loss may be transient or permanent or monocular or binocular. Visual loss is the most feared complication of GCA because it is usually irreversible. Blindness can develop abruptly but more often is preceded by episodes of blurred vision or amaurosis fugax. Rarely is visual loss the first manifestation of GCA; on average, visual loss develops 5 months after the onset of other GCA symptoms. The direct cause of visual loss in GCA is usually occlusion of the posterior ciliary artery, a branch of the ophthalmic artery, which is a branch of the carotid artery. The posterior ciliary artery supplies blood to the optic nerve head. Interruption of that flow leads to anterior ischemic optic neuropathy.

When visual loss occurs, it usually is profound. Patients often cannot detect a hand waving directly in front of the affected eye. In the first few hours after infarction, the disc generally appears normal on funduscopic examination, even in the presence of profound visual loss. Later, disc pallor (Figure 31–2) and swelling, cotton-wool spots, and flame-shaped intraretinal hemorrhages may develop. Over weeks or months, the disc becomes atrophic. Most patients with visual loss also demonstrate a relative afferent pupillary defect, demonstrated by moving a shining light from the normal eye to the blind eye and noting that both pupils dilate. Not all patients with GCA have the same risk of developing blindness. Multiple studies reveal that those who experience fever or other manifestations

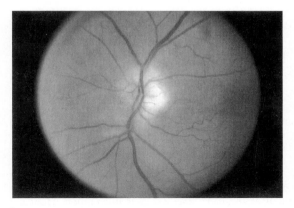

Figure 31–2. Early funduscopic appearance in a patient with giant cell arteritis in whom blindness has developed.

Table 31–2. Atypical Manifestations of Giant Cell Arteritis

Fever of unknown origin
Respiratory tract symptoms
  Dry cough
  Throat pain
  Tongue pain
Neurologic symptoms
  Mononeuritis multiplex
  Stroke
  Transient ischemic attack
  Dementia
  Hallucinations
Large artery involvement
  Claudication in arms or legs
  Unequal arm blood pressures
  Thoracic aortic aneurysm
Tumorlike lesions
  Especially of the breasts and ovaries
Syndrome of inappropriate antidiuretic hormone secretion

of a strong inflammatory response are less likely to experience visual loss. Fever and other inflammatory features correlate with high serum levels of interleukin-6. About three-quarters of all blindness occurs before treatment is begun, and another quarter develops during treatment, usually within the first month. Blindness rarely develops thereafter.

5. Other features—Almost all patients with the classic features of GCA also have nonspecific manifestations such as malaise, fatigue, and loss of appetite. Weight loss of 2–10 kg is common. Some patients also experience depression.

B. ATYPICAL MANIFESTATIONS

GCA presents with atypical features in 40% of cases. Awareness of these atypical presentations (Table 31–2) maximizes the physician's chance of diagnosing GCA before blindness develops.

1. Fever of unknown origin—Fever develops in about 40% of patients with GCA; of those, 10–15% are fevers of unknown origin. Although GCA causes only 2% of all cases of fever of unknown origin, it accounts for 16% of all cases of fever of unknown origin in patients over the age of 65. Fevers in GCA may reach nearly 40°C, and average about 39°C. About two-thirds of patients with fevers also have rigors and drenching sweats. Despite these manifestations of a robust inflammatory response, the white blood cell count is almost always normal (at least before prednisone is started).

2. Respiratory—Respiratory symptoms develop in 1 of 10 patients and constitute the presenting complaint in 1 of 25. The most common symptom is a dry cough, resembling that seen in some patients taking angiotensin-converting enzyme inhibitors. The cause of the cough is obscure because chest imaging studies are normal. The cough may reflect inflammation within the arteries adjacent to cough centers, which are distributed throughout various sites in the respiratory apparatus, including the diaphragm, the bronchi, and the mid-brain. Other respiratory or otolaryngeal manifestations include tongue pain, glossitis, dental pain, and posterior or anterior pharyngeal pain. These symptoms reflect ischemia caused by arteritis of nearby vessels; tongue ulceration and gangrene may also occur.

3. Neurologic—The most common neurologic manifestation of GCA is mononeuritis multiplex. Unlike mononeuritis multiplex in other forms of vasculitis, which most commonly affects the foot or the hand, mononeuritis multiplex in GCA most commonly affects the shoulder, producing sudden weakness and pain that mimics a C5 radiculopathy. Central nervous system disease, outside of the eye, also occurs. Delirium, dementia, transient ischemic attacks, and cerebrovascular accidents have been reported. GCA preferentially affects the posterior circulation of the brain; whereas the ratio of anterior to posterior circulation cerebrovascular accidents is about 3:2 in the general population, the ratio is reversed in GCA. Intracranial disease does not occur in GCA, perhaps because arteries lose their elastic lamina almost as soon as they penetrate the dura. Therefore, transient ischemic attacks and cerebrovascular accidents complicating GCA are attributed to occlusion of extracranial vessels or to thromboemboli.

4. Large-artery disease—Clinically evident involvement of large arteries—the aorta and its major branches—develops in at least 25% of patients. Positron emission tomography scans reveal subclinical inflammation of large arteries in over 80% of patients. The most commonly affected vessels include the vertebral, carotid, subclavian, and axillary arteries, and the aorta. Involvement of large arteries in the lower extremities has also been described. Presenting symptoms may include transient ischemic attack, cerebrovascular accident, hand ischemia, and arm or leg claudication. Aortic involvement may lead to thoracic aortic aneurysm, which is increased 17-fold in patients with GCA. Thoracic aortic aneurysm develops an average of 7 years after the diagnosis of GCA. Thoracic aortic aneurysm may be asymptomatic or cause aortic regurgitation, myocardial infarction, or dissection. Abdominal aortic aneurysms, although less common than thoracic lesions, also occur. Involvement of the pulmonary or mesenteric arteries virtually never occurs.

5. Other atypical manifestations—The protean manifestations of GCA include tumorlike lesions localized to the breast or ovaries, mimicking cancer at those sites. Other manifestations include the syndrome of inappropriate antidiuretic hormone secretion and hemolytic anemia (see Table 31–2).

C. LABORATORY FINDINGS

The laboratory hallmarks of GCA and PMR are a markedly elevated ESR and anemia (see Table 31–1). An ESR >30 mm/h is present in 96% of patients with GCA, and an ESR of >50 mm/h is seen in 87% of patients with GCA. A normal ESR may be seen in a slightly higher percentage of patients with PMR. The ESR averages about 100 mm/h in GCA and slightly lower in isolated PMR. The C-reactive protein is also usually elevated and may be more sensitive than the ESR in detecting flares. The anemia, typically normochromic and normocytic, is usually mild with a hematocrit often in the 32–35 range. Occasionally, the anemia may be profound with hematocrits in the 20s. Approximately 20% of patients with GCA demonstrate a mildly elevated alkaline phosphatase (of liver origin). The platelet count, often elevated nonspecifically by inflammatory disorders, is frequently increased in GCA and PMR.

D. IMAGING STUDIES

Radiographs of shoulders and hips are invariably unhelpful. However, magnetic resonance imaging and ultrasonography of shoulders and hips in patients with PMR show inflammation of the bursa and the synovium of nearby joints. Color duplex ultrasonography of affected temporal arteries can show a characteristic "halo" of edema or stenosis, but this technology is no more sensitive for the diagnosis of GCA than a careful physical examination of the temporal artery. Magnetic resonance angiography or computed tomography angiography can provide noninvasive assessment of larger-artery disease. Positron emission tomography scanning can demonstrate occult large-vessel inflammation, but the practical value of this technique is not established.

Making the Diagnosis

The diagnosis of PMR rests almost entirely on clinical grounds, namely symptoms of proximal limb stiffness associated with an elevated ESR and a dramatic response to prednisone. While magnetic resonance imaging and ultrasonographic images are abnormal in PMR, their sensitivity and specificity have not been established, and usually these studies are not obtained.

Classification criteria have also been proposed for GCA, but their predictive value in clinical settings is not well established. Since GCA is uncommon, clinicians have to maintain a high index of suspicion for the diagnosis. Among its classic symptoms, only jaw claudication

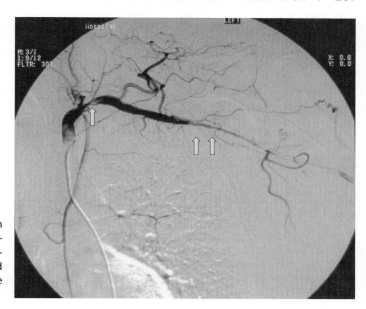

Figure 31–3. Large-artery involvement in GCA. Angiogram in a patient with GCA showing tight stenosis of the proximal left subclavian artery (single arrow) with diffuse, marked narrowing of the axillary artery (double arrows). (Courtesy of Dr. Elliott Levy.)

has been shown to increase the odds (by about threefold) that a patient in whom GCA is suspected actually has the disease. The only physical finding with a high positive predictive value for diagnosing GCA is an abnormal temporal artery. Although a strikingly elevated ESR (eg, >100 mm/h) strongly suggests the diagnosis in the proper setting, moderate elevations of the ESR are quite nonspecific. A normal ESR substantially reduces the likelihood of GCA, but does not eliminate it altogether.

Two guidelines may help determine when to suspect GCA. First, one should consider the composite clinical picture when trying to decide whether a patient could have GCA. A comprehensive review of systems may be especially helpful since most patients with GCA have multiple symptoms. For example, vasculitis should not be suspected in most patients with a dry cough, one of the atypical symptoms of GCA. However, GCA should be considered in a 72-year-old patient with a dry cough, PMR, headache, weight loss, fever, anemia, and an ESR of 105 mm/h. Second, because many of the atypical symptoms involve some type of pain above the neck—headache, or vague discomfort around the jaw, throat, ear, tongue, or teeth—it may be prudent to consider the diagnosis of GCA in any patient over the age of 50 who has pain in any of these areas without another explanation. Thus, the elderly patient with ear pain and a normal ear examination does not benefit from a diagnosis of otitis media and antibiotics, but may benefit from a comprehensive review of systems and an ESR.

In practice, then, the diagnosis of GCA is suggested by the clinical picture combined with an elevated ESR, and proven by a positive temporal artery biopsy. Infrequently, patients with large-artery involvement, such as subclavian disease, are diagnosed by magnetic resonance imaging, computed tomography angiography, or conventional angiography showing long, smooth arterial taperings uncharacteristic of atherosclerosis (Figure 31–3). Although some have proposed using color duplex ultrasonography of the temporal artery, experience with that technique is not sufficient for it to replace temporal artery biopsy as the gold standard for diagnosing GCA.

Differential Diagnosis

It is important to distinguish patients who have PMR alone from those who have PMR plus GCA. Patients are classified as having PMR alone if they have no "above-the-neck" symptoms, namely headache, jaw claudication, scalp tenderness, or visual symptoms. Although about 20% of patients with symptoms of PMR have positive temporal artery biopsy results, practice has shown that patients who have symptoms of PMR alone respond well to low-dose prednisone (see the following section on treatment).

Distinguishing PMR from rheumatoid arthritis in an older person can be difficult, especially in those patients with PMR who have distal polyarthritis. Severe erosive arthritis, rheumatoid nodules, and a positive rheumatoid factor make rheumatoid arthritis the more likely diagnosis. Because both conditions can respond well to low-dose prednisone, differentiating the two disorders may not be possible during the early months of treatment.

Polymyositis causes much more proximal weakness than pain. In contrast, patients with PMR always rate their pain greater than any weakness. The creatine phosphokinase is usually elevated in polymyositis but normal in PMR. Proximal limb pain or stiffness can occur with a variety of endocrine disorders, including hypothyroidism and panhypopituitarism. PMR is usually easily distinguished from fibromyalgia, which is a condition of diffuse pain—both proximal and distal—typically occurring in young women in the absence of objective findings or abnormal laboratory tests. Solid tumors, especially renal cell carcinoma, can produce musculoskeletal pain that resembles PMR. However, patients with malignancy usually have some atypical feature such as pain that affects the distal limbs as much as the proximal portions, clubbing, or a requirement for more than 20 mg of prednisone per day.

Other conditions that can mimic PMR include early Parkinson disease, amyloidosis, late-onset systemic lupus erythematosus, endocarditis, myelodysplastic syndrome, and drug reactions (eg, myositis from statin drugs). Since absence of shoulder involvement is rare in PMR, patients thought to have "below the waist" PMR are more likely to have lumbar spinal stenosis, which can cause stiffness and pain restricted to the hip-girdle region.

Transient nonocular loss of vision (amaurosis fugax) or permanent nonocular blindness can also occur from atherosclerotic cerebrovascular or cardiovascular disease. The nonarteritis patients may be distinguished by their lack of other symptoms and a normal ESR. Both atherosclerosis and GCA can also cause upper or lower extremity claudication. Angiography can usually differentiate these conditions. GCA produces isolated long segments of smooth narrowing in the mid-portions of arteries, whereas atherosclerosis tends to be diffuse and favors branch points.

Some of the clinical features of GCA can be produced by other forms of systemic vasculitis. Wegener granulomatosis and polyarteritis nodosa, for example, can cause jaw claudication. Takayasu arteritis can affect the large vessels as GCA does, but Takayasu arteritis is usually seen in young women. Multiple myeloma, Waldenström macroglobulinemia, and osteomyelitis can produce systemic features with markedly elevated ESRs. Endocarditis should also be considered in a patient with symptoms resembling GCA and a new heart murmur. Many patients with diabetes in whom proteinuria has developed feel poorly and have very high ESRs, as do patients with other forms of renal failure. For example, about 20% of all patients receiving hemodialysis have ESRs > 100 mm/h. Although many of these patients also suffer from malaise, they rarely have symptoms strongly suggestive of GCA. Those who do have symptoms suggesting GCA will require temporal artery biopsy. Other mimickers of GCA include myelodysplastic syndromes and systemic amyloidosis.

Treatment

Prednisone (40–60 mg/d) should be given to any patient in whom GCA is strongly suspected. Then the patient should be referred for a temporal artery biopsy. Temporal artery biopsy has almost zero mortality and very low morbidity. It is the only test that can confirm the diagnosis of GCA, so it is recommended in all suspected cases. Although it is traditional to obtain the temporal artery biopsy quickly, evidence suggests that the pathologic features persist for at least 2 weeks after the start of glucocorticoid treatment. GCA does not involve arteries contiguously, so skip areas may occur. Consequently, the greatest yields will come from biopsies of large segments of artery (eg, 3–5 cm) that have multiple sections examined pathologically. Positive biopsy results demonstrate chiefly mononuclear cells infiltrating all the layers of the artery with varying degrees of intimal proliferation and disruption of the internal elastic lamina. About 50% of positive specimens show multinucleated giant cells. It is intuitively appealing to biopsy the temporal artery that is abnormal on physical examination or that corresponds to the side of the head with symptoms. Unilateral temporal artery biopsy is about 90% sensitive and bilateral biopsies are about 95% sensitive. These figures come from centers where GCA is studied frequently and percentages may not be as high in other communities. In any setting, some patients with a convincing picture of GCA may have a negative biopsy result.

Patients with suspected GCA who have experienced transient visual loss for a few hours should be admitted and given high-dose intravenous methylprednisolone (eg, 1000 mg/d) for 3–5 days, as a few patients have recovered some vision with this regimen. Visual loss of more than 1 day's duration is almost always permanent.

There is increasing evidence that optimal treatment of GCA includes not only prednisone but also low-dose aspirin (ie, 80–100 mg/d). Several retrospective studies have shown that the addition of aspirin reduces by fivefold the risk of blindness or stroke in GCA.

Patients with PMR alone are usually treated with 10–20 mg/d of prednisone. Nonsteroidal anti-inflammatory drugs can help alleviate PMR symptoms but rarely obviate the need for glucocorticoids.

Patients with PMR or GCA respond dramatically to initial treatment. Some report improvement within hours of taking the first dose of prednisone, and most describe a "miraculous" improvement within 2 days. However, about 10% will require a week of therapy before feeling better. Dividing the dose of prednisone into a morning and evening dose for the first 1–2 weeks helps some patients. If the patient does not improve within the first week, doubt should be cast on the diagnosis of PMR or of biopsy-negative GCA. Every-other-day prednisone is not effective initial treatment.

The best studied glucocorticoid-sparing drug for GCA or for PMR is methotrexate. The effectiveness of methotrexate (10–15 mg orally once per week) for GCA is controversial: two randomized, double-blind, controlled trials came to opposite conclusions about methotrexate's efficacy. One study suggests that methotrexate is modestly glucocorticoid-sparing for isolated PMR. The role of biological therapies such as tumor necrosis factor inhibitors is unknown.

To prevent osteoporosis, patients starting prednisone therapy should take 1500–1800 mg of calcium daily with 400–800 U of vitamin D. Bone density scans should be performed, and those with osteopenia or osteoporosis should be started on bisphosphonates.

After the first month of treatment, almost all patients will have a normal ESR. At this point, the prednisone can begin to be tapered by 10% every week or two. The rate of prednisone tapering should be determined by the total clinical picture produced by the patient's symptoms (most important), physical findings, and some laboratory measure of inflammation, such as the ESR or C-reactive protein (least important). Once patients with GCA reach 15 mg of prednisone or patients with PMR reach 10 mg, decrements of 1 mg every 2 or so weeks may reduce the chance of flare.

Complications

Unfortunately, 50–80% of patients with PMR or GCA relapse during the first year as prednisone is tapered. Flares are defined clinically; isolated elevations of ESR or CRP do not require alteration of therapy. The only exception to this rule is that very rare case when visual loss develops in a patient with biopsy-proven GCA in the absence of other symptoms. Patients who experience renewed symptoms usually respond to increasing the prednisone dose 5–10 mg above the last dose at which the patient was asymptomatic. Most patients are unable to completely taper off of prednisone for 1–2 years, and a substantial minority will require some prednisone—usually in the range of 5–10 mg—for longer periods. No glucocorticoid-sparing agent has been proved consistently effective. Reports of the efficacy of methotrexate for GCA have been conflicting.

Complications from prednisone therapy develop in most patients being treated for PMR or GCA (Table 31–3). For example, diabetes or osteoporosis is 2–5 times more likely to develop in patients treated with prednisone than in others of the same age not receiving therapy. Important measures for limiting the toxicity of prednisone therapy include slow but steady tapering of prednisone as suggested above, protecting against early osteoporosis, and avoiding manipulating the dose

Table 31–3. Possible Side Effects of Long-Term Glucocorticoid Therapy

Weight gain
Diabetes
Cataracts
Insomnia
Fluid retention
Hypertension
Proximal weakness
Alopecia
Sweats
Osteoporosis
Infection
Psychiatric disturbance (eg, depression, mania, psychosis)
Easy bruising of the skin
Stress
Tremor
Peptic ulcer disease

of prednisone because of an isolated ESR or CRP elevation.

REFERENCES

Blockman D, et al. Repetitive ^{18}F-fluorodeoxyglucose positron emission tomography in giant cell arteritis: a prospective study of 35 patients. *Arthritis Rheum.* 2006;55:131. [PMID: 16463425]

Caporali R, Cimmino MA, Ferraccioli G, et al. Prednisone plus methotrexate for polymyalgia rheumatica: a randomized, double-blind, placebo-controlled trial. *Ann Intern Med.* 2004; 141:493. [PMID: 15466766]

Huston KA, Hunder GG, Lie JT, Kennedy RH, Elveback LR. Temporal arteritis: a 24-year epidemiologic, clinical, and pathologic study. *Ann Intern Med.* 1978;88:162. [PMID: 626444]

Levine SM, Hellmann DB. Giant cell arteritis. *Curr Opin Rheumatol.* 2002;14:3. [PMID: 11790989]

Miller NR. Visual manifestations of temporal arteritis. *Rheum Dis Clin North Am.* 2001;27:781. [PMID: 11723764]

Salvarani C, Cantini F, Boiardi L, Hunder GG. Polymyalgia rheumatica and giant-cell arteritis. *N Engl J Med.* 2002;347:261. [PMID: 12140303]

Relevant World Wide Web Sites

[The Cleveland Clinic Foundation Center for Vasculitis]
http://www.clevelandclinic.org/arthritis/vasculitis/default.htm
[The International Network for the Study of the Systemic Vasculitides]
http://www2.ccf.org/inssys/
[The Johns Hopkins Vasculitis Center]
http://vasculitis.med.jhu.edu
[The National Institute of Allergy and Infectious Diseases]
http://www.niaid.nih.gov/dir/general.htm
[Vasculitis Foundation]
http://www.wgassociation.org/

Takayasu Arteritis

32

David B. Hellmann, MD

Takayasu arteritis, named for the Japanese ophthalmologist who first described the ocular manifestations in 1908, is a large-vessel vasculitis of unknown cause that chiefly affects women during their reproductive years. The disease often presents two challenges. First, the diagnosis can be delayed for months or even years due to the rarity of the disease, the young age of the (typical) patient, and the protean presenting manifestations. Second, treatment is a challenge. Although Takayasu arteritis is a chronic disease, it usually pursues a waxing and waning course that requires careful monitoring to determine when the disease is active and medical therapy is needed. Treatment with glucocorticoids usually succeeds in halting progression of the vasculitis. Indeed, because of the advances in medical therapy and surgical treatment of vascular complications, such as aortic regurgitation, survival of patients with Takayasu arteritis has increased dramatically.

ESSENTIALS OF DIAGNOSIS

- *Causes vasculitis of the aorta and its major branches.*
- *Preferentially affects young women.*
- *Often presents with absent pulse, bruit, claudication, hypertension, or fever of unknown origin.*
- *Erythrocyte sedimentation rate is usually elevated.*
- *Most patients respond to prednisone.*

General Considerations

Although Takayasu arteritis has been most extensively reported in Japan, Korea, China, Southeast Asia, and Mexico, cases have been described worldwide. In North America, the annual incidence is about 1–3 cases per million people. Takayasu arteritis affects women eight times more frequently than men. The average age of diagnosis is in the mid-20s but the disease may begin as early as age 7 or as late as age 70. Symptoms develop before age 20 in nearly one-third of patients and after age 40 in about 10%. The age of onset tends to be later in European countries.

Pathogenesis

The cause of Takayasu arteritis remains elusive. The geographic clustering of cases suggests important genetic or environmental factors, but few have been identified. Human leukocyte antigen associations have been found in Japanese patients (who preferentially express Bw52, DR2, Dw12, and DQw1), but not in other populations. The predominance of Takayasu arteritis in women of childbearing age suggests that female hormones may play a permissive role, as in systemic lupus erythematosus. An animal model of Takayasu arteritis has been produced with a herpes virus. In that model, the media of the aorta provides an immunoprivileged site for persistent herpes virus infection, which results in chronic inflammation (arteritis).

However initiated, Takayasu arteritis appears to be propagated by a T-cell–driven immune response that results in a granulomatous inflammation affecting all layers of the vessel. Indeed, the histopathology of Takayasu arteritis cannot be distinguished from that of temporal arteritis (also called giant cell arteritis; see Chapter 31). The inflammatory injury mediated by activated T cells, macrophages, and cytokines often results in proliferation of the intima and of smooth muscle cells in the media, leading to occlusion and stenosis of the artery. Transmural inflammation can also cause aneurysmal dilation of the vessel. Overproduction of inflammatory cytokines, such as interleukin-6, results in fever and other constitutional symptoms.

Clinical Findings

A. SYMPTOMS AND SIGNS

Although the presenting features of Takayasu arteritis vary greatly, they can be categorized into two broad groups: those caused by vascular damage (ie, occlusion, stenosis, or dilation of blood vessels), and those caused by systemic inflammation (Table 32–1). The separation of these presenting features is not always neatly maintained; many patients have both vascular complications and constitutional symptoms, and others have a biphasic presentation, with constitutional symptoms dominating early and vascular features becoming more salient later.

Table 32–1. Clinical Features of Takayasu Arteritis

Feature	At Presentation (%)	Ever Present (%)
Vascular	50	100
Bruit		80
Claudication (upper extremity)	30	62
Claudication (lower extremity)	15	32
Hypertension	20	33
Unequal arm blood pressures	15	50
Carotodynia	15	32
Aortic regurgitation		20
Central nervous system	30	57
Light-headedness	20	35
Visual abnormality	10	30
Stroke	5	10
Musculoskeletal	20	53
Chest wall pain	10	30
Joint pain	10	30
Myalgia	5	15
Constitutional	33	43
Malaise	20	30
Fever	20	25
Weight loss	15	20
Cardiac	15	38
Aortic regurgitation	8	20
Angina	2	12
Congestive heart failure	2	10

(Data based on studying 60 patients reported by Kerr GS, Hallahan CW, Giordano J, et al. Takayasu arteritis. *Ann Intern Med.* 1994;120:919. With permission.)

Among the vascular manifestations, bruit, claudication, hypertension, light-headedness (associated with vertebral or carotid artery disease), unequal blood pressures in the extremities, carotodynia, aortic regurgitation, and loss of a pulse are most common. Bruits develop most frequently over the carotid arteries, but also often develop in the supraclavicular or infraclavicular space (reflecting subclavian disease), along the flexor surface of the upper arm (from axillary artery disease), or in the abdomen (from renal or mesenteric artery vasculitis). Many patients have multiple bruits. Upper extremity claudication—commonly manifested in young women by fatigue and pain in the arm while exercising or blow-drying hair—develops more often than lower extremity claudication. A widened pulse pressure and diastolic murmur along the right sternal border may signal the aortic regurgitation that develops in 20% of patients. Stroke, angina, and congestive heart failure affect a significant minority of patients.

The visual symptoms that were first described in 1908 occur rarely today. When present, visual symptoms chiefly result from retinal ischemia produced by narrowing or occlusion of the carotid arteries. Some patients may have such limited blood flow through their carotids and vertebral arteries that merely turning and tilting their head causes light-headedness, dizziness, or visual loss.

Almost half of patients experience constitutional or musculoskeletal symptoms. These constitutional and musculoskeletal features dominate the presentation in approximately one-third of all cases of Takayasu arteritis. Asthenia, weight loss, fever, myalgia, and arthralgia occur commonly. Prominent back pain, especially in the thoracic region, develops in a few patients. This pain resembles that seen in older patients with thoracic dissection and probably results from stimulation of nociceptive nerve fibers along the inflamed aorta.

B. LABORATORY FINDINGS

Takayasu arteritis does not cause any specific blood test or urinary abnormalities but usually produces nonspecific findings of inflammation. Nearly 80% of patients have elevated erythrocyte sedimentation rates or C-reactive protein values, especially during phases of active disease. Anemia develops in 50% of patients, with hematocrits typically in the high 20s or low 30s. Anemic patients commonly have slightly low mean corpuscular volume (eg, high 70s). Thrombocytosis, which develops in one-third of patients, is often mild but may exceed 800,000/μL. Fewer than 10% of patients with Takayasu arteritis have an elevated serum creatinine. About one-quarter will have mild proteinuria or hematuria. Renal abnormalities usually result from hypertension; glomerulonephritis from Takayasu arteritis very rarely occurs.

C. IMAGING STUDIES

Magnetic resonance imaging, computed tomography, vascular ultrasonography, and conventional aortography will be abnormal in virtually all patients with Takayasu arteritis. Magnetic resonance imaging appears most sensitive in that it can detect the inflammatory thickening

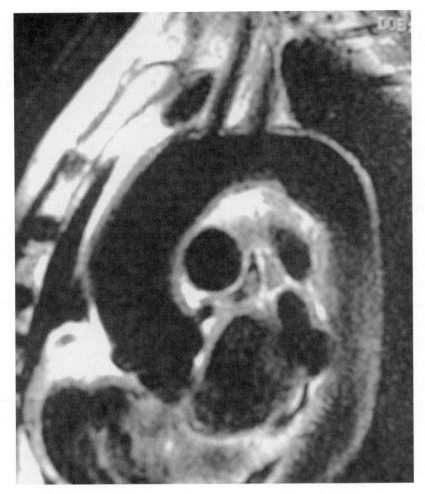

Figure 32–1. Magnetic resonance image showing thickening of the wall of the ascending and descending thoracic aorta in a 26-year-old woman with Takayasu arteritis.

of the aorta or its branches (Figure 32–1) that precedes changes in the caliber of the vessels' lumen. Conventional angiography, although unhelpful in determining the thickness of the vessel wall, provides the most detailed images of the stenoses, occlusions, dilatation, and other vascular wall irregularities characteristic of Takayasu arteritis (Figure 32–2). Advances in computed tomography and three-dimensional image reconstruction have allowed computed tomography angiography to replace the more invasive conventional angiograms.

The most frequently affected vessels are the subclavian arteries, carotid arteries, and aorta (Table 32–2). Involvement of the aorta above and below the diaphragm occurs most commonly. In the extra-aortic vessels, long segments of stenosis are more frequent than dilation or aneurysm. Takayasu arteritis is one of the few forms of vasculitis that can affect, albeit rarely, the pulmonary arteries. Positron emission tomography scanning offers the theoretical advantage of allowing quantification of the degree of vascular inflammation. The role of positron emission tomography scanning in diagnosis and management of patients with Takayasu arteritis has not yet been defined.

D. SPECIFIC TESTS

Biopsies of the aorta or other actively affected arteries show a granulomatous vasculitis with giant cells.

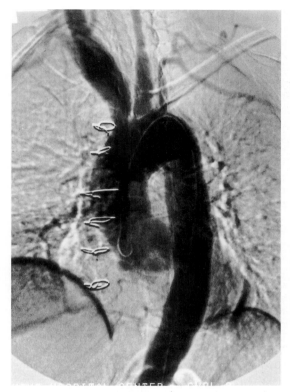

Figure 32–2. Angiogram showing multiple changes of Takayasu arteritis, including dilatations of the ascending aorta (with surgical wires from aortic valve replacement surgery) and the brachiocephalic and proximal right common carotid arteries. The left common carotid artery is occluded distal to its origin. (From Hellmann DB, Flynn JA. Clinical presentation and natural history of Takayasu's arteritis and other inflammatory arteritides. In: Perler BA, Becker GJ, eds. *Vascular Intervention. A Clinical Approach.* Thieme Medical, 1998:249–256. With permission.)

Differential Diagnosis

The biggest impediment to diagnosing Takayasu arteritis is that few physicians are familiar enough with this rare disease to recognize its presenting manifestations. The American College of Rheumatology has developed six criteria for classification of Takayasu arteritis (Table 32–3). In practice, the diagnosis of Takayasu arteritis requires demonstrating vasculitis of the aorta or its major branches by imaging tests (Figure 32–3; also see Figures 32–1 and 32–2) or biopsy, and excluding the diseases that can produce similar abnormalities (Table 32–4).

Of the other vasculitides, temporal arteritis (see Chapter 31) is the form most likely to be confused with

Table 32–2. Frequency of Blood Vessel Involvement in Takayasu Arteritis

Blood Vessel	% Abnormal
Aorta	65
Aortic arch or root	35
Abdominal aorta	47
Thoracic aorta	17
Subclavian artery	93
Common carotid artery	58
Renal artery	38
Vertebral artery	35
Celiac axes	18
Common iliac artery	17
Pulmonary artery	5

(Data based on studying 60 patients reported by Kerr GS, Hallahan CW, Giordano J, et al. Takayasu arteritis. *Ann Intern Med.* 1994;120:919. With permission.)

Takayasu arteritis. Both diseases cause a granulomatous panarteritis and an elevated erythrocyte sedimentation rate. In contrast to Takayasu arteritis, temporal arteritis exclusively affects patients over the age of 50 and chiefly involves extracranial branches of the carotid artery (such as the temporal artery). Cogan syndrome is a rare disease characterized by vestibular-auditory abnormalities (often producing deafness and vertigo) and ocular inflammation (especially keratitis or inflammation of the cornea). A minority of patients with Cogan syndrome have

Table 32–3. American College of Rheumatology Classification Criteria for Takayasu Arteritis[a]

1. Onset at age <40 years
2. Limb claudication
3. Decreased brachial artery pulse
4. Unequal arm blood pressures (>10 mm Hg)
5. Subclavian or aortic bruit
6. Angiographic evidence of narrowing or occlusion of the aorta or its primary branches, or large limb arteritis

[a]The presence of three or more of the six criteria was sensitive (91%) and specific (98%) for the diagnosis of Takayasu arteritis.
(From Arend WP, Michel BA, Bloch DA, et al. The American College of Rheumatology 1990 criteria for the classification of Takayasu Arteritis. *Arthritis Rheum.* 1990;33:1129. With permission.)

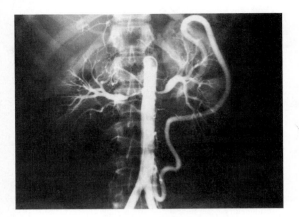

Figure 32–3. Angiogram showing bilateral renal artery stenosis in Takayasu arteritis. A large left colic branch of the inferior mesenteric artery provides collateral circulation. (From Hellmann DB, Flynn JA. Clinical presentation and natural history of Takayasu's arteritis and other inflammatory arteritides. In: Perler BA, Becker GJ, eds. *Vascular Intervention. A Clinical Approach.* Thieme Medical, 1998:249–256. With permission.)

medium- or large-vessel vasculitis, or both. A few other diseases can affect the aorta or its branches, but almost never do they convincingly mimic Takayasu arteritis (see Table 32–4). Relapsing polychrondritis, which results in characteristic changes in cartilage, may also affect the aorta. Rheumatoid arthritis and ankylosing spondylitis rarely affect the thoracic root. Buerger disease—a form of medium-vessel vasculitis associated with smoking—may affect the femoral, brachial, and axillary arteries, as can ergotism. Syphilitic aortitis can be excluded by appropriate serologic studies. Neurofibromatosis and con-

Table 32–4. Differential Diagnosis of Takayasu Arteritis: Other Diseases That Can Affect the Aorta

Rheumatic diseases	Temporal arteritis, Cogan syndrome, relapsing polychrondritis, ankylosing spondylitis, rheumatoid arthritis, systemic lupus erythematosus, Buerger disease, Behçet disease
Infectious disease	Syphilis
Other	Atherosclerosis, inflammatory abdominal aortic aneurysm, ergotism, radiation-induced damage, retroperitoneal fibrosis, inflammatory bowel disease, sarcoidosis, neurofibromatosis, congenital coarctation, Marfan syndrome

genital coarctation may affect the abdominal aorta and mesenteric great vessels. Radiation-induced damage can affect any vessel including the aorta. Atherosclerosis of the aorta and major branches rarely develops before age 50 and does not produce the long, smoothly tapered and stenotic segments of arteries that are so characteristic of Takayasu arteritis. Inflammatory abdominal aortic aneurysm is an unusual form of atherosclerosis characterized by marked thickening of the abdominal aorta, often associated with retroperitoneal inflammation. Almost all of the patients with this disorder are smokers. Patients with inflammatory abdominal aortic aneurysm often have mild anemia and modest elevations of the erythrocyte sedimentation rate. Marfan syndrome does not produce inflammatory symptoms or signs.

Patients with predominantly constitutional symptoms are often evaluated for other conditions. For example, a woman with a hematocrit of 28, a mean corpuscular volume of 78 (reflecting anemia of chronic disease), and a platelet count of $980,000/\mu L$ (nonspecifically reflecting inflammation)—not uncommon findings in Takayasu arteritis—will often unproductively undergo evaluation for gastrointestinal hemorrhage, iron deficiency anemia, or another hematologic disorder. Fatigue and weight loss might erroneously suggest a diagnosis of depression. Transient ischemic attacks in a young woman can be wrongly attributed to migraine. Fever and aortic regurgitation may initially suggest bacterial endocarditis. Measuring blood pressure in both arms, carefully palpating pulses in all extremities, and listening for bruits in the abdomen and chest and along the carotids and supraclavicular and axillary areas provide the best clinical tools in early diagnosis of Takayasu arteritis.

Treatment

Although glucocorticoid therapy for Takayasu arteritis has not been tested in controlled trials, it appears very effective in suppressing vascular inflammation. Initial therapy consists of prednisone (1 mg/kg) for 1 month and then tapered to 10 mg/d over 4–6 months. This treatment nearly universally succeeds in eliminating constitutional and musculoskeletal symptoms within days to a few weeks. Anemia, thrombocytosis, and elevated erythrocyte sedimentation rates also usually respond promptly. Remission, defined as resolution of signs, symptoms, and laboratory markers of inflammation, as well as lack of progression of angiographic abnormalities, is seen in most patients who receive glucocorticoid therapy. Unfortunately, many patients with Takayasu arteritis experience relapses of symptoms or progression of vascular disease that necessitate restarting high-dose prednisone therapy. Open studies suggest that methotrexate plus prednisone or mycophenolate mofetil plus prednisone may be more effective than prednisone alone in some patients. Small open trials also suggest that inflix-imab, an inhibitor of tumor necrosis factor, is an effective glucocorticoid-sparing agent. Because of its toxicity, cy-clophosphamide is rarely used to treat Takayasu arteritis.

Complications of Takayasu arteritis, such as hyperten-sion, congestive heart failure, angina, or aortic regurgita-tion, may benefit from other forms of medical therapy. Treating hypertension is especially tricky in patients with extensive Takayasu arteritis who may have two or more arterial beds with substantially different blood pressures. Reducing blood pressure to achieve a "normal" blood pressure in the legs may aggravate or cause upper ex-tremity claudication. Often the physician must accept compromises in blood pressures that sustain perfusion of critical organs or tissues. Other complications that can be prevented or treated include osteoporosis. Patients tak-ing prednisone long term can guard against osteoporo-sis by performing weight-bearing exercises and taking 400–800 U of vitamin D and 1200–1800 mg of calcium daily, and a bisphosphonate (see Chapter 57).

Interventional radiologists and surgeons also often play important roles in treatment. Angioplasty and stent-ing have been successful in treating some cases of hyper-tension caused by renal artery stenosis. However, resteno-sis is common. Aortic valve replacement, replacement of severely damaged vessels with Dacron grafts, and coro-nary artery bypass surgery can be life-saving. Whenever possible, angioplasty or vascular surgery should be de-ferred until medical therapy has suppressed the inflam-mation.

Prognosis

Most patients have a chronic relapsing and remitting course requiring careful monitoring and adjustment of suppressive therapy. Judging the level of inflammation can be difficult and requires monitoring symptoms, signs, and laboratory markers of inflammation (eg, hemat-ocrit and erythrocyte sedimentation rate). Some experts advocate annual magnetic resonance imaging of the aorta and its branches since some patients show progression in the absence of obvious symptoms or signs of active dis-ease. Pregnancy appears surprisingly well tolerated if the patient has inactive disease, is taking low doses of pred-nisone (ie, <15 mg), and has normal renal function.

Almost all patients experience permanent morbidity from Takayasu arteritis. Because of the morbidity, only about half of the patients are able to work. Survival rates have increased greatly recently so that 10-year survival rates of 80–90% have become common. Advances in di-agnosis, medical and surgical treatment, and monitoring augur even better prognosis in the near future. Mortality has been caused chiefly by renal failure, stroke, cardiac failure, or infectious complications of immunosuppres-sive treatment.

REFERENCES

Hoffman GS, Merkel PA, Brasington RD, Lenschow DJ, Liang P. Anti-tumor necrosis factor therapy in patients with difficult to treat Takayasu arteritis. *Arthritis Rheum.* 2004;50:2296. [PMID: 15248230]

Kerr GS, Hallahan CW, Giordano J, et al. Takayasu arteritis. *Ann Intern Med.* 1994;120:919. [PMID: 7909656]

Kobayashi Y, Ishii K, Oda K, et al. Aortic wall inflammation due to Takayasu arteritis imaged with 18F-FDG PET coregis-tered with enhanced CT. *J Nucl Med.* 2005;46:917. [PMID: 15937300]

Salvarani C, Cantini F, Boiardi L, Hunder GG. Polymyalgia rheu-matica and giant-cell arteritis. *N Engl J Med.* 2002;347:261. [PMID: 12140303]

Weyand CM, Goronzy JJ. Medium- and large-vessel vasculitis. *N Engl J Med.* 2003;349:160. [PMID: 12853590]

Relevant World Wide Web Sites

[Johns Hopkins Vasculitis Center]
http://vasculitis.med.jhu.edu
[Vasculitis Foundation]
http://www.wgassociation.org/

Wegener Granulomatosis

John H. Stone, MD, MPH

ESSENTIALS OF DIAGNOSIS

- *Three pathologic hallmarks of Wegener granulomatosis (WG) are granulomatous inflammation, vasculitis, and necrosis.*
- *Classic clinical features include persistent upper respiratory tract and ear "infections" that do not respond to antibiotic therapy.*
- *Nonspecific constitutional symptoms, such as fatigue, myalgias, weight loss, and fevers.*
- *Migratory pauciarticular or polyarticular arthritis.*
- *Orbital pseudotumor, nearly always associated with chronic nasosinus conditions.*
- *Nodular or cavitary lung lesions that are misdiagnosed initially as malignancies or infections.*
- *Rapidly progressive glomerulonephritis.*
- *Antineutrophil cytoplasmic antibodies (ANCAs) are helpful in diagnosis if positive (by both immunofluorescence and enzyme immunoassay), but a significant number of patients with WG are ANCA-negative.*

General Considerations

WG is one of the most common forms of systemic vasculitis, with a reported annual incidence of 10 cases per million. The disease involves small- to medium-sized blood vessels (small-sized vessels more often than medium-sized vessels). WG affects both the arterial and venous circulations. The cause of WG is not known, but the prominence of upper and lower airway involvement suggests a response to an inhaled antigen. The disease is the prototype of conditions associated with ANCAs. ANCAs are believed to amplify rather than initiate the inflammatory process. WG occurs in people of all ethnic backgrounds but demonstrates a strong predominance for whites, particularly those of northern European ancestry. The male:female ratio is approximately 1:1. Although the mean age at diagnosis is 50 years, the disease also affects the elderly and (occasionally) children.

WG typically presents in a subacute fashion. Patients complain of apparently innocuous symptoms such as nasal stuffiness, "sinusitis," and decreases in hearing. During this prodrome, attentive primary care physicians may suspect and diagnose the disease before the onset of generalized WG. Such early recognition of WG may prevent the disfiguring and devastating end-organ complications of this disorder, such as collapse of the nasal bridge, renal failure, diffuse alveolar hemorrhage, and widespread infarctions of peripheral nerves.

Therapies for WG are associated with substantial treatment-induced morbidity in both the short and long term (see the following section on Complications and the cyclophosphamide section in Chapter 67). Careful follow-up and monitoring of basic laboratory tests (eg, regularly obtaining complete blood cell counts) may prevent some adverse effects of treatment or minimize their impact.

Because of the remitting and relapsing nature of many WG cases and the disease's tendency to recur during or after the taper of treatment, primary care physicians play an important role in the early detection of disease flares.

Clinical Findings

A. SYMPTOMS AND SIGNS

1. Nose, sinuses, and ears—Approximately 90% of patients with WG have nasal involvement, often as the first manifestation of disease. The typical symptoms include persistent rhinorrhea, unusually severe nasal obstruction, epistaxis, and bloody or brown nasal crusts (Table 33–1). Cartilaginous inflammation may lead to perforation of the nasal septum and collapse of the nasal bridge (saddle-nose deformity) (Figure 33–1). Bony erosions of the sinus cavities are characteristic of WG but only develop after long-standing disease (months).

Both conductive and sensorineural forms of hearing loss occur in WG. Conductive hearing loss results from granulomatous involvement of the middle ear, most often leading to serous otitis media. Granulomatous inflammation in the middle ear may also compress the seventh cranial nerve as it courses through the middle ear cavity, leading to a peripheral facial nerve palsy. Sensorineural hearing loss results from inner ear (cochlear) involvement and may also be associated with vestibular dysfunction

Table 33–1. Major Clinical Manifestations of Wegener Granulomatosis

Organ	Manifestation
Nose	Persistent rhinorrhea; bloody, brown nasal crusts; nasal obstruction; nasal septal perforation; saddle-nose deformity
Sinuses	Sinusitis with radiologic evidence of bony erosions
Ears	Conductive hearing loss due to granulomatous inflammation in the middle ear; sensorineural hearing loss; mixed hearing loss common
Mouth	Strawberry gums; tongue or other oral ulcers; occasional purpuric lesions on palate
Eyes	Orbital pseudotumor; scleritis (often necrotizing); episcleritis; conjunctivitis; keratitis (risk of corneal melt); uveitis (anterior)
Trachea	Subglottic stenosis
Lungs	Nodular, cavitary lesions; nonspecific pulmonary infiltrates; alveolar hemorrhage; bronchial lesions
Heart	Occasional valvular lesions, usually not evident during life; pericarditis
Gastrointestinal	Mesenteric vasculitis uncommon; splenic involvement quite common but usually subclinical (detected as splenic infarcts on cross-sectional imaging)
Kidneys	Glomerulonephritis (small-vessel vasculitis of the kidney). Medium-vessel vasculitis occasionally evident on renal biopsy.
Skin	Palpable purpura, subcutaneous nodules (Churg-Strauss granulomas), ulcers, vesiculobullous lesions, splinter hemorrhages
Joints	Migratory pauciarthritis or polyarthritis or arthralgias. Arthritis is nondestructive.
Peripheral nerve	Sensory or motor mononeuritis multiplex
Central nervous system	True central nervous system vasculitis rare but reported. More common is granulomatous involvement of the meninges, with a clinical picture of chronic meningitis.

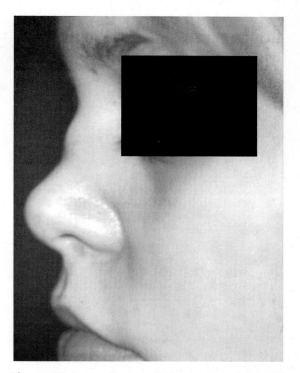

Figure 33–1. Cartilaginous inflammation of the nose in Wegener granulomatosis may lead to nasal septal perforation and ultimately to collapse of the nasal bridge (saddle-nose deformity).

(eg, nausea, vertigo, and tinnitus). "Mixed" hearing loss, the simultaneous occurrence of both conductive and sensorineural hearing loss, is common in WG. (Additional information about sensorineural hearing loss is found in Chapter 64.)

2. Eyes—WG may present with a variety of inflammatory lesions of the eye (Figure 33–2). Orbital pseudotumors behind the eye may lead to proptosis and visual loss through ischemia of the optic nerve. Scleritis causes photophobia and painful, often raised, scleral erythema. If unchecked, necrotizing scleritis may lead to scleral thinning, scleromalacia perforans, and visual loss. Peripheral keratitis may cause ulcerations on the margin of the cornea and lead to the syndrome of "corneal melt." Although episcleritis and conjunctivitis constitute less serious ocular complications, they are very common in WG. Their occurrence may be the presenting symptom of the disease or the first manifestation of a flare. Other ocular complications of WG are anterior uveitis and nasolacrimal duct obstruction. Retinal lesions (posterior uveitis) are rare in WG.

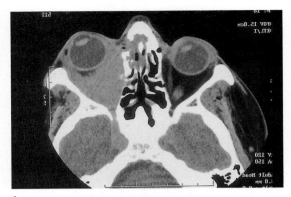

A

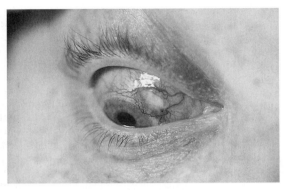

B

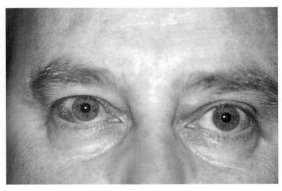

C

Figure 33–2. **A:** Computed tomography scan of the orbit showing an orbital pseudotumor, leading to proptosis and visual loss. **B:** Scleritis with a marginal corneal ulceration. **C:** Painless erythema of the superficial surface of the eye—episcleritis—the most common ocular complication of Wegener granulomatosis.

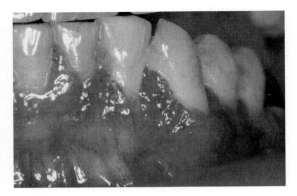

Figure 33–3. Wegener granulomatosis patient with intense inflammation of the gums, a physical finding known as "strawberry gums."

3. Mouth—Two classic mouth lesions of WG are gum inflammation ("strawberry gums" [Figure 33–3]) and tongue ulcers. The gum inflammation of WG, which derives its name from the resemblance of the dental papillae to strawberries, is quite distinctive among rheumatologic conditions. Both of these lesions, which are quite painful, respond promptly to glucocorticoids.

4. Trachea—Subglottic stenosis, the result of tracheal inflammation and scarring below the vocal cords, is a potentially disabling manifestation largely specific to WG (relapsing polychondritis can also cause this lesion). Subglottic involvement is often asymptomatic and may manifest itself only as a subtle hoarseness. With time, however, airway scarring and profound tracheal narrowing may occur. Supraglottic disease, though substantially less common than subglottic stenosis, may also occur in WG.

5. Lungs—Approximately 80% of patients with WG have pulmonary lesions during the course of their disease. Pulmonary symptoms include cough, hemoptysis, dyspnea, and sometimes pleuritic chest pain. Lung lesions are often asymptomatic, however, and may be detected only if chest imaging is performed. The most common radiographic findings are pulmonary infiltrates and nodules. The infiltrates, which may wax and wane, are often misdiagnosed initially as pneumonia. Single large pulmonary nodules may often be misdiagnosed as lung cancer. Nodules are usually multiple and bilateral and often cavitary. Pulmonary capillaritis may lead to hemoptysis and rapidly changing alveolar infiltrates. Finally, venous thrombotic events (particularly deep venous thromboses) and pulmonary emboli are now known to be a common complication of WG. Pulmonary emboli should be considered in the WG patient who develops dyspnea, pleuritic chest pain, or other compatible symptoms.

6. Kidneys—Renal disease is the most ominous clinical manifestation of WG. Renal involvement, present in approximately 20% of patients with WG at the time of diagnosis, develops eventually in a substantially higher portion of patients (up to 80%) during the course of the disease. The clinical presentation of renal disease in WG is rapidly progressive glomerulonephritis: hematuria, red blood cell casts, proteinuria (usually non-nephrotic), and rising serum creatinine. Without appropriate therapy, loss of renal function may ensue within days or weeks.

7. Other organs—Nonspecific arthralgias and frank arthritis often occur early in the course of WG. The arthritis of WG is migratory in nature and may assume a variety of joint patterns, from a pauciarticular syndrome of lower extremity joints to a polyarthritis of the small joints of the hands. Digital ischemia and gangrene resulting from inflammation in medium-sized digital arteries are occasionally the presenting feature of WG. The skin manifestations of WG include the full array of findings associated with cutaneous vasculitis: palpable purpura, papules, ulcers, and vesiculobullous lesions. Examination of the skin should include careful inspection for the nodular lesions of "Churg-Strauss granulomas" (cutaneous extravascular necrotizing granulomas), typically located on the extensor surfaces of the elbows and other pressure points (Figure 33–4). Splinter hemorrhages may occur in WG, raising diagnostic confusion with endocarditis. Lesions resembling pyoderma gangrenosum may also occur. Although involvement of the brain parenchyma with WG has been reported, meningeal inflammation (presenting as excruciating headaches and cranial neuropathies) is a more typical central nervous system disease manifestation. Mononeuritis multiplex may also accompany WG

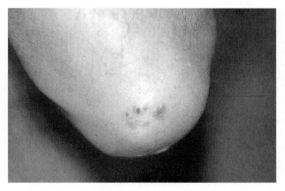

Figure 33–4. This patient has Wegener granulomatosis and has a positive test result for rheumatoid factor. The nodule over the extensor surface of the elbow was initially misdiagnosed as a rheumatoid nodule instead of a "Churg-Strauss granuloma" (cutaneous extravascular necrotizing granuloma).

but is less characteristic of this disease than others (eg, polyarteritis nodosa, microscopic polyangiitis, and Churg-Strauss syndrome).

B. Laboratory Findings

The results of routine laboratory tests and more specialized assays in WG are shown in Table 33–2. All of these tests are appropriate at the initial evaluation of a patient with possible WG. The exclusion of renal disease through the careful performance of a urinalysis is essential in the evaluation and follow-up of all patients with WG. The erythrocyte sedimentation rate and serum C-reactive protein level are useful (albeit imperfect) biomarkers in the longitudinal evaluation of disease activity.

C. Imaging Studies

Up to one-third of patients with WG have asymptomatic pulmonary lesions on radiologic imaging. Computed tomography is superior to chest radiography in demonstrating the extent of pulmonary disease (Figure 33–5). Consequently, patients with confirmed or strongly suspected diagnoses of WG should have computed tomography scans of the chest as baseline studies. Virtually any finding (with the rare exception of hilar and mediastinal adenopathy) may be present on chest imaging in WG, including pleural effusions and nonspecific infiltrates. Lung nodules are typically multiple and bilateral and have a tendency to cavitate. The pulmonary lesions are often located in the periphery of the lung and may appear to be wedge-shaped and pleural-based. They may therefore be mistaken for pulmonary emboli or lung malignancies.

D. Special Tests

1. Biopsy—Because of the numerous potential mimickers of WG and the frequent shortcomings of ANCA (see next section on ANCA testing), the diagnosis of WG is most secure when established through biopsy of an involved organ. Among the organs commonly involved in WG, those most likely to yield tissue that permits a diagnosis are (in descending order): lung, kidney, and upper respiratory tract (nose or sinuses). The tissue necrosis associated with WG is frequently so extensive within diseased tissues that it is termed "geographic necrosis." Even when all three pathologic hallmarks (granulomatous inflammation, vasculitis, and necrosis) are present, the diagnosis of WG requires the careful integration of pathologic findings with clinical, laboratory, and radiologic data. Acid-fast and fungal pathogens must be excluded by special stains and cultures.

Biopsies of the upper respiratory tract (nose, sinuses, and subglottic region) are frequently nondiagnostic, yielding only nonspecific acute and chronic inflammation. Upper respiratory tract biopsies demonstrate the complete diagnostic triad in only about 15% of cases. However, these biopsies are generally safer

Table 33–2. The Laboratory Evaluation in Wegener Granulomatosis

Test	Typical Result
Complete blood cell count	• Normochromic, normocytic anemia; acute, severe anemias possible in alveolar hemorrhage • Mild to moderate leukocytosis common, usually not exceeding $18 \times 10^9/L$ • Moderate to pronounced thrombocytosis typical, ranging from platelet counts of $400 \times 10^9/L$ to occasionally $>1000 \times 10^9/L$
Electrolytes	Hyperkalemia in the setting of advanced renal dysfunction
Liver function test	Hepatic involvement is quite unusual in WG; when present, there can be elevations of transaminases (AST/ALT) in excess of 1000 mg/dL
Urinalysis with microscopy	• Hematuria (ranging from mild to so high that red blood cells are too numerous to count) • Red blood cell casts • Proteinuria (nephritic range proteinuria in a small minority)
Erythrocyte sedimentation rate/C-reactive protein	Dramatic elevations of acute phase reactants are typical, generally with good correlation to disease activity
ANA	Negative
Rheumatoid factor	Positive in 40–50% of patients, often leading to diagnostic confusion with rheumatoid arthritis
C3, C4	Complement levels are normal to elevated in WG, in contrast to systemic lupus erythematosus, cryoglobulinemia, and other diseases in which immune complexes appear to play major roles
ANCA	Positive in 60–90% of patients with WG
Anti-GBM	A minority of patients with WG also have anti-GBM antibodies

WG, Wegener granulomatosis; AST/ALT aspartate aminotransferase/alanine aminotransferase; ANA, antinuclear antibody; ANCA, antineutrophil cytoplasmic antibody; anti-GBM, antiglomerular basement membrane antibody.

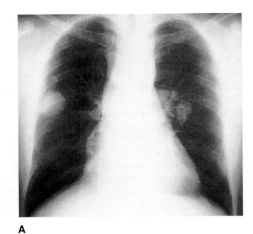

A

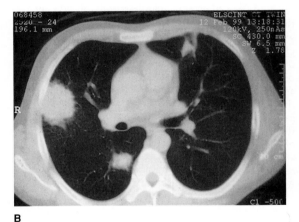

B

Figure 33–5. Chest radiograph and computed tomography scan show multiple bilateral nodules. **A:** Posteroanterior view of the chest shows bilateral lung nodules. **B:** Computed tomography scan of the chest in the same patient shows additional lesions not evident on the radiograph.

than lung or kidney biopsies, and the finding of even parts of this triad in a nose or sinus biopsy may serve as compelling evidence for the diagnosis of WG, provided that other manifestations of the disease are present elsewhere.

WG finds its fullest pathologic expression in the lung, where the large amounts of tissue obtained at open or tho-racoscopic lung biopsy may capture the entire spectrum of disease. Transbronchial and radiologically guided needle biopsies usually fail to yield diagnostic tissue specimens. The leukocytoclastic vasculitis of WG may involve arteries, veins, and capillaries, with or without granulomatous features. Vascular necrosis begins as clusters of neutrophils within the blood vessel wall (microabscesses) that degenerate and become surrounded by palisading histiocytes. Coalescence of such neutrophilic microabscesses leads to geographic necrosis.

Although renal biopsy findings are not specific for WG (other pauci-immune forms of glomerulonephritis may have identical findings), renal biopsy results are sufficiently characteristic to establish the diagnosis in appropriate clinical settings. The typical renal lesion of WG is segmental necrotizing glomerulonephritis, with or without crescent formation. Thrombotic changes in the glomerular capillary loops are among the earliest histologic lesions. Immunofluorescence studies of renal biopsies in WG confirm the "pauci-immune" nature of the renal involvement (ie, the relatively sparse immunoglobulin and complement deposition found in this disorder compared with such diseases as systemic lupus erythematosus, Henoch-Schönlein purpura, and Goodpasture syndrome).

2. Serologic testing for ANCAs—ANCAs are directed against antigens that reside within the primary granules of neutrophils and monocytes. Positive ANCA assays are often instrumental in suggesting the diagnosis. Titers of these antibodies, however, often correlate poorly in time with disease flares and should never be used as the sole guide to the use of immunosuppression. The two types of ANCA tests now in common use are immunofluorescence assays and enzyme immunoassays. These two tests are complementary in the diagnosis of WG, and both should be used in evaluating patients in whom this disease is suspected. Negative ANCA assays do not preclude the diagnosis of WG; most series indicate that up to 10% of patients with active, "disseminated," untreated WG are ANCA-negative. Among patients with "limited" disease (see section on Treatment), 30% or more may lack ANCA.

With immunofluorescence, three principal patterns are recognized: cytoplasmic (C-ANCA), perinuclear (P-ANCA), and atypical. Immunofluorescence testing alone has low specificity and a low positive predictive value for WG. Hence the diagnosis of WG should never rest primarily on a positive immunofluorescence assay, regardless of whether the pattern is C-ANCA or P-ANCA. In patients with vasculitis, the C-ANCA pattern usually corresponds to the presence of antiproteinase-3 antibodies (PR3-ANCA), detected by enzyme immunoassay. The presence of both a C-ANCA pattern on immunofluorescence testing and PR3-ANCA by enzyme immunoassay has a high positive predictive value for WG.

The P-ANCA pattern, which (in patients with vasculitis) usually corresponds to the presence of antimyeloperoxidase antibodies, occurs in approximately 10% of patients with WG but is more typical of microscopic polyangiitis, the Churg-Strauss syndrome, and necrotizing crescentic glomerulonephritis. Atypical immunofluorescence ANCA patterns, which may occur in association with a wide variety of diseases such as inflammatory bowel disease and connective tissue disorders, are not directed against either PR3 or MPO and do not imply the presence of a primary vasculitis.

Differential Diagnosis

The protean nature of WG dictates that an all-inclusive differential diagnosis for the varied presentations of this disease is enormously broad. It encompasses sinusitis and pneumonia caused by microbial pathogens, other forms of vasculitis often associated with ANCA, and the confluence of several common medical problems in the same patient (eg, the simultaneous occurrence of pneumonia and interstitial nephritis caused by antibiotics). The major disease entities in the differential diagnosis of WG are shown in Table 33–3.

WG may smolder in the upper respiratory tract for months or even years before becoming a generalized, life-threatening illness. Recognition of the systemic disorder underlying the repeated "ear infections," allergies, musculoskeletal symptoms, and other complaints is often delayed. Before the correct diagnosis, patients with WG frequently endure multiple courses of antibiotics, myringotomies, and other interventions that are largely ineffectual or provide only temporary relief. WG should be suspected when mundane complaints persist long enough to become unusual.

Table 33–3. Differential Diagnosis of Wegener Granulomatosis

Other vasculitides
Polyarteritis nodosa
Microscopic polyangiitis
Churg-Strauss syndrome
Henoch-Schönlein purpura
Mixed cryoglobulinemia
Goodpasture syndrome
Giant cell arteritis

Infections
Mycobacterial diseases
Fungal infections (histoplasmosis, blastomycosis, coccidioidomycosis)
Streptococcal pneumonia with glomerulonephritis

Malignancies
Nasopharyngeal carcinoma
Hodgkin disease
Non-Hodgkin lymphoma
Angiocentric lymphoma ("lymphomatoid granulomatosis")
Castleman disease

Granulomatous disorders
Sarcoidosis
Berylliosis

Systemic autoimmune conditions
Systemic lupus erythematosus
Rheumatoid arthritis
Relapsing polychondritis

Limited WG may pose difficult diagnostic problems. The destructive upper airway disease that occurs in limited WG may also be caused by infection (eg, mycobacteria, fungi, actinomycosis, and syphilis), malignancy (eg, squamous cell carcinoma and extranodal lymphoma), or illicit drug use (eg, intranasal cocaine or smoking crack). The sinus destruction of WG may be mimicked by nonvasculitic disorders such as "lethal midline granuloma," now known to be an angioproliferative T-cell lymphoma.

Chronic infections such as those caused by mycobacterial and fungal pathogens are essential to exclude through special stains and cultures of tissue biopsies. Because granulomatous infections of the lung may also cause vasculitis and necrosis, special stains and cultures for infection should show negative results before the diagnosis of WG is made. Infections are especially important to consider in patients with established diagnoses of WG who have been treated with immunosuppressive medications.

Rheumatoid arthritis is a common misdiagnosis because arthritis is a frequent finding at presentation. Furthermore, approximately half of all patients with WG have positive test results for rheumatoid factor, and Churg-Strauss granulomas often occur at precisely the most frequent sites for rheumatoid nodules—the elbows—further heightening the diagnostic confusion. (Patients are usually unaware of these lesions, as they may be unaware of rheumatoid nodules.) Other systemic inflammatory conditions associated with autoimmunity (eg, lupus) also affect multiple organ systems and must be distinguished from WG. Sarcoidosis is an excellent mimicker of WG because of the frequency with which it involves many of the same organs.

Finally, many other forms of systemic vasculitis are high on the differential diagnosis for WG. Accurate distinction among WG, polyarteritis nodosa, giant cell arteritis, Goodpasture syndrome, microscopic polyangiitis, Churg-Strauss syndrome, Henoch-Schönlein purpura, relapsing polychondritis, and cryoglobulinemia is essential because their complications, treatments, and prognoses vary widely. ANCA-associated vasculitis can also be induced by certain medications, particularly propylthiouracil and hydralazine. Cutaneous vasculitis is usually the predominant manifestation of drug-induced ANCA-associated vasculitis, and the type of ANCA typically found is MPO- rather than PR3-ANCA.

Treatment

The management of WG should be stratified according to whether the patient has severe or limited disease. Severe disease (defined as an immediate threat to either the function of a vital organ or to the patient's life) requires treatment with cyclophosphamide and high doses of glucocorticoids. The combination of cyclophosphamide (2 mg/kg/d for those with normal renal function) and glucocorticoids (1 mg/kg/d of prednisone, perhaps preceded by a 3-day intravenous "pulse" of methylprednisolone) leads to excellent initial therapeutic responses (and dramatic improvement) in 90% or more of patients and to complete remission in 75%. Daily cyclophosphamide administration is more likely to result in durable remissions than intermittent (ie, monthly) dosing.

By definition, limited disease includes all cases of WG that are not severe. Because patients with limited WG are more likely to have nasosinus disease, arthritis, nodular pulmonary lesions, cutaneous findings, minor ocular complications, and mild renal disease as their principal manifestations, they may benefit from a less dangerous approach to therapy. Patients with limited WG may respond to the combination of methotrexate (up to 25 mg/wk) and glucocorticoids, thus sparing patients the potential side effects of cyclophosphamide. Methotrexate is not an appropriate first-line treatment for patients with severe involvement of the kidney, lung, or other vital organs and should not be used in patients with significant renal dysfunction (eg, a serum creatinine of >2.0 mg/dL). Regardless of whether cyclophosphamide or methotrexate is used in the remission induction regimen, all patients with WG should receive prophylaxis against *Pneumocystis jiroveci* pneumonia with either single-strength trimethoprim-sulfamethoxazole or 100 mg/d of dapsone. The higher doses of prednisone and methotrexate used to treat WG (compared with other systemic inflammatory conditions) justify the use of *P. jiroveci* pneumonia prophylaxis in WG.

Contrary to widespread beliefs, the induction of neutropenia is not necessary for the achievement of remission and control of the disease. By opening the door to opportunistic infections, the induction of neutropenia is far more likely to cause harm than good. One strategy for the avoidance of such infections is to keep the white blood cell count $>4.0 \times 10^9$/L. Reducing the dose of cyclophosphamide, azathioprine, or methotrexate is appropriate when the total white blood cell count begins to decline.

In attempting to control the disease and avoid the side effects of long-term cyclophosphamide therapy, shorter courses (eg, 3–6 months) of induction treatment with cyclophosphamide are now used followed by longer-term treatment for the maintenance of remission with either azathioprine (up to 2 mg/kg/d) or methotrexate. A wide array of other therapies (eg, plasmapheresis and intravenous immune globulin) have been considered as adjunct approaches for the induction of remission. These treatments have been used in small numbers of patients, so data are insufficient to judge their efficacy.

Patients with subglottic stenosis comprise a unique subset of WG, with a disease complication that often responds better to mechanical interventions (eg, surgical dilatation accomplished through noninvasive approaches and glucocorticoid injections) than to immunosuppressive therapy. Laser techniques should be avoided during these procedures because they may exacerbate tissue injury. Otolaryngologists frequently use mitomycin C injections to help prevent the proliferation of scar tissue following dilatations of subglottic stenoses.

Complications

Regimens of cytotoxic agents and glucocorticoids have converted this once nearly always fatal disease into one that responds well to treatment and enters remission (for variable lengths of time) in most cases. Unfortunately, WG is marked by a pronounced tendency to flare during the tapering of medications or after the cessation of treatment. The requirement of treating disease flares with additional courses of therapy frequently leads to mounting treatment-related morbidity.

Under the original regimen established by the National Institutes of Health, patients were treated with cyclophosphamide for a mean period of approximately 2 years (for 1 full year after the achievement of remission). Although many patients had remissions that lasted for up to several years, less than 40% of the patients in the National Institutes of Health series achieved "cures" following their initial courses of therapy. Repeated administration of these potentially toxic treatments to patients with disease recurrences led to substantial long-term morbidity. Forty-two percent of patients treated under the National Institutes of Health regimen suffered permanent medication-induced morbidity. The major complications of treating WG with cytotoxic agents (not including the multiple and often severe side effects of prolonged glucocorticoid treatment) follow:

- Bone marrow suppression
- Myelodysplastic syndromes
- Opportunistic infection
- Drug-induced injury to the lungs, bladder, and liver
- Infertility
- Long-term risk of malignancies, particularly lymphoma and bladder cancers

When to Refer to a Specialist

The overall disease process frequently appears to accelerate once renal involvement becomes evident. Thus the finding of an active urine sediment or a rise in serum creatinine in WG signals a matter of utmost urgency.

Gross hematuria may indicate drug-induced cystitis in patients treated with cyclophosphamide. This complication may be associated with dysuria but not always. Cystoscopy is required to confirm the diagnosis in patients with drug-induced cystitis. Upon the diagnosis of cyclophosphamide-induced bladder injury, further treatment with this medication is contraindicated. Alternatively, gross hematuria is sometimes a presenting feature of active glomerulonephritis. The occurrence of hematuria months to years after a course of cyclophosphamide may indicate the development of bladder cancer and should prompt a cystoscopic evaluation by a urologist.

Hemoptysis, shortness of breath, rapidly changing pulmonary infiltrates, and abrupt declines in hematocrit may all indicate active pulmonary capillaritis. Hemoptysis may be an insensitive indicator of diffuse alveolar hemorrhage. This WG complication requires rapid intervention with immunosuppressive medications (cyclophosphamide and glucocorticoids) and perhaps observation or management in an intensive care unit.

The occurrence of thrush should prompt reevaluation of the patient's immunosuppressive regimen.

A fever in a patient who is receiving therapy for WG signals a potential medical emergency, indicating the possibility of infection in immunocompromised patients.

The complaint of ocular pain, photophobia, or visual loss should prompt a swift referral to an ophthalmologist. Orbital pseudotumor, necrotizing scleritis, and marginal ulcers of the cornea may all lead quickly to vision-threatening ocular events.

Voice huskiness and subtle signs of stridorous breathing may indicate impending critical stenosis of the subglottic region. Some patients present with subacute respiratory stridor. Severe cases may require tracheostomies. Pulmonary function tests (flow-volume loops) provide a useful noninvasive means of quantifying and following the degree of extrathoracic airway obstruction. However, thin-cut computed tomography scans of the trachea are more sensitive for these lesions. In some cases, direct visualization with fiberoptic laryngoscopy is required to make the diagnosis.

Sensorineural hearing loss, which is often associated with other symptoms of inner ear dysfunction such as vertigo, tinnitus, and nausea, may proceed quickly to irreversible hearing loss. The cochlea should be regarded (along with the glomerulus) as an integral part of a vital organ that may suffer permanent damage in relatively short order. Sensorineural hearing loss requires the prompt institution of treatment and consultation with an otolaryngologist to ensure that no other causes of hearing loss are present.

REFERENCES

Hoffman G, Kerr GS, Leavitt RY, et al. Wegener granulomatosis: an analysis of 158 patients. *Ann Intern Med*. 1992;116:488. [PMID: 1739240] (Report of the long-term follow-up of patients treated under the National Institutes of Health regimen of daily cyclophosphamide and glucocorticoids.)

Hoffman G, Specks U. Antineutrophil cytoplasmic antibodies. *Arthritis Rheum.* 1998;41:1521. [PMID: 9751084] (Still the classic summary article on ANCA).

Seo P, Stone JH. The anti-neutrophil cytoplasmic antibody-associated vasculitides. *Am J Med.* 2004;117:39. [PMID: 15210387] (Detailed review of the clinical, pathological, radiological, and treatment issues in this spectrum of disease).

Wegener's Granulomatosis Etanercept Trial (WGET) Research Group. Etanercept plus standard therapy for Wegener's granulomatosis. *N Engl J Med.* 2005;352:351. [PMID: 15673801]. (This is the first randomized, controlled trial of Wegener granulomatosis in the U.S. Etanercept was ineffective in remission maintenance. High rates of disease flares and a high incidence of adverse effects with conventional therapy were emphasized.)

Relevant World Wide Web Sites

[The Johns Hopkins Vasculitis Center]
http://vasculitis.med.jhu.edu
[The Vasculitis Foundation]
http://www.wgassociation.org/
[Vasculitis Clinical Research Consortium]
http://rarediseasesnetwork.epi.usf.edu/vcrc/

Microscopic Polyangiitis

34

Geetha Duvuru, MD, & John H. Stone, MD, MPH

ESSENTIALS OF DIAGNOSIS

- *Microscopic polyangiitis (MPA) is the most common cause of the pulmonary-renal syndrome of alveolar hemorrhage and glomerulonephritis, and is several times more common, for example, than antiglomerular basement membrane disease (Goodpasture disease).*
- *Usually includes combinations of two or more of the following:*
  - *Nonspecific constitutional symptoms, including fatigue, myalgias, weight loss, and fevers.*
  - *Migratory arthralgias or arthritis, either pauciarticular or polyarticular.*
  - *Palpable purpura, sometimes with skin ulcerations.*
  - *Sensorimotor mononeuritis multiplex.*
  - *Alveolar hemorrhage associated with hemoptysis and respiratory compromise.*
  - *Glomerulonephritis.*
- *Antineutrophil cytoplasmic antibodies (ANCAs) are an important adjunct to diagnosis, but serologic testing for these antibodies has several potential pitfalls. The majority of patients with MPA who are ANCA-positive have antibodies directed against myeloperoxidase (MPO-ANCA).*
- *ANCA tests seldom obviate the need to confirm the diagnosis by tissue biopsy.*

General Considerations

Microscopic polyangiitis (MPA) is a form of systemic vasculitis that may affect many major organs in a crippling or even fatal fashion. Seventy percent of patients with MPA have antineutrophil cytoplasmic antibodies (ANCAs). There has been increasing recognition of this

disorder in the United States since the 1994 Chapel Hill Consensus Conference on the nomenclature of systemic vasculitides. Many cases before then were considered to be forms of polyarteritis nodosa, a disease with which MPA shares substantial characteristics. An even closer disease relative is Wegener granulomatosis, which is often very difficult to distinguish from MPA on clinical grounds alone. However, there are significant differences among MPA, polyarteritis nodosa, and Wegener granulomatosis in organ involvement, treatment, response to therapy, and prognosis; thus it is important to distinguish among these major forms of systemic vasculitis. Table 34–1 compares the features of MPA with these other two diseases.

The term "polyangiitis" is preferred to "polyarteritis" for MPA because of the tendency of the disease to involve veins as well as arteries. The Chapel Hill Consensus Conference defined MPA as a process that (1) involves necrotizing vasculitis with few or no immune deposits; (2) affects small blood vessels (capillaries, arterioles, or venules) and possibly medium-sized vessels, as well; and (3) demonstrates a tropism for the kidneys and lungs. With an estimated incidence of 4 cases per million per year, MPA is more common than classic polyarteritis nodosa but slightly less common than Wegener granulomatosis.

MPA occurs in people of all ethnic backgrounds, but epidemiologic studies in the United States demonstrate a predilection for whites. The male:female ratio is approximately 1:1. The typical patient is middle-aged, but the disease may affect people of all ages. Several epidemiologic studies have tried to elucidate environmental factors associated with the onset of vasculitis. Some authors have found associations with silica and solvent exposure. The strongest link between an exposure and MPA relates to the use of propylthiouracil for the treatment of hyperthyroidism (a handful of other drugs for other indications have also been implicated, but not as strongly). Anti-MPO antibodies are detected frequently in propylthiouracil-treated patients, albeit the development of overt vasculitis occurs in only a small minority. Drug-induced ANCA-associated vasculitis is discussed further in Chapter 43).

Table 34–1. Comparison of the Features of MPA, WG, and PAN

	MPA	WG	PAN
Vessel size	Small to medium	Small to medium	Medium
Vessel type	Capillaries, venules, and arterioles; sometimes arteries and veins	Capillaries, venules, and arterioles; sometimes arteries and veins	Muscular arteries
Granulomatous inflammation	No	Yes	No
Lung involvement	Yes (pulmonary capillaritis)	Yes (pulmonary nodules, often cavitary)	No
Glomerulonephritis	Yes	Yes	No
Renin-mediated hypertension	No	No	Yes
ANCA-positive	75%	60–90%	No
Hepatitis B association	No	No	Yes (<10% of cases now)
Microaneurysms	Rarely	Rarely	Typically
Mononeuritis multiplex	Commonly (60%)	Occasionally	Commonly (60%)
Likelihood of disease recurrence	33%	>50%	≤10%

MPA, microscopic polyangiitis; WG, Wegener granulomatosis; PAN, polyarteritis nodosa; ANCA, antineutrophil cytoplasmic antibody.

Clinical Findings

A. SYMPTOMS AND SIGNS

Although MPA is classified appropriately as a "pulmonary-renal syndrome," regarding this disorder exclusively as a disease that affects the kidneys and lungs is a major potential clinical error. The five most common clinical manifestations of MPA are glomerulonephritis (nearly 80% of patients), weight loss (>70%), mononeuritis multiplex (60%), fevers (55%), and a variety of cutaneous findings (> 60%). Alveolar hemorrhage, in contrast, occurs in a comparative minority: 12%. The major clinical manifestations of MPA are shown in Table 34–2.

1. Head, eyes, ears, nose, and throat—Upper respiratory tract involvement in MPA is limited to rhinitis or mild cases of nondestructive sinusitis. Serous otitis media may occur in MPA but unlike in Wegener granulomatosis, granulomatous inflammation is absent. Some vasculitis experts regard the presence of any upper respiratory tract involvement as evidence that the diagnosis is Wegener granulomatosis, not MPA. Ocular lesions in MPA (eg, episcleritis, conjunctivitis, keratitis, and occasionally scleritis) have been reported.

2. Lungs—The principal pulmonary manifestation of MPA is capillaritis, which leads to alveolar hemorrhage and often to hemoptysis (although the latter may be only a late indication of bleeding). The typical radiologic features of alveolar hemorrhage are shown in Figure 34–1.

Table 34–2. Major Clinical Manifestations of Microscopic Polyangiitis

Organ	Manifestation
Constitutional	Weight loss, anorexia, fevers
HEENT	Rhinitis, tongue or other oral ulcers; occasional purpuric lesions on palate; ocular inflammation (eg, sclerouveitis) reported but rare
Lungs	Alveolar hemorrhage; nonspecific infiltrates; pulmonary fibrosis; pleural effusions
Gastrointestinal	Mesenteric vasculitis with microaneurysms in some patients
Kidneys	Glomerulonephritis (small-vessel vasculitis of the kidney); medium-vessel vasculitis occasionally evident on renal biopsy or demonstrated by cross-sectional imaging studies (renal infarcts)
Skin	Palpable purpura, ulcers, vesiculobullous lesions, splinter hemorrhages
Joints	Migratory pauciarthritis or polyarthritis or arthralgias; arthritis is nondestructive
Peripheral nerve	Sensory or motor mononeuritis multiplex
Central nervous system	True central nervous system vasculitis rare but reported

HEENT, head, eyes, ears, nose, throat.

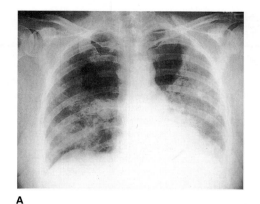

A

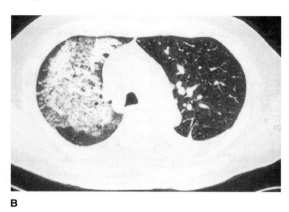

B

Figure 34–1. Radiologic features of alveolar hemorrhage. **A:** Chest radiograph. **B:** Computed tomography scan of the chest.

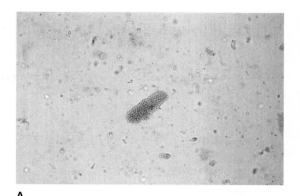

A

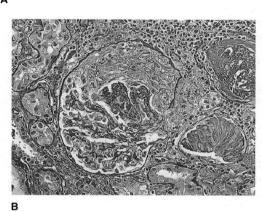

B

Figure 34–2. Renal manifestations of microscopic polyangiitis. **A:** Red blood cell cast in a patient with glomerulonephritis secondary to microscopic polyangiitis. (From Stone JH, Calabrese LH, Hoffman GS, et al. Vasculitis. A collection of pearls and myths. *Rheum Dis Clin North Am.* 2001;27:677. With permission.) **B:** Glomerular crescent in a patient with microscopic polyangiitis.

Alveolar hemorrhage, observed in up to 30% of patients, is associated with a worse prognosis. Interstitial fibrosis and pleuritis occur in some patients with MPA. Pulmonary fibrosis resembling usual interstitial pneumonitis in clinical presentation is increasingly recognized as a disease manifestation of MPA. Many cases of pulmonary fibrosis are associated with previous alveolar hemorrhage, but the precise relationship between alveolar hemorrhage and fibrosis is not clear.

3. Kidneys—Renal involvement is seen in at least 80% of patients with MPA. The classic presentation of renal disease in MPA is a rapidly progressive glomerulonephritis reminiscent of Wegener granulomatosis (Figure 34–2A). Some patients, however, have renal deterioration that progresses more slowly, over many months. Renal involvement may also present with urinary abnormalities such as proteinuria, microscopic hematuria, and red cell casts detected during investigation of other features of the illness. Up to 40% of patients have 24-hour uri-

nary protein excretion of more than 3 g. Proteinuria of this severity is regarded as a poor prognostic factor for renal outcome. The pathologic features of renal disease in MPA are indistinguishable from other forms of pauci-immune glomerulonephritis: namely a necrotizing, crescentic lesion (Figure 34–2B). Compared with biopsies from patients with ANCA directed against proteinase 3, those with MPO-ANCA have a more chronic pattern of renal injury, with more glomerulosclerosis, tubular atrophy, and interstitial fibrosis.

4. Nervous system—Vasculitic neuropathy may be a devastating complication of MPA. The nerve involvement typically occurs in the pattern of a distal, asymmetric, axonal polyneuropathy (mononeuritis multiplex). The first symptoms of vasculitic neuropathy are usually

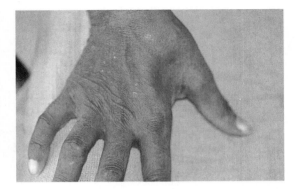

Figure 34–3. Muscle wasting caused by vasculitic neuropathy (mononeuritis multiplex) associated with microscopic polyangiitis.

sensory, with numbness, tingling, and dysesthesias. Muscle weakness and wasting follow the infarction of motor nerves (Figure 34–3). Recovery from vasculitic neuropathy may take months; some patients have residual nerve damage after the disease is controlled. Although peripheral nerve lesions tend to dominate the neurologic features of MPA, central nervous system involvement by vasculitis is also described in this disease.

5. Skin—The skin manifestations of MPA include all of the cutaneous lesions associated with small-vessel vasculitis (palpable purpura, papules, vesiculobullous lesions, and splinter hemorrhages). In the presence of medium-vessel involvement, ulcers, nodules, livedo reticularis, and digital gangrene may occur. As with most forms of cutaneous vasculitis, the lesions favor the lower extremities.

6. Musculoskeletal system—Nonspecific arthralgias and frank arthritis usually present early in the course of MPA and respond very quickly to therapy. Musculoskeletal symptoms may also herald disease flares. The arthritis of MPA is migratory in nature and may assume a variety of joint patterns, from a pauci-articular syndrome of large joints to a polyarthritis of small joints. Destructive joint lesions do not occur in MPA.

B. LABORATORY FINDINGS

The results of routine laboratory tests and specialized assays in MPA are shown in Table 34–3. All of these tests are appropriate at the initial evaluation in patients who demonstrate features consistent with MPA. The exclusion of renal disease through the careful performance of a urinalysis is essential in the evaluation and follow-up of all patients with MPA. The erythrocyte sedimentation rate and serum C-reactive protein level are useful in the longitudinal evaluation of disease activity. Positive ANCA assays are often instrumental in suggesting the diagnosis, but the titers of these antibodies correlate poorly

Table 34–3. The Laboratory Evaluation in Microscopic Polyangiitis

Test	Typical Result
Complete blood cell count	• Normochromic, normocytic anemia; acute, severe anemias possible in alveolar hemorrhage • Mild to moderate leukocytosis common, usually not exceeding 18×10^9/L • Moderate to pronounced thrombocytosis typical, ranging from platelet counts of 400×10^9/L to occasionally $>1000 \times 10^9$/L
Electrolytes	Hyperkalemia in the setting of advanced renal dysfunction
Liver function tests	Hepatic involvement unusual in MPA When present, there can be elevations of transaminases (AST/ALT) in excess of 1000 mg/dL
Urinalysis with microscopy	• Hematuria (ranging from mild to so high that red blood cells are too numerous to count) • Red blood cell casts • Proteinuria (nephritic range proteinuria in a small minority)
Erythrocyte sedimentation rate/C-reactive protein	• Dramatic elevations of acute phase reactants are typical, generally with good correlation to disease activity
ANA	Negative
Rheumatoid factor	Positive in 40–50% of patients, often leading to diagnostic confusion with rheumatoid arthritis
C3, C4	Usually normal (or increased, because complement proteins are acute phase reactants)
ANCA	Positive in 70% of patients with MPA (and probably a higher percentage of patients with generalized disease)
Anti-GBM	A small number of patients have both ANCA and anti-GBM antibodies

MPA, microscopic polyangiitis; AST/ALT, aspartate aminotransferase and alanine aminotransferase; ANA, antinuclear antibody; ANCA, antineutrophil cytoplasmic antibody; anti-GBM, antiglomerular basement membrane antibodies.

in time with disease flares. Moreover, approximately 30% of patients with MPA diagnosed on a clinical basis are ANCA-negative (see section on serologic testing, below). The diffusion capacity of carbon monoxide may be used as an indicator of alveolar hemorrhage, because bleeding into the alveoli leads to elevated diffusion capacity measurements. However, because of the increased sensitivity of thin-cut computed tomography scans, the diffusion capacity of carbon monoxide has largely been supplanted as a screen for active lung hemorrhage.

C. SPECIAL TESTS

1. Tissue biopsy—By definition, MPA involves small blood vessels: arterioles, venules, and capillaries. Glomerulonephritis is considered the renal equivalent of small-vessel vasculitis (akin to palpable purpura in the skin and capillaritis in the lung). Renal biopsy findings, although not specific for MPA, are sufficiently characteristic to establish the diagnosis in appropriate clinical settings. Immunofluorescence studies of renal biopsies in MPA confirm the "pauci-immune" nature of the renal involvement. MPA may also involve medium-sized arteries and veins, but such medium-vessel involvement is not essential to the diagnosis.

MPA is high on the differential diagnosis of leukocytoclastic vasculitis within the small blood vessels of skin lesions. The presence of extracutaneous findings and ANCA (particularly if directed against MPO) increases the likelihood of MPA. If sufficiently deep, skin biopsies may also demonstrate the involvement of medium-sized vessels in the deep dermis subcutaneous tissue layer. The finding of medium-vessel involvement eliminates certain forms of cutaneous vasculitis limited to small-vessel disease (eg, hypersensitivity vasculitis [cutaneous leukocytoclastic angiitis]) and Henoch-Schönlein purpura. The involvement of both veins and arteries distinguishes MPA from classic polyarteritis nodosa, which is confined to arterial lesions.

2. Nerve conduction studies—Nerve conduction studies are an important part of the work-up for patients with neuropathic symptoms. Nerve conduction studies may reveal the characteristic asymmetric, axonal sensorimotor neuropathy. Nerves such as the sural nerve, shown to be involved in this fashion are prime candidates for biopsy, with simultaneous sampling of adjacent muscle (eg, the gastrocnemius). In some cases, histopathology diagnostic of vasculitis is confined to the muscle as opposed to the nerve, or vice versa.

Although lung involvement can be a florid manifestation of MPA, demonstration of vasculitis on thoracoscopic or open lung biopsy is often challenging; frank capillaritis may be difficult to demonstrate. Nevertheless, lung biopsies are often essential to exclude other processes (eg, infections or malignancies) if no other tissue options exist for biopsy.

3. Serologic testing for ANCA—Three fourths of all patients with clinical diagnoses of MPA are ANCA-positive. A full discussion of ANCA is found in the chapter on Wegener granulomatosis (see Chapter 33). In MPA, the classic pattern of serum reactivity upon immunofluorescence testing (with human neutrophils as the substrate) is perinuclear staining (P-ANCA). In

Table 34–4. Differential Diagnosis of Microscopic Polyangiitis

Other vasculitides
Polyarteritis nodosa
Wegener granulomatosis
Churg-Strauss syndrome
Henoch-Schönlein purpura
Hypersensitivity vasculitis
Mixed cryoglobulinemia
Goodpasture disease
Giant cell arteritis
Drug-induced ANCA-associated vasculitis
Infections
Endocarditis
Pulmonary conditions
Interstitial pulmonary fibrosis
Idiopathic pulmonary hemosiderosis
Systemic autoimmune conditions
Systemic lupus erythematosus
Rheumatoid arthritis
Miscellaneous nonvasculitic conditions associated with P-ANCA
Inflammatory bowel disease
Autoimmune hepatitis
Sclerosing cholangitis

ANCA, antineutrophilic cytoplasmic antibody; P-ANCA, perinuclear antineutrophilic cytoplasmic antibody.

MPA, the P-ANCA pattern is usually caused by antibodies to MPO, a constituent of the primary granules of neutrophils. A variety of nonvasculitic conditions (Table 34–4) can also cause P-ANCA immunofluorescence, but these results are usually caused by antibodies to antigens not associated with vasculitis (eg, lactoferrin).

The combination of both a P-ANCA pattern on immunofluorescence testing and MPO-ANCA demonstrated by enzyme immunoassay has a high positive predictive value for ANCA-associated vasculitis, most commonly MPA. The other type of ANCA found in MPA is PR3-ANCA, directed against proteinase 3. This type of ANCA is usually associated with a cytoplasmic (C-ANCA) pattern of immunofluorescent staining. Despite advances in ANCA testing techniques, histopathology remains the cornerstone of diagnosis in MPA. When the diagnosis is unconfirmed, all reasonable attempts to obtain a "tissue diagnosis" should be pursued.

Differential Diagnosis

The greatest mimickers of MPA are other forms of vasculitis (see Table 34–4). Henoch-Schönlein purpura and hypersensitivity vasculitis (also known as cutaneous leukocytoclastic angiitis) can cause identical skin lesions, as can Wegener granulomatosis, the Churg-Strauss syndrome, mixed cryoglobulinemia, and polyarteritis nodosa. The delineation of MPA from these disorders comes from the pattern recognition of extracutaneous involvement (kidneys, lung, and nerve), the biopsy of involved organs, and ANCA testing. The difficulties of distinguishing MPA from Wegener granulomatosis and from polyarteritis nodosa are illustrated in Table 34–1. Goodpasture disease, which may present in an identical fashion, may benefit from plasmapheresis or plasma exchange in addition to glucocorticoids and cytotoxic agents. MPA may mimic temporal (giant cell) arteritis both clinically and pathologically (leading to lymphoplasmacytic infiltrates within the adventitia). In contrast to "true" temporal arteritis, MPA involving the temporal artery is not associated with giant cells. In addition, some medications, particularly propylthiouracil (used to treat thyroiditis), can cause a drug-induced ANCA-associated vasculitis associated with high titers of antibodies to MPO.

A variety of pulmonary, renal, and peripheral nerve disorders must be distinguished from MPA by imaging studies, tissue biopsy, nerve conduction studies, and serologic testing. Systemic autoimmune conditions such as systemic lupus erythematosus and rheumatoid arthritis are also prone to imitating MPA because of their abilities to involve multiple organ systems and cause positive P-ANCA results on immunofluorescence testing of serum (see above).

Treatment

The essentials of management for MPA are shown in Table 34–5. MPA is one of a handful of vasculitic conditions that usually requires both glucocorticoids and a cytotoxic agent to control. The usual regimen to induce remission in those patients with severe organ involvement includes high doses of prednisone (often preceded by a 3-day "pulse" of methylprednisolone, 1 g/d) plus cyclophosphamide. Cyclophosphamide may be adminis-

Table 34–5. Essentials of MPA Management

- Because most patients with MPA have major organ involvement such as glomerulonephritis, alveolar hemorrhage, or vasculitic neuropathy, the combination of cyclophosphamide and glucocorticoids is the cornerstone of most treatment regimens.
- Cyclophosphamide may be administered on either a daily or intermittent basis.
- "Pulse" methylprednisolone (1 g/d for 3 days) may be considered for patients with severe organ involvement at diagnosis.
- Altenative medications such as azathioprine or methotrexate should be considered after 3–6 months of cyclophosphamide therapy.

MPA, microscopic polyangiitis.

tered either daily (orally) or intermittently (eg, monthly). A meta-analysis of several small trials demonstrated no difference in the induction of remission between two basic cyclophosphamide regimens: intermittent treatments (eg, monthly intravenous pulse) versus daily therapy (smaller doses administered orally). The rate of relapse, however, appeared higher among patients treated with intermittent pulses. Both regimens of cyclophosphamide administration are successful in the induction of remission if used carefully. The important points are that the medication be used promptly when indicated, and with appropriate cautions (see section on cyclophosphamide in Chapter 67). All patients who are receiving treatment for MPA should be given either single-strength trimethoprim-sulfamethoxazole or 100 mg/d of dapsone as prophylaxis against *Pneumocystis jiroveci* (formerly *P carinii*) pneumonia.

Following the induction of remission, patients may be switched to either azathioprine (up to 2 mg/kg/d) or methotrexate (up to 25 mg/wk, assuming that residual renal dysfunction does not preclude this medication). The optimal duration of these remission maintenance agents is not clear. In general, the continuation of azathioprine or methotrexate for a period of 1 year after the achievement of remission is a reasonable recommendation.

Once the inflammatory process has been controlled with immunosuppressive therapy, primary care physicians may institute renal preservation therapies for patients with renal damage (blood pressure control, angiotensin-converting enzyme inhibition, and salt restriction).

Complications

If MPA is diagnosed early and treated promptly, patients have a high likelihood (>90%) of achieving disease remissions. Approximately one-third of patients suffer disease flares after the achievement of remission. In general, MPA is considered less likely than Wegener granulomatosis to flare. Unfortunately, significant damage frequently ensues before recognition of the disease. One study indicated that the 5-year renal survival for patients with this disease was only 55%, but this prognosis may have improved somewhat since the widespread availability of ANCA testing. The renal prognosis in MPA may be worse than that of Wegener granulomatosis, perhaps because of a greater likelihood of delay in diagnosis in MPA, attributable to the involvement of fewer organ systems. Another major disability associated with MPA results from nerve damage and consequent muscle weakness caused by vasculitic neuropathy. Finally, Wegener granulomatosis, closely related to MPA along the spectrum of ANCA-associated vasculitis, is now known to be associated with a high risk of venous thrombotic events. Heightened suspicion for this complication, possibly caused by involvement of the veins by the vasculitic process, should also be maintained in MPA.

REFERENCES

Goek ON, Stone JH. Randomized controlled trials in vasculitis associated with anti-neutrophil cytoplasmic antibodies. *Curr Opin Rheumatol.* 2005;17:257. [PMID: 15838233] (Review of recent major clinical trials in ANCA-associated vasculitis.)

Guillevin L, Durand-Gasselin B, Cevallos R, et al. Microscopic polyangiitis: clinical and laboratory findings in eighty-five patients. *Arthritis Rheum.* 1999;42:421. [PMID: 10088763] (Seventy percent of patients with microscopic polyangiitis are ANCA-positive, but only 12% have alveolar hemorrhage.)

Guillevin L, Lhote F. Treatment of polyarteritis nodosa and microscopic polyangiitis. *Arthritis Rheum.* 1998;41:2100. [PMID: 9870866] (Because of its propensity to cause glomerulonephritis, pulmonary hemorrhage, and other life- or organ-threatening complications, microscopic polyangiitis should be treated with cyclophosphamide and prednisone.)

Jennette JC, Falk RJ, Andrassy K, et al. Nomenclature of systemic vasculitides. Proposal of an international consensus conference. *Arthritis Rheum.* 1994;37:187. [PMID: 8129773] (This paper framed the current thinking about vasculitis classification, and clearly differentiated microscopic polyangiitis from classic polyarteritis nodosa.)

Relevant World Wide Web Sites

[The Johns Hopkins Vasculitis Center]
http://vasculitis.med.jhu.edu
[Vasculitis Clinical Research Consortium]
http://rarediseasesnetwork.epi.usf.edu/vcrc/

Churg-Strauss Syndrome

35

Philip Seo, MD, MHS, & John H. Stone, MD, MPH

ESSENTIALS OF DIAGNOSIS

- *Asthma, eosinophilia, and systemic vasculitis are the hallmarks of the Churg-Strauss syndrome.*
- *Classic clinical features include the following:*
  - *Allergic rhinitis and nasal polyposis.*
  - *Reactive airway disease.*
  - *Peripheral eosinophilia (10–60% of all circulating leukocytes).*
  - *Fleeting pulmonary infiltrates and occasional alveolar hemorrhage.*
  - *Vasculitic neuropathy.*
  - *Congestive heart failure.*
- *Approximately 50% of patients with Churg-Strauss syndrome have antineutrophil cytoplasmic antibodies (ANCAs), usually with a specificity for myeloperoxidase (MPO).*

General Considerations

In 1951, Churg and Strauss reported a series of 13 patients with "periarteritis nodosa" (see Chapter 36) who demonstrated severe asthma and an unusual constellation of other symptoms: "fever. . . hypereosinophilia, symptoms of cardiac failure, renal damage, and peripheral neuropathy, resulting from vascular embarrassment. . . ." The investigators termed this new disease "allergic angiitis and allergic granulomatosis," and specified three histologic criteria for the diagnosis: (1) the presence of necrotizing vasculitis, (2) tissue infiltration by eosinophils, and (3) extravascular granuloma.

In 1990, an American College of Rheumatology panel liberalized the criteria for the classification of this disease, dropping the requirements for histopathologically proven vasculitis and granuloma (Table 35–1). The Chapel Hill Consensus Conference on nomenclature of the vasculitides subsequently defined the Churg-Strauss syndrome (CSS) as a disorder characterized by eosinophil-rich, granulomatous inflammation of the respiratory tract and necrotizing vasculitis of small- to medium-sized vessels, associated with asthma and eosinophilia.

CSS is a rare disease—significantly more uncommon than the other forms of ANCA-associated vasculitis. The annual incidence of CSS is approximately 2.4 cases per million individuals. The distribution of cases is roughly equal between men and women. In recent years, associations between the use of leukotriene antagonists and CSS have been reported. Rather than causing the disease, however, it is more likely that these medications permit the tapering of glucocorticoids, thereby "unmasking" the vasculitic phase CSS.

Clinical Findings

A. SYMPTOMS AND SIGNS

After the diagnosis of CSS has been made, three disease phases are often recognizable:

- *Prodrome:* Characterized by the presence of allergic disease (typically asthma or allergic rhinitis). This phase often lasts for several years.
- *Eosinophilia/tissue infiltration:* Striking peripheral eosinophilia may occur. Tissue infiltration by eosinophils is observed in the lung, gastrointestinal tract, and other tissues.
- *Vasculitis:* Systemic necrotizing vasculitis affects a wide range of organs, ranging from the heart and lungs to the peripheral nerves and skin (Figure 35–1).

1. Nose and sinuses—Upper airway disease in CSS usually takes the form of nasal polyps or allergic rhinitis. A surprisingly high percentage of patients with CSS have histories of nasal polypectomies, usually long before suspicion of an underlying disease is raised. Although pansinusitis occurs frequently, destructive upper airway disease is not characteristic of CSS.

2. Ears—Middle ear granulation tissue with eosinophilic infiltrates occurs in some patients, leading to conductive hearing loss. Cases of sensorineural hearing loss have also been reported.

Table 35–1. American College of Rheumatology 1990 Criteria for the Classification of Churg-Strauss Syndrome[a]

Criterion	Definition
Asthma	History of wheezing or diffuse high-pitched rales on expiration
Eosinophilia	Eosinophilia >10% on white blood cell differential count
Mononeuropathy or polyneuropathy	Development of mononeuropathy, multiple mononeuropathies, or polyneuropathy (ie, stocking/glove distribution)
Pulmonary infiltrates, nonfixed	Migratory or transitory pulmonary infiltrates on radiographs
Paranasal sinus abnormality	History of acute or chronic paranasal sinus pain or tenderness, or radiographic opacification of the paranasal sinuses
Extravascular eosinophils	Biopsy including artery, arteriole, or venule, showing accumulations of eosinophils in extravascular areas

[a] To be classified as having Churg-Strauss syndrome, a patient must have at least four of these six criteria. Among patients with various forms of systemic vasculitis, the sensitivity of these criteria for the classification of an individual patient as having Churg-Strauss syndrome was estimated to be 85%. (Adapted from Masi AT, Hunder GG, Lie TT, et al. The American College of Rheumatology 1990 criteria for the classification of Churg-Strauss syndrome [allergic granulomatosis and angiitis]. *Arthritis Rheum.* 1990;33:1094. With permission.)

3. Lungs—More than 90% of patients with CSS have histories of asthma. Typically, the asthma represents either adult-onset reactive airway disease, or less commonly, a significant worsening of long-standing disease. Upon encroachment of the vasculitic phase of CSS, patients' asthma may improve substantially, even before therapy for vasculitis has begun. Following successful treatment of the vasculitic phase, however, glucocorticoid-dependent asthma persists in many patients.

The pathologic features of lung disease in CSS vary according to the disease phase. In the early phases, there may be extensive eosinophilic infiltration of the alveoli and interstitium. During the vasculitic phase, necrotizing vasculitis and granuloma may be evident. In the current era, when many patients with asthma are treated with varying doses of systemic glucocorticoids, lung biopsy specimens showing all three histologic hallmarks of this disease are unusual.

4. Peripheral nerves—Mononeuritis multiplex occurs with remarkable frequency in CSS, often with devastating effects. Vasculitic neuropathy was evident in 74 (77%) of the 96 patients in one series. Nerve infarctions may appear several weeks after the start of appropriate treatment, but do not always indicate the need to intensify therapy, particularly if patients are already on both high-dose prednisone and cyclophosphamide. This may be due to continued disease activity, but is more likely secondary to thrombosis of vessels that have become severely compromised by previously active inflammation. Nerve infarctions clinically are heralded by the abrupt occurrence of a foot drop, wrist drop, or some other focal nerve lesion. Muscle wasting secondary to nerve infarctions may continue to appear for weeks after the disease has been brought under control (Figure 35–2).

5. Heart—Cardiac involvement also occurs with a disproportionate frequency in CSS, and is a common cause of death. Some form of cardiac involvement occurred in 12.5% of patients in one large series. Congestive heart failure is the most common cardiac manifestation, although coronary arteritis and valvular abnormalities have also been reported.

6. Skin—Skin disease in CSS takes many forms, none of which is specific. Palpable purpura, papules, ulcers, and vesiculobullous lesions are common. Nodular skin lesions are usually "Churg-Strauss granuloma" (cutaneous extravascular necrotizing granuloma). These tend to occur on the extensor surfaces of the elbows and other pressure points. Skin biopsy specimens in CSS reveal eosinophilic infiltration of blood vessel walls. Splinter hemorrhages, digital ischemia, and gangrene associated with inflammation in medium-sized digital arteries are often present at the time of diagnosis.

7. Kidneys—CSS is less likely to cause end-stage renal disease than other forms of ANCA-associated vasculitis. When glomerulonephritis does occur, however, the histopathologic findings are often indistinguishable from those of other forms of pauci-immune vasculitis (eg, Wegener granulomatosis, microscopic polyangiitis, and renal-limited vasculitis).

8. Joints—Nonspecific arthralgias and frank arthritis often occur early in the course of CSS. The arthritis of CSS is migratory in nature and may assume a variety of joint patterns, from a pauciarticular syndrome of lower extremity joints to a polyarthritis of the small joints of the hands.

B. Laboratory Findings

Eosinophilia (before treatment) is a *sine qua non* of CSS. Eosinophil counts may comprise as much as 60% of the total white blood cell count. Eosinophil counts are usually sensitive markers of disease flares, but generally

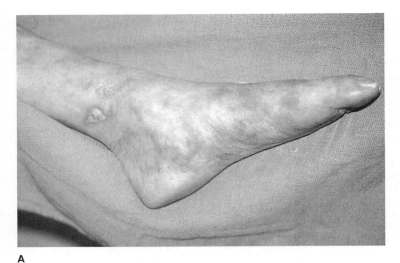

A

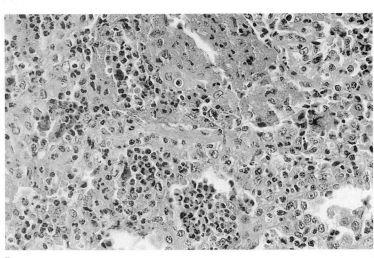

B

Figure 35–1. **A:** Foot of a patient with Churg-Strauss syndrome showing livedo reticularis and a cutaneous ulcer just superior to the medial malleolus. The patient's foot is held in extension because of a left foot drop (vasculitic neuropathy of the left peroneal nerve). **B:** Eosinophilic pneumonia in a patient with Churg-Strauss syndrome. Biopsy shows dense clusters of eosinophils within the lung parenchyma.

respond very quickly to treatment with high doses of glucocorticoids. Most patients with CSS also have elevated serum IgE levels. Serum complement levels are usually normal. Immune complexes are not believed to play a primary role in this disease. The erythrocyte sedimentation rate, serum C-reactive protein level, and eosinophil count can be useful in the longitudinal evaluation of disease activity. The reported percentages of CSS patients with ANCA are somewhat variable, with most figures in the literature in the range of 50% (see Chapter 33 on Wegener granulomatosis for a full discussion of ANCA). Antibodies to either proteinase-3 or MPO (but not to both) may be found. Of the two vasculitis-specific ANCAs, which include antibodies to MPO and

proteinase-3, those to MPO are more common in CSS. MPO-ANCAs usually produce a perinuclear-ANCA pattern on serum immunofluorescence testing. Patients who are ANCA-negative tend to have more cardiopulmonary complications, while patients who are ANCA-positive tend to have more of the classic vasculitic manifestations of this disease, although there is considerable overlap between these two groups.

C. IMAGING STUDIES

Pulmonary infiltrates are evident in approximately one-third of patients with CSS. These lesions are usually migratory infiltrates that occur bilaterally. Pulmonary hemorrhage is unusual, but has been reported. Nodular or

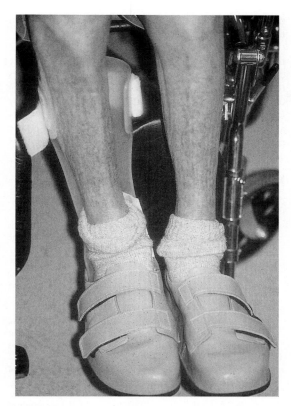

Figure 35–2. The ravages of vasculitic neuropathy. Bilateral ankle-foot orthoses are required because of bilateral foot drop. Note severe muscle wasting in both legs.

Table 35–2. Differential Diagnosis of the Churg-Strauss Syndrome

Eosinophilic Disorders	Other Vasculitides
Löffler syndrome	Wegener granulomatosis
Chronic eosinophilic pneumonia	Microscopic polyangiitis
Eosinophilic gastroenteritis	Polyarteritis nodosa
Hypereosinophil syndrome	Mixed cryoglobulinemia
Eosinophilic leukemia	Goodpasture syndrome
Eosinophilic fasciitis	

cavitary lesions suggest the alternative diagnoses of Wegener granulomatosis or an infection. Among patients with cardiac involvement, echocardiography may confirm poor cardiac function consistent with cardiomyopathy or demonstrate findings compatible with regional myocardial fibrosis.

Differential Diagnosis

The major disease entities in the differential diagnosis of CSS are shown in Table 35–2. There are many diseases in which patients occasionally demonstrate mild eosinophilia (eg, a peripheral blood eosinophilia on the order of 10% or so in asthma or parasitic infections). In contrast to CSS, however, only a handful of diseases can cause eosinophilia as high as 20–60%, as occasionally observed with CSS and its related conditions. *Strongyloides* infection, which can cause both high levels of eosinophilia and asthma, should be considered in endemic areas. CSS must also be distinguished from

other hypereosinophilic disorders: Löffler syndrome, chronic eosinophilic pneumonia, eosinophilic gastroenteritis, hypereosinophilic syndrome, eosinophilic fasciitis, and eosinophilic leukemia.

The fleeting pulmonary infiltrates of the Löffler syndrome and the peripheral infiltrates of chronic eosinophilic pneumonia may both mimic CSS closely.

However, differentiating CSS from hypereosinophilic syndrome may be the biggest challenge. Clinically, hypereosinophilic syndrome is rarely associated with reactive airway disease. Laboratory tests for the F1P1L1-PDGFR gene translocation or elevated serum tryptase levels (both of which are associated with hypereosinophilic syndrome) may also be helpful in the evaluation of such patients.

Many other forms of systemic vasculitis are high on the differential diagnosis for CSS. Wegener granulomatosis, polyarteritis nodosa, microscopic polyangiitis, Goodpasture syndrome (antiglomerular basement membrane disease), cryoglobulinemia, and other vasculitic disorders have clinical features that overlap with those of CSS. However, the finding of eosinophilia superimposed upon a history of allergy or asthma usually permits the clear distinction of CSS from these other disorders.

Treatment

In contrast to other forms of ANCA-associated vasculitis, many patients with CSS may be treated effectively with glucocorticoids alone. Nevertheless, certain disease complications, particularly the presence of vasculitic neuropathy or glomerulonephritis, should trigger the use of cyclophosphamide (2 mg/kg/d, decreased in the setting of renal dysfunction or advanced age) as part of the remission induction strategy. Cyclophosphamide should also be considered with other complications of CSS that pose immediate threats to the function of vital organs (eg, the heart). Appropriate cautions are paramount when using this medication (see Chapter 67). Whenever possible, the duration of cyclophosphamide therapy should be limited to 6 months or less. Milder cases may be treated with azathioprine (2 mg/kg/d), methotrexate

(15–25 mg/wk), or mycophenolate mofetil (2–3 g/d in divided doses) provided that appropriate precautions are observed (see Chapter 67). For patients whose disease remains active despite the combination of glucocorticoids and a cytotoxic agent, interferon-α has been used with some success in a limited number of cases, but may be difficult to tolerate. The bronchospastic component of this disease rarely responds to steroid-sparing agents, and should be managed with conventional bronchodilators, and if necessary, glucocorticoids.

Complications

Substantial morbidity and death may result from CSS. The major sources of morbidity are the disease itself and its therapies. Because the disease begins with a long prodrome of comparatively mundane problems (eg, atopic symptoms and asthma), the diagnosis is often overlooked until the occurrence of significant damage. The complications of vasculitic neuropathy are particularly devastating in this regard. Crippling nerve dysfunction occurs to varying degrees in all four distal extremities, leading to enormous disabilities. The recovery of function in infarcted nerves generally requires months, and in many cases the return of function is minimal. Recovery is likely dependent partly on the age of the patient and on the severity and extent of nerve damage.

Treatment regimens for CSS that include prolonged courses of high-dose glucocorticoids and (often) cyclophosphamide are associated with a high incidence of adverse effects, some of which may be permanent or fatal. Following the remission of vasculitis, many patients have persistent, glucocorticoid-dependent asthma. The long-term use of even moderately low-dose glucocorticoids brings many unwanted side effects. More dangerous, however, is the intensive immunosuppression associated with the combination of glucocorticoids and cytotoxic agents. Even with careful monitoring, opportunistic infections, myelosuppression, infertility, bladder toxicity, and (in the long term) an increased risk of certain malignancies are all major concerns.

Although clinical remissions may be obtained in more than 90% of patients with CSS, disease recurrences are common upon cessation of therapy. In the largest series reported to date, flares were detected in more than 25% of the patients. In most cases, relapses are heralded by the return of eosinophilia. In an even higher percentage of patients, following the resolution of the vasculitic phase of CSS, glucocorticoid-dependent asthma remains an issue requiring ongoing management.

REFERENCES

Churg A. Recent advances in the diagnosis of Churg-Strauss syndrome. *Mod Pathol.* 2001;14:1284. [PMID: 11743052] (Enlightened discussion of the pathologic approach to diagnosis in the modern era of glucocorticoid therapy and leukotriene antagonists.)

Guillevin L, Cohen P, Gayraud M, et al. Churg-Strauss syndrome. Clinical study and long-term follow-up of 96 patients. *Medicine (Baltimore)*. 1999;78:26. [PMID: 9990352] (Largest and most comprehensive clinical report on this disease to date.)

Sable-Fourtassou R, Cohen P, Mahr A, et al. Antineutrophil cytoplasmic antibodies and the Churg-Strauss syndrome. *Ann Intern Med.* 2005;143:632. [PMID: 16263885] (One of two recent manuscripts examining the relationship between ANCA-status and clinical manifestations of CSS.)

Masi AT, Hunder GG, Lie TT, et al. The American College of Rheumatology 1990 criteria for the classification of Churg-Strauss syndrome (allergic granulomatosis and angiitis). *Arthritis Rheum.* 1990;33:1094. [PMID: 2202307] (Discussion of clinical and laboratory features that distinguish CSS from other forms of vasculitis.)

Relevant World Wide Web Sites

[The Cleveland Clinic Foundation Center for Vasculitis]
http://www.clevelandclinic.org/arthritis/vasculitis/default.htm
[The Johns Hopkins Vasculitis Center]
http://vasculitis.med.jhu.edu
[Vasculitis Clinical Research Consortium]
http://rarediseasesnetwork.epi.usf.edu/vcrc/

Polyarteritis Nodosa

36

John H. Stone, MD, MPH

ESSENTIALS OF DIAGNOSIS

- *Subacute onset of constitutional complaints (eg, fever, weight loss, malaise, arthralgias), lower extremity nodules and ulcerations, mononeuritis multiplex, and intestinal angina (postprandial pain caused by the involvement of mesenteric vessels).*

- *Cutaneous polyarteritis nodosa (PAN) is a variant of the systemic disease in which vasculitis is limited to the skin, usually presenting as nodules that break down into ulcers.*

- *Angiogram or biopsy of an involved organ required for diagnosis.*

- *Angiography may reveal microaneurysms in the kidneys or gastrointestinal tract.*

- *Biopsies of the skin and peripheral nerves (with sampling of the adjacent muscle) are the least invasive ways of confirming the diagnosis histopathologically.*

General Considerations

Classic PAN is a disorder characterized by necrotizing inflammation of small or medium arteries that spares the smallest blood vessels (eg, arterioles or capillaries) and is not associated with glomerulonephritis. Two additional features that distinguish PAN from other forms of systemic vasculitis are confinement of the disease to the arterial rather than the venous circulation, and the absence of granulomatous inflammation.

Reported annual incidence rates of PAN range from 2–9 cases per million people per year. A higher incidence (77 cases per million) was reported in an Alaskan area hyperendemic for hepatitis B virus (HBV). With the availability of the HBV vaccine, however, the percentage of cases associated with HBV has declined substantially (now <10% of all cases in the developed world). PAN appears to affect men and women with approximately equal frequency and to occur in all ethnic groups.

Clinical Findings

A. SYMPTOMS AND SIGNS

PAN can involve virtually any organ system, with the exception of the lungs. The disease, however, demonstrates a predilection for certain organs, particularly the skin, peripheral nerves, gastrointestinal tract, and kidneys. A nearly universal complaint among patients is pain caused by myalgias, arthritis, peripheral nerve infarction, testicular ischemia, or mesenteric vasculitis.

1. Constitutional symptoms—Fevers are a common feature of PAN. The characteristics of the fever vary substantially among patients, ranging from periods of low-grade temperature elevation to spiking febrile episodes accompanied by chills. Tachycardia with or without fever may be another feature of PAN. Malaise, weight loss, and myalgias are also common.

2. Skin and joints—Vasculitis of medium-sized arteries may produce several types of skin lesions. These cutaneous findings include livedo reticularis, nodules, papules, ulcerations, and digital ischemia leading to gangrene. All of these findings or combinations of them may occur in the same patient. The livedo reticularis, which may have a diffuse distribution over the extremities and buttocks, does not blanch with the application of pressure to the skin. Nodules, papules, and ulcers tend to occur on the lower extremities, particularly near the malleoli, in the fleshy parts of the calf, and over the dorsal surfaces of the feet. Nodules frequently evolve into ulcerations that have scalloped borders (Figure 36–1) and heal with scarring. Although the principal skin manifestations relate to disease caused by arteritis in medium-sized muscular arteries and arterioles, crops of purpura (caused by the involvement of smaller blood vessels) occur in a minority of patients. Digital ischemia, often accompanied by splinter hemorrhages, sometimes leads to tissue loss. Arthralgias of large joints (knees, ankles, elbows, and wrists) occur in up to 50% of patients; however, true synovitis is seen in many fewer patients.

3. Peripheral nerves—Mononeuritis multiplex, the infarction of named nerves by inflammation in the vasa nervorum, occurs in approximately 60% of patients with PAN. The most commonly involved nerves are the sural, peroneal, radial, and ulnar. Vasculitic neuropathy tends

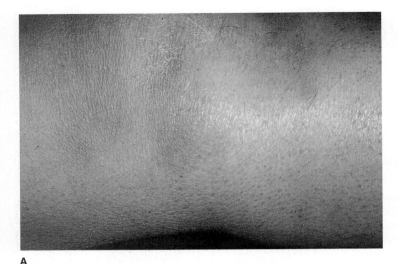

A

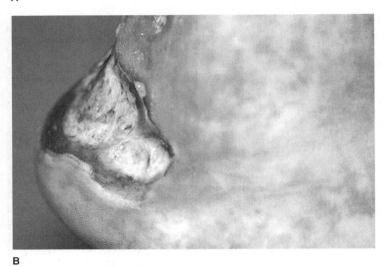

B

Figure 36–1. Cutaneous manifestations of polyarteritis nodosa. **A:** A nodular lesion. **B:** An ulcer with scalloped borders. (From Williams & Wilkins. With permission.)

to involve the longest (ie, distal) nerves first and usually begins asymmetrically. Thus the first motor symptoms of vasculitic neuropathy may be a foot or wrist drop (resulting from infarctions of the peroneal and radial nerves, respectively). In advanced stages, the neuropathy may mimic a confluent, symmetric polyneuropathy. Careful history taking, however, may unmask its initial asymmetry.

4. Gastrointestinal tract—The gastrointestinal manifestations of PAN occur in approximately half of all patients and are among the most challenging symptoms to diagnose correctly because of their nonspecific nature. Postprandial abdominal pain ("intestinal angina") is common. Involvement of the mesenteric arteries in PAN

may lead to the disastrous complications of mesenteric infarction or aneurysmal rupture, each of which is associated with a high mortality rate. Angiography of the mesenteric vessels reveals multiple microaneurysms (Figure 36–2A). These range in size from lesions that are barely visible to the naked eye to several centimeters in diameter. Sometimes PAN is detected at cholecystectomy or appendectomy in the absence of other disease manifestations. In such cases, surgical removal of the involved organ may be curative.

5. Intraparenchymal renal inflammation—This major feature of PAN is found in 40% of patients. The inflammatory process targets the renal and interlobar arteries (the medium-sized, muscular arteries within the

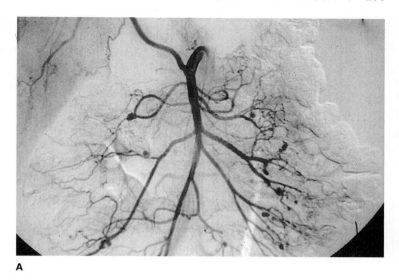

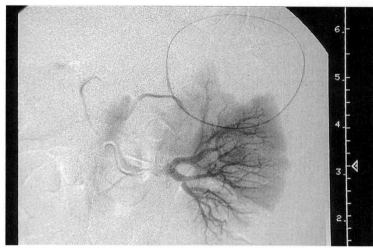

Figure 36–2. Angiographic features of polyarteritis nodosa. **A:** Mesenteric angiogram showing multiple microaneurysms. **B:** A wedge-shaped renal infarction. (From Elsevier. With permission.)

kidney) and occasionally also involves the smaller arcuate and interlobular arteries. Angiography may reveal microaneurysms within the kidney or large, wedge-shaped renal infarctions (Figure 36–2B). Renal artery involvement or involvement of intra-renal arterioles in PAN may lead to renin-mediated hypertension. Red blood cell casts on urinalysis imply glomerulonephritis and thus usually implicate another disease (eg, microscopic polyangiitis). However, both proteinuria and hematuria may be observed in PAN.

6. Cardiac symptoms—Patchy necrosis of the myocardium caused by subclinical arteriolar involvement is a frequent finding. Tachycardia may reflect either di-rect cardiac involvement or a general inflammatory state. Congestive heart failure and myocardial infarction sometimes occur. Specific heart lesions are rarely diagnosed while the patient is alive; however, autopsy series indicate that cardiac involvement is present in a majority of patients with PAN.

7. Miscellaneous—Central nervous system involvement occurs in a small percentage of patients with PAN. The usual presentations are encephalopathy and strokes. Renin-mediated hypertension may contribute to both of these neurologic complications. Other unusual presentations of PAN include involvement of the eyes (scleritis), pancreas, testicles, ureters, breasts, and ovaries.

B. LABORATORY FINDINGS

Although the laboratory features of PAN are often strikingly abnormal and help characterize the disease process as inflammatory, they do not distinguish PAN from a host of other inflammatory diseases. Anemia, thrombocytosis, and elevation of acute phase reactants are typical (Table 36–1). Erythrocyte sedimentation rate and C-reactive protein are often useful in longitudinal evaluations of disease activity but are imperfect for this purpose. Assays for antinuclear antibodies and rheumatoid factor are also generally negative in patients with PAN, but low titers of these antibodies are detected in a few patients. Patients with HBV-associated PAN are generally hypocomplementemic, regardless of whether they have demonstrable cryoglobulins. When associated with HBV, PAN usually develops within weeks to months of the acute viral infection.

When tested by immunofluorescence, the serum of some patients with PAN is positive for antineutrophil cytoplasmic antibodies (ANCAs). However, specific enzyme immunoassays for antibodies to proteinase-3 or myeloperoxidase (the two antigens known to be associated with systemic vasculitis) are negative. Thus, PAN is not considered to be an ANCA-associated vasculitis. The fact that PAN is "seronegative"—not associated with a particular autoantibody—is one of the issues that makes the disease so difficult to diagnose in many cases.

C. SPECIAL TESTS

The diagnosis of PAN requires either a tissue biopsy or an angiogram that demonstrates microaneurysms.

1. Biopsy—In the skin, medium-sized arteries lie within the deep dermis and in the subdermal adipose tissue. Thus, the diagnosis of PAN can be made by obtaining biopsy specimens of the skin that capture lobules of subcutaneous fat. Biopsies of nodules, papules, and ulcer edges have higher yields than biopsies of livedo reticularis. Nerve conduction studies are useful in detecting the typical axonal pattern of nerve injury and identifying involved nerves for biopsy. Because muscle tissue is highly vascular and may harbor involved vessels even in the absence of symptoms or signs of muscle involvement, biopsies of adjacent muscle should be performed simultaneously (eg, the gastrocnemius, if the sural nerve is biopsied). Blind biopsies of asymptomatic organs such as the testicle, however, are rarely diagnostic.

2. Angiography—PAN is a panarteritis characterized by transmural necrosis and a homogeneous, eosinophilic appearance of the blood vessel wall (fibrinoid necrosis). The cellular infiltrate is pleomorphic, with both polymorphonuclear cells and lymphocytes present in varying degrees at different stages. Degranulation of neutrophils within and around the arterial wall leads to leukocytoclasis. The vascular wall inflammation in PAN may be

Table 36–1. Laboratory and Radiologic Evaluation in PAN

Test	Typical Results
Complete blood cell count	• Normochromic, normocytic anemia. • Mild to moderate leukocytosis common, usually not exceeding 18×10^9/L. • Moderate to pronounced thrombocytosis typical, ranging from platelet counts of 400×10^9/L to occasionally >1000×10^9/L.
Renal function	Renal artery involvement may cause elevated serum creatinines, and occasionally, end-stage renal disease.
Serum hepatic transaminases	Hepatic artery involvement common in PAN. Can lead to mild to moderate elevations in serum hepatic transaminases.
Urinalysis with microscopy	• Hematuria (ranging from mild to severe). • Red blood cell casts suggest glomerulonephritis and are therefore atypical. • Proteinuria (nephritic range proteinuria distinctly unusual).
ESR/CRP	Dramatic elevations of acute phase reactants are typical. ESRs in excess of 100 mm/h are frequently found.
ANA	Negative.
Antiprecipitin antibodies (anti-Ro, -La, -Sm, -RNP)	Negative.
Rheumatoid factor	Negative.
C3, C4	Low in patients with PAN associated with HBV. In patients with idiopathic PAN, serum complement levels may be elevated (as acute phase reactants).
ANCA	Occasionally positive on immunofluorescence testing (low titers of perinuclear [P-ANCA] immunofluorescence, but specific antibodies to serine proteinase-3 and myeloperoxidases are negative).
Hepatitis B and C serologies	Hepatitis B causes a minority of cases (<10% in the developed world).
Chest radiography	Normal. PAN spares the lungs.

PAN, polyarteritis nodosa; ESR, erythrocyte sedimentation rate; CRP, C-reactive protein; ANA, antinuclear antibody; HBV, hepatitis B virus; ANCA, antineutrophil cytoplasmic antibody.

strikingly segmental, affecting only part of the circumference of a given artery. Segmental necrosis, in turn, leads to aneurysm formation. During later stages, complete occlusion may occur secondary to endothelial proliferation and thrombosis. Throughout involved tissues, the coexistence of acute and healed lesions is typical. Even in patients without gastrointestinal symptoms, mesenteric angiography may demonstrate telltale microaneurysms.

Differential Diagnosis

Even when flagrant inflammation is present, PAN may elude diagnosis for weeks or months. Except for evidence obtained from angiography or biopsy, the disease has no individual features that are pathognomonic. Many connective tissue diseases must be considered in the differential diagnosis of PAN (Table 36–2). However, systemic lupus erythematosus, mixed connective tissue disease, and undifferentiated connective tissue disorders usually can be distinguished from PAN by the presence of autoantibodies (eg, anti-Ro/SS-A, anti-La/SS-B, anti-Sm, and anti-RNP). These are absent in PAN.

In its early phases, rheumatoid arthritis may mimic PAN, but the arthritis of PAN is usually migratory and always nondestructive. Rheumatoid vasculitis, which has features very similar to PAN, almost always occurs in patients with severe, long-standing, destructive joint disease, not simultaneously with or before the arthritis. Similarly, although the fever pattern of PAN may recall Still disease, the evanescent, salmon-colored rash in that disorder is atypical of PAN. Moreover, diffuse polyarthritis develops in 95% of patients with Still disease within 1 year (or earlier) of disease onset. The catastrophic antiphospholipid syndrome, which causes digital ischemia, strokes, and other arterial thrombotic events, may be confused with PAN. However, venous events, which are even more common than arterial events in most patients with the antiphospholipid syndrome, are not characteristic of PAN.

The lack of pulmonary involvement in PAN helps distinguish it from most cases of ANCA-associated vasculitis. The occurrence of pulmonary lesions (pulmonary nodules, cavities, infiltrates, or alveolar hemorrhage) in combination with systemic vasculitis shifts the differential diagnosis in favor of other vasculitides, such as Wegener granulomatosis, microscopic polyangiitis, and Churg-Strauss syndrome. In addition, features of small-vessel disease (eg, purpura) are generally absent in PAN. Isolated peripheral nervous system vasculitis, a form of vasculitis that involves the peripheral nervous system alone, may mimic PAN and require similar therapy. In addition, in a subset of cases, the predominant features of PAN imitate the presentation of giant cell arteritis (eg, headache, jaw claudication, fever, and polymyalgias). Findings of histopathologic features of PAN on temporal artery biopsy specimens have been reported.

The multi–organ-system inflammatory nature of PAN may be mimicked by numerous bacterial, mycobacterial, or fungal infections. These must be excluded with great caution before beginning a treatment course for vasculitis. Finally, a host of other systemic or single-organ diseases may mimic PAN in their individual organ features. These include inflammatory bowel disease, sarcoidosis, erythema nodosum, atrophie blanche (livedoid vasculitis), cholesterol emboli, fibromuscular dysplasia, and malignancies (particularly lymphoma). PAN may occur as a complication of hairy cell leukemia.

Table 36–2. Differential Diagnosis of Polyarteritis Nodosa

Systemic disorders associated with autoimmunity
Systemic lupus erythematosus
Mixed connective tissue disease
Catastrophic antiphospholipid antibody syndrome
Rheumatoid arthritis (with rheumatoid vasculitis)
Still disease
Systemic vasculitides
Wegener granulomatosis
Microscopic polyangiitis
Churg-Strauss syndrome
Cryoglobulinemia
Isolated vasculitis of peripheral nerves
Infections
Endocarditis
Deep fungal infections (histoplasmosis, coccidioidomycosis, blastomycosis)
Miscellaneous
Inflammatory bowel disease
Sarcoidosis
Erythema nodosum
Atrophie blanche
Cholesterol emboli
Fibromuscular dysplasia
Lymphoma

Treatment

In patients with idiopathic PAN, glucocorticoids and cytotoxic agents remain the cornerstones of treatment. Approximately half of patients with PAN achieve remissions or cures with high doses of glucocorticoids alone. Cyclophosphamide (eg, 2 mg/kg/d orally or $0.6 \, g/m^2/mo$ intravenously, decreased in the setting of renal dysfunction) is indicated for patients whose disease is refractory to corticosteroids or who have serious involvement of major organs. Prophylaxis against *Pneumocystis jiroveci* (formerly *P carinii*) pneumonia is an important consideration in patients treated with these medications.

Treatment of HBV-associated PAN with immunosuppressive agents has deleterious long-term effects on the liver. Fortunately, the availability of effective antiviral agents has revolutionized the treatment of HBV-associated cases in recent years. One effective strategy involves the initial use of prednisone (1 mg/kg/d) to suppress the inflammation. Patients begin 6-week courses of plasma exchange (approximately three exchanges per week) simultaneously with the start of prednisone. The doses of glucocorticoids are tapered rapidly (over approximately 2 weeks), followed by the initiation of antiviral therapy (eg, lamivudine 100 mg/d)

Complications

Advanced mononeuritis multiplex can be a severely disabling problem from which recuperation is measured in months or years, if at all. Residual nerve dysfunction in the form of muscle weakness or painful neuropathy is common. The patient's ultimate degree of recovery is difficult to predict. The occurrence of bowel perforation and rupture of a mesenteric microaneurysm are potentially catastrophic events in PAN, requiring emergency surgical intervention and associated with high mortality rates. Patients treated with levels of immunosuppression required for PAN are at substantial risk for opportunistic infection and other complications of treatment (see

Chapter 67 sections about cyclophosphamide and glucocorticoids).

Prognosis

In contrast to the ANCA-associated vasculitides, which are more prone to recurrences, PAN is generally considered to be a "one-shot" disease. For patients with HBV-associated PAN, seroconversion to anti-HB$_e$ antigen antibody usually signals the end of the active phase of vasculitis. Among those with idiopathic PAN, disease recurrences are observed in perhaps 10% of cases.

REFERENCES

Colmegna I, Maldonado-Cocco JA. Polyarteritis nodosa revisited. *Curr Rheumatol Rep.* 2005;7:288. [PMID: 16045832]

Guillevin L, Mahr A, Callard P, et al. Hepatitis B virus-associated polyarteritis nodosa: clinical characteristics, outcome, and impact of treatment in 115 patients. *Medicine (Baltimore)* 2005;84:313. [PMID: 16148731]

Stone JH. Polyarteritis nodosa. *JAMA.* 2002;288:1632. [PMID: 12350194]

Relevant World Wide Web Sites

[The Johns Hopkins Vasculitis Center]
http://vasculitis.med.jhu.edu

[Vasculitis Clinical Research Consortium]
http://rarediseasesnetwork.epi.usf.edu/vcrc/

Mixed Cryoglobulinemia

Geetha Duvuru, MD & John H. Stone, MD, MPH

ESSENTIALS OF DIAGNOSIS

- *Vasculitis associated with mixed cryoglobulinemia (MC) involves both small- and medium-sized vessels. The skin is the most commonly involved organ.*
- *Other frequently affected organs include the joints, peripheral nerves, and kidneys. The central nervous system, gastrointestinal tract, and lungs are involved rarely or very rarely in MC.*
- *Virtually all patients are rheumatoid factor positive.*
- *Lower survival rates are observed with age over 60 years, male gender, and renal involvement.*

General Considerations

Cryoglobulins are immunoglobulins (Ig) that precipitate from the serum at low temperatures (see method of collection under Laboratory Findings). Cryoprecipitates are comprised most commonly of IgG and IgM (either singly, or in the case of mixed cryoglobulinemia, together). Occasionally IgA may be associated with clinically relevant cryoglobulin syndromes as well. Cryoglobulinemia is divided into three clinical subsets—types I, II, and III (Table 37–1)—based on two features: the clonality of the IgM component and the presence of rheumatoid factor (RF) activity. RF activity, by definition, is the reactivity of an IgM component with the Fc portion of IgG. This chapter focuses on cryoglobulinemia types II and III. (Type I cryoglobulinemia is usually not "mixed," being associated with only a monoclonal IgG or IgM in the setting of a malignancy.)

Formerly referred to as "essential" MC, hepatitis C virus (HCV) infections are now known to be associated with approximately 90% of all cases of MC. Latency periods of up to 15 years between the occurrence of HCV infection and the development of clinical signs of MC have been reported. In some cases, the presentation of HCV may be the development of the clinical features of MC (usually palpable purpura). Cryoglobulins also occur in the setting of other types of infections as well as in connective tissue disorders and hematopoietic malignancies.

The presence of cryoglobulins is not always associated with clinical disease, but these proteins may result in a wide variety of immune complex–mediated complications. The term "mixed cryoglobulinemia" was coined to differentiate types II and III (both of which contain mixtures of both IgG and IgM) from type I (which contains only a single monoclonal antibody).

When an underlying infection, autoimmune disorder, or malignancy can be identified, the preferred treatment approach is to direct therapy toward the underlying condition. Occasionally, in patients with rampant systemic vasculitis, generalized immunosuppression or measures designed to remove immune complexes (ie, plasmapheresis) may be required for limited periods.

Clinical Findings

The symptoms and signs of MC-associated vasculitis are caused by the vascular deposition of cryoprecipitate components. In type II MC, the cryoprecipitate contains polyclonal IgG, a highly restricted monoclonal IgM that has RF activity, low-density lipoprotein, and in cases of HCV-associated disease, HCV RNA. In general, the diagnosis of MC is made by some combination of the following: (1) recognition of a compatible clinical syndrome, accompanied nearly invariably by cutaneous vasculitis of small blood vessels (Figure 37–1); (2) isolation of cryoglobulins from serum; (3) detection of antibodies to HCV or HCV RNA; and (4) biopsy of other apparently involved organs as necessary to exclude other diagnoses. Because assays for cryoglobulins are not 100% sensitive and because HCV does not cause all cases of MC, all four of these conditions are not required.

A. SYMPTOMS AND SIGNS

1. Skin—A major hallmark of MC is a small-vessel vasculitis of the skin. Medium-vessel vasculitis may also be present, but this type of involvement generally does not occur without small-vessel disease. Biopsy of the skin with immunofluorescence studies shows an immune complex–mediated leukocytoclastic vasculitis, with deposition of IgG, IgM, C3, and other immunoreactants in and around the walls of small- and medium-sized vessels.

Table 37–1. Types of Cryoglobulinemia

Subtype	Rheumatoid Factor Positivity	Monoclonality	Associated Diseases
Type I	No	Yes (IgG or IgM)	Hematopoietic malignancy (multiple myeloma, Waldenström macroglobulinemia)
Type II	Yes	Yes (polyclonal IgG, monoclonal IgM)	Hepatitis C (other infection, Sjögren syndrome, systemic lupus erythematosus)
Type III	Yes	No (polyclonal IgG and IgM)	Hepatitis C (other infection, Sjögren syndrome, systemic lupus erythematosus)

Vascular thrombi are also prominent in many cases. Palpable purpura with a predilection for the lower extremities is the typical skin rash, but the rash is also found sometimes on the upper extremities, trunk, or buttocks. In addition, a host of other types of vasculitic rashes may be encountered, depending on the size of blood vessel involved. Such findings may include macules, papules, vesiculobullous lesions, urticarial lesions in the setting of small-vessel involvement, and ulcers above the malleoli—potentially extensive—in the context of medium-vessel disease.

2. Rheumatologic—Arthralgias are a prominent symptom in most cases of MC. The typically involved joints are the proximal interphalangeal and metacarpophalangeal joints and the knees. Frank arthritis is much less common than arthralgias but does occur. When present, the arthritis of MC is nondeforming. Raynaud phenomenon and acrocyanosis may also complicate MC.

3. Peripheral nerve—In the peripheral neuropathy of MC, sensory involvement predominates over motor nerve disease. The typical presentation is an axonal sensory neuropathy, associated with pain and paresthesias for years before the development of motor deficits. Motor mononeuritis multiplex may also occur, but never in the absence of sensory symptoms. HCV-induced vasculitis of the vasa nervorum is the pathogenetic mechanism of this peripheral nerve dysfunction.

4. Kidney—Renal involvement is present in up to 20% of patients at diagnosis. The most frequent manifestations are asymptomatic microscopic hematuria, proteinuria, and variable degrees of renal insufficiency. A small proportion may present as acute nephrotic syndrome and acute nephritic syndrome. The most frequent histologic picture is membranoproliferative glomerulonephritis, which can mimic lupus nephritis. Three specific histologic findings serve to distinguish glomerulonephritis secondary to mixed cryoglobulinemia: intraluminal thrombi composed of precipitated cryoglobulins; diffuse IgM deposition in the capillary loops; and subendothelial deposits presenting a crystalloid aspect on electron microscopy. MC-related renal disease may lead to nephrotic-range proteinuria, but progression to end-stage renal disease is uncommon. Rapidly progressive glomerulonephritis occurs in only a small number of patients.

5. Liver—Although HCV is obviously a hepatotropic virus, the clinical manifestations of liver disease in MC are few. Moreover, correlations between clinical liver disease and histology are poor. Most patients with HCV-related MC have various degrees of periportal inflammation, fibrosis, and even cirrhosis on liver biopsy. The formation of lymphoid follicles in the liver is a characteristic histologic feature of chronic HCV infection. Within these follicles (and in the bone marrow), most of the IgM RF is formed. Immunophenotyping of mononuclear cells within liver biopsy specimens from patients with HCV-associated MC reveals that they are mostly B cells that express IgM.

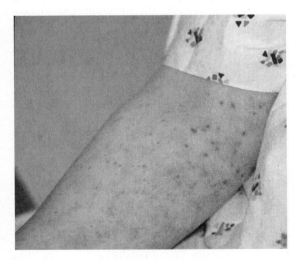

Figure 37–1. Small- and medium-vessel vasculitis in a patient with mixed cryoglobulinemia. Palpable purpura, a feature of small-vessel vasculitis, coexists with florid livedo reticularis, a manifestation of medium-vessel disease.

6. Hematopoietic system—In many cases, MC is truly a lymphoproliferative condition. In addition to its hepatotropism, HCV also tends to infect lymphocytes. Infection of these cells often leads to lymphoproliferation and a type III (polyclonal) MC. If a dominant B-cell clone emerges, a type II (monoclonal) MC is produced. In some cases, the emergence of a dominant B-cell clone results from a genetic alteration that favors B-cell survival, eg, a *bcl-2* gene mutation (translocation of the *bcl-2* gene from chromosome 18 to chromosome 14). Such a mutation leads to overexpression of the antiapoptotic *bcl-2*. B-cell lymphoma is the most frequent form of malignancy complicating MC. Hepatocellular carcinoma is also found with an increased incidence among patients with MC, almost certainly related to the effects of underlying viral hepatitis infections in most cases.

7. Central nervous system—Central nervous system disease in MC usually results from hyperviscosity and symptoms secondary to "sludging" of blood within the brain. Hyperviscosity, a rare complication of types II or III MC, is more common in type I cryoglobulinemia, a condition in which the cryoglobulin levels are often substantially higher. The occurrence of a hyperviscosity syndrome is an indication for plasmapheresis. In addition to hyperviscosity syndromes, true central nervous system vasculitis also occurs in a very small number of patients with MC.

8. Gastrointestinal tract—Clinically evident gastrointestinal tract involvement is uncommon, but patients with MC present occasionally with acute abdomen. Acute cholecystitis and mesenteric vasculitis secondary to MC have both been reported.

9. Miscellaneous organ involvement in MC—Pulmonary disease, consisting chiefly of interstitial lung lesions, has been described in MC. This manifestation remains poorly understood; cases are usually mild or even asymptomatic. Dryness of the mouth and eyes caused by lymphocytic salivary gland infiltration is not uncommon in MC. This type of organ involvement occurs in the absence of specific serologic evidence of Sjögren syndrome, ie, the finding of anti-Ro/SS-A or anti-La/SS-B antibodies. Bilateral parotid swelling and lymphadenopathy have also been described.

B. LABORATORY FINDINGS

MC is associated with a number of laboratory findings that offer clues to the diagnosis. These tests are of limited value in the assessment of disease activity, however, because in general their levels correlate very poorly with disease. An overview of laboratory test results is shown in Table 37–2.

1. Cryoglobulins—Assays for cryoglobulins are associated with a high false-negative rate, caused principally

Table 37–2. Laboratory and Radiologic Evaluation in Possible Mixed Cryoglobulinemia (MC)

Test	Typical Results
Complete blood cell count	Mild anemia common. Thrombocytopenia may be present if liver disease is advanced.
Renal and hepatic function	Renal function may be impaired in patients with glomerulonephritis. Hepatic dysfunction often subclinical but evident in most cases on liver biopsy. Liver transaminases may be normal.
Urinalysis with microscopy	Abnormal in cases with renal involvement. Proteinuria may reach nephritic range.
Erythrocyte sedimentation rate/C-reactive protein	Moderate to severe elevations common, generally reflecting disease activity when very high.
ANA	Positive in the majority of cases.
Rheumatoid factor	Positive in types II and III.
C3, C4	Low, particularly C4 levels.
ANCA	Negative.
Hepatitis B and C serologies	Hepatitis C serologies positive in approximately 90% of patients.
Antiphospholipid antibodies	Negative rapid plasma reagin and anticardiolipin antibody assays. Normal Russell viper venom time (for lupus anticoagulant).
Blood cultures	Negative.

ANA, antinuclear antibody; ANCA, antineutrophil cytopiasmic antibody.

by insufficient care in handling. After phlebotomy, the blood sample must be transported to the laboratory at 37°C and allowed to clot at that same temperature. Specimens are then centrifuged at 37°C and stored at 4°C for up to 1 week. The presence of cryoglobulins is indicated by the development of a white precipitate at the bottom of the tube.

2. Cryocrit—The percentage of serum comprised by cryoglobulins may be determined by the centrifugation of serum at 4°C. The cryocrit may then be measured in precisely the same fashion as a hematocrit. As with other laboratory indicators, the cryocrit correlates poorly with clinical status and treatment. Cryocrit levels should not dictate therapeutic decisions, which are driven more appropriately by the clinical condition of the patient.

3. Hypocomplementemia—Because complement proteins are involved in the formation of immune complexes, C3 and C1q are often found on specific immunofluorescence testing of biopsy specimens. Serum complement levels—C3, C4, and CH50—are also low in MC. The finding of a very low serum C4 level in the setting of a normal or only moderately reduced level of C3 is a strong clue to the presence of MC.

4. Rheumatoid factor positivity—Eighty percent of the monoclonal IgMs found in HCV-associated MC share a major complementarity region termed "WA." ("WA" refers to the initials of the patient in whom it was initially reported.) This cross idiotype has a high degree of RF activity. Virtually all patients with type II MC are RF positive.

5. Anti-HCV antibodies and quantification of HCV RNA—Anti-HCV assays are typically performed by enzyme immunoassay or immunoblotting. Levels of HCV RNA may be used to follow the treatment response to specific antiviral therapies. HCV genotyping may also be performed by polymerase chain reaction, but no specific viral genotype has been associated with a predisposition to the development of MC.

Differential Diagnosis

MC develops in up to one-third of patients with Sjögren syndrome, but manifestations of vasculitis are present in only a small subset of these patients. Clinical and laboratory features of MC and Sjögren syndrome also overlap. In both disorders, patients may have sicca symptoms of the eyes and mouth and have RF, antinuclear antibodies, and hypocomplementemia. In general, patients with MC not associated with SS do not have antibodies to the Ro- and La-antigens.

Patients with systemic lupus erythematosus and MC patients share tendencies for antinuclear antibody positivity and hypocomplementemia, as well as the clinical features of Raynaud phenomenon, joint complaints, and an immune complex–mediated glomerulonephritis. The two disorders are usually distinguishable through the presence of other clinical and laboratory features (eg, specific antibody testing for antibodies to double-stranded DNA or precipitins). Some patients with systemic lupus erythematosus have positive test results for cryoglobulins, but the attribution of disease to these proteins in the setting of systemic lupus erythematosus is often difficult. RF positivity and joint complaints among patients with MC often lead to the misdiagnosis of rheumatoid arthritis. True synovitis in MC is the exception, however, and when MC is associated with arthritis the joint disease is nondestructive.

Other forms of systemic vasculitis must also be distinguished from MC. There may be considerable overlap in the clinical features of polyarteritis nodosa (see Chapter 36), microscopic polyangiitis (see Chapter 34), Wegener granulomatosis (see Chapter 33), and Henoch-Schönlein purpura (see Chapter 40). The reader is referred to these specific chapters for further details.

Treatment

Although certain laboratory tests (see above) are useful in making the diagnosis, there remain no laboratory values—apart from acute phase reactants such as the erythrocyte sedimentation rate and C-reactive protein levels—that are generally reliable in attempts to ascertain levels of disease activity. As a rule, treatment decisions must be based on the presence of other clinical manifestations of the disease and on the determination by the physician that the symptoms or signs are the result of active disease rather than damage.

MC is characterized by periods of remission and exacerbation. There is also a wide range of disease severity, from mild purpura to severe necrotizing vasculitis. Consequently, all treatment decisions must be individualized based on the patient's particular circumstances, considerations of organs at risk, and the potential for adverse effects of therapy. The tendency for cutaneous vasculitis to develop in dependent areas may be exacerbated by venous stasis. Support stockings may reduce the number of cutaneous vasculitis flares.

Under ideal circumstances, the treatment of MC is based on the identification and treatment of the underlying cause, such as a viral infection. For HCV, the sustained response rates to interferon-α are poor (15–20%) but improved somewhat by the addition of ribavirin. Pegylated preparations of interferon-α are more effective for the treatment of HCV, and presumably therefore for HCV-associated MC as well. Pegylated interferon-α and ribavirin currently comprise the therapeutic regimen of choice in patients with HCV who require therapy.

When direct antiviral approaches are not possible or not sufficiently effective, treatment options include nonsteroidal anti-inflammatory drugs for arthralgias and arthritis, low-dose glucocorticoids for cutaneous vasculitis and peripheral neuropathy, and higher-dose glucocorticoids plus cytotoxic therapy for necrotizing vasculitis involving vital organs in a dangerous fashion. Patients with severe necrotizing vasculitis may also benefit from plasmapheresis. Based on the demonstration of B-cell clonal expansion in MC, innovative strategies have been proposed. Rituximab, an anti-CD20 monoclonal antibody, modifies the dynamics of B cells by deleting expanded clones and may protect against factors potentially involved in the pathogenesis of malignant B-cell transformation. Because of heightened rates of viral replication among patients treated with immunosuppression, these treatment approaches should be used for circumscribed periods.

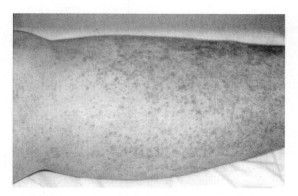

Figure 37–2. Hyperpigmentation of the lower extremities resulting from recurrent bouts of purpura in a patient with mixed cryoglobulinemia.

Complications

Hyperpigmentation over the involved areas of skin often develops in patients with long-standing, recurrent cutaneous vasculitis (Figure 37–2). Cutaneous ulcers may heal with scarring. End-stage renal disease results in glomerulonephritis in a small number of patients, particularly those who are not treated adequately. Vasculitic neuropathy may lead to permanent sensory or motor neurologic sequelae. In 10% or less of type II MC cases, the disease evolves into a malignant B-cell lymphoma. The portion of HCV-related non-Hodgkin lymphomas ranges widely in different studies, from 0% to 40%. Low-grade B-cell lymphomas may regress with effective treatment of the underlying HCV infection (ie, interferon), but high-grade malignancies require chemotherapy.

REFERENCES

Della Rossa A, Tavoni A, Baldini C, Bombardieri S. Treatment of chronic hepatitis C infection with cryoglobulinemia. *Curr Opin Rheumatol.* 2002;14:231. [PMID: 11981318] (Aggressive use of cytotoxic agents is discouraged in favor of treatments related to the underlying cause, eg, HCV.)

Ferri C, Sebastiani M, Giuggioli D, et al. Mixed cryoglobulinemia: demographic, clinical and serologic features and survival in 231 patients. *Semin Arthritis Rheum.* 2004;33:355. (The risk of death was three times higher among MC patients with renal disease than among those without. The most common causes of death in MC were nephropathy [33%], malignancies [23%], liver disease [13%], and diffuse vasculitis [13%].)

Kjaergard LL, Krogsgaard K, Gluud C. Interferon alfa with or without ribavirin for chronic hepatitis C: systematic review of randomized trials. *BMJ* 2001;323:1151. [PMID: 11711405] (Compared with interferon-α alone, the combination of that agent plus ribavirin reduced the risk of not having a sustained virologic response for 6 months by 26% in naïve patients, 33% in relapsers, and 11% in previous nonresponders.)

Sansonno D, Dammacco F. Hepatitis C virus, cryoglobulinemia, and vasculitis: immune complex relations. *Lancet Infect Dis.* 2005;5:227. (B-cell clonal expansion, which occurs primarily in the liver, correlates with intrahepatic viral load.)

Relevant World Wide Web Sites

[The Johns Hopkins Vasculitis Center]
http://vasculitis.med.jhu.edu

Hypersensitivity Vasculitis

John H. Stone, MD, MPH

ESSENTIALS OF DIAGNOSIS

- *Small-vessel vasculitis of the skin, with no apparent involvement of other organs (with the exception of joint symptoms in many patients).*
- *Known by a variety of other names, including cutaneous leukocytoclastic angiitis.*
- *Primary forms of vasculitis such as Henoch-Schönlein purpura, microscopic polyangiitis, or Wegener granulomatosis must be excluded. Similarly, well-recognized forms of secondary vasculitis such as mixed cryoglobulinemia caused by hepatitis C must also be eliminated from the differential diagnosis.*
- *Precipitants such as medications and infections are often identifiable, but approximately 40% of cases have no definable cause.*
- *Most cases are self-limited if the precipitant can be identified and removed. Colchicine, dapsone, or glucocorticoids are required in other cases.*

General Considerations

Hypersensitivity vasculitis refers to small-vessel vasculitis that is restricted to the skin and not associated with any other form of primary or secondary vasculitis. Implicit in this definition is that the condition is not associated with medium- or large-vessel disease at other sites, nor with small-vessel disease in other organs (eg, the glomeruli or pulmonary capillaries). In many cases, an identifiable precipitant such as a drug or an accompanying infection is present—hence the term "hypersensitivity." In up to 40% of cases, however, no specific cause is identified.

The term "hypersensitivity vasculitis" has been associated with much confusion ever since it was incorporated into the first vasculitis classification scheme in the early 1950s. The condition's name derives from the fact that by the 1950s, both human and animal models of hypersensitivity to foreign antigens had been shown to cause small-vessel vasculitis involving the kidneys, lungs, and other organs besides the skin. Consequently, even microscopic polyangiitis (see Chapter 34), a disorder that commonly affects internal organs as well as the skin and is often associated with antineutrophil cytoplasmic antibodies, was grouped initially under the heading of hypersensitivity vasculitis. Because of the confusion surrounding its name, many clinicians have suggested that hypersensitivity vasculitis be replaced, but no entirely suitable alternative has been found. Terms used synonymously with hypersensitivity vasculitis have included **leukocytoclastic vasculitis, cutaneous leukocytoclastic angiitis,** and **cutaneous small-vessel vasculitis,** among others. In evaluating patients with small-vessel vasculitis of the skin, it is critical to remember that skin findings may only herald an underlying disorder involving other organs, as well. Extracutaneous involvement, which mandates reconsideration of the diagnosis, must be excluded with appropriate tests.

In most cases of hypersensitivity vasculitis, the problem is believed to have an immune complex–mediated pathophysiology. Histopathology generally shows a leukocytoclastic vasculitis, with features of necrosis in some cases but not granulomatous inflammation. Biopsies very early in the course of disease may show a lymphocytic predominance.

Clinical Findings

Table 38–1 outlines the classification criteria for hypersensitivity vasculitis established in 1990 by the American College of Rheumatology.

A. Symptoms and Signs

1. Skin—The lesions of small-vessel vasculitis of the skin include purpura (either palpable or nonpalpable) (Figure 38–1), papules, urticaria/angioedema, erythema multiforme, vesicles, pustules, ulcers, and necrosis. The lesions typically occur first and most prominently in dependent regions, ie, the lower extremities or buttocks. The lesions tend to occur in cohorts or "crops" that are the same age. The occurrence of the lesions may be asymptomatic but is usually accompanied by a burning or tingling sensation.

2. Joints—Hypersensitivity vasculitis is sometimes accompanied by arthralgias and even frank arthritis, with a predominance for large joints.

Table 38–1. American College of Rheumatology 1990 Criteria for the Classification of Hypersensitivity Vasculitis[a]

1. Age at disease onset >16 years
2. Medication at disease onset
3. Palpable purpura
4. Maculopapular rash
5. Biopsy including arteriole and venule, showing granulocytes in a perivascular or extravascular location

[a]For purposes of classification, hypersensitivity vasculitis may be diagnosed if the patient meets at least three of these five criteria. Sensitivity = 71%; specificity = 83.9%.
(From Calabrese LH, Michel BA, Bloch DA, et al. The American College of Rheumatology 1990 criteria for the classification of hypersensitivity vasculitis. *Arthritis Rheum.* 1990;33;1108. With permission.)

B. LABORATORY FINDINGS

The results of routine laboratory tests and more specialized assays in hypersensitivity vasculitis are shown in Table 38–2. All of these tests are appropriate at the time of initial patient evaluation, primarily for the purpose of excluding other forms of vasculitis that may mimic hypersensitivity vasculitis.

C. SPECIAL TESTS

1. Biopsy—The pleiomorphic lesions of cutaneous vasculitis and the large number of vasculitis mimickers make histopathologic confirmation of the diagnosis by skin biopsy important in most cases. A biopsy specimen of an active lesion (<48 hours old, if possible) usually demonstrates leukocytoclastic vasculitis of the postcapillary venules. Direct immunofluorescence studies show variable quantities of immunoglobulin and complement deposition, with a nondiagnostic pattern. The perfor-

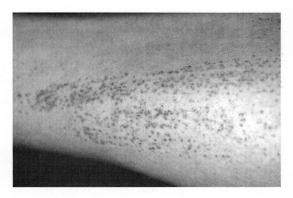

Figure 38–1. Palpable purpura.

Table 38–2. Laboratory and Radiographic Work-up of Patients with Possible Hypersensitivity Vasculitis

Test	Typical Result
Complete blood cell count, with differential	Normal
Electrolytes	Normal
Liver function tests	Normal
Urinalysis with microscopy	Normal
Erythrocyte sedimentation rate/ C-reactive protein	Mild to moderate elevations in <50% of patients
ANA	Negative
Rheumatoid factor	Negative
C3, C4	Normal
ANCA	Negative
Antihepatitis B and C assays	Negative
Cryoglobulins	Negative
Chest radiography	Normal

ANA, antinuclear antibody; ANCA, antineutrophil cytoplasmic antibody.

mance of direct immunofluorescence studies, however, is an important (and often neglected) part of the work-up, critical for the exclusion of Henoch-Schönlein purpura, cryoglobulinemia, and other conditions.

Differential Diagnosis

The differential diagnosis of hypersensitivity vasculitis is shown in Table 38–3. Hypersensitivity vasculitis must be distinguished primarily from other small-vessel vasculitides, from autoimmune inflammatory conditions

Table 38–3. Differential Diagnosis of Hypersensitivity Vasculitis

Other vasculitides
Henoch-Schönlein purpura
Microscopic polyangiitis
Churg-Strauss syndrome
Wegener granulomatosis
Mixed cryoglobulinemia
Polyarteritis nodosa

Systemic autoimmune conditions
Systemic lupus erythematosus (including urticarial vasculitis)
Rheumatoid arthritis

Miscellaneous
Acute hemorrhagic edema of infancy
Other types of drug eruptions

associated with joint disease and rashes, and from other cutaneous reactions to medications.

Treatment

Treatment strategies for hypersensitivity vasculitis are largely empiric. The type, intensity, and duration of therapy are based on the degree of disease severity in individual cases. For patients in whom a precipitant can be identified, removal of the offending agent usually leads to resolution of the vasculitis within days to weeks. Mild cases may be treated simply with leg elevation and the administration of nonsteroidal anti-inflammatory drugs (or H_1 antihistamines). For persistent disease that does not lead to cutaneous ulcers or gangrene, colchicine (0.6 mg two or three times daily), hydroxychloroquine (200 mg twice daily), or dapsone (100 mg/d) may be used. For refractory or more severe cases, immunosuppressive agents may be indicated, generally beginning with a moderate dose of glucocorticoids (eg, prednisone 20–40 mg/d). When a patient cannot tolerate a glucocorticoid taper over weeks or even several months, the addition of an immunosuppressive agent may be necessary. Azathioprine (2 mg/kg/d) is used most commonly for this purpose (see Chapter 67 for appropriate precautions before prescribing this drug).

Complications

Most cases with a clearly identified precipitant resolve over 1–4 weeks, often with some residual hyperpigmentation or (in the case of ulcerated lesions) scars. Some patients, however, have recurrent disease that remains confined to the skin and requires prolonged therapy.

REFERENCES

Fiorentino D. Cutaneous vasculitis. *J Am Acad Dermatol.* 2003;48: 311. [PMID: 12637912] (A comprehensive review that places hypersensitivity vasculitis in the context of other causes of small-vessel vasculitis of the skin.)

Relevant World Wide Web Sites

[The Johns Hopkins Vasculitis Center]
http://vasculitis.med.jhu.edu
[The Cleveland Clinic Foundation Center for Vasculitis]
http://www.clevelandclinic.org/arthritis/vasculitis/default.htm

Behçet Disease

David B. Hellmann, MD

ESSENTIALS OF DIAGNOSIS

- *Recurrent attacks of oral aphthous ulcers, genital ulcers, uveitis, and skin lesions.*
- *Onset usually in young adults, aged 25–35 years.*
- *Prevalent in parts of Asia and Europe; rare in North America.*
- *Blindness, central nervous system disease, and large-vessel events are the most serious complications.*
- *Glucocorticoids, immunosuppressive drugs, or both are required for severe disease.*

General Considerations

Behçet disease, a form of vasculitis of unknown cause, is named for the Turkish dermatologist who in 1937 described the syndrome as a triad of recurrent oral aphthous ulcers, genital ulcers, and ocular inflammation. Although these features are often the most salient, Behçet disease can cause inflammation in almost any organ. Indeed, involvement of the central nervous system, gastrointestinal tract, and large vessels can be life-threatening. Except for eye disease, most of the manifestations of Behçet disease do not persist chronically but recur in attacks, which usually become less frequent over time. Disability stems most often from ocular inflammation, which causes blindness, and less often from central nervous system disease. Mortality results chiefly from major vascular events, including thrombosis, aneurysm, and rupture of large vessels.

Epidemiology

One of the most striking features of Behçet disease is how common it is in countries along the ancient Silk Road and how rarely it develops elsewhere. Most prevalent in Turkey (up to nearly 400 cases per 100,000 people), Behçet disease also occurs frequently in Iran, Saudi Arabia, Greece, Japan, Korea, and China. In contrast, Behçet disease rarely develops in Western countries such as the United States, where the disease affects about 1 out of every 170,000 people.

Behçet disease is chiefly a disease of young people; typically, patients are in their 20s or 30s when symptoms first develop. Although males are more commonly affected than females in the Middle Eastern countries, female patients predominate in Japan.

Etiology & Pathogenesis

Although the cause of Behçet disease is unknown, the distinct geographic clustering of cases suggests the importance of environment, genes, or both. Genetic studies have revealed a strikingly high prevalence of the human leukocyte antigen (HLA)-B51 allele in patients living along the Silk Road, reaching nearly 80% of Asian patients. However, this allele is not associated with Behçet disease in Western countries.

Much of the damage in Behçet disease results from blood vessel inflammation, justifying the disease's classification as a form of vasculitis. Although Behçet disease typically affects the small- and medium-sized vessels, it is one of the rare forms of vasculitis capable of also affecting large arteries. Arterial inflammation can lead to occlusion, aneurysm, or rupture. Behçet disease joins Wegener granulomatosis and Buerger disease in being a form of vasculitis that has a predilection for involving veins and causing venous thrombosis.

Vasculitis does not appear to account for all of the pathologic changes in Behçet disease. Many of the pathologic changes—including ulceration of the mouth and gut—may be more attributable to an abnormal reactivity of neutrophils and lymphocytes.

Clinical Findings

A. SYMPTOMS AND SIGNS

Oral ulceration is the hallmark of the disease, tends to be the earliest manifestation, and is required for the diagnosis of Behçet disease (Table 39–1). Oral ulcers are painful, shallow or deep, round or oval, with a white or yellow base and red halo (Figure 39–1). They vary in size from 1–20 mm. The ulcers most frequently affect the buccal mucosa, tongue, lips, gingivae, palate, tonsils, uvula, or pharynx. During an attack, patients usually have two to five lesions, but some patients may have a

Table 39–1. Frequency of Clinical Manifestations of Behçet Disease

Feature	Frequency (%)
Oral ulcers	100
Genital ulcers	75
Skin lesions	60–90
Arthritis	50
Gastrointestinal disease	25
Thrombophlebitis	20
Central nervous system disease	10–20
Epididymitis	5

single ulcer or too many to count. The aphthae may be so painful that the patient has trouble eating or drinking. Usually the aphthous lesions heal without scarring over 10–20 days.

Genital aphthae occur slightly less often than oral ulceration (Table 39–1). However, genital ulcers tend to be larger and deeper, and often heal with scarring. In men, the ulcers develop most commonly on the scrotum and less commonly on the shaft of the penis, and in women ulcers affect the vagina and vulva. Genital lesions in men are often associated with epididymitis.

Cutaneous manifestations of Behçet disease, which develop in 60–90% of patients, are protean. Erythema nodosum occurs most commonly, especially in women. Erythema nodosum in Behçet disease tends to ulcerate and heal with scarring and hyperpigmentation, compared with erythema nodosum associated with sarcoidosis and inflammatory bowel disease, which does not ulcerate and heals without scarring. In men, pseudofolliculitis and acneiform nodules develop frequently over the neck and face. Pathergy—the phenomenon of developing an aseptic nodule or ulcer larger than 2 mm in diameter 24–48 hours following a sterile needle prick to the forearm—occurs frequently in Japanese and Turks but in only approximately one-third of Americans with Behçet disease. Migratory thrombophlebitis also commonly occurs in Behçet disease.

Ocular inflammation, one of the hallmark manifestations of Behçet disease, tends to occur early in the course. Recurrent or persistent ocular inflammation frequently leads to visual loss, making eye inflammation one of the most common causes of disability in Behçet disease. Behçet disease is one of the few autoimmune diseases that can cause both anterior and posterior uveitis. Anterior uveitis typically presents with a red eye, intense photophobia, and blurred vision. The anterior uveitis may be so intense that a grossly visible layer of pus in the anterior chamber (hypopyon) develops. The posterior uveitis and vasculitis of the carotid and retina occur less commonly but pose a greater threat to vision.

Peripheral arthritis or spondylitis develops in approximately half of patients with Behçet disease. The peripheral arthritis may be monarticular or polyarticular, while the spondylitis usually presents as sacroiliitis (with low back or buttock pain). The peripheral arthritis is usually not deforming.

Gastrointestinal involvement develops in about one-quarter of patients. Although gastrointestinal involvement can appear at any time, it typically emerges several years after the onset of oral ulcers. Behçet disease of the gastrointestinal tract most commonly presents as aphthous ulcers affecting the ileum and cecum. However, any portion of the gut from the mouth to the anus can be involved. The most frequent manifestations of bowel involvement are pain, anorexia, rectal bleeding, vomiting, and diarrhea. In American patients, esophageal

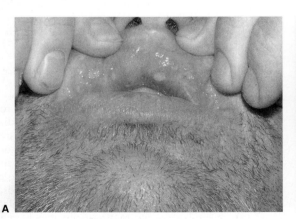
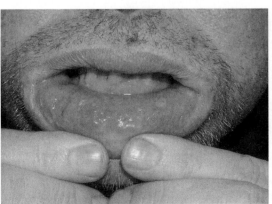

A   **B**

Figure 39–1. **A & B:** Multiple aphthous ulcers behind the lower and upper lips of a man with Behçet disease.

ulceration appears especially common. In addition, ischemia of the bowel may result from vasculitis of the medium- and large-sized mesenteric arteries. The unusual predilection for Behçet disease to involve veins explains why the Budd-Chiari syndrome develops in some patients.

Central nervous system disease, which develops in 10–20% of patients, resembles gastrointestinal involvement in following oral ulceration by 3–5 years. The neurologic features are variable and include headache and confusion (from recurrent sterile meningitis) and meningoencephalitis. Other complications are thrombotic or hemorrhagic hemispheric stroke, dural venous thrombosis, seizures, hearing and vestibular involvement, progressive dementia, and psychiatric disease including personality changes.

Large-vessel vasculitis explains why bruits develop in some patients' chest or abdomen. Affected vessels—especially in the pulmonary and mesenteric circulation—may occlude, develop aneurysm swelling, or rupture. Clinically important cardiac disease develops infrequently, and renal disease occurs rarely.

B. LABORATORY FINDINGS

Behçet disease produces no specific blood test abnormalities. Nonspecific markers of inflammation, such as anemia, mild leukocytosis, and an elevated erythrocyte sedimentation rate, are common during attacks of active inflammation. Patients with active Behçet disease also often show elevated levels of serum IgD. Cerebrospinal fluid analysis in patients with meningoencephalitis usually reveals elevations of protein and IgG and a pleocytosis of either polymorphonuclear cells or lymphocytes.

C. IMAGING STUDIES

Patients with neurologic disease can have abnormalities evident on computed tomography or magnetic resonance imaging. The most frequent magnetic resonance imaging abnormalities are seen with T2 weighting and consist of multiple high-intensity focal lesions that are widely distributed. Angiograms or magnetic resonance angiography can demonstrate large-artery thrombosis and aneurysm, typically seen in the chest or abdomen.

D. SPECIAL TESTS

Biopsies of mucocutaneous lesions and gastrointestinal ulcers reveal a neutrophilic vascular reaction. True vasculitis is rare. The pathergy phenomenon is uncommon in Americans.

Diagnosis & Differential Diagnosis

Since Behçet disease produces no pathognomonic laboratory finding, the diagnosis rests upon clinical criteria, which have been refined by an international study group (Table 39–2).

Table 39–2. Criteria for the Diagnosis of Behçet's Disease

Clinical Feature	Definition
Recurrent oral ulceration	Minor aphthous, major aphthous, or herpetiform ulcerations observed by physician or patient that recurred at least three times over a 12-month period
Plus two of the following criteria:	
Recurrent genital ulceration	Aphthous ulceration or scarring observed by patient or physician
Ocular lesions	Anterior uveitis, posterior uveitis, or cells in vitreous on slitlamp examination, or retinal vasculitis observed by ophthalmologist
Skin lesions	Erythema nodosum observed by patient or physician, pseudofolliculitis or papulopustular lesions, or acneiform nodules observed by physician in a postadolescent patient not taking glucocorticoids
Positive pathergy test	Interpreted by physician at 24–48 hours

(From International Study Group for Behçet's Disease. Criteria for diagnosis of Behçet's Disease. *Lancet.* 1990;335:1078. With permission.)

The differential diagnosis of recurrent oral and genital aphthous ulceration includes complex aphthosis (the label given to patients who suffer from almost constant mouth ulcers or recurrent oral and genital ulcers in the absence of Behçet disease), herpes simplex virus infection, Crohn disease, gluten-sensitive enteropathy, HIV disease, various vitamin or other nutrient deficiencies (including iron, zinc, folate, and vitamins B_1, B_2, B_6, or B_{12}), cyclic neutropenia, Reiter syndrome, and factitious disease. Medications, especially nonsteroidal anti-inflammatory drugs, can cause recurrent oral ulcerations. Another cause of recurrent oral lesions is systemic lupus erythematosus. The oral and pharyngeal lesions of Wegener granulomatosis and histoplasmosis are not usually recurrent. Stevens-Johnson syndrome, pemphigoid, and lichen planus can involve the mouth, genitals, and eye, but do not produce aphthous lesions.

Erythema nodosa has many causes besides Behçet disease, including sarcoidosis and inflammatory bowel disease. As noted, only erythema nodosa associated with Behçet tends to ulcerate. Some of the skin lesions in Behçet can mimic those of Sweet syndrome.

Syphilis and sarcoidosis are two diseases that, like Behçet disease, can cause both anterior and posterior

Table 39–3. Treatment for Behçet Disease

Treatment	Dose	Used as First-Line Therapy	Used as Alternative Therapy
Topical glucocorticoids			
Triamcinolone acetonide	3 times a day topically	Oral ulcers	
Betamethasone ointment	3 times a day topically	Genital ulcers	
Betamethasone drops	1–2 drops 3 times daily topically	Anterior uveitis, retinal vasculitis	
Dexamethasone	1–1.5 mg injected below tenon capsule for an ocular attack	Retinal vasculitis	
Systemic glucocorticoids			
Prednisone	5–20 mg/d orally		Erythema nodosum, anterior uveitis, retinal vasculitis, arthritis
	20–100 mg/d orally	Gastrointestinal lesions, acute meningoencephalitis, chronic progressive central nervous system lesions, arteritis	Retinal vasculitis, venous thrombosis
Methylprednisolone	1000 mg/d for 3 days intravenously	Acute meningoencephalitis, chronic progressive central nervous system lesions, arteritis	Gastrointestinal lesions, venous thrombosis
Other agents			
Tropicamide drops	1–2 drops once or twice daily topically	Anterior uveitis	
Tetracycline	250 mg in water solution once a day topically		Oral ulcers
Colchicine	0.5–1. 5 mg/d orally	Oral ulcers,[a] genital ulcers,[a] pseudofolliculitis,[a] erythema nodosum, anterior uveitis, retinal vasculitis	Arthritis
Thalidomide	100–300 mg/d orally		Oral ulcers,[a] genital ulcers,[a] pseudofolliculitis[a]
Dapsone	100 mg/d orally		Oral ulcers, genital ulcers, pseudofolliculitis, erythema nodosum
Pentoxifylline	300 mg/d orally		Oral ulcers, genital ulcers, pseudofolliculitis, erythema nodosum
Azathioprine	100 mg/d orally		Retinal vasculitis,[a] arthritis,[a] chronic progressive central nervous system lesions, arteritis, venous thrombosis

(continued)

Table 39–3. Treatment for Behçet Disease (*Continued*)

Treatment	Dose	Used as First-Line Therapy	Used as Alternative Therapy
Chlorambucil	5 mg/d orally		Retinal vasculitis, acute meningoencephalitis, chronic progressive central nervous system lesions, arteritis, venous thrombosis
Cyclophosphamide	50–1000 mg/d orally		Retinal vasculitis, acute meningoencephalitis, chronic progressive central nervous system lesions, arteritis, venous thrombosis
	700–1000 mg/mo intravenously		Retinal vasculitis, acute meningoencephalitis, chronic progressive central nervous system lesions, arteritis, venous thrombosis
Methotrexate	7.5–15 mg/wk orally		Retinal vasculitis, arthritis, chronic progressive central nervous system lesions
Cyclosporine[b]	5 mg/kg of body weight/day orally	Retinal vasculitis[a]	
Interferon-α	5 million U/day intramuscularly or subcutaneously		Retinal vasculitis, arthritis
Indomethacin	50–75 mg/d	Arthritis orally	
Sulfasalazine	1–3 g/d orally	Gastrointestinal lesions	Arthritis
Warfarin[c]	2–10 mg/d orally	Venous thrombosis	Arteritis
Heparin[c]	5000–20,000 U/d subcutaneously	Venous thrombosis	Arteritis
Aspirin[d]	50–100 mg/d orally	Arteritis, venous thrombosis	Chronic progressive central nervous system lesions
Dipyridamole	300 mg/d orally	Arteritis, venous thrombosis	Chronic progressive central nervous system lesions
Surgery	—		Gastrointestinal lesions, arteritis, venous thrombosis

[a]The efficacy of this drug for this use has been reported in controlled clinical trials.
[b]Cyclosporine is contraindicated in patients with acute meningoencephalitis or chronic progressive central nervous system lesions.
[c]This drug should be used with caution in patients with pulmonary vascular lesions.
[d]Low-dose aspirin is used as an antiplatelet agent.
(From Sakane T, Takeno M, Suzuki N, Inaba G. Behçet's Disease. *N Engl J Med*. 1999;341:1284. With permission.)

uveitis. Anterior uveitis can also be caused by inflammatory bowel disease, ankylosing spondylitis, and Reiter syndrome.

It can be virtually impossible to distinguish Behçet disease from Crohn disease unless the patient has bowel biopsies showing granulomatous lesions (supporting the diagnosis of Crohn disease).

Neurologic disease can sometimes mimic multiple sclerosis.

All patients with unexplained recurrent oral and genital ulcers should have the following tests performed or considered: cultures or polymerase chain reaction testing for herpes simplex virus infection; complete blood count with differential; comprehensive metabolic panel; erythrocyte sedimentation rate; urinalysis; HIV antibody test; serum levels of iron, folate, zinc, and vitamin B_{12}; antiendomysial or antigliadin antibodies; and antinuclear antibody. Patients with visceral symptoms may require imaging with magnetic resonance imaging or CT scanning, or invasive testing including lumbar puncture or upper and lower endoscopy. Consultation by a rheumatologist, gynecologist, ophthalmologist, neurologist, dermatologist, or gastroenterologist may also be helpful in establishing the diagnosis of Behçet disease or conditions that can mimic it.

Treatment

Treatment—like the disease itself—runs the gamut in intensity and illustrates how important it is to ensure that the treatment fits the disease manifestation. Recurrent oral ulcers, although painful, can be treated with topical glucocorticoids or dapsone. Vision-threatening uveitis or life-threatening meningoencephalitis requires high-dose systemic glucocorticoids and immunosuppressive agents such as chlorambucil. Interferon is effective in treating refractory mucocutaneous manifestations. The tumor necrosis factor inhibitor infliximab is effective for severe ocular disease. Other treatments and their indications are listed in Table 39–3.

Course & Prognosis

Behçet is a chronic disease characterized by recurrent attacks. Most manifestations, except for eye disease and large-vessel inflammation, tend to burn out over 1–2 decades. Disability most commonly results from uveitis (causing blindness), central nervous system disease (causing stroke and dementia), and gastrointestinal disease. Mortality results from central nervous system disease, rupture of arterial aneurysms, and infectious and oncologic complications of immunosuppressive therapy.

REFERENCES

Alpsoy E, Durusoy C, Yilmaz E, et al. Interferon alfa-2a in the treatment of Behcet disease: a randomized placebo-controlled and double-blind study. *Arch Dermatol.* 2002;138:467. [PMID: 11939808]

Letsinger JA, McCarty MA, Jorizzo JL. Complex aphthosis: a large case series with evaluation algorithm and therapeutic ladder from topicals to thalidomide. *J Am Acad Dermatol.* 2005;52:500. [PMID: 15761429]

Sakane T, Takeno M, Suzuki N, Inaba G. Behçet's disease. *N Engl J Med.* 1999;341:1284. [PMID: 10528040]

Tugal-Tutkun I, Mundun A, Urgancioglu M, et al. Efficacy of infliximab in the treatment of uveitis that is resistant to treatment with the combination of azathioprine, cyclosporine, and corticosteroids in Behçet's disease: an open-label trial. *Arthritis Rheum.* 2005;52:2478. [PMID: 16052571]

Yurdakul S, Hamuryudan V, Yazici H. Behcet syndrome. *Curr Opin Rheumatol.* 2004;16:38. [PMID: 14673387]

Relevant World Wide Web Site

[The Johns Hopkins Vasculitis Center]
http://vasculitis.med.jhu.edu

Henoch-Schönlein Purpura

Geetha Duvuru, MD, & John H. Stone, MD, MPH

ESSENTIALS OF DIAGNOSIS

- *Nonthrombocytopenic purpura, caused by inflammation in blood vessels of the superficial dermis, is the sine qua non of Henoch-Schönlein purpura (HSP).*

- *The pathologic hallmark of HSP is the deposition of immunoglobulin (Ig) A in the walls of involved blood vessels.*

- *The tetrad of purpura, arthritis, glomerulonephritis, and abdominal pain is often observed; however, all four elements are not required for the diagnosis.*

- *More than 90% of cases occur in children. The disease is self-limited most of the time, resolving within a few weeks. Adult cases are sometimes more recalcitrant.*

- *Renal insufficiency develops in fewer than 5% of patients with HSP. The long-term renal prognosis depends mainly on the degree of initial damage to the kidney.*

- *HSP can be mimicked by other forms of systemic vasculitis that are more often life-threatening. For example, Wegener granulomatosis and microscopic polyangiitis (see Chapters 33 and 34, respectively) may also present with purpura, arthritis, and renal inflammation. Both of these disorders have the potential for serious involvement of other organs (eg, the lungs and peripheral nerves) and carry more dire renal prognoses.*

General Considerations

Henoch-Schönlein purpura (HSP) is the most common form of systemic vasculitis in children, with an annual incidence of 140 cases per million persons. The peak incidence is in the first and second decades of life (90% of patients are younger than 10 years of age), with a male:female ratio of 2:1. The incidence is significantly lower in adults, with a mean age at presentation of 50 years. Males and females are affected equally and although HSP affects all ethnic groups, it is reportedly

less common among African Americans. Some epidemiologic studies suggest that HSP is more prevalent in the winter months.

HSP may be misdiagnosed as another form of vasculitis—most commonly hypersensitivity vasculitis (see Chapter 38)—because of the frequent failure to perform direct immunofluorescence testing on skin biopsy specimens. In two-thirds of the cases, the disease follows an upper respiratory tract infection, with onset an average of 10 days after the start of respiratory symptoms. Despite this association, no single microorganism or environmental exposure has been confirmed as an important cause of HSP. The American College of Rheumatology 1990 criteria for the classification of HSP are shown in Table 40–1. The Chapel Hill Consensus Conference on the nomenclature of vasculitides defined HSP as a form of vasculitis characterized by: (1) IgA-dominant immune deposits within vessel walls; (2) small-vessel involvement (ie, capillaries, venules, or arterioles); and (3) skin, gut, renal, and joint manifestations.

The skin histopathology of HSP shows a leukocytoclastic vasculitis of small blood vessels within the superficial dermis. Necrosis is often present, but features of granulomatous inflammation are not. Immunofluorescent staining of biopsy specimens shows coarse, granular IgA staining in and around small blood vessels. In the kidney, the renal inflammation is indistinguishable from IgA nephropathy. There is a predilection for IgA deposition within the mesangium. However, in HSP nephritis, capillary wall staining for IgA is more frequently found and may be even more prominent than IgA in the mesangium. Most patients have increased serum IgA levels and circulating immune complexes that contain IgA, as well as IgA deposition in inflamed blood vessels.

Clinical Findings

A. SYMPTOMS AND SIGNS

The classic full presentation includes the acute onset of fever, palpable purpura on the lower extremities and buttocks (Figure 40–1), abdominal pain, arthritis, and hematuria. However, all components of this presentation are not required for the diagnosis. Conversely, even classic presentations are not diagnostic of this disorder. The diagnosis should be confirmed by biopsy (direct

Table 40–1. American College of Rheumatology 1990 Criteria[a] for the Classification of Henoch-Schönlein Purpura (HSP)

1. Palpable purpura
2. Age at onset <20 years
3. Bowel angina
4. Vessel wall granulocytes on biopsy

[a] The presence of two criteria classified HSP with a sensitivity of 87% and specificity of 88% in a group of individuals with forms of systemic vasculitis.

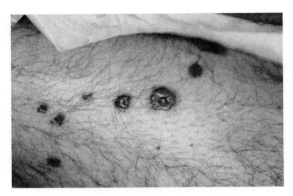

Figure 40–2. A bullous lesion with a purpuric component in a patient with Henoch-Schönlein purpura.

immunofluorescence as well as conventional hematoxylin and eosin staining) in most cases.

1. Skin—The cutaneous findings of HSP include purpura (usually palpable, although sometimes not), urticarial papules, and plaques. Among adults, 60% of patients have bullous or necrotic lesions (Figure 40–2), but these are uncommon in children. Lesions are concentrated over the buttocks and lower extremities and tend to involve the small blood vessels in the superficial dermis. Medium-sized vessels are rarely involved in HSP except in the setting of HSP associated with IgA paraproteinemia. Localized edematous swelling of the subcutaneous tissues of the lower extremities is frequently observed and does not correlate with the presence or degree of proteinuria. Persistent rash over a period longer than 1 month is a significant predictor of disease relapse and renal sequelae in children with HSP.

2. Joints—Joint disease, which occurs in more than 80% of patients with HSP, manifests itself as arthralgias or arthritis in large joints, especially the knees and ankles, and to a lesser degree the wrists and elbows. Migra-

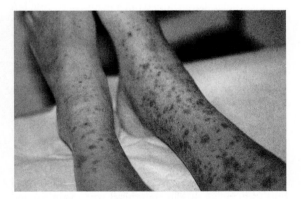

Figure 40–1. Palpable purpura with some superficial ulcerations in a patient with Henoch-Schönlein purpura. Note also the presence of right ankle swelling due to arthritis.

tory patterns of joint involvement are common. Lower-extremity involvement among patients with HSP and arthritis is nearly universal; up to one-third of patients have upper-extremity involvement as well. The pain associated with HSP arthritis may be incapacitating. The arthritis is nondeforming in nature.

3. Gastrointestinal tract—Approximately 60% of patients with HSP have abdominal pain and 33% have evidence of gastrointestinal bleeding. Abdominal symptoms result from edema of the bowel wall as well as hemorrhage induced by mesenteric vasculitis. Abdominal pain may precede the appearance of purpura by up to 2 weeks, often leading to diagnostic confusion and occasionally to invasive testing. The abdominal pain is typically colicky and may worsen after eating (ie, intestinal angina). Some patients experience nausea, vomiting, and upper or lower gastrointestinal bleeding. Mesenteric ischemia in HSP rarely leads to gut perforation. Massive gastrointestinal hemorrhage occurs in only 2% or so of patients. Purpuric lesions may be seen on endoscopy, commonly in the descending duodenum, stomach, and colon.

Gastrointestinal involvement in children with HSP can cause intussusception, a rare complication in adults. In contrast to idiopathic intussusception, which typically is ileocolic, HSP-associated intussusception is usually ileoileal. Other rare complications include pancreatitis, cholecystitis, and a protein-losing enteropathy.

4. Kidney—Renal involvement is the most potentially debilitating complication of HSP. Forty percent of patients with HSP have renal disease. In general, renal involvement is more frequent and tends to be persistent in adults, who have a higher risk than children of developing end-stage renal disease. In a retrospective study of 134 children with HSP, age >4 years, persistent purpura, and severe abdominal symptoms increased the likelihood of renal involvement.

In contrast to gastrointestinal disease and arthritis, both of which occasionally precede the onset of purpura, glomerulonephritis almost always appears after the development of skin manifestations. The occurrence of glomerulonephritis may be delayed by several weeks in up to 25% of all patients with this complication. The clinical hallmark of nephritis in HSP is hematuria, often macroscopic, but more typically microscopic. The hematuria can be transient, persistent, or recurrent. Proteinuria never occurs in the absence of hematuria. Even in cases in whom the renal disease resolves spontaneously, many patients have persistent urinary abnormalities (eg, proteinuria).

The most common renal lesion (60% of cases) is a focal, proliferative endocapillary glomerulonephritis. Crescents are present in up to 40% of biopsies. Direct immunofluorescence studies characteristically demonstrate IgA deposition in the mesangium. Regardless of age, the degree of proteinuria, the presence of renal insufficiency at presentation, the number of crescents, and the degree of interstitial fibrosis on biopsy correlate with outcome. Histologic recurrences of HSP nephritis in renal allografts occur in 50% of patients who undergo renal transplantation. Allograft recurrences are associated with clinically significant disease in 20%, allograft failure in 12%, and allograft loss in 9% of cases.

5. Other organs—Pulmonary and central nervous system complications of HSP have been described, but these are very rare. When present, the usual lung manifestation of the disease is alveolar hemorrhage. Seizures are the usual central nervous system manifestation of HSP; the precise mechanism is obscure. Testicular involvement occurs in up to 10% of boys with this disease and may mimic torsion.

B. LABORATORY FINDINGS

The results of routine laboratory tests and more specialized assays in HSP are shown in Table 40–2. All of these tests are appropriate at the initial evaluation of a patient with possible HSP. The exclusion of other forms of vasculitis that may mimic HSP in presentation is essential. Sixty percent of patients have an elevated serum IgA. Although there are two subclasses of IgA, HSP is associated with serum elevations and tissue deposits of IgA1 only. The reason for the preferential elevation of IgA1 is not clear.

C. IMAGING STUDIES

Chest radiography should be performed to rule out pulmonary lesions. The presence of pulmonary involvement, unusual in HSP, raises the possibility of other diagnoses that may require other treatment approaches (see section below on Differential Diagnosis).

Table 40–2. The Laboratory Evaluation in Henoch-Schönlein Purpura

Test	Typical Result
Complete blood cell count with differential	Mild to moderate leukocytosis common, but otherwise the complete blood count is usually normal
Electrolytes	Hyperkalemia in the setting of advanced renal dysfunction
Liver function tests	Hypoalbuminemia can occur with nephrotic proteinuria; otherwise the liver function tests are normal
Urinalysis with microscopy	Hematuria (ranging from mild to too numerous to count red blood cells)
	Red blood cell casts
	Proteinuria (nephrotic range proteinuria in a small minority)
Erythrocyte sedimentation rate/C-reactive protein	Modestly elevated acute phase reactants may be observed; approximately one-third of patients have abnormal erythrocyte sedimentation rates
Serum IgA level	60% of patients have an elevated serum IgA; although there are two subclasses of IgA, HSP is associated with increases only in IgA1
ANA	Negative
Rheumatoid factor	Negative
C3, C4	Even though immune complexes containing IgA are essential to the pathophysiology of HSP, serum complement levels are usually normal
ANCA	Negative (both IgG and IgA ANCA)
Cryoglobulins	Negative

ANA, antinuclear antibody; ANCA, antineutrophil cytoplasmic antibody.

D. SPECIAL TESTS

Direct immunofluorescence studies of skin biopsies can only be performed on fresh samples, and therefore must be planned at the time the biopsy is performed. The usual procedure is to biopsy one skin lesion for hematoxylin and eosin staining and another for immunofluorescence.

Differential Diagnosis

The differential diagnosis of HSP is shown in Table 40–3. HSP must be distinguished from other small-vessel vasculitides, from autoimmune inflammatory conditions associated with joint disease and rashes, and from infections. Other disorders may be associated occasionally

Table 40–3. Differential Diagnosis of Henoch-Schönlein Purpura

Other vasculitides
    Hypersensitivity vasculitis
    Microscopic polyangiitis
    Churg-Strauss syndrome
    Wegener granulomatosis
    Mixed cryoglobulinemia
    Polyarteritis nodosa
Systemic autoimmune conditions
    Systemic lupus erythematosus
    Rheumatoid arthritis
Renal disorders
    IgA nephropathy
Infections
    Acute viral or bacterial infections
Malignancies
    Childhood leukemias
Miscellaneous
    Acute hemorrhagic edema of infancy

with mild IgA deposition in blood vessels, but the process is rarely so florid as with HSP. IgA nephropathy is pathologically indistinguishable from the renal disease associated with HSP (including the preferential deposition of IgA1), but it has a typically chronic course and is not associated with disease in other organ systems.

A particularly crucial distinction is between HSP and the antineutrophil cytoplasmic antibody–associated conditions, primarily Wegener granulomatosis and microscopic polyangiitis. (Churg-Strauss syndrome may be distinguished more readily by the presence of eosinophilia.) The antineutrophil cytoplasmic antibody–associated vasculitides often present with purpura, migratory arthritis, and renal inflammation, but in contrast to HSP, do not typically have self-limited courses. Organ manifestations that are atypical for HSP, such as pulmonary involvement, symptoms or signs compatible with vasculitic neuropathy, or inflammatory eye disease, should broaden the differential diagnosis. Misdiagnoses of HSP because of failure to perform direct immunofluorescence testing on skin biopsies and antineutrophil cytoplasmic antibody assays on serum can lead to poor outcomes.

Treatment

Nonsteroidal anti-inflammatory drugs may alleviate arthralgias but can aggravate gastrointestinal symptoms and should be avoided in any patient with renal disease. Dapsone (100 mg/d) may be effective in cases of HSP, perhaps through interference with the interactions of IgA and neutrophils. Although glucocorticoids have not been evaluated rigorously in HSP, they appear to ameliorate joint and gastrointestinal symptoms. Glucocorticoids do not appear to improve the rash, however, and their effectiveness in renal disease is controversial. Uncontrolled trials suggest that high-dose methylprednisolone followed by oral prednisone or high-dose prednisone combined with azathioprine or cyclophosphamide may help patients with severe nephritis (ie, nephrotic syndrome and >50% crescents).

Complications

In most cases, HSP follows a self-limited course, resolves without substantial morbidity, and does not recur. The vast majority of cases resolve within 6–8 weeks. Recurrences, found in 33% of patients, usually develop within the first few months after resolution of the first bout. Even when associated with small ulcerations, the cutaneous lesions are usually so superficial that they heal without scarring. A small percentage of patients have progressive renal insufficiency and long-term follow-up of all patients with severe renal symptoms at onset is needed.

REFERENCES

Fervenza FC. Henoch-Schönlein purpura nephritis. *Int J Dermatol.* 2003;42:170. [PMID: 12653909]

Pillebout E, Thervet E, Hill G, et al. Henoch-Schönlein purpura in adults: outcome and prognostic factors. *J Am Soc Nephrol.* 2002;13:1271. [PMID: 11961015] (In a retrospective study of 250 adults with HSP nephritis, approximately one-third developed at least moderate renal insufficiency and 11% suffered end-stage renal disease.)

Saulsbury FT. Henoch-Schönlein purpura in children. Report of 100 patients and review of the literature. *Medicine (Baltimore).* 1999;78:395. [PMID: 10575422] (Well-characterized cohort of pediatric patients evaluated and followed at one center.)

Tancrede-Bohin E, Ochonisky S, Vignon-Pennamen MD, et al. Schönlein-Henoch purpura in adult patients. Predictive factors for IgA glomerulonephritis in a retrospective study of 57 cases. *Arch Dermatol.* 1997;133:438. [PMID: 9126006] (Adults are more likely to have persistent disease and serious renal involvement.)

Relevant World Wide Web Site

[The Johns Hopkins Vasculitis Center]
http://vasculitis.med.jhu.edu

Vasculitis of the Central Nervous System

David B. Hellmann, MD

Central nervous system (CNS) vasculitis is not a single disease but a collection of conditions that cause inflammatory damage of blood vessels in the brain and spinal cord. About half of the cases have no known cause and are therefore classified as *primary* vasculitis of the CNS. The other half of the cases arise in the setting of some other disorder, often a rheumatic disease such as systemic lupus erythematosus, and are classified as secondary forms of CNS vasculitis. Primary vasculitis of the CNS has been referred to by many names. Bowing to tradition, this chapter will use the term "primary angiitis of the CNS" (PACNS).

CNS vasculitis presents a two-handed clinical challenge. On the one hand, clinicians need to recognize and treat those rare patients whose strokes and other neurologic deficits result from CNS vasculitis. On the other hand, clinicians need to avoid overdiagnosis of CNS vasculitis and must realize that the angiographic and magnetic resonance imaging (MRI) abnormalities observed in CNS vasculitis can be mimicked by infection, tumor, and other conditions.

ESSENTIALS OF DIAGNOSIS

- *Common presentation includes headache, encephalopathy, and multiple strokes.*
- *Brain MRI sensitive but not specific.*
- *Most patients in whom PACNS is suspected have some other disorder.*
- *Angiographic abnormalities are suggestive but not specific.*
- *Definitive diagnosis requires brain biopsy.*

General Considerations

PACNS is a disease of unknown cause characterized by vasculitis limited to the brain and spinal cord. PACNS is rare; at large medical centers PACNS constitutes only about 1% of all cases of systemic vasculitis. Evidence suggests that PACNS is not one disease. Indeed, the clinical picture of PACNS that emerges from reviewing the literature depends a great deal on whether the analysis focuses on biopsy-proven cases (BP-PACNS) or cases defined by angiography (AD-PACNS) without biopsy proof. Some clinicians have speculated that AD-PACNS may be caused by spasm rather than by inflammation. The term "benign angiography of the CNS" is sometimes applied to cases of AD-PACNS. Table 41–1 outlines the clinical pictures of both BP-PACNS and AD-PACNS.

Clinical Findings

A. SYMPTOMS AND SIGNS

BP-PACNS chiefly affects middle-aged men. The initial presentation is typically headache and encephalopathy, and multifocal strokes develop later. BP-PACNS usually develops insidiously, unfolding with additive neurologic deficits over weeks or months before the diagnosis is suspected. Strokes in the absence of diffuse cortical dysfunction would be most unusual for BP-PACNS. However, the presentation of BP-PACNS is highly variable. Some patients may appear to have had one stroke, but PACNS is suspected after an MRI reveals multiple strokes of varying age. In other patients, headache may be the dominating feature. In some patients who have headache and what appear to be mass lesions on MRI, a brain tumor is suspected. Diffuse cortical dysfunction can manifest as either a decline in cognitive ability or an alteration in consciousness. The English teacher who can no longer spell accurately or the bank teller who cannot count change exemplifies how cognitive changes from diffuse cortical dysfunction may present. Seizure and brainstem or cranial nerve dysfunction develops in approximately one-third of patients. Spinal cord involvement occurs less commonly. Isolated dementia is a very rare presentation of BP-PACNS. It is a common misconception that BP-PACNS is associated with systemic symptoms such as fever, weight loss, or sweats. In reality, such symptoms develop in fewer than 20% of cases.

Table 41–1. Clinical and Laboratory Features of PACNS Based on the Method of Diagnosis[a]

Feature	BP-PACNS	AD-PACNS	*p* Value
Sex, no. (%)			
Males	78 (69.0)	17 (30.8)	<.001
Females	38 (31.0)	38 (69.1)	<.001
Age, mean ± SD	46 ± 17	33 ± 14	
Headache, no. (%)			
Yes	63 (55.8)	43 (78.2)	
No	50 (44.3)	12 (21.8)	
Stroke, no. (%)			
Yes	83 (86.5)	15 (32.6)	
No	13 (13.5)	31 (67.4)	<.008
Seizure, no. (%)			
Yes	29 (30.2)	11 (23.9)	
No	67 (69.8)	35 (76.1)	
Cerebral hemorrhage, no. (%)			
Yes	13 (11.5)	5 (9.1)	
No	100 (88.5)	50 (90.9)	
Diffuse neurologic dysfunction, no. (%)			
Yes	77 (68.1)	26 (47.3)	
No	36 (31.9)	29 (52.7)	<.009
Decreased cognition, no. (%)			
Yes	64 (83.1)	20 (76.9)	
No	13 (16.9)	6 (23.1)	
Days from symptom onset to diagnosis, mean ± SD	170 ± 261	46 ± 73	<.001
Abnormal CSF/total tested (%)	90	50	<.005

[a]An abnormal cerebrospinal fluid (CSF) sample had >5 cells/μL or protein >55 mg% or both.
PACNS, primary angiitis of the central nervous system; BP-PACNS, biopsy-proven PACNS; AD-PACNS, angiographically-defined PACNS.
(From Calabrese LH, Duna GF, Lie JT. Vasculitis in the central nervous system. *Arthritis Rheum.* 1997;40:1189. With permission.)

The clinical picture of AD-PACNS differs in several important ways. AD-PACNS preferentially affects women four times more commonly than men. The average age of onset is 40, the onset is sudden, and the most prominent presenting symptom is a severe headache. Focal findings of seizure or stroke develop in approximately 60% of patients (see Table 41–1). Diffuse cortical abnormalities develop less commonly. In AD-PACNS, as in BP-PACNS, systemic symptoms and signs are usually absent. As will be discussed in greater detail below, AD-PACNS patients also differ from BP-PACNS patients by having fewer cerebrospinal fluid abnormalities and responding to relatively short courses of corticosteroids.

B. LABORATORY FINDINGS

In BP-PACNS, about one-fifth of the patients have anemia (usually mild), one-half have an elevated white blood cell count, and two-thirds have an elevated erythrocyte sedimentation rate. The hematocrit and erythrocyte sedimentation rate are less frequently abnormal in AD-PACNS cases. The cerebrospinal fluid (CSF) is abnormal in nearly 90% of BP-PACNS cases and in about 50% of AD-PACNS cases. The most common abnormalities are an elevated CSF protein (with a mean of 177 mg/dL and a median of 100 mg/dL) and a CSF lymphocytosis (with a mean of 77 cells/μL). A CSF cell count exceeding $250/\mu$L almost never occurs in PACNS. In AD-PACNS, the CSF abnormalities are typically very mild. CSF protein levels are usually below 60 mg/dL and the CSF white blood cell count is usually less than 10 cells/μL. Fewer than 10% of AD-PACNS patients have CSF with a protein >70 mg/dL or a white blood count >$10/\mu$L.

C. IMAGING STUDIES

MRI is the most sensitive imaging method for detecting PACNS, being abnormal in approximately 90% of cases.

However, the abnormalities are not specific for vasculitis. On average, patients with PACNS have multiple lesions that are predominantly bilateral and supratentorial. The most commonly affected areas are the subcortical white matter, the deep gray matter, the deep white matter, and the cortex. The lesions appear most commonly as infarcts but can also appear as mass lesions or areas of signal change. Hemorrhagic lesions are uncommon. MRI angiograms are normal in the vast majority of cases. Even though PACNS is classified as a vasculitis of medium-sized vessels, MRI angiography lacks the resolution to detect the size of arteries usually affected by PACNS.

Computed tomography of the brain is much less sensitive in PACNS, detecting abnormalities in only about two-thirds of the cases. However, computed tomography is more sensitive than MRI at detecting hemorrhagic lesions.

Traditional angiography is abnormal in 50–80% of patients with PACNS. The classic finding in PACNS of "beading" of the small intracranial arteries caused by dilations interspersed with normal areas of artery (Figure 41–1). Slow flow, threadlike thinning of arteries, and occlusion are other angiographic (albeit nonspecific) abnormalities found in PACNS. Microaneurysms occur much less commonly in PACNS than in polyarteritis nodosa. The small branches of the middle anterior arteries and the posterior cerebral arteries are the most commonly affected. Angiographic abnormalities of larger, more proximal arteries are unusual. Angiographic abnormalities are usually bilateral and more widespread than the MRI lesions. None of the angiographic abnormalities are absolutely specific for PACNS. In patients in whom CNS vasculitis is suspected, angiography carries an 11.8% risk of transient neurologic deficit and a 0.8% risk of permanent stroke.

The role of positron emission tomography scanning in PACNS has not been defined.

D. SPECIAL TESTS

Brain biopsy, required for definitive diagnosis of PACNS, carries a risk of serious morbidity of 0–2%, and will be falsely negative in at least one-quarter of cases. Sampling the tip of the nondominant temporal lobe can reduce the chance of neurologic deficits from biopsy. Biopsy should include the leptomeninges, as this tissue is often involved by PACNS. Biopsies should be processed for histologic examination and cultures and should be stained for bacteria, fungi, and viruses. PACNS affects chiefly small- and medium-sized arteries and arterioles of the brain and spinal cord. Affected vessels are infiltrated chiefly with lymphocytes. A minority of biopsies will show granulomatous inflammation. Thrombosis and rupture can lead to infarction and hemorrhage of the surrounding tissue.

E. EVALUATION

Most patients in whom CNS vasculitis is suspected will need to undergo a battery of tests. Since MRI is the most sensitive noninvasive imaging method overall, it is preferred over computed tomography unless hemorrhage is a concern. After MRI has excluded mass lesion, the patient should undergo lumbar puncture. The CSF analysis can help support the diagnosis of CNS vasculitis, as noted above, and can help exclude the many infections and tumors that can mimic CNS vasculitis (see below). Angiograms can be done to exclude other causes of the patient's symptoms and to add support to the diagnosis of vasculitis. However, repeated studies have emphasized that the classic beading pattern of angiographic changes is not specific for vasculitis. Indeed, in one recent series of 35 patients who had undergone angiography and leptomeningeal biopsy, none of the patients whose angiogram was considered positive for vasculitis had a brain biopsy positive for vasculitis. Conversely, the only patients with brain biopsies positive for vasculitis did not have classic angiographic changes. Whether all patients in whom PACNS is suspected should undergo brain biopsy is controversial. Few centers have a large experience with either PACNS or brain biopsy. It is reasonable to recommend brain biopsy for those who have a slow onset, severe neurologic impairment, and striking cerebrospinal fluid abnormalities, or for others who have failed to respond to corticosteroid therapy. Other laboratory evaluations will depend on the patient's presentation and differential diagnosis (see below).

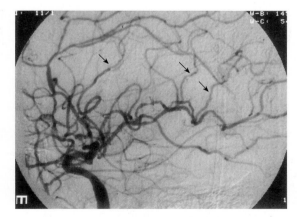

Figure 41–1. Angiogram of intracranial arteries showing segmental narrowing typical of central nervous system vasculitis.

Diagnostic Criteria

A definite diagnosis of PACNS requires the following:

1. Symptoms and signs of an acquired neurologic deficit consistent with the diagnosis of PACNS (eg, headache, confusion, and multiple strokes).
2. No evidence of a systemic vasculitis or another disorder that could cause the clinical picture, despite a thorough investigation.
3. A brain or spinal cord biopsy demonstrating vasculitis in the absence of infection.

The diagnosis of PACNS should be regarded as *possible* if, in the absence of a positive biopsy, the patient meets the first two criteria and has an angiogram with classic changes of vasculitis in multiple intracranial vessels.

Differential Diagnosis

Since most patients in whom CNS vasculitis is suspected have some other disorder, the differential diagnosis should be reviewed meticulously (Table 41–2). Among the rheumatic diseases, systemic lupus erythematosus, polyarteritis nodosa, and Wegener granulomatosis are the disorders that most often cause secondary CNS vasculitis. Rarely, however, are these conditions confused with PACNS. Almost all patients with those conditions have other organs involved (eg, skin in systemic lupus erythematosus) and have other characteristic laboratory abnormalities (eg, positive antineutrophil cytoplasmic antibodies in Wegener granulomatosis).

Infection can be more difficult to distinguish from PACNS. HIV, herpes zoster virus, syphilis, and histoplasmosis are among the infections that can closely mimic PACNS. Most patients affected are immunosuppressed by HIV, alcoholism, or cancer chemotherapy. Many of the infections, especially fungi, preferentially affect the base of the brain. Infection should also be considered whenever the number of cells in the CSF exceeds $250/\mu L$.

The possibility of herpes zoster virus–related vasculitis should be considered in a person who is immunosuppressed or who has had shingles in a V_1 distribution in the last few weeks. Angiographic abnormalities seen with infection can perfectly mimic the changes seen with PACNS. Because of the difficulty of recognizing when infection is causing vasculitis, cerebrospinal fluid and brain biopsies should be cultured and stained for infection. Blood cultures, HIV testing, and CSF Venereal Disease Research Lab tests should also be routinely performed when evaluating a patient for PACNS. Special tests (eg, polymerase chain reaction assay) for other infections may be warranted if the patient is immunosuppressed.

Cocaine, amphetamines, and ephedrine derivatives are the drugs that most commonly produce CNS vasculopathy. There is some evidence that these drugs can

Table 41–2. Differential Diagnosis of Primary Angiitis of the Central Nervous System

Category	Examples
Rheumatic disorders	Systemic lupus erythematosus, Wegener granulomatosis, polyarteritis nodosa, Takayasu arteritis, temporal arteritis, Behçet disease, Sjögren syndrome, Cogan syndrome
Infections	Bacteria (eg, endocarditis, bacterial meningitis, tuberculosis, syphilis, Lyme disease), fungi (eg, histoplasmosis, *Aspergillus*), viruses (eg, herpes zoster, HIV, hepatitis C)
Drugs	Cocaine, ephedrine, amphetamine, allopurinol, phenylpropanolamine, heroin
Vasculopathies	Atherosclerosis, antiphospholipid antibody syndrome, cerebral amyloid angiopathy, moya moya, radiation-induced vasculopathy, vasospasm associated with severe hypertension or hemorrhage, arterial fibromuscular dysplasia, cardiac myxoma, embolism, cholesterol embolism, pregnancy- and postpartum-associated vasculopathy, sickle cell anemia, thrombotic thrombocytopenic purpura
Malignancy	Vascular lymphoma, Hodgkin disease, small-cell lung cancer
Heritable disorders	Cerebral autosomal dominant arteriopathy with subcortical infarcts and leukoencephalopathy (CADASIL)
Other inflammatory disorders	Sarcoidosis, inflammatory bowel disease, celiac disease
Metabolic disorders	Pheochromocytoma

(From Hellmann DB, Stone J. Vasculitis of the central nervous system. In: Asbury AK, McKhann GM, McDonald WI, Goadsby PJ, McArthur JC, eds. *Disease of the Nervous System: Clinical Neuroscience and Therapeutic Principles.* 3rd ed. Cambridge University Press, 2002:1547. With permission.)

produce vasculitis itself and not just a vasculopathy that imitates PACNS. Most patients with cocaine-induced vasculitis are men in their 20s. However, profiling for PACNS is an inexact science, so detailed drug histories and toxicology screens should be used routinely.

Atherosclerosis should always be considered because it is so common, especially if the patient is over the age of 50 and has hypertension, hypercholesterolemia, or diabetes. No angiogram should be interpreted as showing vasculitis if atherosclerosis is evident in the carotid siphon or other vessels. Cerebral amyloid should be considered if the patient is over the age of 65 and has cerebral hemorrhages. Other conditions that can resemble PACNS are listed in Table 41–2.

Treatment

Patients with BP-PACNS should be treated with glucocorticoids. The role of immunosuppressive drugs such as cyclophosphamide is not yet established. Patients who have declined rapidly should be started on methylprednisolone 1000 mg intravenously daily for 3–5 days, followed by prednisone (or equivalent) 1 mg/kg/d. Patients who have not progressed rapidly can begin treatment with prednisone. The rarity of PACNS means that no large, detailed studies are available to guide tapering. Prednisone should not be reduced until the patient has stabilized and after all manifestations of inflammation (erythrocyte sedimentation rate, hematocrit, and CSF abnormalities) have resolved. Typically this takes a month. Thereafter, prednisone can be tapered by 10% every 1–2 weeks until 20 mg is reached, at which time the reduction schedule is slowed further. New symptoms or signs or new imaging abnormalities will require an increase in prednisone dose. Cyclophosphamide or other immunosuppressive drugs should be considered if the patient has severe deficits or if the disease progresses despite glucocorticoid therapy.

Treatment of AD-PACNS is also not well defined. However, studies suggest that some cases result more from spasm of the arteries than from true inflammation. Spasm appears to be especially likely in young women who have an abrupt onset of headache and focal deficits and who have no or minimal abnormalities of the CSF. There is growing evidence that these patients infrequently require immunosuppressive drugs. Some experts advocate treating these cases with a calcium channel blocker such as verapamil (to reduce spasm) and prednisone (1 mg/kg/d). Following resolution of the acute illness, the prednisone is tapered over 6–12 weeks. Failure to demonstrate substantial angiographic improvement should cast doubt on spasm as a major component and should suggest true vasculitis that will require a slower tapering of prednisone. All patients with PACNS should be instructed to avoid drugs that cause vasoconstriction or thrombosis (such as birth control pills, ephedrine, nicotine, and cocaine). All patients who take prednisone for more than 2 months should be evaluated and treated to minimize the risks of osteoporosis.

Prognosis

In the absence of treatment, almost all patients with BP-PACNS die of progressive neurologic deficits. Treatment has reduced mortality in the first year to 5%. The prognosis of AD-PACNS appears to be better. More than 90% of patients in whom spasm is suspected will recover.

REFERENCES

Calabrese LH, Duna GF, Lie JT. Vasculitis in the central nervous system. *Arthritis Rheum.* 1997;40:1189. [PMID: 9214418]

Hajj-Ali RA, Furlan A, Abou-Chebel A, Calabrese LH. Benign angiopathy of the central nervous system: cohort of 16 patients with clinical course and long-term followup. *Arthritis Rheum.* 2002;47:662. [PMID: 12522842]

Hellmann DB, Stone J. Vasculitis of the central nervous system. In: Asbury AK, McKhann GM, McDonald WI, Goadsby PJ, McArthur JC, eds. *Diseases of the Nervous System: Clinical Neuroscience and Therapeutic Principles.* 3rd ed. Cambridge University Press, 2002:1547.

Kadkhodayan Y, Alreshaid A, Moran CJ, et al. Primary angiitis of the central nervous system at conventional angiography. *Radiology.* 2004;233:878. [PMID: 15498898]

Relevant World Wide Web Site

[The Johns Hopkins Vasculitis Center]
http://vasculitis.med.jhu.edu

Buerger Disease

John H. Stone, MD, MPH

ESSENTIALS OF DIAGNOSIS

- *Active tobacco use, typically moderate to heavy.*
- *Severe digital ischemia without evidence of internal organ involvement.*
- *Angiography reveals segmental involvement of medium-sized arteries, with abrupt vascular cutoffs and corkscrew collaterals. The major vessel involvement occurs at the levels of the ankle and wrist.*

General Considerations

In Buerger disease, also called thromboangiitis obliterans, the classic patient is a young male smoker. The mean age of onset is approximately 40 years, with a broad age range that includes both late teens and the elderly. Although the patients described initially were men, the disease may afflict women as well, probably in direct proportion to the number of women in any particular society who smoke. The precise mechanism underlying the relationship between Buerger disease and cigarette smoking is unknown; autoimmune reactions to constituents of tobacco have been postulated. Cases may present several years after the start of smoking, but Buerger disease does not occur in the absence of ongoing tobacco exposure.

The diagnosis of Buerger disease is made by recognition of the compatible clinical findings—digital ischemia without involvement of other organs—identification of the typical pattern of vascular involvement by angiography, exclusion of diseases that may mimic Buerger disease (Table 42–1), and confirmation that the major risk factor, ongoing tobacco exposure, is present. Because of difficulty in accessing medium-sized vessels for biopsy, the diagnosis is rarely confirmed histologically. The exceptions to this rule are superficial thrombophlebitis, which seldom comes to medical attention, and amputation specimens, by which time medical attention is (at least in some senses) too late. When biopsy is possible, acute Buerger disease is characterized by a highly inflammatory thrombus composed of a variety of cell types: lymphocytes, neutrophils, giant cells, and occasional microabscesses. Fibrinoid necrosis, a hallmark of most systemic vasculitides, is absent in Buerger disease.

Clinical Findings

A. SYMPTOMS AND SIGNS

1. Extremities—A major hallmark of Buerger disease is its confinement to the extremities. The initial symptoms may be nonspecific pains in the calf, foot, or toes. The progression of thrombosis and vasculitis can lead to horrific pain in the digits and limbs and ultimately to gangrene and tissue loss, through either autoamputation or elective amputation. For unknown reasons, however, other vascular beds (eg, the cardiac, pulmonary, renal, and mesenteric vasculature) are nearly always spared in Buerger disease. Although Buerger disease has a predilection for the feet and toes, the hands and fingers may also be affected prominently. More than 60% of patients have abnormal Allen tests, indicating compromise of circulation to the hand; many demonstrate obliterations of the radial or ulnar artery pulses on physical examination. In contrast to atherosclerosis, which is a disease of the proximal vasculature, Buerger disease is characterized by inflammation and thrombosis of medium-sized, distal blood vessels (both arteries and veins), most intense at the levels of the ankles and wrists.

2. Skin—The earliest lesion may be a superficial thrombophlebitis. This complaint is often disregarded by the patient or misdiagnosed as deep varicosities. Histologic examination of these lesions reveals an acute thrombophlebitis with marked perivascular infiltration. This herald lesion is then followed by progressive occlusion of the deeper veins and arteries, leading the patient to seek medical attention. Patients with Buerger disease may have splinter hemorrhages, arousing suspicions of infective endocarditis. Most cutaneous features of disease are those of a process involving the medium-sized vessels exclusively (purpura, for example, a manifestation of small-vessel disease, is absent). Gangrene occurs in the most distal tissues, ie, the toes and fingers, first (Figure 42–1). If the process remains undiagnosed or if the patient continues to smoke even after the diagnosis, larger portions of the extremities become compromised. In advanced cases, the

Table 42–1. Differential Diagnosis of Buerger Disease

Cardiovascular conditions
 Atherosclerosis
 Cardiogenic emboli (eg, infective endocarditis)
Systemic disorders associated with autoimmunity
 Systemic lupus erythematosus
 Antiphospholipid antibody syndrome
 Systemic sclerosis (particularly limited scleroderma, or CREST syndrome)
 Mixed connective tissue disease
Systemic vasculitides
 Rheumatoid vasculitis
 Polyarteritis nodosa
 Wegener granulomatosis
 Microscopic polyangiitis
 Churg-Strauss syndrome
 Cryoglobulinemia
Miscellaneous
 Paraproteinemia
 Ergotism

CREST, calcinosis, Raynaud phenomenon, esophageal motility, sclerodactyly, and telangiectasias.

major arterial supplies to the hands and feet may become occluded, leading to coolness and pain of the entire distal extremity, necessitating amputation (Figure 42–2).

3. Peripheral nerve—Early in the disease, nonspecific pains in the calf, foot, or toes may imply a primary neuropathic process. These sensory symptoms may result from thickening of the tissues immediately surrounding the veins and arteries, leading to connective tissue proliferation around the nerve bundles that are intimately connected with the vasculature. True vasculitic neuropathy, however, does not occur in Buerger disease.

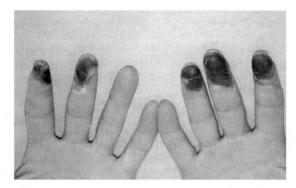

Figure 42–1. Digital ischemia with gangrene in Buerger disease.

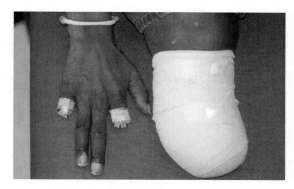

Figure 42–2. The consequence of failure to stop smoking: multiple amputations. This patient proceeded to amputations of every finger on both hands and bilateral below-the-knee amputations.

4. Gastrointestinal tract and other organs—Extremely rare cases of Buerger disease involving the gastrointestinal tract and other organs have been reported.

B. LABORATORY FINDINGS

There is no single diagnostic test for Buerger disease. The demonstration of "corkscrew collaterals" (Figure 42–3)

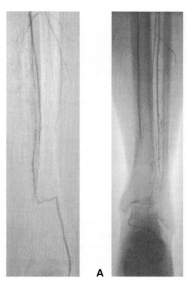

B A

Figure 42–3. Angiographic findings in Buerger disease. **A:** Attenuation of the anterior tibial artery in the mid-calf. This artery forms a collateral at the site of occlusion with the peroneal artery. The posterior tibial artery is occluded superiorly. **B:** Abrupt arterial cutoffs several centimeters above the ankle, with minimal blood flow distal to the cutoffs.

Table 42–2. Laboratory and Radiologic Evaluation in Possible Buerger Disease

Test	Typical Results
Complete blood cell count	Normal. Mild elevations of the white blood cell and platelet count would not be unexpected.
Renal and hepatic function	Normal
Urinalysis with microscopy	Normal
Erythrocyte sedimentation rate (ESR)/ C-reactive protein	Mild to moderate elevations in patients with severe digital ischemia. Dramatically elevated acute phase reactants (eg, an ESR >100 mm/h) unusual.
ANA	Negative
Rheumatoid factor	Negative
C3, C4	Normal
ANCA	Negative
Hepatitis B and C serologies	Negative
Antiphospholipid antibodies	Negative rapid plasma reagin and anticardiolipin antibody assays. Normal Russell viper venom time (for lupus anticoagulant).
Blood cultures	Negative
Echocardiography (or TEE)	No cardiac valvular vegetations. Normal aortic root.
Angiography	Corkscrew collaterals (see Figure 42–3). Abrupt cutoffs of medium-sized arteries at levels of the ankles and wrists, and often higher. Segmental areas of involvement, with diseased regions interspersed with normal-appearing arterial stretches

ANA, antinuclear antibody; ANCA, antineutrophil cytoplasmic antibody; TEE, transesophageal echocardiography.

on angiography is highly characteristic but not pathognomonic. Such vessels may also be observed in polyarteritis nodosa and other forms of medium-vessel vasculitis. Laboratory and radiologic investigations are important in Buerger disease, both to identify the typical vascular lesions and to exclude conditions that require other approaches to management. Table 42–2 lists the results of routine laboratory tests and specialized assays that are done to rule out disorders masquerading as Buerger disease.

The erythrocyte sedimentation rate and C-reactive protein levels are generally lower than observed in many other types of diffuse systemic vasculitis, but most pa-tients have at least moderate elevations of these acute phase reactants. Routine hematology, serum chemistry, and urinalysis studies are normal in Buerger disease; abnormalities in these tests suggest other diagnoses. Markers of hypercoagulable states that may be associated with widespread arterial thromboses, eg, antiphospholipid antibodies, should be investigated.

C. IMAGING STUDIES

Echocardiography (possibly including a transesophageal study) should examine the heart valves and aortic root. Comprehensive angiographic studies that define the vasculature of the extremities, proximal aorta, gastrointestinal tract, and renal arteries should be considered. Such studies are critical in identifying vascular involvement typical of Buerger disease and excluding atheroembolic sources as well as findings more typical of other vasculitides (eg, microaneurysms). The arterial involvement in Buerger disease is highly segmental, with abrupt vascular occlusions interspersed with regions of vessels that appear angiographically normal (see Figure 42–3). In advanced cases, the thready appearance of vessels distal to the wrists and ankles may resemble a disorganized spider web. The most commonly involved vessels are the digital arteries of the fingers and toes as well as the palmar, plantar, tibial, peroneal, radial, and ulnar vessels.

Differential Diagnosis

The major conditions in the differential diagnosis of Buerger disease are cardiovascular diseases, autoimmune disorders, and systemic vasculitides (see Table 42–1). Among the cardiovascular diseases, atherosclerosis and cardiogenic emboli are the principal considerations. Echocardiography (including transesophageal echocardiography) and angiography may be helpful in distinguishing Buerger disease from cardiovascular conditions. Careful imaging of the proximal aorta is essential. In contrast to Buerger disease, atherosclerotic disease characteristically affects the proximal vessels. Sources of cardiogenic emboli must be excluded by echocardiography and blood cultures.

Among the autoimmune disorders, systemic lupus erythematosus, the antiphospholipid antibody syndrome, and scleroderma all may present with digital ischemia. Limited scleroderma (the CREST syndrome [*c*alcinosis, *R*aynaud phenomenon, *e*sophageal dysmotility, *s*clerodactyly, and *t*elangiectasias]; see Chapter 26) may pose special diagnostic challenges because of its propensity to cause digital loss, particularly when associated with anticentromere antibodies. Careful examination of the vasculature in the nailbeds, where dilated capillary loops appear in scleroderma and other connective tissue disorders, may help distinguish these conditions from Buerger disease. Buerger disease, in contrast to connective tissue diseases, is not associated with a significant autoantibody response.

The systemic vasculitides commonly associated with distal ischemia and gangrene are rheumatoid vasculitis, polyarteritis nodosa, Wegener granulomatosis, microscopic polyangiitis, Churg-Strauss syndrome, and cryoglobulinemia. In general, the lack of visceral involvement in Buerger disease helps distinguish it from other vasculitides. For example, ulcerations of the shins, calves, and malleolar regions are atypical of Buerger disease but common among the other forms of vasculitis listed above. Vasculitic neuropathy, often striking in the other forms of systemic vasculitis, does not occur in Buerger disease.

Treatment

The only effective intervention in Buerger disease is complete smoking cessation. Despite the similarities of Buerger disease to systemic vasculitides that affect medium-sized blood vessels and to hypercoagulable states, there is no role for immunosuppressive interventions or anticoagulation in this condition. Moreover, because of the obliterative nature of the vascular inflammatory and thrombotic processes, the vasculature distal to the lesions generally offers no blood vessels large enough to sustain bypass grafts. Thrombolysis, which has not been studied in substantial numbers of patients, carries with it significant risks and perhaps a low likelihood of success, given the length of thromboses present in Buerger disease. Effective pain control is important during periods of intense pain from digital ischemia (without it, patients may only smoke more).

Complications

Without smoking cessation, Buerger disease progresses inexorably through an obliterative vascular process, leading to coolness of the digits, hands, and feet; paresthesias; intermittent claudication symptoms; skin ulcerations over the fingers and toes; and gangrenous infarctions of the extremities. Once established, the disease may be maintained by even small exposures to tobacco (even smokeless tobacco or second-hand smoke). Failure to stop smoking is associated with a dramatic increase in the risk of limb loss by amputation. The angiogram often looks far worse than the patient does; the extent of vascular obliteration may hold out little hope for preserving the patient's extremities, but complete abstinence from tobacco may be remarkably successful in saving limbs.

REFERENCES

Buerger L. Thromboangiitis obliterans: a study of the vascular lesions leading to presenile spontaneous gangrene. *Am J Med Sci.* 1908;136:567. (Perceptive, detailed summaries of the first cases described and recognized to be a new disease.)

McKusick VA, et al. Buerger's disease: A distinct clinical and pathological entity. *JAMA.* 1962;181:93.

Mill JL, Sr. Buerger's disease in the 21st century: diagnosis, clinical features, and treatment. *Semin Vasc Surg.* 2003;16;179. [PMID: 12975757] (Smoking cessation remains the mainstay of treatment.)

Relevant World Wide Web Site

[The Johns Hopkins Vasculitis Center]
http://vasculitis.med.jhu.edu

Miscellaneous Forms of Vasculitis

Philip Seo, MD, MHS & John H. Stone, MD, MPH

RHEUMATOID VASCULITIS

ESSENTIALS OF DIAGNOSIS

- *Rheumatoid vasculitis usually occurs in patients with severe, long-standing, nodular, destructive rheumatoid arthritis, especially when the joint disease is "burnt out."*
- *Palpable purpura, cutaneous ulcers (particularly in the malleolar region), digital infarctions, and peripheral sensory neuropathy are common manifestations.*
- *Tissue biopsy helps establish the diagnosis of rheumatoid vasculitis. Nerve conduction studies can identify involved nerves for biopsy. Muscle biopsies should be performed simultaneously with nerve biopsies to increase the diagnostic yield of the procedure.*

General Considerations

Rheumatoid vasculitis (RV) is a medium-vessel vasculitis that occurs in patients with "burnt-out" but previously severe rheumatoid arthritis (RA). The typical patient has long-standing RA characterized by rheumatoid nodules, destructive joint disease, and high titers of rheumatoid factor. The diagnosis of RV should be considered in any patient with RA in whom new constitutional symptoms, skin ulcerations, serositis, digital ischemia, or symptoms of sensory or motor nerve dysfunction develop. RV resembles polyarteritis nodosa because it leads to multiorgan dysfunction in the skin, peripheral nerves, gastrointestinal tract, and other organs. Manifestations of RV include cutaneous ulcerations, digital ischemia, mononeuritis multiplex, and mesenteric vasculitis (see Chapter 36).

Pathogenesis

Immune complex deposition and antibody-mediated destruction of endothelial cells both appear to contribute to RV. Certain human leukocyte antigen (HLA)-DR4 alleles that predispose patients to severe RA may also heighten patients' susceptibility to RV. Cigarette smoking increases the risk of RV. However, the inciting events leading to the development of RV among patients with previously destructive arthritis are not known. Factors in addition to vasculitis (eg, diabetes, atherosclerosis, and hypertension) likely play an important adjunctive role in promoting vascular occlusion, but the central issue in RV is necrotizing inflammation of blood vessels.

Clinical Findings

A. SYMPTOMS AND SIGNS

1. Skin—Dermatologic findings, the most common manifestation of RV, may include palpable purpura, cutaneous ulcers (particularly in the malleolar region), and digital infarctions (Figure 43–1).

2. Nervous system—A peripheral sensory neuropathy is a common manifestation of RV. A mixed motor-sensory neuropathy or mononeuritis multiplex may also be seen. Central nervous system manifestations (such as strokes, seizures, and cranial nerve palsies) are considerably less common.

3. Eyes—Retinal vasculitis as a manifestation of RV is common but frequently asymptomatic. Necrotizing scleritis and peripheral ulcerative keratitis (Figure 43–2) pose threats to vision and require aggressive immunosuppressive therapy.

4. Serositis—Pericarditis and pleuritis may occur in association with RV. Other cardiopulmonary manifestations of RV are unusual.

B. LABORATORY FINDINGS

Most laboratory findings in RV (such as elevations in the erythrocyte sedimentation rate) are nonspecific, and merely reflect the presence of an inflammatory state. Hypocomplementemia, antinuclear antibodies, atypical antineutrophil cytoplasmic antibodies (ANCAs) (by immunofluorescence testing but not enzyme immunoassay; see Chapter 33 on Wegener granulomatosis), and anti-endothelial cell antibodies are all detected more frequently in patients with RV than in those with RA alone.

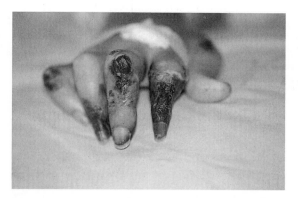

Figure 43–1. Digital infarctions in rheumatoid vasculitis.

The usefulness of these findings for diagnosing RV, however, is not well established.

C. IMAGING STUDIES

The presence of bony erosions is a risk factor for the development of RV, but plain radiographs and other imaging studies have no consistent role in the evaluation of this disorder.

D. SPECIAL TESTS

Because the treatment implications for RV are so severe, the diagnosis must be established by tissue biopsy whenever possible. Deep skin biopsies (full-thickness biopsies that include some subcutaneous fat) taken from the edge of ulcers are very useful in detecting the presence of medium-vessel vasculitis. Nerve conduction studies help identify involved nerves for biopsy. Muscle biopsies (eg, of the gastrocnemius muscle) should be performed simultaneously with nerve biopsies.

Differential Diagnosis

Patients with erosive RA are at increased risk for infections. When patients with RA seek medical attention for the new onset of nonspecific systemic complaints, the possibility of infection must be considered first. Cholesterol emboli may cause digital ischemia and a host of other signs and symptoms that mimic vasculitis. Diabetes mellitus is another major cause of mononeuritis multiplex, but multiple mononeuropathies occurring over a short period of time are unusual in that condition. Many clinical features of RV mimic those of polyarteritis nodosa and other forms of necrotizing vasculitis.

Treatment

Therapy must reflect the severity of organ involvement. Small, relatively painless infarctions around the nailbed develop in some patients with nodular RA (Figure 43–3). Although such lesions are caused by a low-grade vasculitis, they do not herald the presence of systemic rheumatoid vasculitis and do not necessarily require any adjustment in patients' therapy. With other disease manifestations, however, such as cutaneous ulcers, vasculitic neuropathy, and inflammatory eye disease, glucocorticoids may be required. Cyclophosphamide, required in many cases of RV, should be employed with appropriate caution, given that many patients with RV suffer substantial disabilities at baseline. Tumor necrosis factor inhibition may be an effective strategy in RV, but the role of tumor necrosis factor inhibitors relative to that of other agents (eg, methotrexate and cyclophosphamide) requires further investigation.

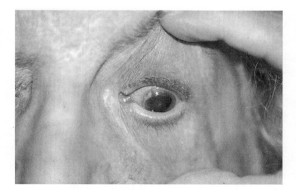

Figure 43–2. Peripheral ulcerative keratitis in a patient with nodular, destructive rheumatoid arthritis and rheumatoid vasculitis.

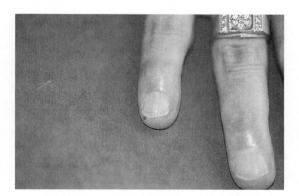

Figure 43–3. Nailbed infarctions in a patient with rheumatoid arthritis. Such lesions do not necessarily herald the onset of systemic rheumatoid vasculitis.

Prognosis

Although RV is a treatable condition, the development of this complication is a poor prognostic indicator.

COGAN SYNDROME

ESSENTIALS OF DIAGNOSIS

- *The hallmark of Cogan syndrome is the presence of ocular inflammation and audiovestibular dysfunction. These findings may be accompanied by evidence of a systemic vasculitis.*
- *Interstitial keratitis is the most common form of ocular involvement.*
- *Audiovestibular dysfunction may lead to the acute onset of vertigo, tinnitus, nausea, and vomiting.*
- *Vasculitis in Cogan syndrome may take the form of aortitis, renal artery stenosis, or occlusion of the great vessels.*

General Considerations

Cogan syndrome (CS), an immune-mediated condition that primarily affects young adults, is associated with ocular inflammation (usually interstitial keratitis) and audiovestibular dysfunction. This syndrome may be accompanied by a systemic vasculitis of large- and medium-sized arteries that may resemble Takayasu arteritis.

Pathogenesis

The onset of CS is frequently preceded by an upper respiratory tract infection. Because many features of CS can be caused by known pathogens (eg, *Treponema pallidum*), CS may be the direct consequence of an unidentified pathogen affecting the eyes, ears, and blood vessels. Alternatively, CS may be the indirect consequence of a pathogen that induces an immune response that continues to attack the host long after the pathogen has been eliminated (a phenomenon known as molecular mimicry). Neither of these theories has been proved.

Clinical Findings

A. SYMPTOMS AND SIGNS

1. Eye—The most common ocular manifestation of CS is interstitial keratitis, which is characterized by the abrupt onset of photophobia, lacrimation, and eye pain.

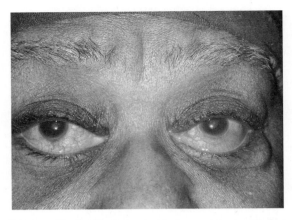

Figure 43–4. Bilateral scleritis in a patient with Cogan syndrome who had suffered the rapid onset of sensorineural hearing loss in both ears.

CS may also be associated with inflammation in other parts of the eye; scleritis (Figure 43–4), peripheral ulcerative keratitis, episcleritis, anterior uveitis, conjunctivitis, and retinal vascular disease are all possible.

2. Ear—Patients with CS frequently suffer the acute onset of vertigo, tinnitus, nausea, and vomiting. These symptoms may be enormously disabling. The audiovestibular symptoms may occur before or after the onset of ocular disease, and are often separated in onset by weeks or months. If not treated promptly and aggressively, permanent hearing loss may ensue. Recurrent attacks, which are common, may cause decremental loss of hearing. Ultimately, complete hearing loss occurs in as many as 60% of patients.

3. Large-vessel vasculitis—The most common manifestation of vasculitis in patients with CS is aortitis. Aortitis may lead to dilatation of the aorta and subsequent incompetence of the aortic valve. Involvement of aortic branches (Figure 43–5) may cause claudication in the arms or legs. Renal artery stenosis or occlusion of the great vessels may also occur. These manifestations may be accompanied by nonspecific constitutional symptoms such as malaise, fever, or weight loss, as well as arthralgias and frank arthritis.

B. LABORATORY FINDINGS

Laboratory findings are nondiagnostic and generally reflect the presence of inflammation. An antibody against a 68-kDa antigen has been identified in cases of autoimmune sensorineural hearing loss but is not found in patients with CS. Exclusion of syphilis with fluorescent treponemal antibody testing (ie, FTA-ABS, not just the rapid plasma reagin) is essential.

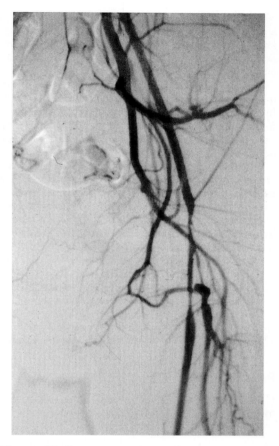

Figure 43–5. Large-vessel vasculitis in Cogan syndrome. Femoral artery disease led to lower extremity claudication.

C. Imaging Studies

Gadolinium-enhanced T1-weighted magnetic resonance imaging studies may demonstrate a hyperintensity in the membranous labyrinth secondary to vessel inflammation in the stria vascularis. This enhancement is not seen in patients with inactive CS and may be useful in identifying the activity of the disease. Brainstem magnetic resonance imaging studies are also essential to exclude tumors of the cerebellopontine angle, which may mimic the audiovestibular features of CS. Angiography may be useful to define the involvement of the great vessels (see Figure 43–5). Magnetic resonance angiography is useful in evaluating vessel wall thickness and edema as well as the degree of luminal stenosis. Serial echocardiography may be used to assess and monitor aortic insufficiency.

Table 43–1. Differential Diagnosis of the Audio-vestibular Complications of Cogan Syndrome

Alternate Diagnoses	Comments
Immune-mediated inner ear disease	Sensorineural hearing loss and vestibular dysfunction in the absence of eye inflammation.
Syphilis	Latent and tertiary forms of this disease. Ordering both rapid plasma reagin and FTA-ABS essential.
Other infections	Lyme disease, mumps
Acoustic neuroma	Performance of brainstem magnetic resonance imaging essential to exclude this tumor.
Ménière syndrome	Inner ear disturbances in Ménière are generally more intermittent, with a waxing/waning character.
Systemic vasculitides	Wegener granulomatosis, giant cell arteritis
Collagen vascular diseases	Sjögren syndrome
Other inflammatory conditions	Sarcoidosis, Susac syndrome
Barotrauma	Other etiologies of perilymph fistula formation
Medications	Aminoglycosides, loop diuretics, antimalarials

FTA-ABS, fluorescent treponemal antibody, absorption test.

D. Special Tests

Formal audiometric testing is important early in the evaluation to distinguish conductive hearing loss from sensorineural hearing dysfunction. In CS, audiometry demonstrates sensorineural hearing loss that preferentially affects the low- and high-range frequencies. This may be a useful way to document response to therapy, although subsequent hearing loss is not always due to active disease.

Differential Diagnosis

The differential diagnosis of immune-mediated inner ear disease (ie, sensorineural hearing loss with or without vestibular dysfunction) is shown in Table 43–1. Inflammatory eye disease may be caused by a variety of pathogens, including bacterial (eg, *Chlamydia* or *Neisseria*), spirochetal (eg, *Borrelia burgdorferi*), viral (eg, herpes simplex or varicella-zoster), and mycobacterial (eg, *Mycobacterium tuberculosis* or *M leprae*).

Treatment

Some manifestations of CS respond well to symptomatic therapy. In general, the ocular manifestations are more amenable to therapy than the auricular complications. Interstitial keratitis may be treated with topical atropine or glucocorticoids. Sensorineural hearing loss in CS is analogous to rapidly progressive glomerulonephritis in other forms of systemic vasculitis: Prompt treatment with cyclophosphamide and glucocorticoids is indicated. For patients with advanced, irreversible hearing loss, hearing aids and cochlear implants may help. Vestibular retraining may be required for some patients with significant cochlear damage.

Complications

The prevention of complications depends directly on the rapid recognition of this diagnosis, and the equally swift institution of therapy. Permanent damage may result early in the course of immune-mediated inner ear disease, and hearing deficits will not respond to therapy if initiated too late. Therefore, a high index of suspicion for this diagnosis must be maintained when evaluating patients with compatible complaints.

Prognosis

Even if the initial event is recognized and responds to the therapy, recurrent bouts of sensorineural hearing loss may cause the gradual loss of hearing. Up to 60% of patients experience some degree of permanent hearing loss. Some patients become completely deaf.

URTICARIAL VASCULITIS

ESSENTIALS OF DIAGNOSIS

- *The lesions of urticarial vasculitis are frequently associated with burning or pain rather than pruritus and require more than 24 hours to resolve.*
- *Immunofluorescence on skin biopsy specimen is the critical test. Intense staining for immunoreactants (ie, IgG, IgM, C3, C4, and C1q) not only in and around small blood vessel walls but also in a ribbon along the dermal/epidermal junction is pathognomonic of hypocomplementemic urticarial vasculitis.*

General Considerations

Urticarial vasculitis (UV) is a leukocytoclastic vasculitis that presents as hives (often associated with pain or dis-

comfort) that last longer than 24 hours. Although UV is occasionally seen in isolation, it most often appears in association with connective tissue disorders such as serum sickness, cryoglobulinemia, and systemic lupus erythematosus (SLE).

UV targets the capillaries and postcapillary venules in the skin, leading to the appearance of hivelike lesions. In approaching patients with this problem, it is critical to distinguish cases associated with hypocomplementia from those in which the serum complement levels are normal.

Hypocomplementemic UV is associated with depressed serum levels of C3 and C4. Such cases often overlap with known connective tissue disorders, particularly SLE. At the severe end of the spectrum of this disorder are patients with a distinct disorder known as the **hypocomplementemic urticarial vasculitis syndrome** (HUVS).

The normocomplementemic form is a subset of cutaneous leukocytoclastic angiitis (see Chapter 38) in which the leukocytoclastic vasculitis manifests clinically as urticaria. In general, these cases are secondary to "hypersensitivity" reactions (usually caused by a medication) and respond to discontinuation of the offending agent. This form of UV is not discussed further in this chapter.

Pathogenesis

Hypocomplementemic UV is mediated at least in part by immune complex deposition. In one model, following an unknown inciting event, the deposition of IgG and C3 leads to further complement activation. The complement cascade activates mast cells and eosinophils, both of which act to form the typical urticarial wheal. The eosinophils are gradually replaced by neutrophils, leading to the leukocytoclastic destruction of capillary walls.

Clinical Findings

A. SYMPTOMS AND SIGNS

The lesions of UV, typically between 0.5 and 2.0 cm in diameter (Figure 43–6), are frequently associated with burning or pain rather than pruritus. In contrast to common urticaria, UV lesions usually require more than 24 hours to resolve, and typically leave small amounts of hyperpigmentation in the skin, caused by red blood cell extravasation.

Like SLE, hypocomplementemic UV may also be associated with malaise, arthralgias, fever, and glomerulonephritis. Unlike SLE, HUVS is characterized not only by recurrent or chronic UV, but also by angioedema. Moreover, severe chronic obstructive pulmonary disease and uveitis—manifestations that are atypical of SLE—often complicate this condition. Jaccoud arthropathy has

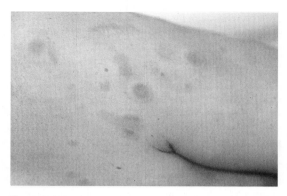

Figure 43–6. Lesions of hypocomplementemic urticarial vasculitis.

been noted in some patients with HUVS and possibly correlates with the presence of cardiac valvular lesions.

B. LABORATORY FINDINGS

Serum C3, C4, and CH50 levels are depressed. Hypocomplementemic UV is generally accompanied by the presence of anti-C1q autoantibodies. The presence of these antibodies is not pathognomonic, since they also may be found in patients with SLE who do not have UV. Patients with hypocomplementemic UV have antinuclear antibodies, and if significant overlap with SLE is present, may also have other autoantibodies (eg, anti-dsDNA, anti-Ro/SS-A, anti-La/SS-B, anti-Sm, and anti-RNP).

C. SPECIAL TESTS

Hematoxylin and eosin staining of skin biopsy specimens reveals a leukocytoclastic vasculitis in the superficial dermis. Older lesions may have a predominantly lymphocytic infiltrate. The critical test is the performance of immunofluorescence on the skin biopsy specimen, which reveals intense staining for immunoreactants (ie, IgG, IgM, C3, C4, and C1q) not only in and around small blood vessel walls, but also in a ribbon along the dermal/epidermal junction. These findings are pathognomonic of hypocomplementemic UV.

Differential Diagnosis

The skin lesions of hypocomplementemic UV must be distinguished from common urticaria (which is characterized by pruritic lesions that resolve completely over 2–8 hours, leaving no traces of the original lesion), neutrophilic urticaria (a persistent, treatment-refractory form of urticaria not associated with vasculitis), and normocomplementic UV (see above).

Treatment

UV may respond to therapies commonly used in SLE, such as low-dose prednisone, hydroxychloroquine, dapsone, or other immunomodulatory agents. There is anecdotal evidence that antihistamines, calcium channel antagonists, doxepin, methotrexate, indomethacin, colchicine, and pentoxifylline are effective in some cases.

HUVS is frequently a therapeutic challenge. Serious cases, particularly those presenting with glomerulonephritis or other organ involvement, may require treatment with high doses of glucocorticoids, cyclophosphamide, or cyclosporine. Angioedema, chronic obstructive pulmonary disease, and cardiac valvular abnormalities may all necessitate other specific interventions.

Prognosis

Hypocomplementemic UV frequently reflects the presence of an underlying disorder, which may influence the prognosis substantially. HUVS may be associated with multiple complications (eg, severe chronic obstructive pulmonary disease) that affect prognosis adversely.

ERYTHEMA ELEVATUM DIUTINUM

 ESSENTIALS OF DIAGNOSIS

- *New lesions come in the form of tender papules, associated with pruritus or a burning sensation.*
- *Lesions develop into red, reddish-brown, or purple papules or nodules.*
- *Lesions may coalesce to form large plaques, usually over the extensor surfaces of joints.*

General Considerations

Erythema elevatum diutinum (EED) is a chronic, recurring cutaneous vasculitis in which tender papules appear on the extensor surfaces of the extremities. The onset of these lesions is usually heralded by the presence of pruritus or stinging, followed by the development of tender papules or nodules that coalesce with others to form plaques. The skin findings are frequently located near joints, such as on the extensor surfaces of the hands and fingers.

Pathogenesis

The pathogenesis of EED is unknown but may involve recurrent immune complex deposition, followed by incomplete attempts at healing. Persistence of an antigen, with a subsequent increase in dendrocyte activity, may also play a role in its pathogenesis. There is an association between EED and multiple infections (including HIV, hepatitis B and C, tuberculosis, and streptococcal infections), autoimmune diseases (such as RA, relapsing polychondritis, and type 1 diabetes mellitus), and the paraproteinemias (such as multiple myeloma).

Clinical Findings

A. Symptoms and Signs

A new lesion is heralded by the presence of pruritus or a burning sensation in the skin, which then leads to the development of a red, reddish-brown, or purple papule or nodule. These lesions may coalesce to form large plaques, usually over the extensor surfaces of joints. With healing, the lesions often assume a yellowish or brown color, resembling xanthomata.

B. Laboratory Findings

Patients in whom EED is suspected should be screened for possible causes, including HIV infection, viral hepatitis, syphilis, cryoglobulinemia, and monoclonal gammopathy. When appropriate, patients may benefit from screening for associated autoimmune diseases as well.

C. Special Tests

Skin biopsy specimens usually show a nonspecific leukocytoclastic vasculitis with C3 deposition and are important for excluding non-vasculitis mimickers. In older lesions, the neutrophils are replaced by histiocytes, and there is marked granulation tissue and fibrosis.

Differential Diagnosis

Biopsy of lesions at various stages of development may demonstrate findings that are also consistent with a wide variety of diagnoses, including Sweet syndrome, pyoderma gangrenosum, drug reaction, erythema multiforme, fibrous histiocytoma, Kaposi sarcoma, xanthoma, and necrobiotic xanthogranuloma. The diagnosis can be established only by clinical judgment, supplemented by supportive findings on pathology.

Treatment

When a cause can be established, EED may respond to treatment of the underlying disorder. It is well established, for instance, that patients with EED as a consequence of HIV infection experience a regression of the cutaneous lesions with institution of highly active antiretroviral therapy. Nonspecific therapies are less successful. Lesions may be suppressed by dapsone but tend to recur when the drug is stopped. Lesions may also respond to tetracycline, colchicine, chloroquine, and glucocorticoids (either topical or systemic).

Complications

Although recurrent and frequently unresponsive to therapy, EED is limited to the skin and does not lead to significant morbidity.

Prognosis

The prognosis associated with EED itself, even when unresponsive to therapy, is generally quite good. The overall prognosis for the patient, however, largely depends on the underlying disease process.

DRUG-INDUCED ANCA-ASSOCIATED VASCULITIS

 ESSENTIALS OF DIAGNOSIS

- *Cutaneous eruptions, such as palpable purpura or a maculopapular rash limited to the lower extremities, are the most common manifestation of the drug-induced AAV.*
- *Frequently associated with very high titers of anti-myeloperoxidase ANCA.*
- *Tissue biopsy provides a definitive diagnosis.*

General Considerations

Drug-induced ANCA-associated vasculitis (AAV) is a form of vasculitis induced by certain medications in some patients. The majority of cases are associated with ANCA directed against myeloperoxidase, often in very high titers. Drug-induced AAV may resolve following discontinuation of the offending agent. Other cases, however, are indistinguishable from idiopathic AAV and require intensive therapy with glucocorticoids and cytotoxic agents.

Many cases of drug-induced AAV are associated with relatively minor symptoms (eg, constitutional symptoms, arthralgias or arthritis, and purpura). Propylthiouracil is a well-documented cause of drug-induced AAV. Other drugs implicated thus far include hydralazine, sulfasalazine, minocycline, D-penicillamine, ciprofloxacin, phenytoin, clozapine, allopurinol, and pantoprazole. Leukotriene inhibitors have been linked to the occurrence of the Churg-Strauss syndrome, but the true direct relationship (if any) between these medications and that condition remains unclear (see Chapter 35).

Pathogenesis

All of the events in the pathogenesis of drug-induced AAV remain undefined. Propylthiouracil is known to accumulate within neutrophil granules and alter myeloperoxidase, an event that may trigger the production of anti-myeloperoxidase ANCA. The presence of this human model of ANCA-associated disease forms one of the strongest arguments for a direct contribution of ANCA to the pathophysiology of other human disorders. Recent mouse models also strongly support the concept that ANCA may be pathogenic in humans.

Clinical Findings

A. Symptoms and Signs

Cutaneous eruptions are the most common manifestation of drug-induced AAV. These often present as palpable purpura or a maculopapular rash limited to the lower extremities. Unlike other types of AAV, the skin lesions in the drug-induced form frequently appear in "crops" (ie, simultaneously). Arthralgias and myalgias are common. The kidneys and upper respiratory tract may also be involved, as with the classic forms of AAV.

B. Laboratory Findings

In drug-induced AAV, very high titers of anti-myeloperoxidase antibodies are characteristic. Reports of cases associated with anti-proteinase 3 antibodies are rare. Even when the vasculitis resolves after discontinuation of the causative agent and initiation of immunosuppression, ANCA titers often remain elevated.

C. Special Tests

Tissue biopsy is usually necessary to provide a definitive diagnosis.

Differential Diagnosis

Drug-induced AAV is frequently slow to resolve after cessation of the offending agent and may be difficult to distinguish from the primary ANCA-associated vasculitides. In general, the manifestations of drug-induced AAV are mild and responsive to short courses of immunosuppression, although this is not always the case.

Treatment

The first step in treatment is the identification of the potential offending agents. Clinicians should take into account all exposures during the 6 months before the onset of symptoms, including nonprescription medications, herbal and dietary supplements, and illicit substances. Withdrawal of the offending agent may result in the resolution of the symptoms, although this may take months and may require the withdrawal of numerous agents simultaneously.

Patients with severe organ involvement may require aggressive immunosuppression with glucocorticoids and cytotoxic agents such as cyclophosphamide. The required length of therapy in drug-induced AAV may be shorter than that recommended for primary AAV.

Prognosis

Overall, the prognosis associated with drug-induced AAV is quite good. Organ involvement is frequently limited to the skin, and even systemic involvement frequently responds to lower doses of immunosuppressive agents administered for shorter periods of time than that required for primary AAV.

REFERENCES

Choi HK, Merkel PA, Walker AM, Niles JL. Drug-associated antineutrophil cytoplasmic antibody-positive vasculitis: prevalence among patients with high titers of antimyeloperoxidase antibodies. *Arthritis Rheum.* 2000;43:405. [PMID: 10693882]

Gibson LE, el-Azhary RA. Erythema elevatum diutinum. *Clin Dermatol.* 2000;18:295. [PMID:10856661]

Gluth MB, et al. Cogan's syndrome: A retrospective review of 60 cases through half a century. *Mayo Clin Proc* 2004;81:483. [PMID: 16610568]

Goronzy JJ, Weyand CM. Vasculitis in rheumatoid arthritis. *Curr Opin Rheumatol.* 1994;6:290. [PMID: 8060764] (Focuses on some of the predisposing factors to this complication of rheumatoid arthritis, particularly on potential genetic risk factors.)

Grasland A, et al. Typical and atypical Cogan's syndrome: 32 cases and review of the literature. *Rheumatology* (Oxford) 2004; 43:1007. [PMID: 15150435]

Gunton JE, Stiel J, Clifton-Bligh P, Wilmshurst E, McElduff A. Prevalence of positive anti-neutrophil cytoplasmic antibody (ANCA) in patients receiving anti-thyroid medication. *Eur J Endocrinol.* 2000;142:587. [PMID: 10822221]

Stone JH, Francis HW. Immune-mediated inner ear disease. *Curr Opin Rheumatol.* 2000;12:32. [PMID: 10647952] (A basic review that quantifies many of the unknowns about this condition.)

Stone JH, Nousari HC. "Essential" cutaneous vasculitis: what every rheumatologist should know about vasculitis of the skin. *Curr Opin Rheumatol.* 2001;13:23. [PMID: 11148712] (A logically ordered review of the approach to cutaneous vasculitis, with an emphasis on diagnosis.)

Vollertsen RS, Conn DL. Vasculitis associated with rheumatoid arthritis. *Rheum Dis Clin North Am.* 1990;16:445. [PMID: 2189161] (Comprehensive description of this disease complication.)

Wisnieski JJ. Urticarial vasculitis. *Curr Opin Rheumatol.* 2000;12:24. [PMID: 10647951] (Thoughtful synthesis of the different clinical forms of this disorder.)

SECTION V

Degenerative Joint Disease & Crystal-Induced Arthritis

Osteoarthritis

44

David T. Felson, MD, MPH

ESSENTIALS OF DIAGNOSIS

- *Joint pain brought on and exacerbated by activity and relieved with rest.*
- *Stiffness that is self-limited upon awakening in the morning or when rising from a seated position after an extended period of inactivity.*
- *Absence of prominent constitutional symptoms.*
- *Examination notable for increased bony prominence at the joint margins, crepitus or a grating sensation upon joint manipulation, and tenderness over the joint line of the symptomatic joint.*
- *Diagnosis supported by radiographic features of joint space narrowing and spur (or osteophyte) formation.*

General Considerations

Osteoarthritis (OA) is the leading cause of arthritis in the adult American population and affects an estimated 20 million people in the United States. Joint pain is a frequent symptom that often prompts a patient to seek medical attention; osteoarthritis figures prominently in the differential diagnosis. The challenge for clinicians is to correctly identify the cause of the patient's pain and to initiate appropriate therapy, both medicinal and non-medicinal. Synonymous with degenerative joint disease, OA is characterized by joint pain related to use, self-limited morning stiffness, an audible grating sound or crepitus on palpation, the presence of tenderness over the affected joint on palpation, and frequently reduction in joint range of motion.

Characteristic sites of involvement in the peripheral skeleton include the hand (distal interphalangeal joint, proximal interphalangeal joint, and first carpometacarpal joint [Figure 44–1]), knee (Figure 44–2), and hip (Figure 44–3). Constitutional symptoms are absent. The diagnosis of OA can usually be made relatively easily and confidently based on the history and examination alone. The bedside diagnosis of OA can be supported by plain radiography.

Epidemiology

At the population level, OA results in substantial morbidity and disability, particularly among the elderly. It is the leading indication for the several hundred thousand knee and hip replacement surgeries performed each year in the United States. Therefore, much effort has been invested in improving the understanding of the epidemiology of this disorder, including identifying the factors that predispose persons to OA, especially those risk factors that are reversible or modifiable.

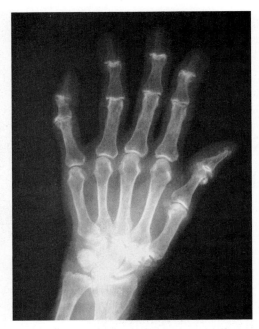

Figure 44-1. Radiograph of a hand showing osteoarthritis of the distal interphalangeal (DIP), proximal interphalangeal (PIP), and first carpometacarpal (CMC) joints. Note the joint space narrowing of the DIP and PIP joints compared to the metacarpophalangeal joints, as well as the bony sclerosis (eburnation) of all joints involved by the osteoarthritis process.

Several factors heighten the risk of incident OA, including age, gender, joint injury, and obesity. Although the clinical manifestations of OA can begin as early as the fourth and fifth decades of life, the incidence of OA continues to increase with each decade of aging. Moreover, women in their 50s, 60s, and 70s have a greater prevalence of OA in the hands and knees than do men. There is evidence that OA among African Americans is more severe and has greater impact on disability than in whites. Genetics probably plays a role in increasing the vulnerability of some joints to disease. The influence of genetics on disease occurrence is significant, for example, in the hips and hands, sites at which OA often runs in families, but appears less important for knee OA, which is more often the consequence of joint injury and loading history.

Trauma to a pristine joint such as a ruptured anterior cruciate ligament or torn meniscus increases the risk of later osteoarthritis at that joint site. Obese women and men are at high risk of knee osteoarthritis and have a modest increase in hip OA risk. This increase in risk is due mostly to the excess load across weight-bearing joints conferred by obesity, and at least for women, the risk is proportional to the degree of overweight. For knee OA, weight loss in middle age may lower this risk.

Pathogenesis

The currently known causes of osteoarthritis are shown in Table 44-1. OA is a disease in which most or all of the joint structures are affected by pathology. The primary tissue affected is the thin rim of hyaline articular cartilage interposed between the two articulating bones. This avascular tissue becomes worn away, especially in areas of injury. There is also sclerosis of underlying bone, growth of osteophytes at the joint margin, weakness and atrophy of muscles that bridge the joint, ligamentous laxity and disruption, and in many joints, synovitis. With focal cartilage loss on one side of the joint and bony remodeling there, malalignment across the joint can develop, increasing focal transarticular loading and causing further damage to cartilage and underlying bone. Both subtle chronic

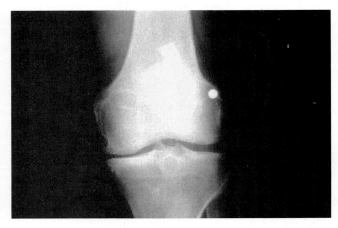

Figure 44-2. Knee osteoarthritis with medial joint space narrowing and osteophytes.

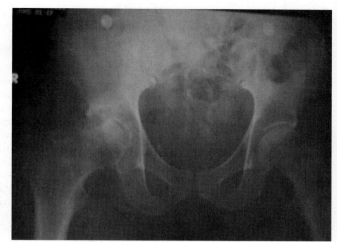

Figure 44–3. Right hip osteoarthritis. Note the joint space narrowing of the superior portion of the involved joint, compared to the same portion of the opposite joint.

and flagrant acute injuries can start this disease process. Cartilage matrix turnover, spurred by daily loading across the joint, can replenish cartilage, but as a consequence of genetic abnormalities, age, and other metabolic factors not yet fully understood, some cartilage is especially vulnerable to loading.

Prevention

At present, there are no proven preventive strategies, but there are some promising measures that can be taken.

Table 44–1. Identifiable Causes of Osteoarthritis

Congenital disorder (hip)
  Legg-Calvé-Perthes disease
  Acetabular dysplasia
  Slipped capital femoral epiphysis
Inborn error of connective tissue
  Ehlers-Danlos syndrome
  Marfan syndrome
Posttraumatic (knee)
  Anterior cruciate ligament tear
  Meniscus tear with or without prior meniscectomy surgery
Metabolic disorders
  Hemochromatosis
  Wilson disease
  Ochronosis (alkaptonuria)
  History of a septic joint
Postinflammatory
  Underlying rheumatoid arthritis
Generalized osteoarthritis
  Predilection for first CMC, DIP, PIP, knee, and hip joints

CMC, carpometacarpal; DIP, distal interphalangeal; PIP, proximal interphalangeal.

Among women who participated in the Framingham Osteoarthritis Study, over a 10-year period, those who had experienced a 5-kg or more reduction in weight had half the risk of developing symptomatic knee osteoarthritis. Such data support the claim that weight reduction can alter the risk of developing OA, and it stands to reason that weight loss may also delay disease progression.

Because major joint injury causes a large proportion of knee OA in the community, avoiding major injuries may prevent disease. This is especially relevant to young women athletes who are at high risk of anterior cruciate ligament tears, injuries associated with a high risk of subsequent knee osteoarthritis. Persons with knees that have already sustained major injuries are at high risk of subsequent injuries and should avoid athletic activities associated with high risk.

Clinical Findings

The signs, symptoms, and diagnostic features of osteoarthritis are shown in Table 44–2.

A. SYMPTOMS AND SIGNS

The patient with osteoarthritis affecting a joint in the peripheral skeleton, such as the finger, knee, or hip, may initially experience relatively minor pain or discomfort with use of the involved joint (see Table 44–2). For example, at the outset of osteoarthritis involving the hip joint, patients may have some difficulty crossing their legs or putting on a pair of shoes or pants; however, once they are dressed and upright, bearing weight and ambulation are still well tolerated. As osteoarthritis progresses, a patient will gradually experience progressively severe joint discomfort and increasing difficulty with activities of daily living.

Table 44–2. Signs, Symptoms, and Diagnostic Features of Osteoarthritis

---

Joint pain that increases with activity

Morning stiffness that is relatively brief and self-limited

Crepitus (a grating sensation with motion)

Bony enlargement at the joint margin

Tenderness to palpation over the joint

Noninflammatory synovial fluid (<1000 WBC/mm^3)

Erythrocyte sedimentation rate normal for age

Radiographic evidence of osteoarthritis (nonuniform joint space narrowing, osteophyte [spur] formation, subchondral cysts, and eburnation [bony sclerosis])

Negative serologic tests for antinuclear antibody and rheumatoid factor

---

With further disease progression, such as an osteoarthritic hand or finger, increasing difficulty with previously routine activities often follows. Thus, such tasks as gripping, holding, or writing with a pen or pencil, putting car keys in and turning the ignition switch, lifting a gallon of milk out of the refrigerator, or removing a pot of water from the stove become difficult tasks. At the extreme end of the disease spectrum, marked impairment in activity follows. Even walking from room to room in one's home may be unbearably painful when advanced osteoarthritis affects the hip or knee joint.

In patients with knee osteoarthritis, joint instability or "giving way" is common, sometimes leading to falling or near-falling events. These pose substantial health risks to the elderly, and can contribute significantly to fear, frailty, and isolation.

B. Laboratory Findings

There is no specific laboratory test used in clinical practice to confirm a diagnosis of osteoarthritis. Instead, routine laboratory blood testing, including complete blood cell counts, acute phase reactants (erythrocyte sedimentation rate and C-reactive protein), and screening autoantibodies (rheumatoid factor and antinuclear antibody) are indicated if inflammatory arthritis such as rheumatoid arthritis is being considered. If joints affected are typical of OA (eg, distal interphalangeal, proximal interphalangeal, and the first carpometacarpal joints) and symptoms in hands and other joints are related to activity, serological evaluation is probably not indicated. However, if the clinical presentation is consistent with rheumatoid arthritis (eg, if the wrists are affected or if prolonged morning stiffness [stiffness lasting >30–60 minutes] is prominent), blood tests may be of diagnostic value to distinguish osteoarthritis from rheumatoid arthritis. Unlike most patients with OA, those with inflammatory arthritis including rheumatoid arthritis will have elevated levels of acute phase reactants and may be anemic.

C. Imaging Studies

Radiographic imaging can confirm the diagnosis of osteoarthritis. In an older patient with bony enlargement on examination and activity-related pain, x-rays (which have imperfect sensitivity, sometimes being negative in the presence of disease), may not be indicated. More than 4 decades ago, Kellgren and Lawrence described characteristic radiographic features of OA—joint space narrowing, osteophytes, subchondral cysts, and bony sclerosis (eburnation) (see Figure 44–1). These remain the radiographic hallmarks of osteoarthritis. Although magnetic resonance imaging may reveal characteristic findings of OA, such findings are universal in older persons, making it a test with poor discriminative power for the diagnosis of OA.

D. Special Tests

An arthrocentesis can be a valuable test when encountering a patient with presumptive osteoarthritis. In OA the synovial fluid white blood cell count is <1000 cells/mm^3; counts >1000/mm^3 suggest the possibility of an inflammatory arthritis (see Chapter 4). In fluids from osteoarthritic joints, crystals visible by light microscopy are absent, but the presence of gout or pseudogout crystals provides diagnostic evidence of other forms of arthritis that occasionally are difficult to distinguish from osteoarthritis. This is particularly true for pseudogout.

Differential Diagnosis

The challenge when evaluating a patient with joint pain is to use the history, physical examination, and sometimes a modicum of additional tests to arrive at the correct diagnosis in an efficient manner. The presence of joint pain brought on by activity and relieved with rest suggests the existence of osteoarthritis. The absence of constitutional signs and symptoms and the presence of bony enlargement and tenderness at the joint margin reinforce this clinical impression. Finally, the pattern of joint involvement is meaningful because osteoarthritis has a predilection for the knees, hips, and distal interphalangeal, proximal interphalangeal, and first carpometacarpal joints of the hands. This distribution of joint involvement distinguishes osteoarthritis from such inflammatory forms of arthritis as rheumatoid arthritis, psoriatic arthritis, and gout, which have different sites of involvement.

It is also worth noting that a variety of secondary disorders represent identifiable causes of osteoarthritis. Several such disorders, including those resulting from inborn errors of metabolism and metabolic derangements, are listed in Table 44–1. Recognition of their distinct features, such as predilection for involvement of the second and third metacarpophalangeal joints in hemochromatosis-associated arthropathy, may identify the underlying cause of the joint pain. Finally, since osteoarthritis is extremely common, its presence does not exclude consideration of an alternate explanation for joint pain, such as an occult malignancy. Such diagnoses should be considered when there is a meaningful change in the pattern of joint pain.

If giving way or buckling occurs, this may indicate a meniscal tear or other internal derangement of the knee. Tears often occur abruptly and memorably. Joint buckling from meniscal tears generally occurs with activities that involve twisting or changing direction, not while walking straight.

Treatment

The goals of medical therapy are to control pain, improve function, minimize disability, and enhance health-related quality of life. A further therapeutic priority is to minimize the risk of drug-associated toxicity, particularly that which may result from nonsteroidal anti-inflammatory drug (NSAID) therapy.

In patients with osteoarthritis, nonpharmacologic treatments are underutilized. They have demonstrated efficacy and can often help relieve pain and improve function. For example, an assistive device, such as a properly-used cane or walker, can unload an affected knee or hip and diminish pain with walking. Similarly, quadriceps strengthening and aerobic exercise are effective in the management of osteoarthritis at the knee. For exercise therapy, referral to a physical therapist is often helpful, as they will evaluate function and craft the right mix of exercises. Adherence to exercise is often poor, and it helps to reinforce the exercise regimen at each visit. For knee osteoarthritis patients with varus deformity and pain, neoprene sleeves have been shown in a randomized trial to diminish pain. If this does not work, fitted valgus braces, designed to decrease the varus malalignment across the knee, have been shown also to decrease pain. Other approaches to realignment of the malaligned knee can also be tried such as wedged shoe insoles, but there is no strong evidence-based support for their efficacy. Weight loss should be encouraged for all persons with knee or hip osteoarthritis.

A front-line approach to medicinal therapy for osteoarthritis includes use of acetaminophen. This drug improves pain and function and has a safer toxicity profile, particularly with regard to the gastrointestinal tract, than NSAIDs. For many years, NSAIDs have been widely used in the management of OA. Via their inhibition of cyclooxygenase, particularly the inducible isoform at sites of joint damage, symptomatic benefit is achieved. Recent studies have demonstrated that NSAIDs are modestly more efficacious than acetaminophen for the pain

of osteoarthritis. Patients are unlikely to respond to acetaminophen if they have already been treated with NSAIDs.

The gastrointestinal toxicity of NSAID therapy remains a major concern. The following factors increase the risk of such toxicity:

- Prior peptic ulcer disease.
- Age over 65 years.
- Concomitant tobacco and alcohol use.
- Co-administration of glucocorticoids or anticoagulation therapy.
- Comorbid *Helicobacter pylori* infection.

Ways to diminish NSAID toxicity include:

- *Gastroprotective drugs.* The two classes of drugs shown to be effective among NSAID users are proton pump inhibitors and misoprostol, although the latter frequently causes bloating and diarrhea.
- *Administration of cyclooxygenase-2 isoenzyme inhibitors.* Although cyclooxygenase inhibitors cause increased risks of heart disease and stroke, celecoxib may be less guilty of this, especially at doses under 400 mg/d.

The efficacy of glucosamine sulfate in the medical management of osteoarthritis is controversial. Glucosamine sulfate is a component of human articular cartilage that is administered orally. A recent multicenter National Institutes of Health trial found no efficacy of glucosamine overall, but suggested a modest effect in those with mild to moderate knee pain. Chondroitin sulfate (also commercially available) is similarly controversial. The same National Institutes of Health trial failed to show efficacy in all treated patients. It is still unclear whether additive benefit can be obtained from concomitant administration of both glucosamine and chondroitin. Intra-articular hyaluronic acid is a controversial FDA-approved treatment for knee OA. Meta-analyses evaluating placebo-controlled trials have reported significant but modest efficacy and have also reported publication bias suggesting that estimates of efficacy from published studies are inflated.

Complications

Table 44–3 displays certain acute complications of osteoarthritis. After a diagnosis of osteoarthritis has been firmly established, subsequent change in symptoms or course will not necessarily be directly attributable to this disease. For example, the abrupt onset of warmth, redness, and swelling in a known yet previously stable osteoarthritic knee may herald the onset of a superimposed microcrystalline arthritis or of a ruptured Baker (or

Table 44–3. Acute Complications of Osteoarthritis

Microcrystalline arthropathy (knee and hand joints)
 Gout
 Pseudogout
Spontaneous osteonecrosis of the knee
Ruptured Baker cyst (pseudothrombophlebitis syndrome
 in the knee)
Bursitis
 Anserine bursitis (knee)
 Trochanteric bursitis (hip)
Symptomatic meniscal tear (knee)

popliteal) cyst. Alternately, new-onset joint locking or giving way may suggest the presence of a loose body or meniscal tear that warrants arthroscopic intervention before a catastrophic fall occurs. The development of new symptoms near the joint may be attributable to active inflammation of adjacent nonarticular tissues, including regional tendons and bursae.

Future Directions

A. BIOMECHANICAL TREATMENTS

Ongoing research in this field is largely directed at identification of factors that predispose some but not all aging adults to the development of osteoarthritis. In addition, there is an intense effort underway to identify biomarkers—of bone and cartilage turnover—that may identify those at risk for osteoarthritis and those at risk for disease progression. In the future, availability of drug therapy that may inhibit the adverse effects of degradative enzymes or promote the growth of deficient cartilaginous structures will be critical to realizing therapies that may effectively control, if not cure, osteoarthritis.

REFERENCES

Felson DT. Clinical practice: osteoarthritis of the knee. *N Engl J Med.* 2006;354:841.

Kirkley A, Webster-Bogaert S, Litchfield R, et al. The effect of bracing on varus gonarthrosis. *J Bone Joint Surg.* 1999;81:539. (A randomized trial showing that for pain in persons with varus knee OA, bracing was more effective than neoprene sleeve use, which was in turn more effective than no treatment.)

Messier SP, Loeser RF, Miller GD, et al. Exercise and dietary weight loss in overweight and obese older adults with knee osteoarthritis: the Arthritis, Diet, and Activity Promotion Trial. *Arthritis Rheum.* 2004;50:1501. (A randomized trial suggesting that the combination of weight loss and exercise was more effective than either alone.)

Pincus T, Koch GG, Sokka T, et al. A randomized, double-blind, crossover clinical trial of diclofenac plus misoprostol versus acetaminophen in patients with osteoarthritis of the hip or knee. *Arthritis Rheum.* 2001;44:1587. (A large multicenter trial showing that diclofenac plus misoprostol were more efficacious than high-dose acetaminophen for pain in knee OA.)

Relevant World Wide Web Sites

[Arthritis Foundation]
http://www.arthritis.org
[Johns Hopkins Arthritis Center]
http://www.hopkins-arthritis.com
[OsteoArthritis Research Society International]
http://www.oarsi.org

Gout

Sherri Sanders, MD, & Robert L. Wortmann, MD

ESSENTIALS OF DIAGNOSIS

- *Caused by deposition of uric acid crystals and usually associated with hyperuricemia.*
- *Usually begins as an intermittent, acute monarthritis, especially of the first metatarsophalangeal joint.*
- *Over time, attacks become more frequent, less intense, and involve more joints.*
- *Diagnosed by demonstrating uric acid crystals in joint fluid.*
- *Extra-articular manifestations include tophi and renal stones.*
- *Arthritis responds to nonsteroidal anti-inflammatory drugs or colchicine.*

General Considerations

The underlying basis for gout is an increased total body urate pool. This is generally manifested as hyperuricemia, which is defined as a serum urate concentration more than 7.0 mg/dL. The concentration of 7.0 mg/dL is important because fluids with urate content greater than that are supersaturated with urate, a condition that favors urate crystal precipitation.

At least 5% of asymptomatic Americans manifest hyperuricemia on at least one occasion during adulthood. Hyperuricemia may be even more common in Europe and in countries in the Far East.

The likelihood of developing symptomatic gout and the age at which that occurs correlates with the duration and magnitude of hyperuricemia. In one study, persons with urate levels between 7.0 and 8.0 mL/dL had a cumulative incidence of gouty arthritis of 3%, while those with urate levels >9.0 mL/dL had a 5-year cumulative incidence of 22%. However, hyperuricemia alone is not sufficient for the diagnosis of gout, and asymptomatic hyperuricemia in the absence of gout is not a disease. It appears that clinical gout will develop in fewer than one in four hyperuricemic persons at any point.

Gout presents predominantly in men with a peak age of onset in the fifth decade. The incidence of gout in women approaches that of men only after they have reached age 60 years. The onset of disease in men prior to adulthood or in women before menopause is quite rare and is almost always due to an inborn error of metabolism or congenital condition. The prevalence of self-reported gout is estimated to be 13.6 per 1000 men and 6.4 per 1000 women.

Hyperuricemia can result from increased urate production, decreased uric acid excretion by the kidneys, or a combination of the two mechanisms. Fewer than 5% of patients with gout are hyperuricemic because of urate overproduction. These persons can be recognized because they excrete more than 800 mg of uric acid in their urine during a 24-hour period. Those who excrete less uric acid than 800 mg are hyperuricemic because of impaired renal excretion. Defining individuals as "overproducers" or "underexcreters" is helpful in predicting whether the hyperuricemia is associated with a variety of acquired or genetic disorders (Table 45–1) and may be useful in some cases in determining the most appropriate treatment.

Clinical Findings

A. SYMPTOMS AND SIGNS

The natural history of gout can be divided into three distinct stages (Figure 45–1):

1. Asymptomatic hyperuricemia.
2. Acute and intermittent (or intercritical) gout.
3. Chronic tophaceous gout.

Although most untreated patients with gout will progress to chronic tophaceous gout, the course varies considerably from one patient to another. Some patients experience only one or two attacks of acute gouty arthritis during their lifetime. It is quite unusual for tophi to develop in a patient with no history of acute gouty arthritis.

The initial episode of acute gouty arthritis usually follows 10–30 years of asymptomatic hyperuricemia, and there is no evidence that damage occurs to any organ system during that time. Just why and when the first

Table 45–1. Classification of Hyperuricemia

Urate overproduction
Primary hyperuricemia
  Idiopathic
  Complete or partial deficiency of HGPRT
  Superactivity of PRPP synthetase
Secondary hyperuricemia
  Excessive purine consumption
  Myeloproliferative or lymphoproliferative disorders
  Hemolytic diseases
  Psoriasis
  Glycogen storage diseases: types 1, 3, 5, and 7
Uric acid underexcretion
Primary hyperuricemia
  Idiopathic
Secondary hyperuricemia
  Decreased renal function
  Metabolic acidosis (ketoacidosis or lactic acidosis)
  Dehydration
  Diuretics
  Hypertension
  Hyperparathyroidism
  Drugs including cyclosporine, pyrazinamide, ethambutol
    and low-dose salicylates
  Lead nephropathy
Overproduction and underexcretion
  Alcohol use
  Glucose-6-phosphatase deficiency
  Fructose-1-phosphate-aldolase deficiency

HGPRT, hypoxanthine guanine phosphoribosyltransferase;
PRPP, 5′-phosphoribosyl-1-pyrophosphate.

attack of gout occurs in susceptible persons remains a mystery. Although some patients experience prodromal episodes of mild discomfort, the onset of a gouty attack is usually heralded by the rapid onset of exquisite pain associated with warmth, swelling, and erythema of the affected joint (Figure 45–2). The pain escalates from the faintest twinges to its most intense level over an 8- to 12-hour period. Initial attacks usually affect only one joint, and in half the patients, the first attack involves the first metatarsophalangeal joint. Other joints frequently involved in the early stage of gout include the midfoot, ankle, heel, and knee. The wrist, fingers, and elbows are more typical sites of attacks later in the course of the disease. The intensity of the pain is such that patients cannot stand even the weight of a bed sheet on the affected part and most find it difficult or impossible to walk when the lower extremities are involved in an acute attack. The acute attack may be accompanied by fever, chills, and malaise. Cutaneous erythema associated with the attack may extend beyond the involved joint and resemble cellulitis. Desquamation of the skin may occur as the attack resolves.

Symptoms resolve quickly with appropriate treatment, but even untreated, an acute attack resolves spontaneously over 1–2 weeks. With resolution of the attack, patients enter an interval termed the "intercritical period" when they are again completely asymptomatic. The rare patient will not experience a second attack of gout but most will. Early in the intermittent stage, episodes of arthritis are infrequent and the intervals between the attacks vary from months to years. Over time, the attacks become more frequent, less acute in onset, longer in duration, and tend to involve more joints.

During the intercritical periods of acute intermittent gout, the previously involved joints are virtually free of

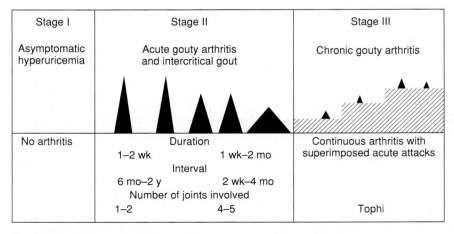

Stage I	Stage II	Stage III
Asymptomatic hyperuricemia	Acute gouty arthritis and intercritical gout	Chronic gouty arthritis
No arthritis	Duration 1–2 wk 1 wk–2 mo Interval 6 mo–2 y 2 wk–4 mo Number of joints involved 1–2 4–5	Continuous arthritis with superimposed acute attacks Tophi

Figure 45–1. The natural history of gout progresses through three stages.

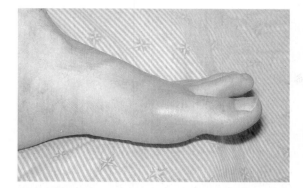

Figure 45–2. Acute gouty attack of the first metatarsophalangeal joint.

symptoms. Despite this, monosodium urate crystal deposition continues. Urate crystals often can be identified in the synovial fluid despite the absence of symptoms and erosive changes indicative of bony tophi begin to appear on radiographs.

Although the reasons why acute gout develops when it does are not clear, attacks tend to be associated with rapid increases, and more often decreases, in the concentration of urate in synovial fluid. These concentrations mirror the fluctuations seen in the serum. Accordingly, a person may experience a sudden drop in the serum urate level leading to an acute attack, and therefore is found to be normouricemic when blood is tested at that time. Trauma, alcohol ingestion, and the use of certain drugs are known to trigger gout attacks as well. Gouty attacks not infrequently occur as a person is recovering from an alcoholic binge. Drugs known to precipitate attacks do so by rapidly raising or lowering serum urate levels. Candidate agents include diuretics, salicylates, and the urate-lowering drugs allopurinol and radiographic contrast agents. It is believed that these fluctuations in urate levels destabilize tophi in the gouty synovium. The sudden addition of urate to them may render them unstable, or the sudden lowering of the urate concentration may cause partial dissolution and instability. As the microtophi break apart, crystals are shed into the synovial fluid and the gouty attack is initiated by the ingestion of these crystals by polymorphonuclear leukocytes.

As gout continues to progress, the patient gradually enters the stage of chronic gouty arthritis. This usually develops after 10 or more years of acute intermittent gout. The transition to chronic gout is complete when the intercritical periods are no longer pain-free. The involved joints are now persistently uncomfortable and may be swollen. Patients report stiffness or gelling sensations as well. Visible or palpable tophi may be detected on physical examination during this stage of gout, even though

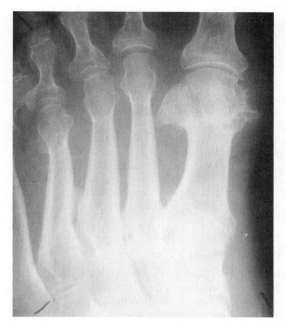

Figure 45–3. Radiographic changes of gout.

they may have been seen on radiographs prior to entry into this stage (Figure 45–3). The development of tophaceous deposits in individual patients varies; in general, they are a function of the duration and severity of the hyperuricemia, with a mean occurrence approximately 12 years after the onset of the first attack of gout in those not treated with urate-lowering drugs.

B. LABORATORY FINDINGS

Hyperuricemia remains the cardinal feature of gout. The usefulness of this laboratory finding in establishing the diagnosis of gout is limited. Whereas most patients with gout will have an elevated serum urate (greater than 7.0 mg/dL), levels may fall within the normal range on occasion; in fact, levels in the normal range are not uncommon during acute attacks, as described above. In addition, during the acute attack, the complete blood cell count may show a leukocytosis with increased polymorphonuclear leukocytes on the differential and elevations of the erythrocyte sedimentation rate and C-reactive protein. The greatest utility of measuring serum urate is in monitoring the effects of urate-lowering therapy.

During an acute attack, the synovial fluid findings are consistent with moderate to severe inflammation (see Chapter 2). The leukocyte count usually ranges between 5 and 80,000 cells/μL with an average between 15,000 and 20,000 cells/μL. The cells are predominantly polymorphonuclear leukocytes.

The definitive diagnosis of gout is made by examination of synovial fluid or tophaceous material with compensated polarized light microscopy and identifying the characteristic monosodium urate crystals. These crystals appear as bright yellow needle-shaped objects when parallel to the access of slow vibration on the first-order compensator. When these crystals are perpendicular to that axis, they are blue. Crystals are usually intracellular and needle-shaped during acute attacks but may be small, blunted, and extracellular as the attack subsides or during intercritical periods.

The 24-hour urine uric acid measurement is not required in all patients with gout but is useful for determining potential causes of hyperuricemia (see above) as well as determining whether uricosuric therapy can be effective, since this form of therapy is effective only in underexcreters.

C. IMAGING STUDIES

No radiographic abnormalities are present early in the disease course. In acute gouty arthritis, the only finding may be soft tissue swelling in the involved joint. Bony abnormalities indicative of deposition of urate crystals (microtophi) develop only after years of disease. These abnormalities are most frequently asymmetric and confined to previously symptomatic joints. The advanced bony erosions of advanced gout are often radiographically distinct. Typically, they are slightly removed from the joint space, have a rounded or oval shape, and are characterized by a hypertrophic calcified "overhanging edge." The joint space may be preserved or show osteoarthritic type narrowing (see Figure 45–3).

D. SPECIAL TESTS

Patients with gout often suffer from hyperlipidemia, glucose intolerance, hypertension, coronary artery disease, and obesity. Accordingly, it is appropriate to measure serum lipids and fasting blood sugars in patients with gout. Because renal dysfunction develops in many patients with hypertension and gout, it is appropriate to monitor serum creatinine levels as well.

Diagnosis & Differential Diagnosis

The definitive diagnosis of gout is made by identifying monosodium urate crystals in polymorphonuclear leukocytes in synovial fluid or from aspirates of tophi (Figure 45–4). The presumptive diagnosis of gout can be made by the presence of the characteristic triad of (1) hyperuricemia, (2) acute monarticular arthritis, and (3) a gratifying clinical response to therapy with colchicine, defined as complete resolution of symptoms within 48 hours and no recurrence for 1 week. Finally, clinicians may also use the criteria proposed by American College of Rheumatology for the diagnosis of gout (Table 45–2).

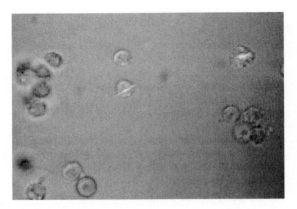

Figure 45–4. Urate crystal ingested by a polymorphonuclear leukocyte in synovial fluid. This finding is pathognomonic for acute gouty arthritis.

Because gouty arthritis often occurs in association with other diseases, those conditions in Table 45–1 should be considered as possible in any person with gout. A variety of conditions can mimic or be confused with gouty arthritis. These include other crystal-induced diseases such as those related to the deposition of calcium pyrophosphate dihydrate crystals (pseudogout) or basic calcium phosphate crystals. The latter may cause a calcific tendinitis that is similar in presentation to gout. Septic arthritis can also mimic gout, although a gouty attack may coexist with an infected joint. The more common

Table 45–2. Criteria for the Diagnosis of Acute Gouty Arthritis

- Presence of characteristic urate crystals in joint fluid, or
- A tophus proved to contain urate crystals by chemical means or polarized light microscopy, or
- The presence of 6 of the following 12 clinical, laboratory, and x-ray phenomena listed below:
  1. More than one attack of acute arthritis
  2. Maximal inflammation developed within 1 day
  3. Attack of monarticular arthritis
  4. Joint redness observed
  5. First metatarsophalangeal joint painful or swollen
  6. Unilateral attack involving first metatarsophalangeal joint
  7. Unilateral attack involving tarsal joint
  8. Suspected tophus
  9. Hyperuricemia
  10. A symptomatic swelling within a joint (radiograph)
  11. Subcortical cysts without erosions (radiograph)
  12. Negative culture of joint fluids for microorganisms during attack of joint inflammation

causes of septic arthritis are gonococcal, staphylococcal, or streptococcal infections. However, infections with fungi or mycobacteria may also be seen. A hemarthrosis or fracture in the joint line may be confused with a gouty attack. Finally, some conditions that are usually considered oligoarticular or polyarticular in presentation may involve only one joint early in the course and be confused with gout. This is particularly true with the peripheral arthritis associated with ankylosing spondylitis, Reiter syndrome, psoriatic arthritis, and the arthritis of inflammatory bowel disease. Rarely, palindromic rheumatism may herald the onset of rheumatoid arthritis and begins with monarticular arthritis.

Occasionally, chronic gouty arthritis and tophi are misdiagnosed as rheumatoid arthritis. The chronic symptoms are polyarticular and symmetric, and the tophaceous deposits mimic rheumatoid nodules. This problem is compounded by the fact that up to 25% of patients with gout have positive tests for rheumatoid factor although these are usually of low titer.

Treatment

The management of gout includes the following:

1. Providing rapid and safe pain relief.
2. Preventing further attacks.
3. Preventing formation of tophi and destructive arthritis.
4. Addressing associated medical conditions.

The goal of treating the acute gout attack is to eliminate the pain and other symptoms caused by the intense inflammation as rapidly as possible. The choices in this situation include nonsteroidal anti-inflammatory drugs (NSAIDs), colchicine, and glucocorticoids. Effective management of the acute attack is not so much determined by which agent is used, but rather by how quickly that agent is initiated after the onset of the attack. If a single dose is given in the first minutes of an attack, it may eradicate the symptoms and terminate the attack. If, however, medication is not taken during the first 48 hours of symptoms, it will probably take at least 2 days before control is gained. Once symptoms have resolved, the particular agent used should be continued at a reduced dose for another 48–72 hours.

NSAIDs have become the most frequently used agents to treat gout because they are so well tolerated. Indomethacin is historically the NSAID of choice for acute gout, but other NSAIDs may be just as effective. The selected NSAID should be started at its recommended maximal dose. The dose may be lowered as symptoms resolve. NSAIDs should be avoided in patients with active or recent peptic ulcer disease and should be used with caution in patients with renal insufficiency or conditions associated with impaired renal blood flow (see Chapter 67).

Colchicine is effective but less well tolerated than NSAIDs. Colchicine is taken in 0.5- or 0.6-mg doses hourly until one of three end points is reached: (1) significant clinical improvement, (2) onset of severe gastrointestinal side effects, or (3) 10 doses are taken without relief (in which case the diagnosis of gout should be questioned). Gastrointestinal side effects include gas, nausea, vomiting, diarrhea, and severe cramping abdominal pain. Gastrointestinal symptoms eventually develop (at a particular dose) in everyone who takes colchicine. However, there is much individual variation in the tolerance to this medication. Often, the development of these side effects coincides with the control of the gouty attack, but they may develop before symptomatic relief.

Intravenous colchicine may be used, particularly in persons who are recovering from surgery or for those in whom oral intake is not possible. Intravenous use of colchicine has the advantages of a rapid onset and no gastrointestinal toxicity, provided oral colchicine is not being used simultaneously. When used, the drug should be diluted in 20–50 mL of normal saline and administered over 15–20 minutes through a secured intravenous line. Extravasation of colchicine into soft tissues results in a severe reaction. A single intravenous dose of colchicine should not exceed 2 mg and the total cumulative dose for an attack should not exceed 3 mg in a 24-hour period. Patients should not receive additional colchicine through any route for 7 days after receiving an intravenous dose. Use of colchicine by the intravenous route is not recommended in the presence of renal or hepatic disease. Absolute contraindications to intravenous colchicine include combined renal and hepatic disease, a glomerular filtration rate less than 25 mL/min, and extrahepatic biliary obstruction. Relative contraindications include significant intercurrent infection, preexisting bone marrow suppression, or the concomitant use of oral colchicine. The improper use of colchicine has led to serious toxicities and even death. All reported cases of death and severe toxicity have involved unusually high doses, or recurrent dosage in patients with renal insufficiency.

Glucocorticoids are usually reserved for patients in whom colchicine or NSAIDs are contraindicated or ineffective. Anecdotal reports suggest early recurrence of gout after treating acute attacks with glucocorticoids, but recent studies have not confirmed that observation. The response time for glucocorticoids is comparable to that for NSAIDs and colchicine. Doses of prednisone of 20–40 mg/d have been used. The dosage is usually tapered over 1–2 weeks after symptoms resolve. Intramuscular or intravenous glucocorticoids provide alternatives for use in the hospitalized patient who can take nothing by mouth. Finally, intra-articular injections with 10–40 mg of prednisone or 10 mg of triamcinolone can also be used.

Most often the gout attack will resolve with the use of one of these agents. However, when this does not occur or in the extremely severe case of gout, these agents may be used in combination. Potent analgesics, including narcotics, may also be added to the regimen.

Once a patient has had an acute gouty attack, the likelihood of further attacks can be reduced by prophylactic therapy with low-dose colchicine or an NSAID on a daily basis. Prophylactic therapy, however, should not be prescribed unless a urate-lowering agent is added to the regimen. The use of prophylactic colchicine without controlling the hyperuricemia only allows tophi and destructive arthritis to continue to develop without the usual warning signs of recurrent acute gouty attacks. The prophylactic use of colchicine in doses of 0.5–0.6 mg 1–3 times a day reduces the frequencies of attacks by 75–85%. These small doses of colchicine rarely cause gastrointestinal side effects and appear to be relatively safe. Long-term colchicine use can cause neuromuscular complications in patients with decreased renal function, especially older patients. It is prudent to avoid using more than 0.6 mg of colchicine daily in a patient with a serum creatinine above 1.5 mg/dL. This toxicity manifests with proximal muscle weakness, painful paresthesias, elevated creatine phosphokinase levels, and abnormalities on electromyograms. This axonal neuromyopathy resolves completely over several weeks after discontinuing the colchicine. Ultimately, specific urate-lowering drugs must be used to eliminate acute attacks and to prevent tophi from forming or cause them to disappear. Although dietary manipulation is essential for control of the comorbid conditions often found with gout, diet cannot reduce serum urate levels sufficiently.

The goal of treatment is to maintain the serum urate level at 5.0 mg/dL or less. Maintaining the serum level at this target allows precipitated crystals to dissolve and be cleared. If the urate level remains above 7.0 mg/dL, supersaturated conditions will persist and urate deposition will continue. In other words, lowering the serum urate from 10.0 mg/dL to 8.0 mg/dL will not reverse the disease; it will only allow it to continue to progress at a slower rate.

The xanthine oxidase inhibitor allopurinol is the agent of choice for most patients with gout. It can effectively lower serum urate levels in those patients with hyperuricemia due to underexcretion and is specifically indicated for those who overproduce urate. Patients with tophi, those with nephrolithiasis, and those who are intolerant of uricosuric therapy are also candidates for xanthine oxidase inhibition. Allopurinol may be used in the presence of renal insufficiency, but its dosage must be reduced to prevent toxicity. Allopurinol at a dose of 300 mg/d adequately controls the serum urate in most patients with normal renal function. If the patient is already taking prophylactic colchicine (which is recommended), then allopurinol can be started at a dose of 300 mg/d. Otherwise, it is recommended that patients start with 100 mg/d for a week and gradually increase the dose until the lowest level of medication that keeps the serum urate level in the target range is reached. Most patients will achieve the desired serum urate level of 5 mg/dL or less while taking 300–400 mg of allopurinol daily. The maximum recommended daily dose is 800 mg. Allopurinol must be used cautiously when the patient is also taking azathioprine or 6-mercaptopurine. Allopurinol reduces the catabolism of these agents, thereby greatly increasing their effective doses.

Side effects and toxicity of allopurinol include fever, headaches, diarrhea, dyspepsia, pleuritis, skin rashes, granulomatous hepatitis, and toxic epidermal necrolysis. The syndrome of allopurinol hypersensitivity is rare but serious with a mortality rate of 20–30%. Allopurinol hypersensitivity reactions are more common in older patients with impaired renal function taking diuretics. The development of a rash in patients taking allopurinol is an indication to stop the medicine. After the rash is cleared, allopurinol may be cautiously reinstituted if the rash was not deemed to be severe. With more severe reactions, hypersensitivity may be overcome through desensitization protocols.

Febuxostat is a potent new xanthine oxidase inhibitor that appears to have certain benefits compared to allopurinol. First, it is metabolized by the liver so febuxostat may be used in patients with mild to moderate renal insufficiency without dose adjustment. Second, it can be used safely even in patients with mild to moderate hepatic insufficiency. Finally, no hypersensitivity reactions have been reported. To date, the use of febuxostat in patients with a history of allopurinol reactions has been safe, effective, and well tolerated. Data from phase II and III clinical trials indicate that doses of 80–120 mg daily are effective in the majority of patients.

Uricosuric agents are also effective in lowering serum urate levels. The patients in whom they are most effective are those who have good renal function (glomerular filtration rate above 60 mL/min), those who have no history of nephrolithiasis, those who can avoid all salicylate ingestions, and those under 65 years of age. Salicylate use in doses in excess of 81 mg/d will interfere with the effectiveness of uricosuric agents. These agents should be avoided in patients with a history of nephrolithiasis because stone formation is more likely due to the flooding of urine with uric acid. Finally, uricosuric agents require good renal function to be effective. Probenecid is started at a dosage of 500 mg twice a day and advanced slowly up to a maximum dosage of 1 g twice a day or until the target urate level is reached. The most common side effects of this agent are rash and gastrointestinal upset. Sulfinpyrazone is the other uricosuric agent available in the United States. This drug is slowly advanced from 100 mg to approximately 800 mg/d in two or three divided doses until the desired level of serum urate is reached. Benzbromarone, an agent available in Europe, is more potent and may be effective in the face of moderate renal insufficiency.

Unfortunately, the treatment of gout is complicated by poor compliance. This is probably related to the difficulty people have in remembering how to take three different medicines on three different schedules. Frequently they become confused about which medicines to take in what situations. An analogy has been developed that may help patients understand and better remember how to take their medications (see the box: Gout is Like Matches).

Hyperuricemia alone is rarely an indication for treatment with specific urate-lowering drugs. Therefore, use of a xanthine oxidase inhibitor or uricosuric agent is not recommended in the treatment of asymptomatic hyperuricemia. On the other hand, the identification of asymptomatic hyperuricemia should not be ignored. First, the cause should be determined (see Table 45–1), and any associated problems, such as hypertension, obesity, alcoholism, diabetes, or hyperlipidemia, should be addressed rigorously.

Complications

As described above, untreated and severe gout leads to visible and palpable tophaceous deposits and a destructive arthropathy. However, these complications are preventable with accurate diagnosis and appropriate therapy.

Nephrolithiasis develops in 10–25% of patients with gout at some time during the disease course. In 40% of these patients, the first episode of renal colic precedes the first attack of acute gouty arthritis. Most of these calculi are composed of uric acid; however, calcium-containing stones are 10 times more common in patients with gout than in the general population. The incidence of nephrolithiasis correlates with the serum urate level, but more strongly with the amount of uric acid excreted in the urine. The likelihood of developing a stone reaches 50% with either a serum urate level above 13.0 mg/dL or a 24-hour urinary uric acid excretion in excess of 1100 mg.

In the past, progressive renal failure has been common in the gouty population with up to 25% of patients with gout dying of renal disease. Today this frequency is much less. Hypertension, diabetes, chronic lead exposure, and chronic atherosclerosis are the most important contributing factors to this complication. In fact, if blood pressure is rigorously controlled, it is very unusual for renal failure to develop in a patient with gout. Chronic urate nephropathy has been described and is a distinct condition caused by the deposition of monosodium urate crystals in the renal parenchyma and pyramids. Although chronic hyperuricemia is thought to be the cause of this urate nephropathy, this form of kidney disease is never seen in the absence of gouty arthritis. Furthermore, with appropriate management, urate nephropathy should easily be prevented.

Hyperuricemia and gout are frequently accompanied by obesity, alcoholism, glucose intolerance related to insulin resistance, and hyperlipidemia. In addition, a very high percentage of patients with gout have hypertension. These associated conditions should be managed aggressively.

GOUT IS LIKE MATCHES

The following paragraph is an analogy that can be used to explain gout to patients.

Gout is caused by uric acid. Everyone has uric acid in their blood but some people have too much of it, and some of those people get gout. In those who get gout, the uric acid accumulates around the joints and acts like matches. When you get a gout attack, one of the matches strikes and catches the joint on fire. When that happens, you should take your indomethacin (or nonsteroidal anti-inflammatory drug of choice). It is important to take it right away. If not, more matches will catch fire and the attack will worsen. Taking indomethacin does not cure the gout because it only puts out the fire. The matches are still there and can light again. A urate-lowering drug will remove the matches. If there are no matches, you cannot get gout. But until the urate-lowering drug has time to work, you can still get gout. Therefore you should take colchicine, one pill twice a day. Colchicine is very good at preventing gout attacks. You can think of colchicine as something that makes the matches damp and harder to strike.

(From Wortmann RL. Effective management of gout: an analogy. *Am J Med*. 1998;105:513. With permission.)

REFERENCES

Agudelo CA, Wise CM. Gout: diagnosis, pathogenesis, and clinical manifestations. *Curr Opin Rheumatol*. 2001;13:234. [PMID: 11333355]

Becker MA, Schumacher HR Jr, Wortmann RL, et al. Febuxostat compared with allopurinol in patients with hyperuricemia and gout. *N Engl J Med*. 2005;353:2450.

Becker MA, Schumacher HR Jr, Wortmann RL, et al. Febuxostat, a novel nonpurine selective inhibitor of xanthine oxidase: a twenty-eight-day, multicenter, phase III, randomized, double-blind, placebo-controlled, dose-response clinical trial examining safety and efficacy in patients with gout. *Arthritis Rheum.* 2005;52:916.

Choi HK, Karlson EW, Willett W, Curham G. Alcohol intake and risk of incident gout in men: a prospective study. *Lancet.* 2004;363:1277.

Terkeltaub RA. Gout. *N Engl J Med.* 2003;349:1647.

Wortmann RL. Gout and hyperuricemia. *Curr Opin Rheumatol.* 2002;14:281. [PMID: 11981327]

Wortmann RL, Schumacher HR Jr. Monosodium urate deposition arthropathy part I: review of the stages and diagnosis of gout. *Adv Stud Med.* 2005;5:133.

Wortmann RL, Schumacher HR Jr. Monosodium urate deposition arthropathy part II: treatment and long term management of patients with gout. *Adv Stud Med.* 2005;5:183.

Pseudogout: Calcium Pyrophosphate Dihydrate Crystal Deposition Disease

Jeffrey S. Alderman, MD, & Robert L. Wortmann, MD

ESSENTIALS OF DIAGNOSIS

- *Calcium pyrophosphate dihydrate (CPPD) crystal deposition disease can mimic gout, rheumatoid arthritis, or osteoarthritis.*
- *Pseudogout causes an intermittent monarthritis, often of the knee or wrist.*
- *Diagnosis of pseudogout is established by demonstrating CPPD crystals in joint fluid.*
- *CPPD crystal deposition disease is associated with other diseases, especially hemochromatosis and hyperparathyroidism.*

General Considerations

Calcium pyrophosphate dihydrate (CPPD) deposition can be asymptomatic or may result in a variety of clinical presentations (Table 46–1). Although the term "pseudogout" is often used to represent the entire spectrum of CPPD, it accurately describes the acute goutlike attacks of inflammation that occur in some patients with CPPD crystal deposition disease. In fact, the name pseudogout was coined when it was discovered that a subset of patients believed to have gout actually had CPPD crystals in their synovial fluid, rather than uric acid crystals. CPPD deposition may give rise to clinical presentations that mimic septic arthritis, polyarticular inflammatory arthritis, or osteoarthritis (see Table 46–1). Additionally, CPPD crystals may coexist in synovial fluid with urate or basic calcium phosphate crystals in inflammatory and osteoarthriticlike diseases, as well as in Charcot joints.

Although the cause of CPPD crystal deposition is unknown, several risk factors have been identified. Perhaps the most important factor is aging. CPPD deposition will probably occur in everyone if they live long enough. Genetic factors also influence crystal formation, given that numerous familial cases of CPPD deposition have been described in many nationalities. Interestingly, the pattern of clinical manifestation differs from family to family. For example, disease may occur in some families at an early age and mimic a spondyloarthropathy. In other families, presentation occurs in later years with sporadic joint distribution. What is notable is that the prevalence of CPPD deposition is greater in people who have suffered orthopedic trauma; symptoms may persist despite attempts to repair affected joints. Finally, several metabolic conditions including hyperparathyroidism, hemochromatosis, hypothyroidism, amyloidosis, hypomagnesemia, and hypophosphatasia have all been associated with an increased frequency of CPPD disease.

Clinical Findings

A. SYMPTOMS AND SIGNS

Approximately 25% of patients with CPPD deposition disease exhibit the pseudogout pattern of disease. Signs and symptoms are characterized by acute, typically monarticular inflammatory arthritis lasting for several days to 2 weeks. These self-limited attacks may vary in intensity, but can occur just as abruptly as an acute gout attack. Between episodes, patients are usually asymptomatic. Nearly half of all attacks involve the knees, although pseudogout can affect other joints, including the first metatarsophalangeal joint, which is the most common site of gouty inflammation. However, attacks of pseudogout may occur spontaneously or be provoked by trauma, surgery, or severe medical illness. Differentiation of gout from joint infection may be difficult, and requires arthrocentesis examination of synovial fluid for crystals and culture. A subset of patients with pseudogout may have fever. Without appropriate analysis of synovial fluid, it may be impossible to differentiate pseudogout from septic arthritis.

Table 46–1. CPPD Crystal Deposition can be Asymptomatic or Cause Clinical Presentations that Mimic Several Conditions

Gout
Septic arthritis
Rheumatoid arthritis
Osteoarthritis
Spondyloarthritis
Meningitis

CPPD, calcium pyrophosphate dihydrate.

Nearly 5% of patients with CPPD deposition manifest symptoms that mimic rheumatoid arthritis. These patients present with low-grade inflammation in multiple, symmetric joints. Moreover, morning stiffness, fatigue, synovial thickening, joint contractures, and an elevated erythrocyte sedimentation rate frequently accompany this form of arthritis. With these misleading findings, this particular variant of pseudogout is often misdiagnosed as rheumatoid arthritis. Making matters more confusing, a small percentage of patients with CPPD deposition have low titers of circulating rheumatoid factor.

Nearly half of patients with CPPD deposition have a progressive, degenerative disease termed "pseudo-osteoarthritis." Although there is some overlap with the pattern of joint involvement in primary osteoarthritis, the distribution of joint degeneration with CPPD deposition may differ. The knees are most commonly affected, followed by the wrists, metacarpophalangeal joints, hips, shoulders, elbows, and ankles. While symmetric involvement is typical, deformities and flexion contractures of affected joints are not uncommon. Several cases have been reported of severe derangement and destruction, mimicking the findings seen in Charcot joint. Valgus deformity of the knees is especially suggestive of underlying CPPD crystal deposition, as is disease localized to the patellofemoral joint. Patients with this pseudo-osteoarthritic pattern may have intermittent episodes of acute joint inflammation of varying severity, superimposed upon their baseline disease state.

Rarely, CPPD crystal deposition occurs in the axial skeleton, which may potentially lead to acute neck pain. The ligamentum flavum has been the most regularly reported site of CPPD crystal deposition in the spine. At times, neck pain may be accompanied by stiffness and fever, mimicking meningitis. Crystal deposits, ligament hypertrophy, and cartilage metaplasia contribute to encroachment of the spinal cord. Infrequently, lumbar spine involvement may give rise to an acute radiculopathy or neurogenic claudication resulting from spinal stenosis. As a result of CPPD deposition and its related changes,

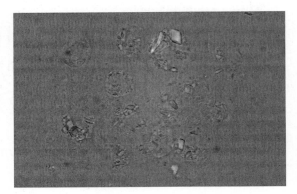

Figure 46–1. Positive birefringent calcium pyrophosphate dihydrate crystals.

signs and symptoms of neurologic long tract disease may develop in some patients.

That being said, many patients with CPPD crystal deposits lack joint symptoms. Even patients with arthritic symptoms in some joints may have other joints with crystal deposition which are completely asymptomatic and clinically normal.

B. Laboratory Findings

The critical laboratory feature of any form of CPPD crystal deposition disease is the demonstration of CPPD crystals. They are most commonly recognized in synovial fluid (Figure 46–1). Their identification requires the use of compensated polarized light microscopy. CPPD crystals are generally rhomboid-shaped and positively birefringent. They appear blue when parallel to the long axis of the compensator and yellow when perpendicular.

Arthrocentesis of patients with pseudogout (and pseudorheumatoid presentations) generally yields cloudy fluid with low viscosity; the white blood cell count typically ranges between 5000 and 25,000 cells/μL. However, white blood cell counts greater than 100,000 cells/μL have been observed, a finding that is more typically associated with septic arthritis. The white blood cells in the synovial fluid in pseudogout (or the pseudoseptic presentation) are most commonly polymorphonuclear leukocytes. Meanwhile, the fluid seen in the pseudo-osteoarthritic form is clear, viscous, and has a very low white blood cell count (generally less than 300 cells/μL). Inflammatory presentation of CPPD crystal deposition disease may be accompanied by a peripheral blood leukocytosis with a shift to the left shift on the differential, along with an elevated erythrocyte sedimentation rate and C-reactive protein.

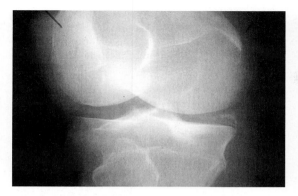

Figure 46–2. Chondrocalcinosis of the knees.

C. IMAGING STUDIES

The radiographic findings of punctate and linear densities in hyaline articular cartilage or fibrocartilaginous tissues are diagnostic of CPPD crystal deposition (Figure 46–2). Other radiographic features include degenerative changes in an uncommon site along with subchondral cyst formation. X-rays most often demonstrate sites of CPPD crystal deposition in the knees, wrist (triangular cartilage of the radiocarpal joint) (Figure 46–3), and the symphysis pubis. The finding of isolated patellofemoral joint space narrowing or degenerative change in the wrist may provide helpful clinical clues to the presence of CPPD deposition-related arthropathy.

When the deposits are typical or unequivocal, the radiographic appearance of pseudogout can be viewed as specific. However, the presence of atypical or calcific deposits can be difficult to interpret, as these changes may be confused with coexisting degenerative findings. Pseudogout can produce severe radiographic changes, marked by subchondral collapse, bone fragmentation, and intra-articular radiodense bodies.

Changes in the metacarpophalangeal joints such as squaring of the bone ends, subchondral cysts, and hook-like osteophytes are characteristic features of the arthritis associated with hemochromatosis. However, these changes can also be observed in patients with CPPD crystal deposition alone or related to another metabolic disorder, such as Wilson disease.

A patient can be screened for CPPD crystal deposition with four radiographs. These include an anteroposterior view of the knees, anteroposterior view of the pelvis, and a posteroanterior view of both hands to include the wrists. If these views show no evidence of crystal deposition, it is unlikely that further study will be fruitful. Tomographic views may be required to identify CPPD deposits surrounding the odontoid process.

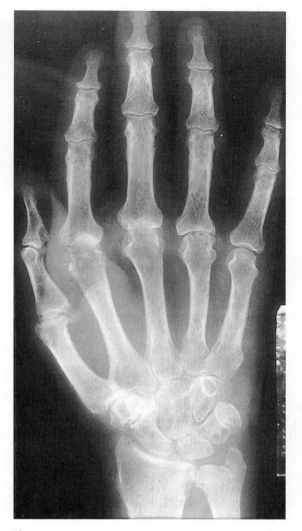

Figure 46–3. Chondrocalcinosis of the radiocarpal triangular cartilage.

D. SPECIFIC TESTS

Because of the recognized association between CPPD deposition and various metabolic diseases, the evaluation of a patient with newly diagnosed CPPD deposition should include tests of serum calcium, phosphorus, magnesium, alkaline phosphatase, and thyroid-stimulating hormone levels. The serum ceruloplasmin levels should also be assessed if Wilson disease is suspected. Hypophosphatasia and Wilson disease need not be considered in patients who become symptomatic after the age of 60 years.

Table 46–2. Diagnostic Criteria for CPPD Crystal Deposition Disease

Criteria
1. Demonstration of CPPD crystals and tissue or synovial fluid by definitive means (for example, characteristic x-ray defraction or chemical analysis)
2A. Identification of monoclinic or triclinic crystals showing no or weakly positive birefringence by compensated polarized light microscopy
2B. Presence of typical radiographic calcifications
3A. Acute arthritis, especially of the knees or other large joints
3B. Chronic arthritis, especially of the knee, hip, wrist, carpus, elbow, shoulder, or metacarpophalangeal joint, especially if accompanied by acute exacerbations. The chronic arthritis shows the following features helpful in differentiating it from osteoarthritis:
    Uncommon site—wrist, metacarpophalangeal, elbow, or shoulder joint
    Radiographic appearance—radiocarpal or patellofemoral joint space narrowing, especially if isolated (patella "wrapped around" the femur)
    Subchondral cyst formation for severity of degeneration—progressive, with subchondral bony collapse and fragmentation with formation of intra-articular radiodense bodies
        Osteophyte formation—variable and inconstant
        Tendon calcifications—especially triceps, Achilles, obturators

Categories
Definite disease: Criteria 1 or 2A must be fulfilled
Probable disease: Criteria 2A or 2B must be fulfilled
Possible disease: Criteria 3A or B should alert the clinician to the possibility of underlying CPPD deposition

CPPD, calcium pyrophosphate dihydrate.

Diagnosis & Differential Diagnosis

The diagnosis of CPPD crystal deposition disease is made through the identification of CPPD crystals in tissue or synovial fluid. These are definitively identified by the means of polarized light microscopy or x-ray diffraction. The radiographic finding of chondrocalcinosis (calcium-containing radiodensities) in articular cartilage is also an indication of CPPD deposition. The criteria for the diagnosis of this disease are outlined in Table 46–2.

Because CPPD crystal deposition disease may present in many different ways, the differential diagnosis can be quite extensive. Acute monarticular attacks of pseudogout can be misdiagnosed as gout, acute basic calcium phosphate crystal arthritis or periarthritis. One must also strongly consider septic arthritis in the differential diagnosis. Polyarticular or oligoarticular inflammatory presentations mirror rheumatoid arthritis and other inflammatory joint diseases. The polyarticular presentation may be difficult to distinguish from primary or posttraumatic osteoarthritis. Uncommonly, an acute inflammatory response to CPPD deposition of the ligament flavum or cervical spine can mimic meningitis.

Treatment of CPPD Crystal Deposition

The recommendations for the management of acute attacks of pseudogout are exactly those that are recommended for the treatment of acute gouty arthritis (see Chapter 45). Therefore, therapeutic options include nonsteroidal anti-inflammatory drugs, oral colchicine, intravenous colchicine, and intravenous or intra-articular glucocorticoids in patients who cannot tolerate oral medications.

Oral colchicine (dosed at 0.5–0.6 mg one to three times daily) is useful in the patient with frequent bouts of pseudogout. However, the efficacy of this prophylactic therapy seems less effective in pseudogout than it is in gout. Nevertheless, colchicine can decrease the frequency of painful attacks in some patients. The management of the pseudo-osteoarthritic form of CPPD deposition disease is similar to that for the management of other forms of osteoarthritis, especially when acute attacks occur infrequently. Activity planning and pacing, assistive devices, analgesic medication (eg, nonsteroidal anti-inflammatory drugs and intra-articular glucocorticoid injections), and eventually surgery have all been proven to be effective tools.

Unfortunately, there is no equivalent to allopurinol or a uricosuric agent for the treatment of CPPD deposition disease. Until the specific cause of this condition is determined, it is unlikely that a specific medicine will be found that removes the crystals from joints. However, in patients with an associated metabolic condition, such as hyperparathyroidism, hemochromatosis, or hypothyroidism, treatment of the underlying disease may decrease the number of attacks, but does not result in resorption of crystals.

Complications

The development of CPPD crystal deposition disease can lead to progressive degenerative damage to the joint. Findings may be severe with joint collapse and Charcot-like degeneration. Fortunately, abnormalities this severe are unusual.

Flares of pseudogout can follow general anesthesia and surgery, occurring most notably after parathyroidectomy. The sudden decline in calcium may precipitate a flare of polyarticular inflammation with fever and mental confusion.

REFERENCES

Canhao H, Fonseca JE, Leandro MJ, et al. Cross-sectional study of 50 patients with calcium pyrophosphate dihydrate crystal arthropathy. *Clin Rheumatol.* 2001;20:119. [PMID: 11346223]

Derfus B, Kurian J, Butler J, et al. The high prevalence of pathologic calcium crystals in pre-operative knees. *J Rheumatol.* 2002;29:570. [PMID: 11908575]

Pons-Estel B, Giminez C, Sacnun M, et al. Familial osteoarthritis and Milwaukee Shoulder associated with calcium pyrophosphate and apatite crystal deposition. *J Rheumatol.* 2000;27:471. [PMID: 10685816]

Reuge L, Van Linthoudt D, Gerster JC. Local deposition of calcium pyrophosphate crystals in evolution of knee osteoarthritis. *Clin Rheumatol.* 2001;20:428. [PMID: 11771528]

Rosenthal AK, Mandel N. Identification of crystals in synovial fluids and joint tissues. *Curr Rheumatol Rep.* 2001;3:11. [PMID: 11177766]

SECTION VI

Infection

Septic Arthritis & Disseminated Gonococcal Infection

47

Monica Gandhi, MD, MPH, & Richard Jacobs, MD, PhD

SEPTIC BACTERIAL ARTHRITIS

ESSENTIALS OF DIAGNOSIS

- *The classic presentation is acute onset of painful, warm, and swollen joint, usually monarticular and affecting large weight-bearing joints.*
- *Synovial fluid white blood cell counts usually >50,000 cells/mm³ with over 80% neutrophils.*
- *Positive synovial fluid culture.*
- *Staphylococcus aureus is the most common cause of septic arthritis in native joints.*

General Considerations

The reported incidence of septic arthritis varies from 2–10 per 100,000 per year in the general population, with substantially higher rates in patients with rheumatoid arthritis (RA) or joint prostheses (both ~30–70 cases per 100,000 per year). The incidence of bacterial arthritis is significantly higher among children than adults.

Septic (bacterial) arthritis is a medical emergency, and delay in diagnosis and treatment can lead to irreversible joint destruction and an increase in mortality. Even with the advent of better antimicrobial agents and techniques of joint incision and drainage, the rate of permanent joint damage from septic arthritis is 25–50%. The case fatality rate for bacterial arthritis also remains high at 5–15%, with increased mortality rates seen in the setting of polyarticular septic arthritis, underlying RA, and in immunocompromised states. Risk factors for the development of bacterial arthritis include chronic arthritic syndromes, prosthetic joints, parenteral drug use, extremes of age, diabetes mellitus, and immunocompromised conditions (Table 47–1).

Pathogenesis

Bacterial pathogens reach the joint spaces by hematogenous spread (>50% of cases), by direct inoculation, or by spread from adjacent bony or soft-tissue infections. Although skin infections are the most common predisposing infections to joint infections, transient bacteremia from respiratory, gastrointestinal, or genitourinary infections can also lead to septic arthritis. Bacteria enter the closed joint space, and within hours the synovium becomes infected, leading to synovial membrane proliferation and infiltration by polymorphonuclear and other inflammatory cells. This inflammatory response in turn leads to enzymatic and cytokine-mediated degradation of the articular cartilage, neovascularization, and the eventual development of granulation tissue. Without appropriate treatment, irreversible subchondral bone loss and

Table 47–1. Risk Factors and Mechanisms of Infection in Bacterial Arthritis

Risk Factor	Mechanism of Infection	Comments
Rheumatoid arthritis (RA)	• Local and systemic factors play a role • Damaged joint serves as nidus for infection • Immunosuppressive medications predispose to infection, especially previous use of oral or intra-articular steroids	• RA is complicated by septic arthritis in 0.3–3% of patients • Polyarticular septic arthritis in RA has >50% mortality rate • *Staphylococcus aureus* most likely organism
Prosthetic joint	• Foreign body serves as nidus for infection, especially for pathogens that lay down biofilms or glycocalyx layer (eg, *Staphylococcus epidermidis*) • No microvasculature in artificial joint	• Rates of infection have decreased over the past 30 years • Higher incidence in revision arthroplasty (see text for details)
Injection drug use; indwelling lines; chronic skin infections	• Recurrent bacteremia with subsequent hematogenous seeding of joints • Patients on chronic hemodialysis, with chronic indwelling lines, with repeated skin injections (eg, insulin), or with chronic skin infections are susceptible	• The knee is the most commonly infected joint in injection drug users, but also see axial joint infections, including sternoclavicular and sacroiliac joint involvement • *S. aureus* (often methicillin-resistant) most common cause in injection drug users • *Pseudomonas aeruginosa* seen in ~10% of cases
Crystal-induced arthritis (gout, pseudogout)	• Local factors • Joint damage from crystals • Synovial fluid acidosis in crystal-induced synovitis promotes cartilage damage	• Crystal-induced arthritis can cause high synovial WBC counts without infection • Presence of crystals does not rule out infection • Infection-mediated destruction of articular cartilage can rarely elicit crystals in synovial space
Severe osteoarthritis, Charcot joint, hemarthroses	• Joint disorganization, chronic synovitis, and blood within synovial space can provide a nidus for infection	• Always send a bloody synovial effusion for culture to exclude infection
Chronic, systemic disease (eg, lupus, cancer, diabetes mellitus, other immunosuppressive conditions, including extremes of age [children <5 or adults >65])	• Impaired host defenses from chronic illness, including phagocytic deficiencies • Medications for chronic illnesses (eg, glucocorticoids in lupus) predispose to infection	• *S aureus* and gram-negative bacilli most common organisms • In lupus, functional hyposplenism may occur, leading to susceptibility to encapsulated organisms (eg, *Neisseria gonorrhoeae, Salmonella, Proteus*)
Intra-articular injection (or arthrocentesis)	• Direct inoculation of the offending organism	• Most common agents are skin flora, including *S epidermidis* and *S aureus*
HIV infection	• Immunosuppression and an increased tendency to develop bacteremia with localized infections	• Even in asymptomatic HIV infection, underlying risk factors for acquiring HIV, such as injection drug use or hemophilia, can predispose
Sexual activity	• Predisposes to localized gonococcal infection, which may disseminate to cause joint and skin disease	• DGI 2–3 times more common in women than men, especially after menses or in postpartum period • Terminal complement deficiencies also predispose to DGI.

DGI, disseminated gonococcal infection; WBC, white blood cell.

cartilage destruction occur within a few days of the initial infection.

Clinical Findings

A. SYMPTOMS AND SIGNS

The classic presentation of bacterial arthritis is the abrupt onset of a painful, warm, and swollen joint. More indolent presentations are seen in patients with preexisting rheumatic illnesses or immunocompromised states. An obvious joint effusion, moderate to severe joint tenderness to palpation, and marked restriction of both passive and active motion are common signs of septic arthritis.

A patient with an acute monarticular arthritis should be considered to have septic arthritis until proven otherwise. Nongonococcal bacterial arthritis is monarticular in 80–90% of cases, with polyarticular involvement (10–20%) carrying a poorer chance of survival. Polyarticular septic arthritis is more likely to occur in patients with RA or other systemic connective tissue diseases or in the syndrome of overwhelming sepsis. Infectious monarthritis typically involves the knee (40–50%), hip (13–20%), shoulder (10–15%), wrist (5–8%), ankle (6–8%), elbow (3–7%), and the small joints of the hand or foot (5%). Bursitis, especially olecranon and prepatellar, may be the first manifestation of septic arthritis in patients with RA.

Septic arthritis manifests with fever in 60–80% of cases, although the temperature elevation is not usually pronounced. Twenty percent of patients with fever have shaking chills that usually correspond to waves of bacteremia. Cough, gastrointestinal symptoms, or dysuria may represent symptoms of the antecedent infection. Indeed, a preceding source of infection, such as pneumonia, otitis, bronchitis, pharyngitis, or cutaneous, gastrointestinal, or genitourinary infection, can be identified in up to 50% of septic arthritis cases.

B. PHYSICAL EXAMINATION

The initial physical examination for septic arthritis should determine whether the source of inflammation and pain is articular or periarticular (specifically, localized to skin, bursae, or tendons). Septic arthritis produces warmth, swelling, and tenderness of the involved joint, and attempts at passive and active motion of the joint usually produce considerable discomfort. Similar findings occur in noninfectious forms of severe inflammatory arthritis, such as acute gout. In contrast, cellulitis and inflammation of bursae and tendons do not cause joint effusions, and passive motion of the adjacent joint usually does not elicit severe pain unless there is stretching of an inflamed tendon. Because septic arthritis can involve more than one joint, all joints should be examined for warmth, swelling, deformity, range of motion, pain on motion, and tenderness.

Septic arthritis of the sacroiliac (SI) joint is often difficult to distinguish from infection in the hip because both present with fever and pain upon ambulation and because examination of the SI joints is difficult (see Chapter 1). Moreover, findings of SI septic arthritis can be subtle and can be mistaken for the syndrome of a protruded disk or a paraspinous muscular strain. Similarly, infection of the shoulder joint is often difficult to identify given the usual lack of a visible effusion. Adults with shoulder infections tend to be elderly, with multiple risk factors for the development of septic arthritis. Infections of the sternoclavicular joint most often occur in injecting drug users; an abscess of the chest wall or in the intrathoracic extrapleural space will develop in 20% of patients with septic arthritis of the sternoclavicular joint. Septic olecranon bursitis is distinguished from infection of the elbow joint by the presence of swelling and erythema overlying the olecranon process and the absence of joint pain with passive extension of the elbow. Infection of the olecranon bursa often follows minor trauma to the region, which leads to inoculation of organisms (usually *S aureus*) into the bursal space.

C. LABORATORY FINDINGS

1. Peripheral counts and cultures—Peripheral white blood cell (WBC) counts are elevated in bacterial arthritis approximately two-thirds of the time. The erythrocyte sedimentation rate and C-reactive protein are usually elevated and may be useful to monitor during treatment, especially in children with septic hip infections. Approximately 40–50% of patients with septic arthritis have associated bacteremia, so blood cultures should be obtained prior to the administration of antibiotics. Targeted cultures from extra-articular sites, such as respiratory, cutaneous, gastrointestinal, or genitourinary sites, should also be collected after a careful history and physical examination.

2. Synovial fluid analysis—Synovial fluid analysis is critical for the definitive diagnosis of septic arthritis. Synovial fluid is usually obtained by emergent arthrocentesis, with fluoroscopic or computed tomographic (CT) guidance if necessary (see Chapter 2). An open surgical procedure may be required to obtain synovial fluid and biopsies for the diagnosis of bacterial arthritis, especially in suspected sternoclavicular, hip, or shoulder infections or in the presence of prosthetic joints. Of note, arthrocentesis is contraindicated if the needle must pass through an area of cellulitis, heavily colonized skin lesions (eg, psoriatic plaques), or infection of any kind because of the risk of introducing bacteria into the joint space. Bacteremia is also a relative contraindication for the performance of arthrocentesis.

Once synovial fluid has been collected, the following analyses should be performed (see Chapter 2):

- *Appearance*: Look for color and clarity of the fluid, since purulence or turbidity or both suggest a septic process.
- *Cell count and differential*: The joint fluid in nongonococcal septic arthritis has more than 50,000 WBC/mm^3 in 50–70% of cases. Low synovial fluid cell counts may be seen early in the process of infectious arthritis, in the setting of partially treated infections, or in immunosuppressed patients. The majority of WBCs in infected synovial fluid are neutrophils (usually >80% polymorphonuclear cells).
- *Gram stain for organisms*: A positive Gram stain is diagnostic for septic arthritis (highly specific), but a Gram stain that is negative for bacteria does not rule out an infected joint. The Gram stain is positive 50–75% of the time in nongonococcal bacterial arthritis, with gram-positive bacterial arthritis more likely to stain positive than gram-negative bacterial arthritis. The Gram stain should be used to guide presumptive therapy.
- *Culture*: Bacterial culture of the synovial fluid is positive in 70–90% of cases of nongonococcal arthritis, depending on the organism. Inoculating synovial fluid into blood culture bottles rather than solid media increases the yield of culture growth and decreases the contamination rate.
- *Microbiology*: Table 47–2 shows the typical pathogens of nongonococcal bacterial arthritis and risk factors for their acquisition. *Staphylococcus aureus* is the most common cause of septic monarthritis in native joints (60–70%) (Figure 47–1). The remaining causes of septic arthritis include streptococcal species, gram-negative rods, and anaerobes in relatively constant proportions. Hematogenous infection can result from transient bacteremia secondary to a remote infection or a surgical procedure, including dental work or respiratory, gastrointestinal, or genitourinary manipulations. Group A streptococci are often isolated from the infected joint after procedures in the oral cavity, whereas gastrointestinal procedures can lead to bacteremia with non–group A streptococcal species, gram-negative bacilli, or anaerobes.

D. Imaging Studies

1. Plain radiographs—Plain radiographs are of little diagnostic usefulness in acute septic arthritis but are often obtained as a baseline and to exclude contiguous osteomyelitis. Radiographs will usually reveal only soft-tissue swelling; in cases of infection with *Escherichia coli* or anaerobic organisms, however, radiographs may demonstrate gas formation within an untapped joint. In late septic arthritis (at least 8–10 days after infection), films may show subchondral bone destruction, periosteal new bone formation, joint space narrowing, or osteoporosis.

2. Computed tomography—Because the hip, shoulder, sternoclavicular, and SI joints are difficult to palpate and to aspirate, evaluation of these joints usually requires CT or magnetic resonance imaging (MRI). CT is preferred for the sternoclavicular joint. CT scans may demonstrate early bone erosions, reveal soft-tissue extension and detect effusions, and facilitate arthrocentesis of the hip, shoulder, sternoclavicular, and SI joints.

3. Magnetic resonance imaging—MRI scans demonstrate adjacent soft-tissue edema or abscesses and may be especially helpful in detecting septic sacroiliitis. MRI can also detect the early bone erosions of incipient contiguous osteomyelitis.

4. Scintigraphy—Scintigraphy makes use of various agents, such as labeled WBCs, technetium colloid, or immunoglobulin, to highlight areas of infection. The drawback of this imaging technique in the diagnosis of septic arthritis is the rate of false-positives with contiguous soft-tissue infections; scintigraphy cannot reliably differentiate septic from aseptic joint inflammation. False-positive scans can also result from underlying fracture or a recent operation. Given this low specificity, scintigraphy is rarely used as the imaging study of choice for the diagnosis of septic arthritis.

5. Gallium scan—Gallium accumulates where there is a extravasation of serum proteins and leukocytes and is better than scintigraphy in distinguishing infection from mechanical damage. Gallium scans have shown increasing utility in the diagnosis of septic arthritis and the identification of concurrent osteomyelitis.

Differential Diagnosis

Septic arthritis usually presents as acute monarthritis, and occasionally as an acute oligoarthritis or a polyarthritis. The differential diagnoses of these syndromes are reviewed in Chapter 4, but several points warrant emphasis here. The diagnosis of acute monarthritis is infection unless proved otherwise. Differentiating infection from crystal-induced arthritis can be particularly difficult, since acute flares of pseudogout or gout can also cause fever, peripheral leukocytosis, and markedly elevated synovial cell counts. Bacterial superinfection can complicate crystal-induced arthritis, although this is rare. A history of recurrent monarthritis, typical podagra, or radiologic evidence of chondrocalcinosis are all suggestive of crystal-induced arthritis. However, only arthrocentesis with culture of the synovial fluid and analysis for

Table 47–2. Major Bacterial Organisms Implicated in Nongonococcal Septic Arthritis and the Percentage of Adult Infections Attributable to Each Pathogen

Organism	% of Adult Infections	Comments
Staphylococcus aureus	60–70%	• Most common pathogen in native joints and late prosthetic joint infections • Rates of methicillin-resistant *S aureus* are increasing in injection drug users and in the community
Streptococcal species	15–20%	• Group A streptococci most common streptococcal species implicated in septic arthritis • Usually preceded by primary skin or soft-tissue infection • Incidence is increasing of non–group A β-hemolytic streptococci (eg, groups B, C, and G streptococci), especially in immunocompromised hosts or following gastrointestinal or genitourinary infections • *S pneumoniae* infectious arthritis is still quite rare
Gram-negative bacilli	5–25%	• Most common in neonates, infants younger than 2 months, the elderly, injection drug users, and the chronically ill (diabetes mellitus, cancer, sickle cell anemia, connective tissue disorders, and renal transplant recipients and other immunosuppressed conditions) • Begin as urinary tract or skin infections, with subsequent hematogenous spread to a single joint • *Haemophilus influenzae* arthritis has decreased markedly since routine *H influenzae* type b childhood vaccination
Anaerobes	1–5%	• Common species include *Bacteroides, Propionibacterium acnes* (skin flora), and various anaerobic gram-positive cocci • 50% of anaerobic arthritis is polymicrobial • Predisposing factors: diabetes mellitus, immunocompromise, or postoperative wound infections, especially following total joint replacement or joint arthroplasty • Suspect if synovial fluid is foul smelling or air is present in the joint space radiologically • Collect cultures under anaerobic conditions and incubate for at least 2 weeks
Staphylococcus epidermidis	Rare in native joints	• Most common agent in early postoperative prosthetic joint infections • Forms glycocalyx layer over foreign surface • Organism often difficult to eradicate without joint removal
Brucella species	Rare	• *B melitensis* most common *Brucella* species implicated • Uncommon in the United States, but more prevalent worldwide • Risk factors: ingestion of unpasteurized milk or cheese or occupational exposures (eg, farmers and meat packers) • Causes monarthritis or an asymmetric peripheral oligoarthritis • Sacroiliitis and spondylitis also common • Diagnose with scintigraphy, computed tomography scan, polymerase chain reaction, and/or positive blood or joint cultures • Treatment courses lengthy and involve antimicrobial combinations
Mycoplasma	Rare	• More common in children than adults • Seen in the immunocompromised, particularly agammaglobulinemia

crystals can definitively distinguish septic arthritis from crystal-induced arthritis.

Treatment

Early diagnosis is the key to successful treatment of septic arthritis; delay in instituting appropriate antibiotic therapy and débridement measures almost invariably leads to poor outcomes. The two mainstays of treatment are drainage and intravenous antibiotic therapy. Progressive joint mobilization will also help prevent some of the long-term complications of septic arthritis.

A. DRAINAGE

The management of septic nongonococcal arthritis requires hospitalization for drainage of the infected joint. The joint must be thoroughly drained to decrease the number of inflammatory cells, which produce cytokines and proteolytic enzymes that cause permanent joint damage. Early arthroscopic lavage, débridement, and drain

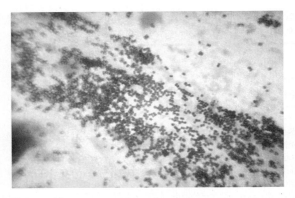

Figure 47–1. Gram stain of an inflammatory exudate showing the clustered gram-positive cocci of *Staphylococcus aureus*. (Image contributed by Dr. Thomas F. Sellers and is in the public domain; from the Centers for Disease Control Public Health Image Library [phil.cdc.gov].)

insertion have largely replaced the standard procedure of performing daily aspirations of the joint. Response to therapy can be gauged by following the synovial fluid cell counts and culture results over the subsequent days of hospitalization.

Open surgical drainage and débridement (arthrotomy) may be required for the following indications:

- Failure to respond to more conservative therapy in 5–7 days.
- Coexistent osteomyelitis that needs surgical intervention.
- Involvement of joints that are difficult to drain using more conservative approaches, such as hips, shoulders, or SI joints.
- Involvement of a prosthetic joint (see section on prosthetic joint infections, below)
- Difficulty in performing adequate drainage of the joint with needle aspiration or arthroscopic manipulations.
- Refusal of the patient to accept repeated needle aspirations or catheter drainage (eg, young children).
- Open drainage is the initial procedure of choice in children with septic arthritis of the hip.

B. Antibiotics

After the initial diagnostic joint aspiration, intravenous antibiotics should be immediately administered. Empiric antibiotic therapy is based on either the initial Gram stain results or the clinical situation (Table 47–3) in suspected bacterial arthritis. Antibiotics are usually administered for a total of 6 weeks for a native joint infection. Intra-articular antibiotic instillation has not been shown to be beneficial and may lead to a chemical synovitis.

C. Mobilization

Management of septic arthritis also includes passive motion exercises to prevent formation of adhesions and to enhance the clearance of purulent exudates after the acute inflammatory response has subsided. Passive mobilization is gradually followed by active strengthening of periarticular structures to help prevent joint contractures.

Complications

The major complications of septic arthritis include osteomyelitis, persistent or recurrent infection, a marked decrease in joint mobility, ankylosis, or persistent pain.

Prognosis

The clinical outcome of septic arthritis is determined by the duration of symptoms before the initiation of effective treatment, the number of infected joints, the age and immune status of the patient, preceding joint disease, the virulence and susceptibilities of the organism, and the particular joint infected. Seventy to eighty-five percent of patients with group A streptococcal infections recover without residual symptoms. Up to 50% of patients with septic arthritis secondary to *S aureus* or gram-negative rods, however, have residual joint damage. Patients with RA and polyarticular infection have a guarded prognosis, with a survival rate <50%.

DISSEMINATED GONOCOCCAL INFECTION

ESSENTIALS OF DIAGNOSIS

- *Sexually active young person without prior joint disease.*
- *Typical presentation is triad of polyarthritis, tenosynovitis, and dermatitis.*
- *Synovial fluid Gram stain and culture are often negative.*
- *Urethral, cervical, pharyngeal, and rectal cultures for Neisseria gonorrhoeae in aggregate are positive in 70–90% of cases.*

General Considerations

Disseminated gonococcal infection (DGI) remains the most common cause of acute septic arthritis in young sexually active persons in the United States and affects persons without prior joint disease. Dissemination of

Table 47–3. Initial Antibiotic Therapy for Septic Arthritis Based on Synovial Gram Stain or Clinical Situation

Synovial Fluid Gram Stain or Clinical Situation	Antibiotic Therapy
Gram-positive cocci	• Use IV vancomycin initially due to increasing rates of methicillin-resistant *S aureus* (MRSA) in the community (dosing: 10–15 mg/kg per dose administered q12h or q8h; typical regimen is 1 g IV q12h initially with doses subsequently adjusted to keep serum vancomycin troughs in the 15–20 μg/mL range) • Switch to high-dose third-generation cephalosporin (eg, ceftriaxone 2 g IV q24h; ceftizoxime 1 g IV q8h) or appropriate penicillin class if methicillin-sensitive *S aureus* (MSSA) or streptococcal growth; if MSSA, can use nafcillin 2 g IV q4h; if penicillin-sensitive streptococcal species, can use penicillin 24 million units qd or 4 million units IV q4h • Oral options: ciprofloxacin (750 mg PO bid) plus rifampin (450 mg PO bid); give bactericidal intra-articular concentrations in combination, but these should be used only for prosthetic joint infections; increasing data are available on linezolid (600 mg PO bid) in MRSA joint infections
Gram-negative bacilli	• Use IV therapy with an aminoglycoside (eg, gentamicin 1 mg/kg IV q8h or tobramycin 1.5 mg/kg IV q8h) in synergistic combination with an antipseudomonal penicillin (eg, ticarcillin 4 g IV q4h or piperacillin 4 g IV q4h) or high-dose third-generation cephalosporin specific for gram-negative organisms (eg, ceftazidime 2 g IV q8h)
Intravenous drug use	• Initial therapy with vancomycin for methicillin-resistant *S aureus*, as well as single or combination therapy for *Pseudomonas* as listed for gram-negative bacilli • Tailor subsequent therapy based on culture results
Immunocompetent normal host	• Initial therapy with IV vancomycin alone • Tailor subsequent therapy based on culture
Chronically ill or immunocompromised	• Initial therapy with broad coverage for gram-positive organisms (eg, vancomycin), gram-negative organisms, and anaerobes if clinically suspected; anaerobic coverage can involve adding a β-lactamase inhibitor to the antipseudomonal penicillin (eg, ticarcillin/clavulanate 3.1 g IV q4h or piperacillin/tazobactam 3.375 g IV q6h) or adding metronidazole 500 mg IV q8h • Tailor subsequent therapy based on culture results
Young adults with negative smear	• Ceftriaxone 1 g IV q24h for suspected gonococcal infection
Neonates and children <2 months old	• Broad-spectrum initial coverage for *H influenzae* (assume ampicillin resistance, so use a third-generation cephalosporin with the doses given above), *S aureus* (vancomycin as above if MRSA; nafcillin if MSSA), group B streptococci (best covered by penicillin, although sensitive to vancomycin, ceftriaxone, and ceftizoxime) and gram-negative bacilli • Combination of vancomycin, an extended-spectrum penicillin (eg, ticarcillin or piperacillin), and an aminoglycoside (eg, gentamicin or tobramycin) often used • Tailor subsequent therapy based on culture results

Neisseria gonorrhoeae occurs in 1–3% of cases of untreated genital gonococcal infections. Women are affected with DGI 2–3 times more commonly than men, with dissemination of *N gonorrhoeae* observed most frequently within 7 days of menses, during pregnancy, or in the postpartum period.

Pathogenesis

The joint and skin manifestations of DGI are mediated by both circulating immune complexes and the direct effects of microbial proliferation. Mucosal infection with *N gonorrhoeae* always precedes the development of DGI,

although this herald infection may be asymptomatic. Inherited deficiencies in either the terminal complement components (C5–C9) or in properdin synthesis result in inefficient outer membrane attack of *Neisseria* species and predispose patients to dissemination of *N gonorrhoeae* from localized sites of infection.

Clinical Findings

A. SYMPTOMS AND SIGNS

The duration from sexual contact to the onset of DGI varies from 1 day to 2 months, although the average duration of symptoms prior to presentation is 5 days. Twenty-five percent of patients with DGI will have the genitourinary or pharyngeal symptoms of the precedent mucosal infection.

DGI usually presents with the clinical triad of polyarthritis, tenosynovitis, and dermatitis. *N gonorrhoeae* accounts for only 20% of cases of monarticular septic arthritis in young adults, since the most common joint presentation of DGI involves an oligoarthritis or polyarthritis. The initial symptoms include fevers, chills, and migratory symptoms of polyarthralgias, which usually progress to frank monarthritis or polyarthritis in the knees, ankles, or wrists. Migratory symptoms of tenosynovitis occur in two-thirds of patients and are most often present over the dorsum of the hand, the wrist, the ankle, or the knee. Skin lesions are seen in approximately two-thirds of patients with DGI, although they are usually painless and patients may be unaware of them. Biopsy of these skin lesions demonstrates perivascular inflammation, leukocytoclastic vasculitis, intra-epidermal neutrophilic infiltration, and microthrombi; *N gonorrhoeae* can be cultured from biopsy specimens of the skin lesions approximately 10% of the time.

Unusual clinical manifestations of DGI include pericarditis, meningitis, aortitis, endocarditis, myocarditis, pyomyositis, and osteomyelitis.

B. PHYSICAL EXAMINATION

Gonococcal suppurative arthritis usually involves one or two joints, with the knees, wrists, ankles, and elbows being involved with decreasing frequency. The physical examination of these joints resembles that of septic nongonococcal arthritis, with warmth, effusion, erythema, and pain with active and passive range of motion. When tenosynovitis is present, there is tenderness to palpation in the periarticular regions of the wrists, fingers, toes, and ankles. The skin lesions of DGI are often asymptomatic and require careful inspection for their detection. Papules or macules are the most common, followed by pustular lesions on an erythematous base, often with a necrotic center (Figure 47–2). The rash is typically found on the trunk and distal extremities (including digits) in a relatively sparse distribution (10–25 lesions are usually found in total). Hemorrhagic bullae, erythema multiforme, and vasculitic lesions have also been reported.

C. LABORATORY FINDINGS

1. Blood and extra-articular cultures—Blood cultures are rarely positive in DGI. If DGI is suspected, however, urethral, cervical, pharyngeal, and rectal cultures should be collected. Genitourinary cultures are positive in 70–90% of patients with DGI.

2. Synovial fluid analysis

- *Cell count and differential:* The synovial fluid in gonococcal septic arthritis generally has lower WBC counts than in nongonococcal infections, with a typical range of 30,000–60,000 WBC/mm^3.

- *Gram stain for organisms:* The Gram stain for gonococcal organisms in synovial fluid is positive <25% of the time in the DGI syndrome (Figure 47–3).

- *Culture:* The culture for *N gonorrhoeae* in synovial fluid is positive in only 20–50% of cases, compared to 70–90% in nongonococcal septic arthritis. Reasons for this low yield of positive synovial cultures in DGI include its pathogenesis, which can involve circulating immune complexes rather than direct infection, and the fastidious growth requirements of the organism. Optimal

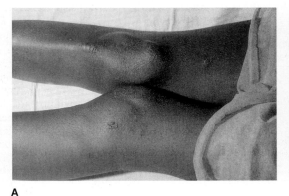

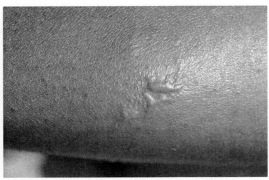

A   **B**

Figure 47–2. **A:** Skin lesions and joint involvement in disseminated gonococcal infection (DGI). **B:** Close-up view of a pustular DGI lesion on the skin of a patient's arm. (Images contributed by Dr. Thomas F. Sellers and are in the public domain; Centers for Disease Control Public Health Image Library [phil.cdc.gov].)

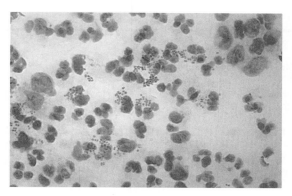

Figure 47–3. Gram stain of purulent fluid sample showing the small intracellular gram-negative diplococci of *Neisseria gonorrhoeae* with surrounding polymorphonuclear cells. (Image is in the public domain; Centers for Disease Control Public Health Image Library [phil.cdc.gov].)

growth conditions for the gonococcus involve the immediate plating of synovial fluid at the bedside on chocolate or Thayer-Martin media with incubation at 5–10% CO_2 concentration. *N gonorrhoeae* organisms may take more than 48 hours of incubation to grow, so the laboratory should be alerted to hold these cultures if DGI is suspected. As these stringent procedures of collection and incubation are not always followed, the yield of recovering *N gonorrhoeae* from any culture site is usually lower than could be optimally achieved. Synovial fluid in DGI is more likely to be positive for gonococcus when the fluid has a high WBC count.

D. IMAGING STUDIES

The uses of imaging studies in acute gonococcal arthritis are the same as those for acute nongonococcal septic arthritis reviewed above. The arthritis associated with DGI can be secondary to immune complex deposition or actual gonococcal infection of the joint; the latter syndrome tends to lead to a more robust inflammatory response that may be more likely to be detected on imaging.

E. SPECIAL TESTS

Various nonculture techniques have been developed for the detection of *N gonorrhoeae* in genitourinary sites. Particularly promising are nucleic acid amplification tests, which given their excellent sensitivity and specificity, are very useful for the diagnosis of patients with clinically typical but culture-negative gonococcal arthritis (Table 47–4). Polymerase chain reaction techniques to identify nongonococcal bacteria in septic and prosthetic joints are still investigational.

Differential Diagnosis

The differential diagnosis for DGI includes nongonococcal polyarticular septic arthritis, bacterial endocarditis, viral arthritis, and meningococcemia. Up to 40% of cases of meningococcemia have articular symptoms; meningococcus-associated arthritides are almost always sterile and present either as monarticular or polyarticular disease. Postinfectious forms of arthritis (acute rheumatic fever and reactive arthritis) also can be difficult to differentiate from DGI early in their course. Both can begin abruptly and be associated with fever; tenosynovitis is often prominent in reactive arthritis, as it is in DGI.

Treatment

A. DRAINAGE

After the initial aspiration procedure to diagnose gonococcal infection in the joint, closed drainage of purulent effusions in DGI is usually only required once or twice given the brisk response of the organism to antibiotics alone. Open drainage of suppurative joints is rarely required except for joints that are difficult to drain percutaneously.

B. ANTIBIOTICS

Penicillin can no longer be used as initial therapy for DGI given increasing rates of penicillinase production or chromosomally mediated resistance to penicillin in the gonococcal organism. Table 47–5 lists the options for initial intravenous or oral therapy for DGI. The initiation of antibiotics for DGI usually results in very rapid

Table 47–4. Sensitivity and Specificity of Various Nonculture-Based Tests for Detection of *Neisseria Gonorrhoeae* in Genitourinary Sites

Method	Sensitivity (%)	Specificity (%)
Antigen detection	70–85	94–99
Nucleic acid amplification tests	85–100	96–100
Ligase chain reaction	94–100	99.7

Table 47–5. Recommended Antibiotic Therapy for Treatment of Gonococcal Arthritis

Antibiotic	Comments
Parenteral third-generation cephalosporin	• Ceftriaxone 1 g IV/IM q24h is the most common third-generation cephalosporin used in DGI • Ceftizoxime or cefotaxime are also used
Spectinomycin	• Reserved for patients with β-lactam allergies • Dose is 2 g IM q12h
Fluoroquinolones	• Resistance is increasing of *N gonorrhoeae* to fluoroquinolones • If susceptible, dose of ciprofloxacin is 500 mg PO bid; dose of ofloxacin is 400 mg PO bid; dose of levofloxacin is 500 mg PO qd • IV formulations can be used initially, but fluoroquinolones have excellent oral bioavailability
Cefixime suspension	• Dose is 400 mg PO bid
Penicillin or ampicillin	• If the *N gonorrhoeae* is penicillin-susceptible, switch to one of the following: ampicillin 1 g IV q6h, penicillin G 12 million units IV qd (divided), amoxicillin 500 mg PO tid, or penicillin VK 500 mg PO qid

improvement (over 24–48 hours) in signs and symptoms, which can be a clue to the diagnosis. Unless complicated by systemic manifestations such as carditis, meningitis, endocarditis, or osteomyelitis, the duration of treatment for DGI is only 10–14 days. Intravenous therapy is usually given for 2–4 days, followed by 7–10 days of oral therapy. Uncomplicated cases of DGI are increasingly being treated in the outpatient setting with oral therapy alone. Given the high prevalence of concurrent chlamydial infections in patients with *N gonorrhoeae* infections, management of DGI usually requires additional treatment for *Chlamydia trachomatis* (eg, azithromycin or doxycycline).

Prognosis

The prognosis of arthritis in DGI is much more favorable than that of nongonococcal septic arthritis, with complete recovery in virtually all patients after the institution of appropriate antibiotic therapy.

PROSTHETIC JOINT INFECTIONS

ESSENTIALS OF DIAGNOSIS

• *Prosthetic joints are at increased risk of developing infectious arthritis.*

• *Prosthetic joint infections that occur <4 weeks after the initial implantation or that are due to hematogenous seeding present with fever, pain, warmth, and swelling.*

• *Infections due to low-virulence organisms introduced at the time of surgery typically present >4*

weeks after implantation with the insidious onset of pain, often without other signs of infection.

• *Early prosthetic joint infections can usually be treated with prosthesis salvage; late infections may require replacement of the joint.*

General Considerations

Septic arthritis in prosthetic joints has unique characteristics in terms of incidence, risk factors, and management. The rate of prosthetic joint infection fell from 10% in the 1960s to <1% by 1990 due to improvements in surgical technique and equipment and the use of preoperative antibiotics. However, prosthetic joint infection is 5–10 times more likely with a revision arthroplasty. Prosthetic joint infections can categorized as "early" or "late," depending on the temporal relationship to the surgical joint replacement. Early postoperative infections reflect contamination of the wound in the perioperative period from skin flora, contaminated equipment, operating room personnel, or airborne bacteria. Risk factors for early postoperative infections include prolonged duration of surgery, an inexperienced primary surgeon, and patient factors such as advanced age, underlying chronic illnesses, RA, or a perioperative nonarticular infection.

Late infections, which occur more than 1 month after the joint replacement, result from hematogenous seeding of the foreign body and damaged native tissue within the prosthetic joints or are due to low-virulence organisms (eg, *Staphylococcus epidermidis*, *Propionibacterium acnes*, or diphtheroids) introduced at the time of surgery. Late indolent infections are typically caused by microorganisms that grow in biofilms. For instance, pathogens such as *Staphylococcus epidermidis* excrete a polysaccharide ("glycocalyx") layer that covers the foreign material, creating a protected environment for further replication. Furthermore, the lack of microvasculature in the prosthetic material limits the penetration of antibiotics and host immune mediators into the joint. As a result, infections in a prosthetic joint require a much lower inoculum of microorganisms than those in a normal joint.

Clinical Findings

A. SYMPTOMS AND SIGNS

Prosthetic joint infections have varying clinical presentations depending on the duration since orthopedic implant. Such infections can present early (≤4 weeks after joint replacement) or late (≥1 month after surgery). Furthermore, prosthetic joints are more susceptible to infection from hematogenous spread than normal joints throughout their lifetime because of the presence of a foreign body. Early prosthetic joint infections and those late infections due to hematogenous seeding are usually due to virulent organisms and typically present with the classic symptoms of acute bacterial arthritis with fever, as well as pain, erythema, effusion, and warmth in the joint persisting beyond the postoperative period. Late infections due to less virulent organisms introduced at the time of surgery usually present with a more indolent course of increasing joint pain, implant loosening, or both, sometimes accompanied by joint drainage, but usually without concurrent fever or peripheral leukocytosis.

B. PHYSICAL EXAMINATION

The physical examination of early prosthetic joint infection or infection due to hematogenous seeding resembles that of acute suppurative arthritis, with warmth, effusion, and erythema in the joint, along with elicitation of pain with passive or active range of motion and fever. Overlying cellulitis and the formation of a sinus tract with purulent discharge may occur in early infections. The physical examination of late prosthetic joint infection is less dramatic and may just reveal moderate pain with movement or joint instability.

C. LABORATORY FINDINGS

1. Peripheral counts and cultures—The blood peripheral leukocyte count may be elevated in early prosthetic joint infections, but can remain normal in late indolent infections. The C-reactive protein level is elevated postoperatively from the surgery itself and should return to normal within weeks if an early postoperative infection does not occur. A combination of a normal erythrocyte sedimentation rate and C-reactive protein has been shown to be a good indicator for the absence of infection.

Blood cultures are rarely positive in late indolent infections, although they may be positive in early infections. If hematogenous spread from an extra-articular infection is suspected, targeted cultures of the involved site should be obtained. Cultures of a superficial wound or sinus tract overlying the prosthetic joint are often contaminated by skin flora and should therefore not be performed.

2. Synovial fluid analysis
- *Cell count and differential*: A synovial fluid white blood cell count of more than 1700 WBC/mm^3 has a sensitivity of 94% and a specificity of 88% for infection in a prosthetic joint in patients without underlying inflammatory joint disease. Alternatively, a neutrophil percentage >65% has 97% sensitivity and 98% specificity for infection in a prosthetic joint.
- *Gram stain for organisms*: As with septic arthritis in a normal joint, a positive Gram stain in a prosthetic joint is diagnostic for the infectious agent (highly specific), but a negative Gram stain does not rule out infection. Gram stains are less frequently positive in prosthetic joints than normal joints, because frank infection can occur with a lower organism burden in the former.
- *Culture*: Cultures in aspirated synovial fluid of prosthetic joints are more frequently positive in early postoperative infections than late infections.
- *Microbiology*: The microbiology of early postoperative infections involves mainly *S aureus* and the coagulase-negative staphylococci introduced at the time of surgical repair. Late prosthetic joint infections that present at least a month after surgery usually evolve from a pathogen of low virulence or of low inoculum introduced at the time of the procedure. These pathogens include skin flora such as *Staphylococcus epidermidis, Propionibacterium acnes,* or diphtheroids, although anaerobes and *S aureus* can also be involved. Hematogenous infection in a prosthetic joint, as in a normal joint, can result from transient bacteremia secondary to a remote infection or a surgical or other invasive procedure and typically involves *S aureus,* streptococci, and gram-negative rods.

3. Histopathological studies—Since most prosthetic joint infections need an open procedure for either débridement and retention of components or removal of the foreign material prior to replacement, tissue is often available for microscopic examination for inflammatory cells, Gram stain, or culture. Cultures of periprosthetic tissue are the most reliable method of detecting the pathogen, with sensitivities reaching 95%. At least three intraoperative tissue specimens should be sampled for Gram stain and culture.

Reasons for negative cultures include prior use of antimicrobials, a low organism count, fastidious organisms, or incorrect specimen handling procedures. Given that most late prosthetic joint infections are low grade, antimicrobial therapy should be discontinued 10 days to 2 weeks before tissue specimens are collected.

D. IMAGING STUDIES

1. Plain radiographs—Plain radiographs are helpful to detect prosthetic joint infections when they are performed serially over time after implantation. New subperiosteal bone growth and transcortical sinus tracts are relatively specific for infection. Radiographs may also show zones of radiolucency at the bone-cement interface to suggest joint loosening, although loosening due to infection is difficult to distinguish from aseptic mechanical loosening.

2. Computed tomography—Prosthetic joints often have distorted joint architecture and CT imaging is better at distinguishing normal from abnormal tissue, but radiologic artifacts caused by metal implants limits its use.

3. Magnetic resonance imaging—MRI scans can only be performed in patients with implants made of safe metals, such as titanium or tantalum. Most of the newer implants are constructed of MRI-safe materials.

4. Scintigraphy—A technetium bone scan can remain positive for more than a year after uncomplicated arthroplasties because of periprosthetic bone inflammation and remodeling. Hence, nuclear scintigraphy is more useful for diagnosing late prosthetic joint infections than early infections.

Differential Diagnosis

Early prosthetic joint infections are usually not subtle, but late prosthetic joint infections can manifest simply as persistent joint pain without any systemic signs of infection. Because joint pain and loosening can occur both in infection and aseptic failure of the joint, it may be difficult to distinguish late prosthetic joint infection from mechanical failure. A diagnosis of prosthetic joint infection may not be made until surgical exploration and cultures reveal purulence and a pathogen.

Treatment

Therapy of prosthetic joint infections varies by the temporal relationship of the infection to the surgical procedure. It is possible to manage infections occurring in the acute postoperative period ($\leq$4 weeks after surgery) with surgical débridement and prolonged antibiotic therapy alone, without subsequent prosthesis removal. This treatment course has been labeled "prosthesis salvage" and has demonstrated up to a 70% success rate for early infections. Infections occurring in the late postoperative period and through hematogenous spread usually require removal of the prostheses for successful cure, although management of late prosthetic joint infections with débridement and prolonged antibiotics alone is becoming more common.

A randomized controlled trial looked at patients with stable orthopedic implants who had culture-proven staphylococcal infection and short durations of infectious symptoms (0–3 weeks). These patients all underwent surgical débridement of the joint without prosthetic material removal, followed by prolonged oral antibiotic therapy (3–6 months) with either oral ciprofloxacin alone or a combination of oral ciprofloxacin and rifampin. The group treated with the oral antibiotic combination had a higher cure rate (100%) than the group treated with ciprofloxacin alone (58%), presumably because of rifampin's superior ability to penetrate tissues and biofilms. Factors associated with cure included stability of the orthopedic implant, a short duration of infections prior to débridement, immediate surgical débridement, and the addition of rifampin to the antibiotic regimen. A recent retrospective study of outcomes of treating prosthetic joint infection with débridement and retention of components followed by prolonged antibiotic therapy demonstrated that the presence of a sinus tract and a prolonged duration of symptoms prior to débridement ($\geq$8 days) predicted treatment failure.

If surgical replacement of the device is necessary, two-stage procedures may be more successful than one-stage exchange. One-stage exchange combines removal of the infected implant, débridement, and replacement of the joint in one procedure, followed by prolonged courses of antibiotics. However, management most often involves a three-stage procedure: (1) removal of the infected joint prosthesis (with concomitant débridement and collection of appropriate diagnostic cultures), often with placement of a temporary cement spacer; (2) administration of appropriate antibiotics for at least 6 weeks; and (3) revision arthroplasty. Pooled data from small studies show a better cure rate with the use of antibiotic-impregnated cement than with regular cement, although randomized controlled trial data on its efficacy are lacking. Other surgical options include resection arthroplasty with permanent removal of the prosthesis and thorough débridement, as well as amputation. As with the management of septic arthritis in native joints, progressive mobilization during and after treatment helps prevent joint contractures.

Complications

The major complication of prosthetic joint infections is failure of the prosthesis and recurrent infection. Even if the patient initially does well with débridement and retention of prosthetic components and does not develop a recurrent infectious process, the joint will most likely require revision arthroplasty sooner than a joint that fails from routine wear and tear.

Prognosis

The same risk factors that predispose to poor clinical outcomes in native joints can affect outcomes with prosthetic joint infections, including age and immune status of the patient, preceding joint disease such as RA, the virulence and susceptibilities of the organism, and the particular joint infected.

REFERENCES

Kaandorp CJ, Van Schaardenburg D, Krijnen P, Habbema JD, van de Laar MA. Risk factors for septic arthritis in patients with joint disease. A prospective study. *Arthritis Rheum.* 1995;38:1819. [PMID: 8849354] (One of a series of prospective community-based trials [all with CJ Kaandorp as the lead author] looking at the incidence, risk factors, and outcomes of septic arthritis.)

Liebling MR, Arkfeld DG, Michelini GA, et al. Identification of *Neisseria gonorrhoeae* in synovial fluid using the polymerase chain reaction. *Arthritis Rheum.* 1994;37:702. [PMID: 8185697] (A case control study of the utility of PCR in the detection of *N gonorrhoeae* in synovial fluid samples.)

Marculescu CE, Berbari EF, Hanssen AD, et al. Outcome of prosthetic joint infections treated with debridement and retention of components. *Clin Infect Dis.* 2006;42:471. (A retrospective cohort analysis of the risk factors for treatment failure with just débridement and retention of prosthesis in 99 episodes of prosthetic joint infection at the Mayo Clinic.)

Ross JJ. Septic arthritis. *Infect Dis Clin North Am.* 2005;19:799. [PMID: 16297733] (A thorough review of the risk factors, clinical presentation, and bacteriology of nongonococcal septic arthritis)

Stengel D, Bauwens K, Sehouli J, Ekkernkamp A, Porzsolt F. Systematic review and meta-analysis of antibiotic therapy for bone and joint infections. *Lancet Infect Dis.* 2001;1:175. [PMID: 11871494] (A meta-analysis that describes the paucity of high-quality data regarding the appropriate use and administration of antibiotics for septic arthritis. Consultation with an infectious diseases specialist may aid in the selection of appropriate antimicrobial therapy for this condition.)

Zimmerli W, Widmer AF, Blater M, Frei R, Ochsner PE. Role of rifampin for treatment of orthopedic implant-related staphylococcal infections: a randomized controlled trial. Foreign-Body Infection (FBI) Study Group. *JAMA.* 1998;279:1537. [PMID: 9605897]. (The results of this important study are reviewed in the text.)

Zimmerli W, Trampuz A, Ochsner PE. Prosthetic-joint infections. *N Engl J Med.* 2004;351:1645. [PMID: 15483283] (An up-to-date and thorough review of the risk factors, pathogenesis, and management of prosthetic joint infections.)

Lyme Disease

Linda K. Bockenstedt, MD

ESSENTIALS OF DIAGNOSIS

Classic clinical features occur in stages:

- *Early localized disease (3–30 days after tick bite): a single hallmark skin lesion (erythema migrans), occasionally associated with fever, malaise, headache, arthralgias, and myalgias; less commonly, these latter symptoms can occur in the absence of erythema migrans.*

- *Early disseminated disease (weeks to months after tick bite): multiple erythema migrans lesions and associated fever, migratory arthralgias, and myalgias; acute pauciarticular arthritis; carditis manifested primarily as atrioventricular nodal block; neurologic features, including cranial nerve (especially facial nerve) palsies, lymphocytic meningitis, and radiculoneuropathies.*

- *Late disease (several months to years after tick bite): primarily neurologic features, especially peripheral neuropathies and chronic mild encephalopathy; arthritis, including monarticular and migratory pauciarticular arthritis.*

- *Supporting serologic evidence of exposure to Borrelia burgdorferi is present in the majority of cases but can be absent in individuals with early infection.*

General Considerations

The multisystem disorder of Lyme disease is due to a tick-transmitted infection with the spirochete *Borrelia burgdorferi*. The diagnosis should be considered in individuals who have a reasonable risk of exposure to infected ticks, such as those who live or vacation in areas endemic for the disorder, and who present with a characteristic complex of signs and symptoms.

Lyme disease is a multisystem disorder caused by infection with spirochetes of the genus *Borrelia burgdorferi sensu lato*: *B burgdorferi sensu stricto*, *B garinii*, and *B afzelii*. Hard-shelled ticks of the *Ixodes* family, primarily *I scapularis* and *I pacificus* in the United States and *I ricinus* in Europe, serve as vectors for infection. In the United States, the disease first came to medical attention in 1975, with the evaluation of a clustering of children with presumed juvenile rheumatoid arthritis around the town of Lyme, Connecticut. Lyme arthritis, as it was initially termed, was soon found to be one manifestation of systemic infection with *B burgdorferi*. Beginning with a characteristic skin lesion, erythema migrans (EM), early infection was either localized to the skin, or disseminated to other sites, with disease most commonly found in the skin, heart, joints, and nervous system. Lyme disease is not a new entity; in Europe, EM had been associated with *I ricinus* tick bites since the early 20th century, and the skin disease was treated successfully with penicillin after spirochetes were visualized in biopsy specimens in the mid-1900s. Other systemic manifestations were occasionally present, especially neurologic disease (Bannwarth syndrome), but the broad clinical spectrum was not fully appreciated until the late 1970s.

Since its emergence in the United States more than a quarter century ago, Lyme disease has become the most common vector-borne infection in this country. In 2002, 23,763 cases from 47 states were reported to the Centers for Disease Control and Prevention, with more than 90% originating from only 9 states: New York, Connecticut, New Jersey, Pennsylvania, Massachusetts, Maryland, Rhode Island, Wisconsin, and Minnesota. Cases of Lyme disease have been reported from 49 states and the District of Columbia, and also occur in other areas of North America as well as in Europe and Asia. In the latter two continents, other *B burgdorferi sensu lato* members—*B garinii* and *B afzelii*—are the main etiologic agents.

Lyme disease begins when humans serve as incidental blood meal hosts for *B burgdorferi*–infected ticks. Although all three forms of ticks—larvae, nymphs, and adults—can harbor *B burgdorferi*, nymphs are more likely to transmit infection to humans because of their promiscuous feeding patterns and small size (see the Centers for Disease Control Lyme disease website for a description of the vector's life cycle and images of ticks). *Ixodes* ticks feed only once per developmental stage, so that the incidence of Lyme disease follows the seasonal feeding patterns of nymphs (late spring, summer, and early fall). Larvae are rarely, if ever, vectors for the disease because they must first acquire infection by feeding on a reservoir host.

Nymphs feed for 3–8 days, during which time spirochetes migrate from the tick midgut to the salivary gland and egress into the host through salivary secretions. Transmission of infection generally requires 24–48 hours of tick feeding, so that tick surveillance and early removal of embedded ticks is a primary preventive strategy in areas endemic for Lyme disease. Spirochetes first establish infection in the skin, where local immune responses give rise to EM, a hallmark of early, localized infection. This rash is present in up to 80% of cases and typically appears within the first month after tick bite. Thereafter, spirochetes can disseminate hematogenously to all areas of the body, but disease primarily manifests in other areas of the skin, the heart, the joints, and the nervous system.

The diagnosis of Lyme disease relies on a characteristic clinical presentation and can be supported by serologic tests showing the presence of antibodies to *B burgdorferi*. Patients early in the course of their treatment or, rarely, those treated early with antibiotics may test negative. The majority of patients with Lyme disease can be treated successfully with antibiotics, with little in the way of long-term sequelae. Misdiagnosis of other conditions as Lyme disease remains the most common reason that patients do not respond to conventional therapy. Oral antibiotics for 2–4 weeks are appropriate initial therapy for all patients except those with severe cardiac or neurologic involvement, who should receive intravenous therapy. One exception may be patients with isolated Bell palsy, because they respond equally well to oral antibiotics. Patients with chronic residual signs and symptoms after treatment for Lyme disease may have irreversible tissue damage, a post-Lyme fibromyalgia syndrome, or possibly infection-induced autoimmunity. Extended courses of oral and/or intravenous antibiotics have not been shown to provide benefit over placebo for this patient population and should be avoided unless clear objective evidence of active infection is present.

Pathogenesis

B burgdorferi survives in nature through alternating infection with ticks and reservoir hosts, including mammals and birds. Ticks feed only once per developmental stage and can lay dormant for years. Thus, spirochetes require that their vertebrate hosts survive in order to increase the probability of transmission back to ticks. In mammals, spirochetes cause disease as they initially infect and disseminate within the host, but inflammation generally resolves even if the organism is not cleared. In humans, *B burgdorferi* is difficult to culture from infected tissues, except for EM lesions, but rare positive cultures have been reported at all stages of the disease, including from blood, cerebrospinal fluid, heart biopsies, and joint fluid. Recently, improved detection of *B burgdorferi* infection by large-volume culture of human plasma has been re-ported, but only in individuals with early signs of Lyme disease, such as EM, suggesting that the blood-borne phase of *B burgdorferi* infection is likely brief. In animal models, few spirochetes can be seen in infected tissues, yet an exuberant inflammatory response arises and then resolves, with spirochetes persisting in tissues. Despite transient sightings of spirochetes within cells, no intracellular phase of *B burgdorferi* infection has been documented. *B burgdorferi* employs several immune evasion mechanisms that are common to extracellular pathogens. Spirochete lipoproteins, which are expressed on internal and surface-exposed pathogen membranes, incite acute inflammation by activating innate immune cells through Toll-like receptor pattern recognition receptors. Downregulation of lipoprotein expression as spirochetes adapt to persist in the host may impede their clearance by innate immune cells and by borrelicidal antibodies targeting specific lipoproteins. Antigenic variation, particularly of the VlsE lipoprotein, has been demonstrated, providing another mechanism whereby the spirochete can evade protective antibodies. *B burgdorferi* also possesses a family of lipoproteins that bind host factor H to impede lysis by complement. Antibiotic therapy may release internally sequestered lipoproteins from dead spirochetes and contribute to the Jarisch-Herxheimer reaction, a febrile response and transient exacerbation of symptoms noted by up to 15% of Lyme disease patients at the start of therapy. Delayed clearance of spirochete inflammatory products may also contribute to lingering symptoms after antibiotic treatment for Lyme disease.

Prevention

The best way to prevent Lyme disease is to reduce the risk of human exposure to *B burgdorferi*–infected ticks through personal preventive behavior and environmental controls. Avoiding physical contact with common tick habitats, such as wooded areas, stone fences, woodpiles, tall grass and brush, helps limit exposure risk of individuals in areas endemic for Lyme disease. Environmental controls such as the removal of tall grass and brush, clearance of woodpiles and the application of insecticides, can reduce the risk of human contact with infected ticks. If entry into tick habitats is anticipated, wearing protective, light-colored clothing such as long-sleeved shirts and long pants tucked into socks allows for ticks to be readily seen and reduces their access to exposed skin. Insect repellants containing DEET (N,N-diethyl-M-toluamide) applied to the clothing and exposed skin surfaces provide added protection. Permethrin can also be sprayed on clothing and kills ticks directly.

Daily tick checks are essential for persons with risk of exposure to ticks. Prompt removal of ticks embedded in the skin can effectively reduce the incidence of Lyme disease in endemic communities. Attached ticks should be removed by grasping the mouthparts with tweezers and pulling steadily up. Use of alcohol, heat, or vaso-occlusive substances will not promote tick detachment. A single 200-mg dose of doxycycline administered within 72 hours of tick bite has been shown to prevent Lyme disease. However, the risk of infection after tick bite is low (~1.4% even in endemic areas), making the routine use of prophylactic antibiotics in individuals bitten by ticks unwarranted. Such persons should be observed for 30 days for the development of a rash at the site of tick bite or for unexplained fever, which may be indicative not only of Lyme disease, but of other tick-borne infections as well.

One effective method for prevention of Lyme disease is vaccination. Two vaccines using the spirochete lipoprotein OspA were developed and tested in humans for safety and efficacy. Although immune responses to OspA that arise after natural infection have been associated with chronic arthritis (see below), the incidence of arthritis in patients undergoing OspA vaccination did not differ from those receiving placebo. One of the two OspA vaccines, LYMErix was approved by the Food and Drug Administration; 76% of adults (aged 18–75) who received three doses of LYMErix were protected from symptomatic Lyme disease. However, limited demand for the vaccine and public concern over potential vaccine-related sequelae led to its discontinuation by the manufacturer.

Clinical Findings

Lyme disease typically occurs in stages that reflect the in vivo biology of the spirochete. After establishing infection in the skin at the site of tick feeding, spirochetes that escape initial immune destruction disseminate through the skin, the blood, and the lymphatics to infect virtually any organ system. The clinical manifestations of Lyme disease thus depend on the stage of the illness at which the patient presents—early localized infection, early disseminated disease, or late disease.

Symptoms & Signs

A. EARLY LOCALIZED INFECTION

The most common early manifestation of Lyme disease is the skin rash EM, present in up to 80% of patients. EM appears within a month after exposure to *B burgdorferi*, with a median of 7–10 days, and first appears at the site of tick bite. Ticks may initially bind to clothing or exposed skin, but typically choose skin folds or creases and areas where clothes are particularly confining (eg, near elastic bands). In adults, the most common sites for EM are the popliteal fossa, gluteal fold, trunk, and axilla; in children, EM often arises near the hairline.

The most characteristic feature of EM is its morphology (Figure 48–1A): it is a flat, macular erythematous lesion that expands rapidly, 2–3 cm/d, and can enlarge

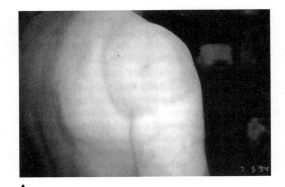

A

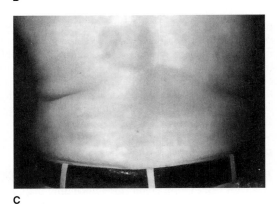

B

C

Figure 48–1. **A:** Erythema migrans rash with central clearing on the shoulder of a patient. Note the central hyperpigmentation at prior tick bite site (punctum). *Borrelia burgdorferi* was isolated from a biopsy culture performed at the periphery of the lesion. **B:** Vesicular erythema migrans lesion. **C:** Multiple erythema migrans lesions on the back of a patient whose primary lesion is depicted in photo **A.** Note absence of central papule or postinflammatory skin change. (From Nadelman RE, Wormser GP. Erythema migrans and early Lyme disease. *Am J Med.* 1995;98:16S. With permission.)

to more than 70 cm in diameter. The lesion should be >5 cm in diameter to fulfill diagnostic criteria. Although central clearing to produce a target or bull's-eye rash can occur in up to 40% of cases, especially when the lesion is large, more often it presents with uniform erythema. Occasionally, the center can be intensely erythematous, vesicular, or even necrotic (Figure 48–1B). Despite its appearance, EM itself rarely produces much in the way of local symptoms other than tingling. Rarely, the lesion is intensely pruritic or painful. Systemic flulike symptoms may be present, including low-grade fever, malaise, neck pain or stiffness, arthralgias, and myalgias; these are particularly severe in individuals with co-infection with another tick-borne pathogen, such as *Babesia microti* or *Anaplasma phagocytophilum,* the agent of human granulocytic ehrlichiosis. In about 18% of cases, Lyme disease can also manifest with a summer flulike syndrome, without respiratory or gastrointestinal involvement, in the absence of EM.

B. Acute Disseminated Disease

Within weeks to months of initial infection, spirochetes can disseminate widely throughout the host. At this stage, infection can be present in multiple tissues but disease most commonly arises in four organ systems: the skin, the heart, the musculoskeletal system, and the nervous system. Patients are generally ill-appearing and complain of debilitating fatigue and malaise. While specific localizing signs and symptoms may be intermittent, persistent fatigue is a hallmark of untreated disseminated Lyme disease.

1. Skin—Multiple EM lesions are a sign of dissemination and arise in about 50% of patients with untreated early, localized infection (Figure 48–1C). Secondary lesions have a random distribution, are smaller than the primary lesion, and less often necrotic or vesicular, although they may exhibit central clearing.

2. Musculoskeletal—A variety of musculoskeletal signs and symptoms may be present in disseminated Lyme disease. Migratory pains in muscles, joints, and periarticular structures, especially tendons and ligaments, that last only hours to days are seen in early localized infection as well as in acute disseminated disease. True inflammatory arthritis usually involves a single joint, particularly the knee, and presents with a large effusion (>50–100 mL) accompanied by stiffness and only mild pain. Other joints involved in order of frequency include the shoulder, ankle, elbow, temporomandibular joint, and wrist. It is rare for Lyme arthritis to involve more than five joints at any one time. Acute Lyme arthritis is usually episodic, with attacks of monarticular or oligoarticular arthritis lasting only weeks, and decreasing in frequency with time. Most patients resolve arthritis completely within 5 years, even without antibiotic therapy. In a minority of patients arthritis can become chronic (see below).

3. Nervous system—Central and/or peripheral nervous system disease occurs in about 15% of patients with early, disseminated Lyme disease. The classic triad consists of aseptic meningitis with cranial neuropathy, especially involving the VIIth nerve, and painful peripheral radiculoneuropathy. Central nervous system involvement most commonly presents as aseptic meningitis, although meningoencephalitis with subtle cognitive deficits can occur. In comparison to other forms of meningitis, the headache may be waxing and waning and neck stiffness is generally mild, so that a high index of suspicion may be required to make the diagnosis. Cranial neuropathy occurs in about 50% of patients with early neuroborreliosis and most often affects the facial nerve. Cerebrospinal fluid (CSF) abnormalities may be present in cases of facial palsy and reflect asymptomatic central nervous system involvement. Although usually unilateral, bilateral facial nerve palsies occur in nearly 30% of patients with VIIth nerve involvement. Peripheral radiculoneuropathy is a mixed motor and sensory neuropathy that presents with sharp, lancinating pain in the distribution of the affected nerves, and later hyporeflexia. Often multiple nerves and nerve roots are involved in an asymmetric fashion. Acute radiculoneuritis is rarely seen in the United States, but is common in Europe where it is also known as Bannwarth syndrome. In untreated patients, neurologic signs and symptoms can have a relapsing, remitting course over many months. Rarely, Lyme disease can be a cause of transverse myelitis.

4. Heart—Lyme carditis is relatively rare, occurring in <10% of patients with disseminated Lyme disease. Conduction system abnormalities with varying degrees of atrioventricular block are the most common cardiac manifestation, with symptomatic third-degree atrioventricular block occurring in about 50% of such patients. Occasionally myocarditis with heart muscle dysfunction and pericarditis can also occur, but valvular disease is not found. Because Lyme carditis is usually self-limited, cardiac involvement in disseminated Lyme disease may be overlooked, especially if it remains clinically asymptomatic in comparison to other features.

5. Other organ system involvement—A variety of other organs can exhibit pathology with disseminated *B burgdorferi* infection. These include the eye (keratitis), the ear (sensorineural hearing loss), the liver (hepatitis), the spleen (necrosis), skeletal muscle (myositis), and subcutaneous tissue (panniculitis). In general, other more classic manifestations of Lyme disease are present concurrently or have been present in the recent past to suggest the diagnosis.

C. Late Persistent Disease

Less than 10% of patients with acute Lyme disease develop chronic manifestations of the disorder, most often in the skin, joints, and nervous system. In Europe, infection with *B afzelii* is associated with the late skin lesion **acrodermatitis chronica atrophicans.** It first appears as an erythematous, hyperpigmented lesion that evolves to a chronic stage of hypopigmentation and atrophic, cellophanelike skin. Antibiotic treatment during the inflammatory phase of this lesion can lead to resolution. Chronic cardiomyopathy has been attributed to Lyme disease in Europe, but this late manifestation has not been documented in the United States.

Late neurologic manifestations include subtle cognitive dysfunction, meningoencephalitis, sensorimotor neuropathies, and rarely, leukoencephalitis. Chronic encephalomyelitis is more commonly found in Europe where the neurotropic spirochete *B garinii* is endemic, and is best documented by CSF examination and neuropsychologic testing.

A small percentage of patients with acute intermittent Lyme arthritis (<10%) may subsequently evolve a pattern of chronic arthritis, usually involving a single joint, often the knee. These patients may fail to respond to antibiotics, particularly if polymerase chain reaction of synovial fluid is negative for *B burgdorferi* DNA. Such "treatment-resistant" Lyme arthritis occurs primarily in patients who possess the human leukocyte antigen (HLA)-DRB1*0401 or *0101 alleles and who have T-lymphocyte and antibody responses to the spirochete lipoprotein OspA. It has been postulated that synovitis can be perpetuated by immune responses to OspA that cross-react with a human protein (LFA-1), which is expressed in inflamed joints, even though the spirochete itself has been eliminated. Animal studies have not supported LFA-1 as a relevant autoantigen, however. Chronic arthritis may also be due to the immune response to poorly degraded spirochete debris or to persistent infection with multiple antigenic variants transmitted by the tick.

Laboratory Findings

A. Routine Studies

Results of laboratory studies of patients with Lyme disease depend on the stage and organ system involved. Routine laboratory tests are nonspecific, with some patients exhibiting a mild elevation in the white blood cell (neutrophil) count, erythrocyte sedimentation rate, and modest abnormalities of liver function tests (Table 48–1). The synovial fluid from patients with acute arthritis is inflammatory. Cell counts range from 2000–100,000 with a predominance of neutrophils. The synovial fluid protein and glucose levels are usually normal. Serum antin-

Table 48–1. Laboratory Tests in Lyme Disease

Test	Result
Complete blood cell count	White blood cell count normal or slightly elevated (neutrophil predominance)
Erythrocyte sedimentation rate	Elevated in 50% of cases
Liver function tests	Mild elevation in GGT and ALT
ANA, rheumatoid factor	Negative
Synovial fluid	Inflammatory, cell counts ranging from 2000 to 100,000 (neutrophil predominance); normal or elevated protein; normal glucose
Cerebrospinal fluid	Lymphocytic pleocytosis; elevated protein; normal glucose; negative oligoclonal bands

GGT, gamma-glutamyl transpeptidase; ALT, alanine aminotransferase; ANA, antinuclear antibody.

uclear antibody and rheumatoid factor tests should be negative. Patients with neurologic Lyme disease, including isolated facial palsy, may have abnormalities in the cerebrospinal fluid. A lymphocytic pleocytosis accompanied by elevated protein and normal glucose is consistent with central nervous system infection, but not specific for Lyme neuroborreliosis. It is debated whether all patients with isolated facial palsy should have a lumbar puncture to exclude central nervous system involvement, since these patients appear to respond well to oral antibiotics.

B. *Borrelia burgdorferi*–Specific Tests

1. Culture—In contrast to other infectious diseases for which isolation of the causative organism is a viable tool for diagnosis, it is rare to culture *B burgdorferi* from tissues and body fluids of patients with Lyme disease. EM provides an exception, with spirochetes readily cultivated from biopsies of the leading margin of the lesion. The morphologic features of EM, however, are sufficiently distinct to make this skin manifestation virtually diagnostic for Lyme disease so that biopsy and culture are rarely performed. While recovery of *B burgdorferi* from the plasma of patients is greatest early in infection when EM is present, the variability of culture medium lots for growing the spirochete make routine use of culture of any blood or tissue specimen impractical other than for research purposes.

2. Serologic tests—Serologic tests that measure antibodies to *B burgdorferi* provide evidence of exposure to the pathogen and can be used to support a clinical diagnosis of Lyme disease. A two-tiered approach to serologic testing utilizes an enzyme-linked immunosorbent assay (ELISA) with *B burgdorferi* antigens as a screening tool for IgM and IgG reactivity to *B burgdorferi*. IgM responses appear within the first 2–3 weeks of infection, whereas IgG responses can usually be detected after 1 month. IgM responses should be used to support a diagnosis of Lyme disease only in patients with ~4 weeks of suggestive signs and symptoms. For individuals with a clinical history of longer duration, IgG responses alone should be considered. A persistently positive IgM ELISA over many months without an IgG response suggests a false-positive test. An immunoblot (Western blot), in which individual proteins of *B burgdorferi* are separated by molecular weight, should be used to confirm specificity of antibodies for all positive or equivocal ELISA tests, but should not be routinely performed on negative ELISA samples. Criteria for positive IgM and IgG immunoblots are listed in Table 48–2. The most commonly detected antigen, the 41-kDa protein flagellin, is not unique to *B burgdorferi* and patients may have detectable antibodies because of past exposure to other bacteria with homologous proteins. Patients with early Lyme disease may initially be seronegative, but the majority will seroconvert after 1 month even with the use of antibiotics. Rarely, patients who receive inadequate antibiotic treatment for early Lyme disease may remain seronegative. False-positive tests are far more frequent than false-negatives, especially among patients whose pretest probability of having the disorder is low. Repetitive testing of an individual when initial acute and convalescent serologies were negative should be avoided, as this increases the risk of obtaining a false-positive result. A history of previous vaccination for Lyme disease, including participation in

Table 48–2. Criteria for Western Blot Interpretation in the Serologic Confirmation of Lyme Disease

Isotype Tested	Criteria for Positive Test
IgM	Two of the following three bands are present: 23 kDa (OspC), 39 kDa (BmpA), and 41 kDa (Fla)
IgG	Five out of 10 bands are present: 18 kDA, 21 kDa, 28 kDa, 39 kDa, 41 kDa, 45 kDa, 58 kDa (not GroEL), 66 kDa, and 93 kDa

(From Centers for Disease Control and Prevention. Recommendations for Test Performance and Interpretation from the Second National Conference on Serologic Diagnosis of Lyme Disease. *MMWR.* 1995;44:590. With permission.)

vaccine trials, should be obtained from patients prior to testing because standard Lyme ELISA and immunoblot tests may be positive in such individuals. Some laboratories offer modified Lyme ELISA and immunoblot tests that have eliminated the vaccine antigen, OspA, from the assays so that infection-induced antibodies can be distinguished from those related to vaccination.

In patients with suspected neuroborreliosis, *B burgdorferi*–specific antibody testing of paired serum and CSF samples can demonstrate the production of intrathecal antibodies. If present, intrathecal *B burgdorferi*–specific antibody production is highly suggestive of central nervous system involvement in Lyme disease.

A peptide-based ELISA has been developed that measures antibodies to a conserved region (C6) of the VlsE protein of *B burgdorferi*. The C6 peptide ELISA has a high specificity (99%) and sensitivity (ranging from 74% in acute Lyme disease to 100% in late Lyme disease), and can be used to distinguish infection-induced antibodies in patients who have received Lyme vaccination. Recent studies suggest that the combination of Lyme ELISA (IgM and IgG) and C6 peptide ELISA may be superior to the currently recommended two-tiered approach, particularly in early infection.

Once present, antibodies to *B burgdorferi* can persist indefinitely and serologic titers should not be used to assess efficacy of antibiotic therapy. In this regard, it should be emphasized that serologic tests at best confirm exposure to the pathogen at some time in the past and are not by themselves indicative of active infection with *B burgdorferi*.

3. DNA tests—The polymerase chain reaction has widespread use in the diagnosis of many infectious diseases, especially for pathogens that are difficult to culture or when rapid diagnosis is critical for management. This technique has been used to detect *B burgdorferi* DNA in synovial fluid and CSF specimens from patients with Lyme disease with variable success. Up to 85% of synovial fluid samples may test positive whereas fewer than 40% of CSF samples from patients with Lyme meningitis yield positive results. The lower sensitivity is believed to be due in part to the preference of spirochetes for connective tissue rather than body fluids.

4. Other laboratory tests—A Lyme urine antigen test has been purported to detect *B burgdorferi* proteins in the urine of patients with chronic symptoms after Lyme disease, and some physicians have used this test to monitor response to treatment. This test, however, has been discredited because of its inconsistent results and marked inter-laboratory variability. Currently there is no *B burgdorferi*–specific test that can be used to monitor efficacy of treatment.

5. Imaging studies—Radiographic studies have limited use in establishing the diagnosis of Lyme disease and serve primarily to eliminate other diagnoses. Plain radiographs of inflamed joints may be normal or show only soft-tissue swelling and effusion. In contrast to septic arthritis due to other bacterial pathogens in which radiographic evidence of infection can be present early, overt changes with periarticular osteoporosis, cartilage loss, and bony erosions are relatively late findings in Lyme arthritis.

Magnetic resonance imaging scans of the brains of patients with central nervous system Lyme disease are generally normal, but 25% of patients with encephalopathy will have white matter lesions that may or may not enhance with gadolinium. The majority of patients with Lyme encephalopathy have multifocal abnormalities in cerebral blood flow on single photon emission computed tomography scans. These findings are not specific for Lyme encephalopathy, however, and can be seen in normal individuals. Abnormalities on these scans alone should not be used as evidence of Lyme disease in the absence of suggestive clinical history and supportive serologic tests.

6. Special tests—Specialized tests for Lyme disease are primarily used to evaluate the extent of cardiac and nervous system involvement. The electrocardiogram can show evidence of conduction system disease (especially varying degrees of atrioventricular block and escape rhythms) or less commonly, more diffuse myocardial involvement with changes consistent with myocardial dysfunction and pericarditis. Electrophysiologic studies reveal a predilection for the atrioventricular node, but any part of the conduction system can be affected.

Patients with radicular symptoms should have nerve conduction testing and electromyography to document changes consistent with axonal polyradiculopathy. For patients with cognitive complaints, neuropsychologic tests are useful to evaluate for depression and to provide objective evidence of memory loss.

Differential Diagnosis

Lyme disease has been called "the new great mimicker" because its protean manifestations resemble those of other diseases. This label is misleading, however, because Lyme disease typically follows a characteristic presentation and clinical course. Accurate diagnosis requires that the patient have an appropriate clinical history and a reasonable risk of exposure to *B burgdorferi*–infected ticks. The hallmark skin lesion EM is a diagnostic criterion for early Lyme disease, but other more common skin disorders can be mistaken for EM (Table 48–3). The seasonal occurrence of EM in late spring and summer months, the size and number of lesions, and the paucity of associated cutaneous symptoms such as itch or pain are useful distinguishing features. Recently, an EM-like rash has been associated with the bite of the soft-shelled tick *Amblyomma americanum* (also known as the Lone Star tick), which

is prevalent in the southeast and south central United States. The etiology of *Southern tick-associated rash illness* (STARI) is unclear, but the disease appears to be localized to the skin. A noncultivatable spirochete named *Borrelia lonestari* has been found in *A americanum*, but individuals with STARI do not develop positive Lyme serology as would be expected with infection with a *B burgdorferi*–related spirochete, and the organism has not been found in skin biopsies of STARI skin lesions.

Although early Lyme disease can less commonly present as a summer flulike illness, headache, myalgia, and arthralgia are nonspecific symptoms of a variety of viral pathogens. The presence of upper respiratory symptoms or gastrointestinal complaints is unusual in Lyme disease. Patients with fibromyalgia and chronic fatigue syndrome often have debilitating fatigue and musculoskeletal complaints in the absence of objective findings or laboratory abnormalities. These syndromes are more insidious in onset than Lyme disease and patients may be symptomatic for many months or years before diagnosis. History of a sleep disturbance and the presence of trigger points on physical examination should suggest a diagnosis of fibromyalgia. Acute Lyme arthritis can mimic other causes of monarticular or pauciarticular arthritis, including reactive arthritis and other seronegative spondyloarthropathies, juvenile rheumatoid arthritis, and systemic lupus erythematosus. Low back pain and spine involvement is commonly seen in the seronegative spondyloarthropathies but is rare in patients with Lyme disease. Lyme arthritis patients generally have strong antibody responses to *B burgdorferi* and negative tests for rheumatoid factor and antinuclear antibodies. Presence of high-titer rheumatoid factor and antinuclear antibodies can lead to false-positive ELISA tests for *B burgdorferi*, emphasizing the need to confirm ELISA results by immunoblot analysis. Other causes of acute monarthritis such as septic arthritis and crystal-induced disease can usually be distinguished by the severity of pain and by examination of joint fluid for infectious microorganisms and crystals.

Even in areas endemic for Lyme disease, isolated facial palsy is more often found to be idiopathic in origin than due to *B burgdorferi* infection. Only a few conditions are common causes of bilateral facial palsy—Guillain-Barré syndrome, HIV infection, sarcoidosis, and other causes of chronic meningitis—and these are readily distinguished from Lyme disease. Acute meningitis due to *B burgdorferi* infection resembles viral meningitis, but most patients at this stage should have positive serologic tests for Lyme disease. The radiculoneuropathy of Lyme disease must be distinguished from neuropathy associated with disc disease or diabetes, or other infections such as herpes zoster. Chronic encephalopathy can be confused with multiple sclerosis when the magnetic resonance imaging scan of the brain shows evidence

Table 48–3. Differential Diagnosis of Erythema Migrans

Differential Diagnosis	Seasonal Occurrence	Associated Symptoms	Location	Size	Evolution	Morphology
Erythema migrans	Yes	Mild systemic symptoms Paucity of pain or itch	Skin folds, central	Large	2–3 cm per day	See text
Tinea corporis	No	Itch	Variable	Variable	Slow progression	Ringlike; may have satellite lesion; scaling much more common
Cellulitis	No	Systemic symptoms Painful	Typically acral	Variable but rarely large except on legs	Grows more in typical cases	Usually a homogeneous erythema; tender to touch
Hypersentivity to insect or tick bite	Yes	No	Variable	Small	Variable	Can be uniform erythema, often with tick still attached
Contact dermatitis	No	Itchy	Variable	Variable	Slow progression	Often linear (rhus) or in an area that suggests the diagnosis
Spider bite	Yes	Painful bite	Acral	Variable	Can develop dependent edema but spreads centrifugally	Often necrotic with eschar
Urticaria	No	Itch	Variable	Individual lesions vary	Individual lesions wax and wane over hours	Raised, multiple, often serpiginous around edges
Pityriasis rosea	More in spring and fall	Mild to moderate itch	Diffuse; usually not on face	Herald patch may be confused with erythema migrans	Tends to stay same day to day when it is expressed	Oval lesions, slightly scaly, with long axis oriented with skin cleavage lines
Fixed drug eruption	No	Variable, but often a burning sensation; recent drug ingestion	Fixed, often in genitals, hands, feet, and face	Variable	Tends to stay fixed	Plaque with deep violaceous hue and well-demarcated borders
Granuloma annulare	No	No	Acral	Several centimeters	Fixed over weeks to months	Tend to spread peripherally; can have central clearing
Erythema multiforme	No	Variable (may be associated with viral syndrome or medication)	Usually diffuse; often palms, soles, mucosa	Most lesions small without a single large one	Slow enlargement or stagnant over days	Target lesion is classic, but these lesions are usually much smaller than erythema migrans; often there is an obvious precipitant

(From Edlow JA. Erythema migrans. *Med Clin North Am.* 2002;86:252. With permission.)

of white matter disease. Oligoclonal bands are generally not found in CSF of patients with Lyme disease, and multiple sclerosis patients have negative serologic tests for Lyme disease. Subtle neurocognitive deficits due to chronic fatigue syndrome, fibromyalgia, or aging are often incorrectly attributed to chronic Lyme encephalopathy. As for any chronic encephalopathy, toxic-metabolic causes should be excluded.

Cardiac manifestations of Lyme disease can resemble those of acute rheumatic fever, except that valvular heart disease is absent. Coronary atherosclerotic disease, structural defects within the heart, and certain medications (especially β-blockers, calcium channel blockers, and digoxin) can lead to conduction system abnormalities characteristic of Lyme carditis. When patients have myocardial dysfunction, other infectious causes should be considered, such as infection with coxsackievirus A and B, echovirus, *Yersinia enterocolitica,* and *Rickettsia rickettsii,* the agent of Rocky Mountain spotted fever.

Treatment

Practice guidelines for the treatment of Lyme disease have been established by the Infectious Disease Society of America (Tables 48–4 and 48–5). Because many of the manifestations of Lyme disease can resolve without specific therapy, the goal of antibiotic treatment is to hasten resolution of signs and symptoms and to prevent later clinical manifestations due to ongoing infection. This is particularly true for facial palsy, in which the rate of recovery is the same as for untreated patients, and for cardiac involvement. Patients with localized or early disseminated disease without neurologic involvement or third-degree atrioventricular block can be treated with oral antibiotics. Although the ideal duration of antibiotics has not been firmly established, administration of oral doxycycline or amoxicillin for 14–28 days is effective therapy for erythema migrans, isolated facial palsy, first- or second-degree heart block, and acute arthritis. For isolated EM, a 10- to 21-day course of doxycycline may be sufficient. Doxycycline has the advantage of also being effective against *Anaplasma phagocytophila* (see below). Parenteral antibiotics should be reserved for patients with other forms of neurologic involvement (central or peripheral), recurrent arthritis after oral antibiotic therapy, or third-degree heart block. This latter group of patients should be hospitalized and monitored by telemetry for the need for temporary pacemaker placement. The rationale for intravenous therapy for high-degree heart block is that intense and/or prolonged inflammation may lead to irreversible cardiac damage. However, no study has directly addressed whether parenteral therapy is more effective than oral therapy in this setting, or whether other means for suppressing inflammation provide added benefit. In this regard, the use of corticosteroids to limit car-

Table 48–4. Recommended Antimicrobial Regimens for Treatment of Patients with Lyme Disease

Recommendation, Drug	Dosage for Adults	Dosage for Children
Preferred oral		
Amoxicillin	500 mg 3 times a day	50 mg/kg/d divided into 3 doses (maximum, 500 mg/dose)
Doxycycline	100 mg twice daily[a]	Age <8 y: not recommended; age >8 y: 1–2 mg/kg bid (maximum, 100 mg/dose)
Alternative oral		
Cefuroxime axetil	500 mg twice daily	30 mg/kg/d divided into 2 doses (maximum, 500 mg/dose)
Preferred parenteral		
Ceftriaxone	2 g IV once daily	75–100 mg/kg IV per day in a single dose (maximum, 2 g)
Alternative parenteral		
Cefotaxime	2 g IV 3 times a day	150–200 mg/kg/d IV divided into 3 or 4 doses (maximum, 6 g/d)
Penicillin G	18–24 million units IV/d divided into doses given every 4 hours[b]	200,000–400,000 units/kg/d, divided into doses given every 4 hours (maximum, 18–24 million units/d)

[a]Tetracyclines are relatively contraindicated for pregnant or lactating women.
[b]The penicillin dosage should be reduced for patients with impaired renal function.
(From Wormser GP, Nadelman RB, Dattwyler RJ, et al. Practice guidelines for the treatment of Lyme disease: The Infectious Disease Society of America. *Clin Infect Dis.* 2000;31 (Suppl 1): 1. With permission.)

diac inflammation may be considered for patients with severe disease who do not respond rapidly to antibiotic therapy.

Pregnant patients and children <8 years of age can be treated in similar fashion to adult patients except that tetracyclines should be avoided.

A puzzling feature of Lyme disease is that patients may experience a delay in resolution of symptoms after antibiotic treatment. This is particularly true for disseminated disease with neurologic abnormalities or arthritis, which may take several months to resolve. For patients with persistent arthritis, a second course of oral antibiotics (generally of 4 weeks' duration) or a single 2- to

Table 48–5. Recommended Therapy for Patients with Lyme Disease

Indication	Treatment	Duration, d
Tick bite	None recommended; observe	
Erythema migrans	Oral regimen[a,b]	14–21
Acute neurologic disease		
Meningitis or radiculopathy	Parental regimen[a,c]	14–28
Cranial-nerve palsy	Oral regimen[a]	14–21
Cardiac disease		
First- or second-degree heart block	Oral regimen[a]	14–21
Third-degree heart block	Parenteral regimen[a,d]	14–21
Late disease		
Arthritis without neurologic disease	Oral regimen[a]	28
Recurrent arthritis after oral regimen	Oral regimen[b] or	28
	parenteral regimen[a]	14–28
Persistent arthritis after two courses of antibiotics	Symptomatic therapy	
Central or peripheral nervous system disease	Parenteral regimen[a]	14–28
Chronic Lyme disease or post-Lyme disease syndrome	Symptomatic therapy[e]	

[a]See Table 48–4.

[b]For adult patients who are intolerant of amoxicillin, doxycycline, and cefuroxime axetil, alternatives are azithromycin (500 mg orally daily for 7–10 days), erythromycin (500 mg orally 4 times per day for 14–21 days), or clarithromycin (500 mg orally twice daily for 14–21 days [except during pregnancy]). The recommended dosages of these agents for children are as follows: azithromycin, 10 mg/kg daily (maximum, 500 mg/d), erythromycin, 12.5 mg/kg 4 times daily (maximum, 500 mg/dose); clarithromycin, 7.5 mg/kg twice daily (maximum, 500 mg/dose). Patients treated with macrolides should be closely followed.

[c]For nonpregnant adult patients intolerant of both penicillin and cephalosporins, doxycycline (200–400 mg/d orally [or IV if oral medications cannot be taken], divided into two doses) may be adequate.

[d]A temporary pacemaker may be required.

[e]See the discussion of chronic lyme disease or post–lyme disease syndrome in the text.

(From Wormser GP, Nadelman RB, Dattwyler RJ, et al. Practice guidelines for the treatment of Lyme disease: The Infectious Disease Society of America. *Clin Infect Dis.* 2000;31 (Suppl 1):1. With permission.)

4-week course of parenteral therapy is reasonable after several months of observation. Repeat treatment is not recommended for chronic neurologic abnormalities unless objective signs of relapse are present.

Complications

Ixodes ticks can carry multiple pathogens simultaneously, some of which are also infectious to humans. These include *Babesia microti,* a protozoan, and *Anaplasma phagocytophila* (formerly *Ehrlichia phagocytophila*), the agent of human granulocytic ehrlichiosis. *B microti* infection presents as a malarialike illness with fever, drenching sweats, and severe constitutional symptoms, especially myalgias, along with hemolytic anemia. Examining the peripheral blood smear for the characteristic ringlike organisms within red blood cells can make the diagnosis. *A phagocytophila* infects granulocytes and leads to leukopenia and thrombocytopenia. The presence of morulae within granulocytes can establish a diagnosis, but polymerase chain reaction of peripheral blood for *A phagocytophila* DNA or antibody testing is more sensitive. Co-infection with these agents should be suspected in Lyme disease patients from endemic areas who present with

severe constitutional symptoms and hematologic abnormalities. In one study of patients with *B microti* infection, 20% also tested positive by serology for exposure to *B burgdorferi*. Co-infection can increase the morbidity associated with Lyme disease; a fatality associated with Lyme carditis was reported in a patient with concomitant *Babesia* infection.

Maternal-fetal transmission of *B burgdorferi* has been reported, but earlier concerns that Lyme disease can cause congenital abnormalities appear unwarranted. Several prospective studies have failed to document an increased prevalence in adverse fetal outcomes (spontaneous abortion, premature delivery, or congenital abnormalities) among pregnant women who were treated with standard therapy for Lyme disease.

Adverse reactions from antibiotic use occur at a frequency comparable to that seen in other infectious diseases. Cholestasis has been reported with intravenous ceftriaxone therapy, so its use should be limited to patients with disseminated disease as described above. About 15% of patients with Lyme disease may experience a Jarisch-Herxheimer reaction (see section on pathogenesis, above) within 24–48 hours of initiation of antibiotic therapy for Lyme disease. This condition is self-limited;

supportive care with reassurance and nonsteroidal anti-inflammatory agents helps to relieve symptoms.

Prognosis

Overall, the majority of patients with Lyme disease respond to antibiotic therapy with little in the way of adverse sequelae. Complete resolution of clinical signs and symptoms may take several months, however, especially in individuals with arthritis or nervous system involvement. In some cases permanent damage may result in residual deficits that do not improve with antibiotic therapy. A small percentage of patients, especially those with HLA-DRB1*0401 or *0101 genotype and/or OspA antibodies, may develop a chronic arthritis unresponsive to antibiotic therapy. These patients are believed to be genetically predisposed to an autoimmune arthritis triggered by the immune response to *B burgdorferi* infection. As for other forms of chronic arthritis, treatment regimens directed toward suppression of the inflammatory response are effective. Arthroscopic synovectomy can achieve clinical remission in 80% of patients.

Patients who receive recommended treatment for Lyme disease can have persistent subjective complaints such as fatigue, memory loss, myalgias, and arthralgias. In such cases, evaluation to exclude entities other than persistent *B burgdorferi* infection should be considered. Rarely, co-infection with *B microti* or *A phagocytophila* may explain unresolved symptoms of patients who acquired Lyme disease from areas in which ticks harbor multiple pathogens. More commonly, fibromyalgia can be seen as a consequence of Lyme disease. A clinical trial evaluating the efficacy of extended courses of antibiotics for patients with chronic unexplained symptoms after standard treatment for Lyme disease failed to show benefit over placebo. Alternative therapeutic approaches should be considered.

REFERENCES

Aguero-Rosenfeld ME, Wang G, Schwartz I, Wormser GP. Diagnosis of Lyme borreliosis. *Clin Microbiol Rev.* 2005;18:484. (Comprehensive review of laboratory tests for Lyme disease and interpretation of ELISA and immunoblot analyses.)

Haass, A. Lyme neuroborreliosis. *Curr Opin Neurol.* 1998;11:253. [PMID: 9642545] (Excellent discussion of the neurologic manifestations of Lyme disease, with a comparison of Lyme disease in Europe versus the United States.)

Klempner MS, Hu LT, Evans J, et al. Two controlled trials of antibiotic treatment in patients with persistent symptoms and a history of Lyme disease. *N Engl J Med.* 2001;345:85. [PMID: 11450676] (Results of the NIH-sponsored multicenter, randomized, placebo-controlled trial of extended antibiotic treatment [IV and oral] for chronic symptoms after Lyme disease. The study was terminated early because of lack of efficacy based on interim analysis of the first 64 patients who received antibiotics versus 65 patients who received placebo.)

Medical Letter. Treatment of Lyme disease. *Med Lett Drugs Ther.* 2005;47:41. [PMID: 15912123] (Most recent update on the treatment of Lyme disease and post-Lyme syndromes.)

Mogilyansky E, Loa CC, Adelson ME, Mordechai E, Tilton RC. Comparison of Western immunoblotting and the C6 Lyme antibody test for laboratory detection of Lyme disease. *Clin Diagn Lab Immunol.* 2004;11:924. [PMID: 15358654] (Provides evidence that the C6 ELISA compares favorably to standard immunoblot tests in the diagnosis of Lyme disease.)

Shapiro ED, Gerber MA. Lyme disease. *Clin Infect Dis.* 2000;31:533. [PMID: 10987718] (Review of Lyme disease along with prevention strategies and recommended treatment regimens.)

Steere AC, Coburn J, Glickstein L. The emergence of Lyme disease. *J Clin Invest.* 2004;113:1093. [PMID: 15085185] (Recent update of the biology of *Borrelia burgdorferi*, clinical manifestations of disease, and pathogenesis. Contains useful algorithms for the diagnosis and treatment of all stages of Lyme disease.)

Wormser GP, Nadelman RB, Dattwyler RJ, et al. Practice guidelines for the treatment of Lyme disease. *Clin Infect Dis.* 2000;31(Suppl 1):1. [PMID: 10982743] (Guidelines from the Infectious Disease Society of America on the treatment of all stages of Lyme disease in adults, children, and pregnant patients. Includes rationale behind recommendations based on quality of evidence and cost considerations.)

Relevant World-Wide Web Sites

[The American Lyme Disease Foundation]
http://www.aldf.com

[American College of Physicians Initiative on Lyme Disease]
http://www.acponline.org/lyme/

[MedlinePlus: Lyme Disease]
http://www.nlm.nih.gov/medlineplus/lymedisease.html

[Centers for Disease Control and Prevention: Lyme disease]
http://www.cdc.gov/ncidod/dvbid/lyme/index.htm

[Centers for Disease Control and Prevention: Southern Tick-Associated Rash Illness]
http://www.cdc.gov/ncidod/dvbid/stari/index.htm

[Centers for Disease Control and Prevention: Caution Regarding Testing for Lyme disease]
http://www.cdc.gov/mmwr/preview/mmwrhtml/mm5405a6.htm

Mycobacterial & Fungal Infections of Bone & Joints

49

Henry F. Chambers, MD, & John B. Imboden, MD

■ INFECTIONS WITH *MYCOBACTERIUM TUBERCULOSIS*

Musculoskeletal infection with *Mycobacterium tuberculosis* accounts for 1–5% of cases of tuberculosis (TB) and can produce spondylitis (Pott disease), arthritis, osteomyelitis, tenosynovitis, bursitis, and pyomyositis. In developing countries, where the prevalence of TB is high, musculoskeletal TB remains an important source of morbidity and mortality, particularly among children. In the developed world, musculoskeletal TB is uncommon and largely affects adults. Immigrants from countries where TB is prevalent account for a substantial proportion of musculoskeletal TB in the United States and Europe. Musculoskeletal infection has been reported in HIV-infected persons and in patients whose TB reactivated in the setting of anti–tumor necrosis factor therapy. Tuberculosis is a reportable disease and suspected or proven cases should be reported to local public health authorities.

SPINAL TUBERCULOSIS (POTT DISEASE)

ESSENTIALS OF DIAGNOSIS

- *Back pain.*
- *Radiographic evidence of spondylitis or spondylodiscitis.*
- *Identification of M tuberculosis in aspirates or biopsy specimens of skeletal lesions.*

General Considerations

Tuberculosis of the spine accounts for approximately 50% of musculoskeletal TB. The thoracic and lumbar vertebrae are most often affected; the cervical spine is involved in fewer than 10% of cases. Organisms reach the vertebrae either by hematogenous spread (at the time of initial infection or during reactivation) or through lymphatic spread from renal, pleural, or other foci of disease. Most patients do not have active TB at sites outside the skeleton. Pulmonary TB, which is the most common form of concomitant extraskeletal disease, occurs in fewer than 20% of cases.

Infection usually begins within the body of a vertebra and then extends to involve adjacent vertebrae and discs; however, "skipping" to noncontiguous vertebrae sometimes occurs. Soft tissue involvement is common, and paravertebral cold abscesses develop in about 75% of cases. Isolated involvement of the posterior elements is unusual (5% in one large series).

Clinical Findings

A. SYMPTOMS AND SIGNS

The most common presenting complaint is pain localized to the spine. The pain typically is not relieved by rest and may be present for months or longer before the patient seeks medical attention. In contrast to pulmonary TB, constitutional symptoms (weight loss, fever, and night sweats) occur in only 50% of cases.

Radicular pain is common. Approximately 50% of patients have lower extremity weakness at presentation; these figures are higher in case series from the developing world. Compression of either the cauda equina or the spinal cord by an inflammatory mass or abscess is the leading cause of neurologic compromise. Meningitis and meningomyelitis are less common. Severe spinal instability can lead to compression or ischemia of the cord.

Destruction of the anterior vertebral body can result in severe angular kyphosis, the gibbus deformity of Pott disease. Paravertebral cold abscesses can track from the lumbar vertebrae along the psoas muscle and present as inguinal masses or can extend from the thoracic spine into the pleural space. Fistulae occur in a small number of patients. In a small percentage of cases, bone can become superinfected with pyogenic organisms.

B. LABORATORY FINDINGS

Routine laboratory investigations are of little diagnostic help. Patients may or may not manifest a peripheral leukocytosis. There usually is a moderate elevation in the erythrocyte sedimentation rate, but in 10% of cases it is <20 mm/h.

C. IMAGING STUDIES

Plain radiographs can be normal early in the course of disease but then demonstrate evidence of spondylitis including osteolysis, a combination of lytic and sclerotic lesions, and bony destruction that classically is confined to the vertebral body. Although initially there may be relative preservation of the intervertebral disc, disc narrowing is common later in the disease course. Computed tomography and magnetic resonance imaging reveal changes earlier than plain radiography, provide greater detail of the extent of bony involvement, and can reveal paraspinal abscesses not suspected on clinical grounds. Magnetic resonance imaging permits prompt detection of compression of the spinal cord or cauda equina and is the preferred imaging technique in cases with signs or symptoms of neurologic compromise.

D. SPECIAL TESTS

Most patients (75–90%) have a positive reaction to purified protein derivative. Cultures of material obtained by percutaneous needle aspiration of paraspinal abscesses, percutaneous needle biopsy of spinal lesions, and open surgical biopsy are positive for *M tuberculosis* in 70–90% of reported cases. Smears of biopsy material reveal acid-fast bacilli in a lower percentage (20–25%) than do smears of aspirates of paraspinal abscesses (60%). Biopsies reveal characteristic caseating granulomas in 70%. These percentages on the yields of culture, staining, and histopathology may be inflated by the relatively strict case definitions of the studies. The bacillary burden in spinal TB is low, and some writers with extensive clinical experience in endemic areas estimate that the false-negative rates of aspirates and biopsies approach 50%. Nucleic acid amplification tests may facilitate earlier diagnosis but have only been studied in small numbers of patients with spinal TB, and these tests are not FDA-approved for diagnosis of extrapulmonary tuberculosis. In patients with extraspinal disease suggestive of tuberculosis, identification of *M tuberculosis* at another site is sufficient to establish the diagnosis of spinal TB.

Differential Diagnosis

Pyogenic or fungal osteomyelitis or neoplasm can cause disease that is clinically indistinguishable from tuberculous spondylitis. Pyogenic vertebral osteomyelitis generally has a more acute presentation and is more often associated with fever and clinical toxicity than spinal TB. Blood cultures are positive for *Staphylococcus aureus,* streptococci, or enteric gram-negative organisms in approximately 50% of cases of pyogenic vertebral osteomyelitis, but in up to 25% of cases, routine bone and blood cultures will not yield an organism. Imaging studies cannot reliably differentiate pyogenic and tuberculous spondylitis. Noncaseating granulomas, which occasionally are the only histologic evidence of spinal TB, can be seen on biopsy specimens of vertebral osteomyelitis due to *Brucella* or fungi (either of which can mimic spinal TB clinically). Certain imaging features, such as the presence of paravertebral abscesses, can help distinguish spinal TB from neoplastic disease, but these are not always present.

Treatment

Antimicrobial therapy is the cornerstone of treatment for spinal TB. Unless there is strong suspicion of resistance to first-line drugs, most authorities recommend a 6- to 9-month total course of therapy with isoniazid, rifampin, pyrazinamide, and ethambutol for 2 months, followed by isoniazid and rifampin for 4–7 months.

When cultures and histopathologic studies fail to yield a definitive diagnosis, empiric therapy for tuberculosis should be considered, especially in foreign-born individuals from areas where *M tuberculosis* is endemic, those with evidence of past tuberculosis, or tuberculin skin test–positive individuals.

The role for surgical intervention is controversial. Uncomplicated cases generally respond well to antituberculous therapy alone. A randomized trial conducted by the Medical Research Council found no additional benefit of surgery over medical therapy alone, but critics of these studies point out that there was a trend toward greater spinal instability in the medically-treated groups and that patients with extensive disease were excluded. Surgery is indicated for patients with persistent neurologic deficits and spinal cord compression, with severe spinal instability, or with ongoing infection despite appropriate antibacterial therapy. A neurosurgeon or orthopedist should evaluate all patients with signs or symptoms of neurologic compromise or with spinal instability or deformity.

Complications

Complications of spinal TB include destruction of vertebral bodies and discs with consequent spinal deformities and instability; paraparesis or paraplegia; and tracking of paravertebral cold abscesses to distant sites in the chest, abdomen, groin, and neck.

TUBERCULOUS ARTHRITIS

ESSENTIALS OF DIAGNOSIS

- *Usually monarticular with predilection for the hip or knee.*
- *Periarticular abscesses and sinus tracts in late stages of disease.*
- *Culture of M tuberculosis from synovial fluid or biopsy.*
- *Demonstration of caseating granulomas on synovial biopsy.*

General Considerations

Tuberculous arthritis is the second most common form of musculoskeletal TB. Tuberculous arthritis is seen mostly in children and young adults who live in developing countries. In nonendemic regions, tuberculous arthritis tends to affect older persons. The hip is most often involved, followed by the knee. Any joint may be infected, however, and infection of non–weight-bearing joints and the sacroiliac joints were prominent in a recent European series. The great majority of cases (85%) of tuberculous arthritis are monarticular; oligoarticular TB is an uncommon but well-recognized condition.

Tuberculous arthritis usually develops from adjacent TB osteomyelitis but also can be initiated by hematogenous spread directly to the synovium. Because *M tuberculosis* does not produce collagenases, joint destruction is more insidious than in septic arthritis due to pyogenic organisms.

Clinical Findings

A. SYMPTOMS AND SIGNS

The classic presentation is that of a monarthritis with pain, stiffness, and gradual loss of function over weeks to months. Some patients seek medical attention after years of symptoms. Approximately 15%, however, have an acute presentation that mimics septic arthritis or microcrystalline disease.

Constitutional symptoms such as fever, night sweats, and weight loss are present in only 50% of patients. Most patients do not have active TB elsewhere, and the chest radiograph may be normal.

On examination there is swelling with or without warmth of the affected joint. Pain limits motion, par-

ticularly when the hip is involved. Cold abscesses and draining sinus tracts may be present in those with long-standing disease.

B. LABORATORY FINDINGS

A mild anemia is common. Peripheral leukocytosis is variable. Most patients have an elevated erythrocyte sedimentation rate.

C. IMAGING STUDIES

The classic radiographic changes of tuberculous arthritis are juxta-articular osteopenia, bony erosions at the periphery of the joint, and gradual narrowing of the joint space (Phemister triad). Computed tomography and magnetic resonance imaging detect changes earlier than plain radiography and can better visualize the extent of bony destruction. Magnetic resonance imaging is superior to computed tomography for the detection of para-articular abscesses, sinus tract formation, and other soft tissue abnormalities.

D. SPECIAL TESTS

The great majority (>90%) of patients have a positive reaction to purified protein derivative, but false-negative tests can occur in immunocompromised patients. Synovial fluid analysis reveals inflammatory fluid; cell counts vary but usually are in the range of 10,000–20,000 cells/mm^3 with a predominance of neutrophils. Smears of synovial fluid reveal acid-fast bacilli in only 20% of cases, but 80% of cultures of synovial fluid grow *M tuberculosis*. Synovial biopsies yield positive cultures (>90%) and compatible histopathology (>90%) and are the test of choice when there is clinical suspicion of tuberculous arthritis and smears of synovial fluid are unrevealing. The sensitivity and specificity of nucleic acid amplification tests are not yet known for tuberculous arthritis.

Differential Diagnosis

Infection with *M tuberculosis* should be suspected in any patient with an unexplained, chronic inflammatory monarthritis. Fungal infections and nontuberculous mycobacterial infections can have a similarly indolent course. The chronic nature of the infection may cause confusion with the spondyloarthropathies, particularly when there is sacroiliac joint involvement or in the unusual patient with oligoarticular involvement. Conversely, acute presentations of tuberculous arthritis can lead to a misdiagnosis of septic arthritis or crystal-induced arthritis. Noncaseating granulomas can be observed in synovial biopsy specimens from patients with sarcoidosis, Crohn disease, foreign body reactions, gout (rarely), brucellosis, and infections due to fungi or atypical mycobacteria.

Treatment

Antimicrobial therapy is the primary treatment. Six- to nine-month total regimens of isoniazid, rifampin, pyrazinamide, and ethambutol for 2 months, followed by isoniazid and rifampin for 4–7 months are recommended for tuberculosis of bones and joints (see the American Thoracic Society web site listed in the references for treatment details). Drainage or joint lavage is necessary if there is thick purulent material in the joint. Occasionally, surgical intervention is required for débridement of extensive foci of osseous infection or for drainage of cold abscesses. Arthroplasty has been successful for patients with joint destruction.

Complications

Untreated infection leads to pannus formation that erodes cartilage and subchondral bone, eventually destroying the joint. Para-articular cold abscesses and draining sinus tracts develop in long-standing disease; the latter can be superinfected with pyogenic organisms.

OTHER FORMS OF MUSCULOSKELETAL TUBERCULOSIS

Spinal TB and tuberculous arthritis account for the great majority of cases of musculoskeletal TB. Although TB can cause tenosynovitis of the hand and wrist, olecranon bursitis, and trochanteric bursitis, infections of tenosynovium and bursae are more common with nontuberculous mycobacterial species than with *M tuberculosis*. Tuberculous osteomyelitis of the phalanges can produce dactylitis, particularly in children. Poncet disease is a polyarthritis seen with extra-articular TB. The failure to isolate *M tuberculosis* from involved joints led to the concept that Poncet disease is a reactive arthritis, but this hypothesis has been questioned. Primary tuberculous myositis is rare and typically affects the psoas muscle. Muscle also can be infected secondarily by sites in joints or bone.

NONTUBERCULOUS MYCOBACTERIA

Nontuberculous mycobacteria can cause bursitis, tenosynovitis, arthritis, and osteomyelitis. The disease is chronic, slowly progressive and indolent with a presentation that is similar to that of tuberculosis except that typically there is a history of surgery, a wound, an injection, or other local trauma leading to direct inoculation of the organism with subsequent infection. Bone or joint infection as a result of hematogenous dissemination is rare except in HIV-infected patients or other immunocompromised individuals. While virtually any nontuberculous mycobacterial species can cause bone or joint infection, *Mycobacterium marinum* and *M avium* complex are most frequent. Rapid growers (*M abscessus*, *M chelonae*, and *M fortuitum*) more typically cause cutaneous infection, which rarely can extend to contiguous bone or joint.

Treatment

Infections caused by nontuberculous mycobacteria respond very slowly, and often poorly, to antimicrobial therapy. Chemotherapy and surgical excision or drainage are often used in combination. Because susceptibilities, and therefore drugs of choice, vary from species to species, establishing a microbiologic diagnosis and susceptibility testing are essential for proper management. Clarithromycin is a particularly useful agent for *M avium* infection as one component of a three-drug combination regimen that is administered for 6–12 months. Consultation with an individual experienced in the treatment of mycobacterial infections is recommended when designing a chemotherapeutic regimen.

■ FUNGAL INFECTIONS

Fungal infections of bones and joints are uncommon in the United States. Histoplasmosis, coccidioidomycosis, blastomycosis, and cryptococcosis are acquired through inhalation. The primary infection is usually asymptomatic but may be associated with transient arthralgias or arthritis, probably on the basis of a hypersensitivity reaction to the pulmonary infection. Osteomyelitis and joint infection are the sequelae of disseminated infection; the clinical presentation is usually that of an indolent process and may mimic skeletal TB. Diagnosis is based on histologic demonstration of organisms on biopsy specimens of affected synovium or bone or on smears and cultures of synovial fluid and biopsy material.

HISTOPLASMOSIS

Primary infection with *Histoplasma capsulatum,* a soil fungus endemic in the midwestern and southeastern United States, can produce a self-limited syndrome of erythema nodosum or erythema multiforme with polyarthralgias or polyarthritis. Disseminated disease is uncommon, and infection of bone and joints is rare. In contrast, African histoplasmosis, due to *H capsulatum* var *duboisii,* frequently leads to osteomyelitis.

COCCIDIOIDOMYCOSIS

Coccidioides immitis is endemic in the southwestern United States. Primary infection is usually asymptomatic, but in a minority of cases results in self-limited arthralgias or arthritis, often in association with erythema nodosum or erythema multiforme. Disseminated disease, which can occur in otherwise healthy persons, commonly produces osteomyelitis and arthritis, due either to direct seeding of synovium or to extension from adjacent infected bone. The clinical presentation can be very similar to that of tuberculosis.

BLASTOMYCOSIS

Blastomyces dermatitidis is endemic in the central and southeastern United States. Polyarthralgias may accompany the primary lung infection. Osteomyelitis develops in most patients with disseminated disease and can lead to cold abscesses and sinus tracts. Vertebral involvement can mimic spinal TB. Arthritis is uncommon and usually due to extension of infection from adjacent osteomyelitis.

CRYPTOCOCCOSIS

Cryptococcus neoformans is ubiquitous. Disseminated disease occurs in immunocompromised persons and leads to osteomyelitis, particularly of the vertebra, in 5–10%

of cases. Cryptococcal arthritis is rare. Documentation of cryptococcal antigenemia strongly suggests the diagnosis.

REFERENCES

Blumberg HM, Burman WJ, Chaisson RE, et al. American Thoracic Society/Centers for Disease Control and Prevention/Infectious Diseases Society of America: treatment of tuberculosis. *Am J Respir Crit Care Med.* 2003;167:603. [PMID: 12588714]

Diagnosis and treatment of disease caused by nontuberculous mycobacteria. *Am J Respir Crit Care Med.* 1997;156:S1. [PMID: 9279284]

Malaviya AN, Kotwal PP. Arthritis associated with tuberculosis. *Best Pract Res Clin Rheumatol.* 2003;17:319. [PMID: 12787528] (Detailed review of peripheral arthritis due to tuberculosis.)

McGill PE. Geographically specific infections and arthritis, including rheumatic syndromes associated with certain fungi and parasites, *Brucella* species and *Mycobacterium leprae. Best Pract Res Clin Rheumatol.* 2003;17:289. [PMID: 12787526]

Relevant World Wide Web Site

[American Thoracic Society TB Treatment Guidelines]

http://www.thoracic.org/sections/publications/statements/resources/tbchild1-16.pdf

Rheumatic Manifestations of Acute & Chronic Viral Arthritis

50

Dimitrios Vassilopoulos, MD

HEPATITIS C VIRUS

ESSENTIALS OF DIAGNOSIS

- *Diagnosis by positive anti–hepatitis C virus (HCV) antibody confirmed by a sensitive, qualitative HCV RNA assay.*
- *Arthralgias and rarely a nonerosive arthritis are seen in patients with chronic HCV infection, with or without associated cryoglobulinemia.*
- *Coexistent rheumatoid arthritis (RA) and HCV infection can create diagnostic and therapeutic problems.*

General Considerations

Chronic hepatitis C is second only to hepatitis B (see next section) as the most common chronic viral infection worldwide, with an estimated 170 million people infected. In the United States, chronic HCV infection affects 2.7 million people and represents the leading cause of liver transplantation and death from liver disease.

HCV, an RNA virus, is transmitted by the parenteral route. The most common causes of HCV transmission are injection drug use and transfusion of blood or blood-derived products before 1992. Infrequent modes of transmission include accidental exposures at work (eg, health care workers), sex, and childbirth. In a number of cases no identifiable risk factor can be found.

Fewer than 20% of patients with acute HCV infections are symptomatic at the time of infection. Most cases of HCV, however, are associated with transition to chronicity (55–85%). The natural history of chronic HCV infection is variable. Between 5% and 20% of chronically infected HCV patients develop cirrhosis within several decades. Among cirrhotic patients, within 10 years 30% develop end-stage liver disease and 10–20%

develop hepatocellular carcinoma. Factors associated with more rapid disease progression include older age, alcohol abuse, co-infection with the human immunodeficiency virus (see Chapter 51), and the presence of hepatic steatosis.

Chronic HCV infection is uniquely associated with a number of extrahepatic rheumatic manifestations including arthralgias, arthritis, sialadenitis (Sjögren-like), and cryoglobulinemic vasculitis.

Pathogenesis

HCV replicates predominantly in hepatocytes after entrance into the circulation. Following acute infection, HCV RNA can be detected in the serum within 1 week. Alanine aminotransferase elevation occurs 2–3 months later. Anti-HCV antibodies can be found 1–2 months after acute infection. Because acute HCV infection is not associated with rheumatic complaints (in contrast to acute hepatitis B), many patients do not know that they are infected.

Chronic HCV infection does not target only the liver, but has a profound effect on the immune system. One of the presumed receptors for HCV in hepatocytes, the CD81, is also expressed on B cells. Mono- and polyclonal B-cell expansions have been found in the liver and bone marrow of chronically infected patients. In approximately half of patients with chronic HCV infections, circulating cryoglobulins can be detected. However, only a minority of these patients (<5%) develop the syndrome of mixed cryoglobulinemia (see Chapter 37). Deposition of immune complexes containing cryoglobulins in different organs is the presumed disease mechanism in mixed cryoglobulinemia, characterized by purpura, arthralgias (or more rarely, arthritis), glomerulonephritis, and polyneuropathy.

Prevention

There is currently no vaccine available for HCV. Screening of blood products has almost eliminated the risk of posttransfusion hepatitis C. The persons at greatest risk for HCV now are injection drug users and persons with high-risk sexual behavior (multiple sexual partners).

Clinical Findings

Arthralgias are observed in approximately 20% of patients with chronic HCV infection and tend to be polyarticular. An inflammatory arthritis with oligo- or polyarticular involvement has been reported in HCV patients (between 2% and 5% of all patients), even in the absence of cryoglobulinemia. Although its pathogenesis remains uncertain, it appears to be related to the underlying infection. The arthritis associated with HCV infections is relatively benign, not leading to bone erosions or joint destruction over time. In the majority of cases (~80%), an RA-like polyarticular involvement of small joints is prominent. In 20% of patients, mono- or oligoarticular involvement of large joints is detected. Morning stiffness is present in two-thirds of patients.

Laboratory Findings

Diagnosis of HCV infection is made initially by the detection of anti-HCV antibodies by enzyme immunoassays. A positive test should be confirmed by a qualitative assay designed to detect serum HCV RNA (by polymerase chain reaction or branched-DNA assays).

Unselected patients with chronic HCV infection display a number of autoantibodies including rheumatoid factor (RF, 40–65%), cryoglobulins (40–55%), antinuclear antibodies (10%), and antithyroid antibodies (<10%). These findings can create a number of diagnostic problems in patients presenting with nonspecific arthralgias or inflammatory arthritis. Antibodies against cyclic citrullinated peptides (CCPs) are helpful in the differential diagnosis between RA and HCV-associated arthritis. It was shown that despite the frequent presence of RF, patients with HCV-associated articular symptoms or cryoglobulinemia were anti-CCP negative, in contrast to RA patients who were usually anti-CCP positive. In patients with HCV-associated mixed cryoglobulinemia, RF positivity (virtually 100%) and low C4 levels (50–85%) are characteristic laboratory findings.

Differential Diagnosis

Differentiating between RA, HCV-associated arthritis, and arthritis in the setting of HCV-associated mixed cryoglobulinemia can be a difficult task. The absence of erosive changes and anti-CCP antibodies are helpful in making this diagnosis. In certain cases, if antin-uclear antibodies are present, the differential diagnosis should be made from systemic lupus erythematosus. It should always be kept in mind that since chronic HCV infection is not uncommon in the general population (~2%), any rheumatic condition can coexist with HCV infection.

Treatment

The treatment of arthritis in the context of HCV infection is always a challenge. Patients with HCV-associated arthritis in the absence of cryoglobulinemia have been treated successfully with nonsteroidal anti-inflammatory drugs, hydroxychloroquine, and low-dose prednisone. Administration of antiviral treatment (interferon-α) has not been associated with significant improvement, and in certain cases has exacerbated the articular symptoms. In a small number of resistant cases, methotrexate was successfully used without significant adverse effects on liver function. Nevertheless, extreme caution with very close monitoring of liver function and viremia levels is needed for patients starting such therapy.

The treatment of RA in patients with coexisting HCV infection is also problematic. First-line disease-modifying drugs such as methotrexate and leflunomide are potentially hepatotoxic and should be used with extreme caution. In mild cases, hydroxychloroquine can be tried first with or without low-dose prednisone (<7.5 mg/d). Tumor necrosis factor-α inhibitors have also been used in patients with HCV infection without significant short-term side effects.

Prognosis

The prognosis of HCV-associated inflammatory arthritis is good. According to a recent study of a large population of patients with HCV-associated cryoglobulinemia, mild disease activity is seen in half of the patients, whereas one-third follow a moderate to severe course. Some patients with cryoglobulinemia can develop non-Hodgkin lymphomas.

Vassilopoulos D, Calabrese LH. Rheumatic manifestations of hepatitis C infection. *Curr Rheum Rep.* 2003;5:200. (A recent review of the most common rheumatic syndromes in patients with chronic HCV infection.)

Rosner I, Rozenbaum M, Toubi E, et al. The case for hepatitis C arthritis. *Semin Arthritis Rheum.* 2004;33:375. (An excellent literature review of HCV-associated arthritis.)

Strader DB, Wright T, Thomas DL, et al. Diagnosis, management and treatment of hepatitis C. *Hepatology.* 2004;39:1147. (The most recent guidelines for the diagnosis and treatment of hepatitis C.)

HEPATITIS B VIRUS

ESSENTIALS OF DIAGNOSIS

- *Symmetric, self-limited polyarthritis accompanied by rash developing during the pre-icteric phase of acute hepatitis B.*
- *Diagnosis by hepatitis B surface antigen and IgM anti–hepatitis B core antigen.*

General Considerations

Hepatitis B virus (HBV) infection is currently the most common chronic viral infection worldwide. It is estimated that 2 billion people have been exposed to the virus and 350 million are chronically infected. Every year 1 million people die from HBV-related complications, including end-stage liver disease and hepatocellular carcinoma.

HBV is an enveloped DNA virus that is transmitted parenterally, sexually, or vertically (during either childbirth or early childhood). HBV infection during the perinatal and early childhood period, though usually asymptomatic, is associated with a high rate of transition to chronicity (30–90%). In contrast, exposure to HBV during adolescence or adulthood leads to the syndrome of acute hepatitis B, followed by clearance of the virus in >95% of the cases (immunocompetent hosts).

During the pre-icteric phase of acute hepatitis B, a symmetric polyarthritis accompanied by skin rash may occur. Joint complaints subside when the symptoms and signs typical of acute hepatitis (eg, jaundice) develop. Polyarthritis has been rarely reported during the course of chronic HBV infection, although it is difficult to establish a clear pathogenetic role for HBV in these cases. Polyarteritis nodosa (see Chapter 36) is a vasculitis affecting medium-sized vessels that can develop during the first few months of acute HBV infection, or more rarely during chronic HBV infection.

Pathogenesis

Both rheumatic syndromes associated with HBV infection are considered to be immune complex–mediated. The composition of the pathogenic immune complexes is a matter of controversy. Circulating HBV antigens (hepatitis B surface antigen and hepatitis B e antigen), their respective antibodies (anti–hepatitis B surface antigen and anti–hepatitis B e antigen), and complement have been detected in joints and involved blood vessels. The reason for the development of polyarteritis nodosa in some patients remains unclear.

Prevention

Through vaccination programs, HBV infection is a preventable disease. Since vaccination of infants is currently utilized in most countries worldwide and screening of blood and blood-derived products is a routine procedure, the most important target groups for hepatitis B prevention are those with high-risk behaviors or occupations (adolescents, injection drug users, men who have sex with men, individuals with multiple sex partners, and health care workers). HBV vaccination is generally very safe.

Clinical Findings

Exposure to HBV is followed by a long incubation period prior to the development of symptoms (6–20 weeks). HBV DNA can be detected by sensitive methods approximately 1 month after infection. During this same period, hepatitis B surface antigen and IgM anti-HBc appear in the circulation (Figure 50–1). Ten to fifteen weeks after infection, serum alanine aminotransferase reaches its higher levels and typical symptoms of acute hepatitis develop.

In a number of cases, 2–3 weeks prior to the onset of jaundice (the pre-icteric phase), acute polyarthritis may develop (see Figure 50–1). In the majority of cases, young adults are affected. The arthritis is characterized by its acute onset and involvement of multiple joints. The proximal interphalangeal joints, knees, and ankles are most commonly affected. An additive or rarely a migratory pattern of involvement is observed.

In 40% of cases, a rash can be detected in an urticarial, maculopapular, or (more rarely) petechial form. Other nonspecific symptoms include myalgias, malaise, and fever. There have been rare case reports of arthropathy developing during the course of chronic HBV infection, although a direct causal association cannot be proven.

Laboratory Findings

Most patients with HBV-associated arthritis have normal white blood cell counts and erythrocyte sedimentation rates. RF has been detected in approximately 25% of the cases. Low C3 and/or C4 can be found in up to 40% of the cases. The diagnosis of acute hepatitis B is made by the highly elevated serum alanine aminotransferase levels and the presence of hepatitis B surface antigen and high titers of IgM anti-HBc in the circulation. Serum HBV DNA and hepatitis B e antigen may be also detected,

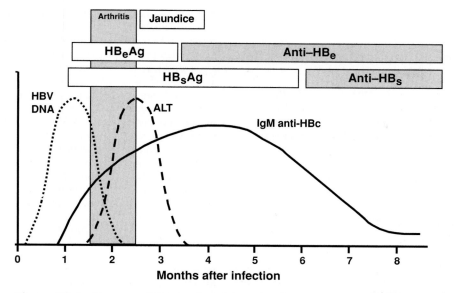

Figure 50–1. The natural history of resolving acute hepatitis B is shown. During the pre-icteric phase, arthritis accompanied by rash can develop. The appearance of the different hepatitis B virus antigens (HB_s Ag and HB_e Ag) and their respective antibodies (anti-HB_s and anti-HB_e) are also illustrated. ALT, alanine aminotransferase; IgM anti-HBc, IgM antibody against the hepatitis B virus core.

although in many cases these have disappeared by the time of diagnosis.

Differential Diagnosis

Serum sickness, other forms of viral infection associated with arthritis (parvovirus, rubella, and HIV), systemic lupus erythematosus, and early RA should be included in the differential diagnosis.

Treatment

Once the diagnosis has been made, no specific therapy is needed. Simple analgesics may be used for pain and fever control while nonsteroidal anti-inflammatory drugs should be avoided. There is usually no need for antiviral treatment in patients with acute hepatitis B. The decision to use antiviral treatment should be made in coordination with a hepatologist. Antiviral therapy can be used either as prophylactic treatment when immunosuppressive medications are administered, or as the main therapy when chronic hepatitis B is diagnosed (defined by elevated aminotransferase levels and moderate to severe hepatitis on liver biopsy). Lamivudine is the only agent that has been used so far as prophylactic treatment in patients receiving immunosuppression. Lamivudine is started a few weeks prior to the initiation of immunosup-

pressive therapy and is continued for several months after treatment discontinuation. For patients with chronic hepatitis B, currently available agents include lamivudine, adefovir, and interferon-α. Interferon-α should be used with extreme caution since it can precipitate or exacerbate autoimmune manifestations.

Complications

There are no long-term sequelae of acute hepatitis B–associated arthritis. Close monitoring of liver function is needed for the rare possibility of fulminant hepatitis B (0.5–1%).

Prognosis

Fewer than 5% of patients with acute icteric hepatitis B undergo transformations to chronic HBV infection. The overall prognosis for the joint disease associated with acute hepatitis B is excellent, with no long-term sequelae.

Inman RD. Rheumatic manifestations of hepatitis B virus infection. *Semin Arthritis Rheum.* 1982;11:406. (Classic review of acute hepatitis B–related arthritis.)

Lok ASF, McMahon BJ. Chronic hepatitis B: Update of recommendations. *Hepatology.* 2004;39:1. (Updated recommendations for the treatment of patients with chronic hepatitis B.)

PARVOVIRUS B19

General Considerations

Human parvovirus infection is caused by parvovirus B19 (B19) a small, nonenveloped, single-stranded DNA virus. B19 infects only humans through binding to its specific receptor, blood group P antigen (globoside or Gb4). This receptor is expressed mainly on erythrocytes and erythroid precursors but also on the following cells and tissues: megakaryocytes, platelets, placental and endothelial cells, synovium, liver, lung, kidneys, and heart. Personal contact, through aerosol or respiratory secretions, is the major mode of virus transmission. Transmission through contaminated blood products (blood or clotting factor concentrate transfusion) and vertical transmission (via pregnancy) has been also documented.

Cyclic outbreaks of B19 infection occur worldwide, especially during the winter and spring seasons. Children represent the major source of transmission and community epidemics. Before the age of 11, <20% of children are seropositive for IgG antibodies to B19. In contrast, 40–70% of the adult population has been exposed to the virus (as demonstrated by serum IgG anti-B19 positivity). Workers at schools or day care facilities (teachers, nurses, and day care staff) who have not been exposed previously represent the population at risk.

The time interval between viral exposure and onset of symptoms is approximately 1 week (Figure 50–2). The majority of infections during childhood remain asymptomatic. B19 infection has been associated with a number of clinical manifestations including erythema infectiosum or fifth disease (mainly in children), arthropathy, pregnancy complications (fetal anemia, spontaneous abortion, and hydrops fetalis), transient aplastic crisis (in patients with chronic hemolytic anemias such as hereditary spherocytosis and sickle cell disease), and chronic anemia in immunocompromised hosts. Other manifestations such as vasculitis, myocarditis, hepatitis, and glomerulonephritis have been reported infrequently.

Pathogenesis

Following the entrance of B19 through the respiratory tract, infection of erythroid precursors occurs. Entry into the cells is accomplished through binding to the P antigen or Gb4. Co-receptors such as $\alpha 5\ \beta 1$ integrin and the Ku80 antigen may be also involved. B19 replicates rapidly in the nucleus of these actively dividing cells, leading to high levels of viremia (10^{10}–10^{12} copies/mL). The viremic phase lasts for approximately 5 days and

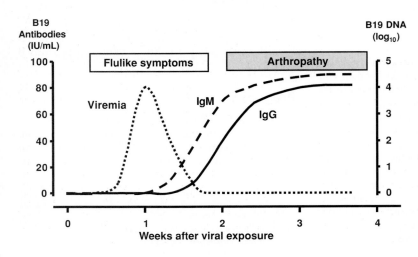

Figure 50–2. The appearance of flulike symptoms and arthritis during the course of acute parvovirus B19 infection is depicted. The timing of serum viremia and detection of IgM and IgG antibodies against B19 is also shown.

is usually accompanied by flulike symptoms (see Figure 50–2).

The appearance of IgM antibodies marks the onset of the late viremic phase and disappearance of B19 from the circulation. IgG antibodies appear 2 weeks after exposure to the virus and indicate the transition to the antibody-response phase (see Figure 50–2). The co-appearance of IgM/IgG antibodies and the characteristic rash and arthropathy of infected individuals are consistent with an immune complex–mediated disease process. Although, the receptor for B19 is expressed in synovial cells, active replication in synovium has not been demonstrated to date.

Long-lasting protection from reinfection is mediated mainly by IgG antibodies. Sustained CD8+ T-cell responses may also contribute to this protective effect.

Prevention

There is currently no vaccine for B19. Avoidance of close contact with infected individuals and isolation of hospitalized patients is recommended.

Clinical Findings

Joint manifestations such as arthralgias or arthritis occur in approximately 8% of children and 50–60% of adult patients with acute B19 infection. The typical arthropathy of B19 infection occurs 2 weeks after viral exposure and 1 week after the onset of flulike symptoms. Females are affected more often than males (60%). Joint manifestations of B10 comprise an acute symmetric polyarthritis that involves the hands and feet and knees and wrists in a distribution that is typical of RA. Joint pain rather than joint swelling dominates the clinical picture. The classic "slapped-cheek" facial appearance occurs in fewer than 20% of patients, although skin rash is common (~75%). The majority of joint symptoms subside in 2–3 weeks. Rarely, joint symptoms (arthralgias) can persist but without evidence of joint destruction.

The role (if any) of parvovirus infection in RA is highly debatable. Although B19 DNA has been found in synovial tissues of patients with chronic arthritis, this has been the case also for healthy seropositive individuals. Furthermore, most epidemiologic studies of patients with early inflammatory arthritides failed to identify B19 infection as an important etiologic factor. Parvovirus infection has been implicated in the pathogenesis or exacerbation of a variety of rheumatic disorders including vasculitis (of small, medium, and large vessels), Raynaud phenomenon, systemic lupus erythematosus, juvenile rheumatoid arthritis, and fibromyalgia. Except for some well-documented cases of small-vessel vasculitis, the evidence for the other diseases is weak.

Laboratory Findings

Although cytopenias (anemia, leukopenia, thrombocytopenia, and pancytopenia) are commonly encountered during acute B19 infection, in the majority of cases of B19-associated arthropathy, blood cell counts are normal. The erythrocyte sedimentation rate and C-reactive protein are usually normal. Antinuclear antibodies and RF are absent. In one study, C4 levels were decreased in one-third of the cases. Transient detection of a number of autoantibodies including antinuclear antibodies, RF, and antibodies against double-stranded DNA or β_2-glycoprotein I have been reported during the course of acute parvovirus infection.

Diagnosis of parvovirus infection is based on the detection of specific B19 antibodies (IgM and IgG) and B19 DNA in the serum. Acute infection is documented by the detection of B19-specific IgM antibodies. These antibodies appear 1 week after acute infection and persist for up to 6 months. Almost all patients with acute B19-associated arthritis demonstrate these antibodies in their serum.

IgG B19 antibodies can be detected simultaneously with the IgM antibodies at the time of arthritis diagnosis. These antibodies are detected also in a large proportion of the general population (40–70%), indicating past infection.

Serum B19 DNA can be detected with various techniques with a sensitivity that ranges between 10^2 (direct DNA hybridization technique) to 10^6 genome copies per milliliter (polymerase chain reaction). During acute infection, serum B19 DNA is usually detected in association with IgM antibodies. The persistence of B19 DNA in the absence of B19 antibodies could indicate chronic B19 infection. This occurs more commonly in immunocompromised hosts (patients receiving chemotherapy or long-term immunosuppression and those with HIV infection), and is usually manifested as chronic anemia. The usefulness of these methods, however, is limited by the frequent detection of B19 DNA in healthy immunocompetent individuals, making the differentiation between acute and past infection problematic. Detection of B19 DNA in tissues such as the synovium, bone marrow, and skin is not diagnostic for acute infection, since this can occur also in healthy individuals with past infection.

Differential Diagnosis

Other diseases that can present with an acute symmetric inflammatory polyarthritis involving the small joints with or without a skin rash should be included in the differential diagnosis. These include RA, systemic lupus erythematosus, other virus-associated arthritides (HCV, HBV, HIV, and rubella), and serum sickness.

Treatment

Given the self-limited course of the disease, only symptomatic therapy is recommended (eg, simple analgesics or nonsteroidal anti-inflammatory drugs). In patients with chronic courses and persistent viremia, intravenous immune globulin at a dose of 0.4 g/kg/d for 5 days can be given. There is no indication for intravenous immune globulin administration during the acute infection or in chronic cases without viremia.

Complications

B19-associated arthritis is a nonerosive arthropathy. No long-term complications are expected.

Prognosis

For cases with B19-associated arthropathy the prognosis is good, without long term sequelae.

Corcoran A, Doyle S. Advances in the biology, diagnosis and host-pathogen interactions of parvovirus B19. *J Med Microbiol.* 2004;53:459. (Review of the pathogenesis and diagnostic tools for parvovirus infection.)

Meyer O. Parvovirus B19 and autoimmune diseases. *Joint Bone Spine.* 2003;70:6. (Review with emphasis on the autoimmune features of B19 infection.)

Young NS, Brown KE. Parvovirus B19. *N Engl J Med.* 2004;350:586. (Recent review of the various clinical manifestations of parvovirus B19 infection in humans.)

OTHER VIRUSES

Alphaviruses

Alphaviruses are RNA viruses that are transmitted by mosquitoes in several areas around the world, leading to specific clinical syndromes characterized by fever, rash, and arthritis. Major Alphavirus epidemics have occurred in different areas of the world. There are 26 members of the Alphavirus genus, but only the ones that have been related to specific articular syndromes are shown in Table 50–1.

After an incubation period that lasts from 2–10 days, the typical clinical syndrome caused by these Alphaviruses begins with general complaints such as fever, myalgias, headache, and nausea. Some of these viruses (Chikungunya, O'nyong-nyong, and Mayaro) can also cause hemorrhagic phenomena such as petechiae, gastrointestinal bleeding, and epistaxis. The rash appears concomitantly or a few days after the constitutional symptoms and lasts for a week. Usually it starts from the trunk and spreads to the extremities and is maculopapular or vesicular. In some cases, itching can be a prominent feature. Desquamation is common when the rash resolves.

Articular symptoms are prominent and incapacitating in patients with Alphavirus infections. Typically, migratory polyarthralgias of the small joints of the hands and feet and wrists and ankles are accompanied by prolonged morning stiffness. In most cases, articular or periarticular swelling is prominent. Although articular symptoms can last only a few weeks, in many cases prolonged debilitating arthralgias lasting for many months or even years are observed. Serologic tests with the isolation of specific IgM antibodies against these viruses are utilized for diagnosis. There is no specific vaccine for these infections. Treatment is symptomatic.

Laine M, Luukkainen R, Toivanen A. Sindbis viruses and other alphaviruses as cause of human arthritic disease. *J Intern Med.* 2004;256:457. (The most recent review on the clinical features of Alphavirus infections.)

Table 50–1. Alphaviruses and Arthritis

Virus	Clinical Syndrome	Main Geographic Distribution
Sindbis	Ockelbo disease	Norway, Sweden
	Karelian fever	Russia
	Pogosta disease	Finland
Chikungunya	Africa, Southeast Asia	
O'nyong-nyong	Africa	
Mayaro	South America	
Ross River	Epidemic polyarthritis	Australia, South Pacific
Igbo-ora	Ivory Coast	
Barmah Forest	Australia	

Rubella Virus

Rubella virus is a togavirus that is transmitted mainly by nasopharyngeal secretions. With the introduction of the live attenuated rubella vaccine, the number of postnatally acquired rubella infections has diminished. In 2001, only 23 cases of rubella infection in adults were reported in U.S. Most cases involve young adults who present with malaise, fever, lymphadenopathy (posterior auricular, occipital, and cervical), and maculopapular rash. The rash begins on the face and spreads to the body. A symmetrical polyarthritis involving hands, knees, and ankles can be observed in association with the appearance of the rash, particularly in female patients. Arthritis can last for several weeks. Diagnosis is made by the detection of specific IgM antibodies and/or by a fourfold increase in serum IgG antibodies obtained in the acute and convalescent period. Prevention of rubella infection is accomplished through administration of the live attenuated vaccine.

Postvaccination arthritis has been occasionally described and in the majority of cases is mild and self-limited.

Human T-Lymphotropic Virus Type I

Human T-lymphotropic virus type I (HTLV-I) is a human retrovirus endemic in Japan. It is the cause of two distinct clinical syndromes: adult T-cell leukemia and HTLV-I–associated myelopathy (HAM, also known as tropical paraparesis). Furthermore, it has been implicated in a number of rheumatic/autoimmune disorders including an RA-like arthritis, a Sjögren like syndrome, uveitis, vasculitis, and polymyositis. In certain cases, an HTLV-I–associated arthropathy has been described. Patients present with symmetric, polyarticular involvement characterized by prominent synovial proliferation. Most patients are RF positive and demonstrate elevation of the acute phase reactants (erythrocyte sedimentation rate and C-reactive protein). Erosive changes are present on x-rays of involved joints.

The virus is transmitted perinatally from the infected mother to the child through sexual activity, and through infected blood or contaminated syringes. Diagnosis is made by serologic assays for HTLV-I (enzyme-linked immunosorbent assay) and confirmed by specific Western blot or polymerase chain reaction techniques. There is currently no treatment for HTLV-I infection. For HTLV-I associated arthropathy, treatment regimens include nonsteroidal anti-inflammatory drugs, corticosteroids, and disease-modifying drugs.

REFERENCES

Manns A, Hisada M, La Grenade L. Human T-lymphotropic virus type I infection. *Lancet.* 1999;353:1951. (Review of the various clinical manifestations of HTLV-I infection.)

Nishioka K, Sumida T, Hasunuma T. Human T lymphotropic virus type I in arthropathy and autoimmune disorders. *Arthritis Rheum.* 1996;39:1410. (Classic review of the characteristic articular manifestations of HTLV-I infection.)

Evaluation of Rheumatic Complaints in Patients with HIV

51

Khalil G. Ghanem, MD, Dimitrios Vassilopoulos, MD, & Kelly A. Gebo, MD, MPH

ESSENTIALS OF DIAGNOSIS

- *Diagnosis of HIV infection is made by serologic tests (enzyme-linked immunosorbent assay) and confirmed by Western blot.*

- *HIV causes nonspecific B-cell activation resulting in a polyclonal hypergammaglobulinemia and a high frequency of false-positive autoantibody tests.*

- *Rheumatologic manifestations include arthralgias, increased severity (and possibly increased incidence) of seronegative spondyloarthropathies, musculoskeletal infections, osteopenia/osteoporosis, and avascular bone necrosis.*

- *Myalgias with minimal laboratory evidence of muscle damage are consistent with several conditions, including fibromyalgia, the HIV wasting syndrome, and antiretroviral toxicity.*

- *Limited data suggest that highly active antiretroviral therapy (HAART) may be associated with several rheumatologic complications including arthralgias, myopathies, and abnormalities in bone mineralization.*

- *Concomitant use of HAART and immunosuppressive agents requires careful consideration of drug interactions, heightened toxicities, and difficulty in monitoring certain clinical HIV-related parameters.*

General Considerations

Human immunodeficiency virus (HIV), a human retrovirus, infects an estimated 39 million people worldwide. Other retroviruses (eg, human T-lymphotropic virus type I) have been reported to be associated with inflammatory arthropathies, so it is not surprising that a number of rheumatologic manifestations have been described in patients with HIV infection (Table 51–1). These include various arthropathies, muscle diseases, bone disorders, symptoms and signs mimicking Sjögren syndrome, and systemic vasculitis. For some of these disorders, a clear pathophysiologic association with HIV has been established. For others, true relationships remain speculative. Geographic predisposition among HIV-infected patients to certain rheumatologic conditions is suggested by a number of recent studies.

Pathogenesis

HIV infection may modulate the host immune response contributing to the development of various rheumatic manifestations. Painful articular syndrome and HIV-associated arthritis represent distinct clinical syndromes that develop during the course of HIV infection, suggesting a direct role for HIV. The role of HIV in reactive arthritides, undifferentiated spondyloarthropathies, and musculoskeletal infections is most likely indirect, either by increasing susceptibility or influencing the clinical course of these diseases in susceptible patient groups. A unique spectrum of rheumatic manifestations has been recently recognized among HIV patients treated with HAART. Immune reconstitution after such therapy may be responsible for some of these manifestations.

JOINT COMPLAINTS: ARTHRALGIAS, ARTHRITIS, & SPONDYLOARTHROPATHIES

HIV Painful Articular Syndrome

This syndrome is characterized by debilitating arthralgias that are often sufficiently severe to precipitate emergency department visits. It has been reported to occur in up to 10% of HIV-infected patients. Symptoms last from 2–24 hours and usually resolve spontaneously. The joint complaints are usually oligoarticular and asymmetric. The affected joints—most commonly the knees, but elbows and shoulders may also be affected—are free of any signs of inflammation on examination. Radiographs often reveal nonspecific findings such as periarticular osteopenia. Targeting symptoms using nonsteroidal anti-inflammatory

Table 51–1. Musculoskeletal Manifestations of HIV Infection

Arthralgias
Painful articular syndrome
HIV-associated arthritis
Spondyloarthropathies
    Reactive arthritis
    Psoriatic arthritis
    Undifferentiated spondyloarthropathy
Musculoskeletal infections
Osteonecrosis
Osteopenia/osteoporosis
    Rheumatic manifestations of HAART-associated IRIS
Myalgias
Noninflammatory myopathies
    NRTI myopathy
    HIV-associated myopathy
    Nemaline rod myopathy
Inflammatory myopathies
    Idiopathic polymyositis
    Pyomyositis

HIV, human immunodeficiency virus; HAART, highly active antiretroviral therapy; IRIS, immune reconstitution inflammation syndrome; NRTI, nucleoside reverse transcriptase inhibitor.

agents or narcotics and reassurance is usually successful. If symptoms do not improve within 1–2 days, reconsidering the diagnosis is mandatory.

HIV-Associated Arthritis

A subacute asymmetric oligoarthritis that usually affects the large joints (most commonly the knees, but ankles and wrists may also be involved), may occur in patients with more advanced HIV infection. This form of arthritis usually has a self-limited course ranging from 1 week up to 6 months. The prevalence has been reported in the range of 3–25% of HIV-infected patients, the higher prevalence coming from a cohort in Zambia, suggesting a possible geographic predisposition. The HIV has been cultured from synovial fluid, consistent with though not diagnostic of an etiologic role for the virus itself in this problem. Suppression of viral replication using HAART may be beneficial for the treatment of this disorder, but controlled trials are lacking. Treatment has centered on nonsteroidal anti-inflammatory drugs and some reports note benefit from low-dose glucocorticoids and hydroxychloroquine.

HIV-Associated Acute Symmetric Polyarthritis

Acute symmetric polyarthritis affects the small joints of the hands, and its manifestations resemble rheumatoid arthritis. Findings include periarticular osteopenia, joint space narrowing, swan-neck deformity, and ulnar deviation. Rheumatoid factor is usually negative. Studies have reported therapeutic success with the use of gold.

Adhesive Capsulitis

There have been several reports of HIV-infected patients presenting with subacute progressive shoulder pain with limited range of motion of the joint. An association with the use of protease inhibitors has been suggested (Table 51–2). Typically, symptoms begin a year after the medications are started and usually resolve within 7–12 months. This is a clinical diagnosis, as radiographic findings are usually lacking. Physical therapy, nonsteroidal

Table 51–2. Rheumatologic Manifestations Reported with Antiretroviral Medications

Medication(s)	Class	Manifestation
AZT (zidovudine); d4T (stavudine)	NRTI	Myopathy, myalgias, rhabdomyolysis
ddC (zalcitabine)	NRTI	Arthralgias
Tenofovir	NRTI	Osteopenia
3TC (lamivudine); FTC (emtricitabine)	NRTI	Arthralgias, myalgias, rhabdomyolysis
Efavirenz	NNRTI	Arthralgias, myopathy, myalgias
Nevirapine	NNRTI	Arthralgias
Nelfinavir; lopinavir; atazanavir	PI	Osteopenia, osteoporosis, aseptic necrosis of bone
Saquinavir; ritonavir	PI	Myalgias, arthralgias, arthritis, cramps, osteopenia, osteoporosis
Indinavir	PI	Adhesive capsulitis of the shoulder, temporomandibular pain syndrome, osteopenia, osteoporosis, aseptic necrosis of bone
Enfuvirtide	FI	Myalgias

NRTI, nucleoside reverse transcriptase inhibitor; NNRTI, non-nucleoside reverse transcriptase inhibitor; PI, protease inhibitor; FI, fusion inhibitor.
The reported association between antiretroviral and the development of bone abnormalities is tenuous.

anti-inflammatory drugs, and the judicious use of intra-articular glucocorticoids (see Chapter 2 on arthrocentesis and joint aspiration) have been successfully used to treat this condition. Although the association with protease inhibitors is far from convincing, physicians may consider switching the HAART regimen to a non–protease inhibitor class (eg, non-nucleoside reverse transcriptase inhibitors). If that is not an option, the data suggest that symptoms tend to resolve despite persistent use of protease inhibitors.

Psoriatic Arthritis

Psoriasis and psoriatic arthritis may be the initial presentation of underlying HIV infection. Prevalence estimates of psoriasis among HIV-infected patients range from 1–32%, with a tendency for appearance or exacerbation in more advanced stages of HIV infection. Arthritis develops in as many as 30% of HIV patients who have cutaneous psoriasis. The pattern of psoriatic arthritis—polyarticular, asymmetric involvement with dactylitis and enthesopathy—differs from that seen in individuals without HIV in that sacroiliac and axial skeleton involvement initially seems less common. As the natural history of HIV has been altered by new treatments, the axial bony changes commonly seen in psoriasis patients without HIV have been observed among patients living longer than 5 years with psoriatic arthritis. These include unilateral sacroiliitis and bulky spondylitis that skips adjacent vertebral bodies. Therapy for this disorder may require immunosuppressive agents and does not differ significantly from the treatment of patients who are HIV-negative.

Reactive Arthritis & Other Spondyloarthropathies

Spondyloarthropathies in the setting of HIV infection may present with the typical form of reactive arthritis or may have atypical features classified as undifferentiated spondyloarthropathy. The characteristic clinical findings are those of a peripheral arthritis involving the lower extremities and prominent enthesopathy (eg, Achilles tendinitis and plantar fasciitis). Extra-articular manifestations including eye inflammation, urethritis, and mucocutaneous lesions are also common. Axial involvement is typically infrequent. The clinical course is unpredictable, although a severe form of erosive polyarthritis has been reported in African patients.

Studies from the late 1980s suggested an increased risk of reactive arthritis in HIV-positive patients. Data from several subsequent cohorts found no change in prevalence between HIV-infected and uninfected patients, suggesting that reactive arthritis was not due to HIV per se, but due to the prevalence of high-risk sexual behaviors

leading to post-venereal reactive arthritis. Recent literature derived from sub-Saharan African patients, however, suggests a more complicated relationship. The prevalence of spondyloarthropathies has clearly risen with the increase in HIV infections, with no apparent change in triggers for reactive arthritis. In contrast to seronegative patients, these HIV-positive patients are predominantly human leukocyte antigen-B27 negative, and seem to have a more aggressive course of arthritis.

Other Considerations

There are other entities that are not directly caused by HIV infection, but should be considered when evaluating HIV-infected patients with rheumatologic complaints:

Septic arthritis: Given the frequency of injection drug use as the primary risk factor for HIV infection, the high incidence of joint infections is not surprising in this subset of HIV patients. As the CD4+ T-cell count drops below 200 cells/mL, the risk of musculoskeletal infections rises. *Staphylococcus aureus* is the most common joint pathogen described.

Malignancies: Rarely, lymphoma may present as arthritis of a large joint. The prevalence of lymphoma among HIV-infected patients ranges from 5–10%. Data suggest a decreased incidence of lymphoma after the introduction of HAART.

DISORDERS OF BONE

Recent data suggest that HIV infection has a significant effect on bone metabolism. Whether this is a direct result of HIV, or an indirect effect (eg, of HAART or injection drug use) is unclear. There are several biological mechanisms that support a direct effect of HIV, including HIV-induced increases in osteoclastic activity. There are also data implicating HAART-mediated mechanisms, including changes in osteoblast activity, osteoclast differentiation, and vitamin D metabolism.

Osteopenia & Osteoporosis

A recent prospective study found a 23–28% prevalence of osteopenia among HIV-infected patients receiving HAART. Recent longitudinal studies suggest that protease inhibitors may be associated with early bone loss that tends to stabilize over time.

Two groups of HIV-infected patients have been found to have significant bone loss: women and children. In one large study, osteopenia was present in 54% of HIV-infected women as opposed to 30% of uninfected controls. However, there was no association between osteopenia and degree of immunosuppression. In HIV-infected children, several studies have documented decreases in bone mineral density, putting these children at higher risk for fractures.

Risk factors for bone disease in HIV-infected patients include history of weight loss and duration of HIV infection. At this time, there is no reason to modify the antiretroviral therapy based on bone mineral density considerations. However, in HIV-infected patients at high-risk for fractures, bisphosphonates have been shown to be a safe and effective therapeutic option.

Osteonecrosis

Osteonecrosis has been frequently reported in both the pre-HAART and the current HAART eras. Recent reports suggest an increased incidence during the current era of HAART. One report of 118 asymptomatic HIV-positive patients showed a prevalence of hip osteonecrosis of 4.4%. The femoral head is the most common site of involvement, but studies from the pre-HAART and current HAART eras have also demonstrated involvement of knees, shoulders, and elbows. Among persons with AIDS, osteonecrosis is frequently bilateral. Studies conflict on the number of involved sites present concurrently as well as the correlation of disease with HIV stage. Initially, protease inhibitors were thought to be causative. More recent evidence suggests that traditional risk factors for osteonecrosis—trauma, smoking, alcohol abuse, glucocorticoid use, and pancreatitis—are also important in HIV-associated osteonecrosis. Evaluation with magnetic resonance imaging is essential for patients with strongly suggestive clinical histories and physical examination findings (eg, pain with internal rotation of the hip) but normal plain films. Prompt diagnosis at an early stage may allow successful core decompression (see Chapter 58). Late-stage disease is treated most effectively with joint replacement.

Other Bone Disorders

A. Osteomyelitis

Relatively rare among patients with HIV (with a prevalence of less than 1%), the onset of persistent discomfort that localizes to the skeleton should raise suspicion for this disease. Although the risk factors for osteomyelitis are similar among HIV-infected and uninfected individuals, specific pathogens merit consideration in the setting of HIV. In addition to *S aureus,* the most common pathogen (particularly among patients who are injection drug users), another commonly encountered pathogen in patients with advanced immunosuppression is *Salmonella*. In the pre-HAART era, *Bartonella* species were found in erosive bone lesions. As the CD4 count declines to <100 cells/mL, the clinician must consider bone infections with atypical mycobacterial organisms, *Candida,* and *Sporothrix,* which rarely cause such problems in immunocompetent patients.

B. Malignancy

Both Kaposi sarcoma and lymphoma may present as bone lesions. Evidence of periosteal reactions and destruction as well as soft tissue masses are not uncommon. The frequent difficulty in distinguishing the presentations of these diseases from infection highlights the importance of obtaining tissue for diagnostic purposes.

DISORDERS OF MUSCLE

Initial Clinical Considerations

Although muscle weakness in HIV/AIDS patients can be the result of severe muscle wasting from infection, nutritional deficiency, or nervous system involvement, skeletal muscle disease is also common in HIV disease. The most common muscle disorders in HIV patients include nucleoside reverse transcriptase inhibitor (NRTI) myopathy, HIV myopathy, and muscle infections. Other muscle disorders including rhabdomyolysis, non-Hodgkin lymphomas, and myasthenia gravis have also been reported.

The distinction between muscle pain and muscle weakness is an important initial step in the evaluation of patients with muscle complaints. Symptoms of acute HIV seroconversion include fever, arthralgias, and myalgias. In the current era of HAART, chronically infected patients who have discontinued HAART medications are at risk for the development of symptoms consistent with HIV seroconversion syndrome as the viral load rebounds. This can occur as early as 1 week after cessation of HAART.

Patients with long-standing HIV infections may have muscle symptoms secondary to autoimmune phenomena, infections, or adverse drug effects. Muscle pain in the setting of elevated levels of serum muscle enzymes should prompt an evaluation of all medications. Statins are a common cause of myositis in HIV patients.

Differential Diagnosis

A. Myalgias

Complaints of muscle pains of varying duration have been reported in as many as 30% of HIV-infected patients in several cohorts. The pathophysiology is unclear. At times these myalgias can be localized. Analgesics are often quite useful. Some clinicians recommend strategies similar to those for patients without HIV who have fibromyalgia.

B. Muscle Weakness

Muscle weakness or evidence of muscle damage identified by elevated serum creatinine kinase may have numerous causes in HIV patients. Biopsy of affected muscles is an important part of the evaluation. The myopathies may be divided into those with biopsy-proven inflammation and those with tissue necrosis accompanied by minimal inflammatory infiltrates.

1. Noninflammatory myopathy—NRTI myopathy was initially described with azidothymidine (zidovudine). This condition resembles HIV myopathy and idiopathic polymyositis. In addition to weakness, patients may first complain of myalgias, muscle tenderness, and proximal muscle weakness. Patients have generally been on NRTI therapy for months prior to symptom onset. Creatinine kinase levels are elevated up to 10-fold. Electromyographic studies may be normal or demonstrate mild myopathic changes. Histopathologic studies indicate that NRTIs disrupt skeletal muscle mitochondrial function, yielding characteristic "ragged-red" fibers on biopsy. The quantity of ragged fibers present correlates loosely with the clinical severity of weakness.

All nucleoside analogues preferentially inhibit reverse transcriptase. Some of these medications also inhibit other DNA polymerases, including mitochondrial DNA polymerases. This type of mitochondrial toxicity can be the cause of myopathy, as well as other drug-induced complications such as a demyelinating polyneuropathy (similar to Guillain-Barré syndrome) and hepatic steatosis. When NRTI myopathy is diagnosed, cessation of therapy leads to normalization of serum creatinine kinase levels within several weeks, presaging return of power to affected muscles in subsequent months. If there is no response to discontinuation of the drug, it is likely that HIV myopathy (see below) is present. For acute symptoms, nonsteroidal anti-inflammatory agents may help to relieve the myalgias. Although there has been some evidence to suggest that carnitine may prevent the development and progression of NRTI myopathy, the clinical efficacy of this treatment is unknown.

2. HIV-associated myopathy—HIV-associated myopathy may resemble idiopathic polymyositis. Typical presentations include myalgias, muscle tenderness, and symmetrical proximal muscle weakness, particularly in the lower extremities. Although this myopathy may be the presenting symptom of HIV, it does not appear to be related to the level of immune suppression, having been described both early and late in the course of HIV infection. One clinical difficulty comes in differentiating HIV myopathy from NRTI-associated myopathy, because the clinical presentations of these two disorders (including elevation of muscle enzymes up to 10-fold) are similar. Electromyography and muscle biopsy demonstrate myopathic changes (ie, increased insertional activity, fibrillation, and polyphasic potentials characteristic of membrane irritability). Histologic changes on biopsy include a mononuclear cell infiltrate accompanied by some perivascular and interfascicular accumulation of inflammatory cells. Some clinicians have posited a causative role for malnutrition, with HIV simply exacerbating the dietary

deficiency. A similar biopsy pattern has been described in patients experiencing clinical signs of HIV-associated wasting syndrome. Several case studies have demonstrated therapeutic benefit from glucocorticoids. Generally, therapy is initiated with prednisone at 1 mg/kg/d. Normalization of muscle enzymes and improvement in strength generally occur in 1–2 months. Upon full recovery, prednisone is gradually tapered and the patient is closely monitored for signs and symptoms of recurrent disease. Alternative diagnoses and steroid myopathy should be considered in patients who do not respond to steroids. In patients who are truly steroid nonresponsive, other therapies including intravenous immune globulin, methotrexate, and azathioprine have all been tried.

3. Nemaline rod myopathy—Finally, the rare condition known as nemaline rod myopathy has been observed in HIV-infected patients as well as in individuals without HIV. Both congenital and acquired forms of this disease exist. Patients present with a slowly progressive proximal myopathy, mildly elevated creatine kinase, and a biopsy revealing type 1 muscle fiber atrophy and small, punctate rods and vacuoles within myocytes. Inflammatory changes, if present, are generally mild. A clear therapeutic strategy for this condition has not been defined, though in some cases a response to glucocorticoids in doses similar to those used for HIV myopathy has been observed.

4. Inflammatory myopathies—An inflammatory muscle disease clinically indistinguishable from polymyositis in HIV-negative persons has been described in HIV-infected persons. Thus the picture of progressive proximal muscle weakness, either subtle or dramatic, with minimal myalgias should prompt consideration of polymyositis. Inflammation-induced necrosis yields elevated serum muscle enzymes. Electromyographic evaluations demonstrate patterns of muscle dysfunction identical to those of idiopathic inflammatory myopathy (see Chapter 28). Confirmation of the diagnosis by muscle biopsy is important because therapy will involve pharmacologic immunosuppression. The electromyogram can direct the clinician to biopsy muscle groups most affected, thus lowering risk of false-negative results due to sampling bias. On biopsy, myositis will manifest as predominantly a CD8+ lymphocytic infiltrate among myofibrils of varying states of destruction and regeneration.

Regardless of the person's state of HIV-induced immunosuppression, immunotherapy with glucocorticoids is a cornerstone of therapy. Patients with CD4 counts <200 cells/mL should receive prophylaxis against *Pneumocystis jiroveci* (formerly *carinii*) when using any immunosuppressive agent. Some patients may require adjunctive therapy either to control symptoms or to facilitate glucocorticoid taper. In these cases, methotrexate or azathioprine are the agents used most often. Patients with

HIV infection are susceptible to bone marrow suppression and may require hematologic growth factors while undergoing immunosuppression.

An infectious myositis (pyomyositis) presents as a deep muscle abscess caused by pyogenic bacteria. Patients complain of focal myalgias, swelling, and tenderness, localizing to the region of the affected muscle, frequently associated with fevers. True weakness is relatively uncommon. Muscle enzymes may not be elevated depending on the volume of muscle involved, but leukocytosis is typical. Persistence of localizing symptoms merits further evaluation with ultrasonography or magnetic resonance imaging. *S aureus* is the most common etiology of pyomyositis, although other bacteria such as *Salmonella, Streptococcus pyogenes, Mycobacterium tuberculosis,* and *Nocardia* have also been described. Surgical incision and drainage or drainage by percutaneous interventional radiology often is necessary as an adjunct to parenteral antibiotics.

5. Non-Hodgkin lymphoma—Non-Hodgkin lymphoma may present as a painful muscle mass that needs to be distinguished from other localized muscle masses including pyomyositis and deep venous thrombosis. Magnetic resonance imaging may be useful in distinguishing infections from neoplasms. A hyperintense ring around a mass on T1-weighted images favors infection due to pyomyositis.

OTHER RHEUMATOLOGIC CONDITIONS

Vasculitis Syndromes

Since the beginning of the HIV epidemic, a wide variety of vascular inflammatory diseases have been described in HIV-infected patients. Given the prevalence of HIV in the general population, it is not surprising that there are case reports of nearly every vascular inflammatory disease in the setting of HIV. In addition, HIV is associated with a number of other co-infections including hepatitis B, hepatitis C, and cytomegalovirus, which can predispose patients to vascular inflammatory syndromes. Currently, there is no clear consensus on whether any distinct vasculitis forms exist in the setting of HIV.

Due to the low prevalence of vasculitis in the general population, extremely large epidemiologic studies would be required to thoroughly evaluate its association with HIV. Because of the prohibitive costs associated with this, most data are obtained from smaller studies. In terms of the primary forms of systemic vasculitis, there are no convincing data suggesting that HIV infection increases the risk of developing any of these diseases. In fact, some evidence indicates that HIV may diminish the chance of developing certain forms of vasculitis, such as polyarteritis nodosa (with or without hepatitis B; see Chapter 36)

or the types of vasculitis associated with antineutrophil cytoplasmic antibodies. Several groups, however, have described clear examples of tissue-confirmed polyarteritis nodosa. Polyarteritis nodosa has been described in patients at all stages of disease and at all CD4 cell count levels.

Secondary vasculitis may result from infection from bacteria, viruses, mycobacteria, fungi, and parasites. Given the immune suppression that occurs in HIV and the resulting higher susceptibility to infections, HIV-infected patients may have higher rates of secondary vasculitis than the general population. Clinicians should perform an extensive evaluation for treatable pathogens that may mediate direct vascular inflammation in HIV-infected patients. Cases of cryoglobulinemia secondary to hepatitis C have been well documented in HIV patients, with cutaneous, neurologic, and renal pathology suggestive of vasculitis. Of note, despite the strong association of hepatitis B infection and development of polyarteritis nodosa and hepatitis C infection with cryoglobulinemic vasculitis, the prevalence of these vasculitides in HIV appears exceedingly low.

Finally, there does appear to be growing clinical, epidemiologic, and pathologic evidence that several distinctive forms of vascular inflammatory disease occur in certain settings. These include aneurysmal disease of the large arteries of the brain occurring in children, and a large-vessel aneurysmal disease primarily affecting the aorta and its branches in young HIV-infected patients from sub-Saharan Africa. Further study of these disorders is necessary to identify specific epidemiologic features and pathogenesis.

Differential Diagnosis

Among the true systemic vasculitides, the most commonly described in HIV patients is a small-vessel vasculitis typically induced by medications (see Chapter 38 on hypersensitivity vasculitis). Palpable purpura is the most common manifestation, with skin biopsy yielding the nonspecific description of leukocytoclastic vasculitis. These lesions may be accompanied by arthritis of wrists, fingers, knees, or ankles, as well as low-grade fevers. Abacavir, β-lactam antibiotics, and sulfa-based medications are the most common offenders in causing hypersensitivity vasculitis in the setting of HIV. Abacavir hypersensitivity, observed in 3–5% of patients, most often presents with a combination of flulike symptoms, fever, rash (usually urticarial or maculopapular), fatigue, and gastrointestinal upset. Symptoms worsen progressively during continued therapy and improve substantially within 24–48 hours of discontinuation. A patient with a presumed abacavir hypersensitivity reaction should never be rechallenged with abacavir due to the possibility of a fatal reaction. Ordinarily, cessation of the drug is sufficient for improvement, which occurs over the ensuing several days to weeks. An identical clinical condition can occur in the weeks following streptococcal infections or subacute bacterial endocarditis, with the sensitizing antigen being a bacterial epitope rather than a medication.

Finally, when the diagnosis of vasculitis is entertained in the HIV patient, the numerous potential mimickers of vasculitis must also be considered. Case reports describe examples of cutaneous and neurologic pathology from infectious pathogens, including the herpesviruses (herpes simplex, varicella-zoster, and cytomegalovirus) and parasites such as *Toxoplasma gondii* and *Pneumocystis jiroveci*. Similarly, hypercoagulable states such as the antiphospholipid syndrome can mimic vasculitis by causing multiorgan system dysfunction. Antiphospholipid antibodies such as the lupus anticoagulant occur with increased frequency in patients with HIV, but their clinical significance is not always clear.

Laboratory Evaluation

The evaluation should include urinalysis with careful attention to the presence of protein, blood, and red blood cell casts. Serum complement levels are often depressed in the setting of immune complex–mediated processes, such as the cryoglobulinemic vasculitis associated with hepatitis C. Comprehensive hepatitis B and C serologies should be obtained. If the partial thromboplastin time is prolonged, antiphospholipid antibodies should be excluded through appropriate serologic testing (see Chapter 24).

Imaging Studies

In the patient with chronic active hepatitis B, complaints of abdominal pain may ultimately require selective mesenteric artery angiography to confirm polyarteritis nodosa.

SICCA SYNDROME

Initial Clinical Considerations

A significant number of patients with HIV complain of dry eyes and dry mouth. These are often assumed to be HAART-related symptoms, yet only indinavir (5% of patients who take the drug), efavirenz, ritonavir, saquinavir, and didanosine (all <2%) are associated with xerostomia. Mycobacterial infections should also be considered but are usually not subtle in presentation. Concurrent symptoms with evidence of a systemic process (eg, arthritis and shortness of breath) may indicate Sjögren syndrome or diffuse infiltrative lymphocytosis syndrome, a condition that occurs exclusively in HIV (see below).

Differential Diagnosis

A. Granulomatous Processes

Chronic granulomatous processes such as mycobacterial infections or sarcoidosis should be considered. Systemic symptoms are expected to accompany mycobacterial infections, but the presentation may be complicated in the setting of HIV. Sarcoidosis, although rare in HIV, has been reported in patients experiencing immune reconstitution. Medication changes may be considered after other conditions have been excluded.

B. Diffuse Infiltrative Lymphocytosis Syndrome

First described in the late 1980s, the prevalence of diffuse infiltrative lymphocytosis syndrome has been reported as 3–7% of outpatient HIV cohorts. Characterized by painless parotid gland swelling with concurrent asymmetric salivary gland enlargement, 60% of patients will also experience sicca symptoms. Tissue biopsy of the minor salivary gland reveals prominent infiltrate of CD8+ lymphocytes, distinctly different from the inflammatory process of Sjögren syndrome. Extraglandular infiltrates also cause visceral organ disease with up to 50% of affected patients experiencing lymphocytic interstitial pneumonitis. Neurologic deficits can include cranial nerve VII palsies, likely secondary to parotid gland compression, and occasionally peripheral neuropathies. Treatments for both glandular and extraglandular manifestations range from moderate doses of prednisone to the use of HAART.

Laboratory Evaluation

A biopsy of the minor salivary gland has a very low risk of morbidity and may contribute significantly to the work-up.

Imaging Studies

Gallium scintigraphy reveals significant signal enhancement in the affected salivary glands. This finding, however, is nonspecific.

RHEUMATOLOGIC MANIFESTATIONS OF HAART

The introduction of HAART in the mid-1990s has led to significant improvements in overall mortality among HIV-infected patients. The effects of HAART on rheumatologic manifestations are still very poorly defined. Whether HAART increases the risk for certain rheumatologic diseases is debatable. Table 51–2 summarizes the reported rheumatologic associations of the various agents used to treat HIV infection. A well-documented association is the myopathy associated with zidovudine. Most NRTIs (eg, zidovudine, stavudine, zalcitabine, didanosine, and lamivudine) have been associated with mitochondrial toxicity leading to lactic acidosis, muscle wasting, myalgias, and myopathies. The association between HAART and bone disease is still controversial. It is unclear whether the use of antiretroviral agents leads to bone demineralization or osteonecrosis. Although listed in Table 51–2, longitudinal data are still needed to verify these associations. Finally, it is still unclear whether the initiation of HAART has beneficial (or untoward) effects on pre-existing conditions such as HIV-associated arthritis, reactive arthritis, or psoriatic arthritis.

The Immune Reconstitution Inflammatory Syndrome

One important diagnosis to consider in the patient who has initiated HAART within the past 1–2 months is the immune reconstitution inflammatory syndrome (IRIS). This syndrome is a paradoxical worsening in clinical status that is caused by an improved capacity of the patient to mount an inflammatory response against persistent microbial antigens or self-antigens. IRIS is usually associated with a response to organisms that were present before the initiation of HAART. The manifestations of IRIS are diverse and depend largely on the particular infectious agent involved. In addition to responses to microorganisms, cases of autoimmunity have also been reported in patients with IRIS.

Following the institution of HAART, suppression of the viral load permits the expansion of memory CD4+ cells within 1–2 weeks. Cytokine production shifts from a Th-2 profile to a Th-1 profile with increases in interferon-γ and interleukin-2, resulting in aggressive immune responses occurring at specific tissue sites. Cessation of HAART is rarely necessary. Short courses of glucocorticoids will mitigate symptoms and may be used in more severe cases.

HAART & Immunosuppressive Medications

The use of immunosuppressive agents in HIV-infected patients on HAART is challenging. There are no published data that offer guidance. The potential for drug interactions must be considered. Several antiretroviral agents have well-documented effects on the cytochrome P450 system. These effects may alter the metabolism of concomitantly-administered immunosuppressive agents. The potential for synergistic toxicities, such as hepatotoxicity and bone marrow toxicity, should also be addressed. Efavirenz, for example, an non-NRTI, is well known to increase the risk of hepatotoxicity. Zidovudine has bone marrow suppressive effects. Because these two common side effects are shared by several immunosuppressive agents, antiretroviral regimens may require tailoring in order to minimize the potential for heightened

toxicity when used in combinations with immunosuppressive agents.

The use of immunosuppressive medications may make it difficult to assess the immunologic response to HAART. Usually, when a patient is started on an effective HAART regimen, suppression of the HIV viral load is followed by an increase in the CD4 count. Immunosuppressives may blunt a CD4 count increase. If feasible, the initiation of HAART prior to the initiation of immunosuppression may make it easier to achieve adequate virologic control. Once the immunosuppressives are added, the HIV viral load should remain undetectable; however, the CD4 count response may be blunted. Finally, it is imperative that prophylaxis against opportunistic infections be initiated. To minimize the risks of untoward events, close collaboration between the rheumatologist and the HIV-care provider is essential.

Laboratory Evaluation: General Concept

Patients with HIV have heightened activation of the B-cell compartment and a high prevalence of polyclonal hypergammaglobulinemia. Partly as a consequence of this, the frequency with which autoantibody production is detected in patients with HIV is increased compared with healthy persons. The interpretation of positive autoantibody assays (eg, antinuclear antibodies, rheumatoid factor, and antineutrophil cytoplasmic antibodies) may be complicated in patients with HIV. Correlation between the laboratory and clinical findings is important.

ACKNOWLEDGMENTS

We are indebted to Drs. Jeffrey Critchfield and Meg Newman, whose chapter for the previous edition we updated. We appreciate Dr. Philip Seo's insightful review of the manuscript.

REFERENCES

Allison GT, Bostrom MP, Glesby MJ. Osteonecrosis in HIV disease: epidemiology, etiologies, and clinical management. *AIDS.* 2003;17:1. (Detailed review of osteonecrosis in HIV-infected patients.)

Amorosa V, Tebas P. Bone disease and HIV infection. *Clin Infect Dis.* 2006;42:108. (The authors summarize all available data on the association between HIV infection and bone demineralization; they also highlight the latest information linking HAART to bone abnormalities.)

Calabrese LH. Infection with the human immunodeficiency virus type 1 and vascular inflammatory disease. *Clin Exp Rheumatol.* 2004;22(6 Suppl 36):S87. (An outstanding review of all available data on HIV and vasculitis.)

Calabrese LH, Kirchner E, Shrestha R. Rheumatic complications of human immunodeficiency virus infection in the era of highly active antiretroviral therapy: emergence of a new syndrome of immune reconstitution and changing patterns of disease. *Semin Arthritis Rheum.* 2005;35:166.

Mody GM, Parke FA, Reveille JD. Articular manifestations of human immunodeficiency virus infection. *Best Pract Res Clin Rheumatol.* 2003;17:265. (Review of the most recent advances in the epidemiology and clinical features of the different osteoarticular manifestations of HIV infection.)

Restrepo CS, Lemos DF, Gordillo H, et al. Imaging findings in musculoskeletal complications of AIDS. *Radiographics.* 2004;24:1029. (Excellent overview of the radiologic manifestations of common diseases that affect HIV-infected patients.)

Relevant World Wide Web Site

[NIH AIDS information site providing the latest information on antiretroviral medications and HIV treatment guidelines]
http://aidsinfo.nih.gov/

Rheumatic Fever

Preeti Jaggi, MD, & Stanford T. Shulman, MD

Acute rheumatic fever (ARF) is a systemic, immune-mediated disease that is triggered by pharyngeal infection with group A streptococci (GAS). Fever, migratory polyarthritis, and carditis are the most common clinical manifestations. ARF is most frequent among 5–15 year olds with a declining incidence in adults. It is extremely rare in children under age 3, prompting speculation that more than one GAS infection is needed before a host acquires the ability to develop ARF. ARF is not considered a sequela of cutaneous GAS infection.

The pathogenesis of ARF is not clearly understood, but appears to involve an immune response to group A streptococcal antigens that then cross-reacts with human tissue through molecular mimicry. Strains of GAS differ in their ability to trigger ARF, and changes in the prevalence of rheumatogenic strains can affect the incidence of ARF. Recent evidence supports the conclusion that ARF has declined in the United States over the past decades because of a decline in rheumatogenic types of GAS causing pharyngitis.

The reported attack rate of ARF among patients with untreated group A streptococcal pharyngitis is 0.4–3% in epidemic circumstances, with a lower rate endemically. Host genetic factors appear to influence the susceptibility to ARF. Observational studies in the 19th century recognized familial tendencies to develop ARF, and, in the early 1940s, studies showed familial clustering of the disease, with greatest risk occurring in children if both parents had rheumatic heart disease. Genetic susceptibility to develop ARF has been characterized as autosomal recessive or autosomal dominant with variable penetrance and has been linked with several human leukocyte antigen types. Significant increases in the frequency of HLA-DRB1*0701, -DR6, and -DQB1*0201 have been observed in several international studies of rheumatic fever. Monozygotic twins, however, are not usually concordant for ARF, indicating that there are also important environmental factors involved in the pathogenesis of the disease.

Clinical Findings

A. DIAGNOSTIC CRITERIA

In 1944 Dr. T. Duckett Jones developed diagnostic criteria for ARF—the "Jones criteria"—based on his observations of hundreds of patients. The Jones crite-

ria have been revised several times, most recently in 1992 (Table 52–1), and continue to form the basis for the clinical diagnosis of ARF. Exceptions to these criteria include patients who present with chorea or indolent carditis; these patients often do not fulfill the requirement for evidence of antecedent GAS infection because their anti-streptococcal antibody levels usually have returned to normal at the time of presentation.

1. Major clinical criteria—Arthritis occurs in approximately 75% of patients with ARF. The arthritis is migratory, which is in contrast to poststreptococcal reactive arthritis, and polyarticular. The arthritis usually affects the larger joints, especially knees, ankles, wrists, and elbows, and less commonly involves the smaller joints of the hands and feet. The axial skeleton is rarely affected. Inflamed joints are often red, hot, swollen, and exquisitely tender—to the point that even minimal contact with the affected joint can cause exquisite pain. Left untreated, inflammation of an individual joint resolves spontaneously over days, but the polyarthritis persists for 1–4 weeks. The arthritis of ARF responds dramatically to salicylates. This response is so characteristic that the lack of response to salicylate therapy within 48 hours should prompt the clinician to doubt the diagnosis of ARF and to consider other possibilities.

Carditis occurs in approximately 50–60% of ARF cases and accounts for significant morbidity and even mortality. When ARF affects the heart, it usually involves the endocardium, myocardium, and pericardium to varying degrees. Endocarditis leading to mitral and/or aortic valvulitis is most characteristic and occurs most frequently; the tricuspid and pulmonary valves are rarely affected. The revised Jones criteria for ARF require auscultation of a new valvular murmur in order to meet the criterion of "carditis"; echocardiographic findings of valvular regurgitation without a murmur do not fulfill either major or minor criteria. When chronic rheumatic heart disease results, valvular regurgitation can be replaced by valvular stenosis. Myocarditis manifests as tachycardia that is disproportionate to the degree of fever and is persistent even in sleep. Pericarditis is the least common finding in rheumatic carditis. It usually manifests as a pericardial effusion and/or friction rub. The presence of pericarditis in the absence of valvular involvement is

Table 52–1. Modified Jones Criteria for Diagnosis of Acute Rheumatic Fever[a]

Major criteria
   Carditis
   Polyarthritis
   Chorea
   Erythema marginatum
   Subcutaneous nodules
Minor criteria
   Fever
   Arthralgia
   Elevated acute phase reactant (C-reactive protein or
      erythrocyte sedimentation rate)
   Prolonged PR interval on electrocardiogram
Supporting evidence of antecedent group A
   streptococcal infection
   Positive throat culture or rapid antigen test
   Elevated or rising streptococcal antibody titer

[a]Diagnosis requires two major criteria or one major and two minor criteria, plus supporting evidence of antecedent group A streptococcal infection.

unlikely to be due to ARF, and other diagnoses should be explored in this circumstance.

Sydenham chorea (St. Vitus dance), which occurs in 10–15% of patients, is usually a later manifestation of ARF. The characteristic features of chorea are purposeless involuntary movements, incoordination, facial grimacing, and emotional lability. Chorea is a self-limited illness, and full recovery takes several months. Rarely, symptoms can occur over years and are exacerbated by stress, pregnancy, oral contraceptives, and intercurrent illnesses. Chorea is thought to be due to antibodies that cross-react with basal ganglia neurons.

Erythema marginatum occurs in less than 2% of patients. It is an erythematous, flat, serpiginous macular rash with pale central clearing. The rash usually occurs on the trunk and extremities and characteristically spares the face. The rash waxes and wanes and may be transient.

Subcutaneous nodules develop in less than 1% of cases of ARF, most often in those with severe carditis. The nodules are firm, nontender, and usually less than 2 cm in diameter. They are typically located over bony prominences or tendon sheaths. Nodules usually resolve spontaneously without permanent sequelae.

2. Minor clinical criteria—The fever in ARF is usually >39.0°C. It is commonly present at the onset of illness and resolves even without treatment over several weeks. In the absence of frank arthritis, arthralgia fulfills a minor criterion in the revised Jones criteria. Arthralgia may be migratory, and the pain may be severe, even without objective signs of arthritis.

B. DIAGNOSTIC TESTS

Approximately one-third of patients presenting with ARF have no history of a recent symptomatic pharyngeal infection, and therefore it is necessary to find laboratory evidence of a recent GAS infection. This can be done either by obtaining a throat culture or a rapid antigen test for GAS from a throat swab, or by documenting an elevated, or rising, serum anti-streptococcal antibody titer. It is important to recognize that anti-streptococcal antibody levels in the normal population vary by patient age, geographic location, and season of the year.

The anti-streptolysin O titer is the most commonly used streptococcal antibody test to establish a recent streptococcal infection. An anti-streptolysin O titer of 240 Todd units or higher in adults or 320 Todd units or higher in children is considered modestly elevated. Anti-streptolysin O titers above 500 Todd units are uncommon in healthy individuals and therefore would serve as evidence of a recent streptococcal infection.

Because anti-streptolysin O titers can be normal in approximately 20% of ARF patients, other streptococcal antibody tests can be used to establish a recent GAS infection; these include anti-deoxyribonuclease B, anti-streptokinase, and anti-hyaluronidase. If all anti-streptococcal antibody titers are normal on initial presentation, it is advisable to repeat these tests a few weeks later to determine whether the antibody titers rise. Low anti-streptococcal antibody titers found in a single test do not exclude a diagnosis of ARF.

C. SPECIAL TESTS

Aspiration of involved joints of ARF patients with polyarthritis reveals sterile inflammatory synovial fluid, typically with 10,000–100,000 white blood cells/mm^3 and a neutrophil predominance.

The nonclinical minor criteria of the revised Jones criteria include an increased PR interval on electrocardiogram and elevated acute phase reactants (C-reactive protein and/or erythrocyte sedimentation rate). Acute phase reactants are almost always elevated in patients presenting with polyarthritis or acute carditis, but are often normal in patients presenting with chorea alone.

Differential Diagnosis

Like ARF, juvenile rheumatoid arthritis, systemic lupus erythematosus, gonococcal arthritis, reactive arthritis, and serum sickness can cause fever and acute polyarticular arthritis in children. Choreiform movements can occur in systemic lupus erythematosus, neoplasms involving the basal ganglia, Wilson disease, and Huntington disease. Chorea can occasionally be encountered in pregnancy ("chorea gravidarum").

Table 52–2. Treatment of Acute Rheumatic Fever

Anti-inflammatory treatment	
Mild or no carditis	Aspirin 50–100 mg/kg/d in 4 divided doses for 2–4 weeks, then taper over 4–6 weeks
Moderate or severe carditis	Prednisone 2 mg/kg/d in 2 doses for 2–4 weeks, then taper with addition of aspirin when prednisone dose is ≤0.5 mg/kg/d
Primary anti-streptococcal therapy	1.2 million units of benzathine penicillin G IM or oral penicillin or erythromycin for 10 days
Prophylaxis of group A streptococcal infection	1.2 million units of benzathine penicillin G IM every 4 weeks, or sulfadiazine 500 mg PO bid (≤27 kg) or 1 g PO bid (>27 kg), or penicillin V 250 mg PO bid
Medications to control cardiac symptoms (if needed)	Diuretic, angiotensin-converting enzyme inhibitor, and/or cautious use of digoxin
Medications to control chorea (if needed)	Haloperidol or phenobarbital
Bacterial endocarditis prophylaxis	As recommended by the American Heart Association

Table 52–3. Recommendations for Duration of Antimicrobial Prophylaxis in Patients with Acute Rheumatic Fever

Patients with rheumatic fever with carditis and residual heart disease	At least 10 years after the last episode and at least until age 40, sometimes lifelong prophylaxis
Rheumatic fever with carditis but no residual heart disease (no valvular disease)	10 years or well into adulthood, whichever is longer
Rheumatic fever without carditis	5 years or until age 21 years, whichever is longer

ciated with increased severity of cardiac disease or with development of cardiac disease not previously present. All patients with ARF should receive antimicrobial prophylaxis with intramuscular benzathine penicillin G every 4 weeks or twice daily oral penicillin or sulfadiazine (give erythromycin if allergic to penicillin and sulfa). The recommendations for the duration of secondary prophylaxis of streptococcal infection are based upon the likelihood of recurrence and the number of years since the last ARF episode (Table 52–3).

Prognosis

The prognosis of patients with ARF is generally attributable to the degree of cardiac involvement and the recurrence of GAS infection. Patients presenting only with chorea or polyarthritis may subsequently develop rheumatic heart disease if they have recurrent ARF, thus emphasizing the importance of prophylactic antibiotics.

POSTSTREPTOCOCCAL REACTIVE ARTHRITIS

General Considerations

Those patients who do not fulfill the diagnostic criteria for ARF but who have arthritis following streptococcal infection are deemed to have poststreptococcal reactive arthritis (PSRA). This arthritis is predominantly associated with GAS infections, but has also been reported after infection with group C and G streptococci. There appears to be a bimodal age distribution of PSRA, with peak incidence at ages 8–14 years and 21–37 years. In Caucasians, PSRA is associated with the class II HLA antigen DRB1*01.

Treatment

Treatment of ARF requires prevention of future streptococcal infections, anti-inflammatory treatment, and symptomatic care (Table 52–2). Upon diagnosis and regardless of the results of throat cultures for GAS, a dose of benzathine penicillin or 10 days of oral penicillin or erythromycin is recommended. Anti-inflammatory treatment includes oral salicylates (50–100 mg/kg/d) in four daily doses. This is continued for 2–4 weeks, then is gradually tapered over 4–6 weeks. Glucocorticoid treatment should be reserved for those patients with congestive heart failure or at least moderate cardiomegaly on chest radiography. Glucocorticoids are tapered slowly over several weeks; during taper of glucocorticoids, salicylates are added. For patients with Sydenham chorea, haloperidol or phenobarbital may be of some benefit.

Prevention of GAS infection is of utmost importance and prevents recurrent attacks of ARF that can be asso-

Table 52–4. Proposed Criteria for Diagnosis of Poststreptococcal Reactive Arthritis

A. Characteristics of arthritis
1. Acute in onset, symmetric or asymmetric, usually nonmigratory
2. Persistent or recurrent symptoms
3. Lack of a dramatic response to nonsteroidal anti-inflammatory drugs
B. Evidence of an antecedent group A streptococcal infection (by throat culture or rapid antigen test or by elevated or rising anti-streptolysin O and/or anti-deoxyribonuclease B titers)
C. Does not fulfill the modified Jones criteria for acute rheumatic fever

Clinical Findings

PSRA is generally acute and nonmigratory and predominantly affects the large joints of the lower limbs. The arthritis may be monarticular or polyarticular, and symmetric or asymmetric. The axial skeleton is affected in about 20% of patients. Tenosynovitis occasionally occurs. During the antecedent GAS infection, fever and a scarlatiniform rash may be present, but they are not usually present during the time of arthritis. The incubation period between the streptococcal infection and the onset of arthritis is generally shorter than that of ARF (onset usually 3–14 days after infection). The symptoms of PSRA resolve slowly within a few weeks to several months (mean duration of symptoms is 2 months). Recurrences have been reported following a subsequent episode of streptococcal pharyngitis. The most concerning sequela is late-onset carditis, which in the original description developed in 31% of patients 1–18 years after PSRA; these patients did not meet the criteria for ARF and did not have a history of ARF. Other extra-articular manifestations of PSRA include glomerulonephritis (which is very rare with ARF) and uveitis in a minority of patients. PSRA patients have a slower response to therapy with nonsteroidal anti-inflammatory drugs than ARF patients, who typically have a dramatic and prompt response to them.

Diagnostic Criteria

The diagnostic criteria for PSRA are not clearly defined, but the criteria proposed by Ayoub and colleagues are detailed in Table 52–4.

Treatment

Although the response is less dramatic than in ARF, aspirin or other nonsteroidal anti-inflammatory drugs are used to treat symptoms of arthritis. Some experts recommend both a baseline echocardiogram and a follow-up echocardiogram 1 year later because of the concern of occult carditis. The American Heart Association currently recommends that patients with PSRA should receive anti-streptococcal prophylaxis for 1 year, that they should be followed for 1 year to assess for evidence of cardiac involvement, and that treatment should be discontinued after 1 year if no evidence of carditis is found. Penicillin is recommended as first-line therapy, and erythromycin is appropriate for penicillin-allergic patients. Some experts suggest that the same prophylaxis recommendations for ARF patients also should apply to PSRA because the onset of documented carditis in PSRA is widely variable, but this recommendation has not been endorsed by the American Heart Association or other organizations.

REFERENCES

Ayoub EM, Ahmed S. Update on complications of group A streptococcal infections. *Curr Prob Pediatr.* 1997;27:90. (Proposed criteria for poststreptococcal arthritis.)

Crea MA, Mortimer EA. The nature of scarlatinal arthritis. *Pediatrics.* 1959;23:879. (Original description of poststreptococcal arthritis.)

Dajani A, Taubert K, Ferrieri P, Peter G, Shulman ST. Treatment of acute streptococcal pharyngitis and prevention of rheumatic fever: a statement for health professionals. *Pediatrics.* 1995;96:758. (American Heart Association guidelines for treatment of rheumatic fever.)

Mackie SL, Keat A. Poststreptococcal reactive arthritis: what is it and how do we know? *Rheumatology.* 2004;43:949. (Review of 188 cases in the medical literature of poststreptococcal arthritis and details clinical and epidemiologic trends in patients.)

Shulman ST, Stollerman G, Beall B, Dale JB, Tanz RR. Temporal changes in streptococcal M protein types and the near disappearance of acute rheumatic fever in the U.S. *Clin Infec Dis.* 2006;42:441.

Special Writing Group of the Committee on Rheumatic Fever, Endocarditis, and Kawasaki Disease of the Council on Cardiovascular Diseases in the Young of the American Heart Association. Guidelines for the diagnosis of rheumatic fever. Jones criteria, 1992 update. *JAMA.* 1992;268:2069. (Most recent American Heart Association revision of the Jones criteria for ARF with detailed clinical descriptions of criteria.)

Stollerman GH. Rheumatic fever in the 21st century. *Clin Infect Dis.* 2001;33:806. (Gives historical perspective on ARF and the diagnostic criteria, and describes the etiology and pathogenesis of ARF.)

SECTION VII

Rheumatic Manifestations of Systemic Disease

Sarcoidosis

53

Edward S. Chen, MD, & David R. Moller, MD

ESSENTIALS OF DIAGNOSIS

- *Systemic disease due to noncaseating epithelioid granulomatous inflammation in affected organs.*
- *Most frequently affected organs are lung, lymph nodes, eyes, skin, liver, joints, heart, muscles, upper airway, kidneys, and central and peripheral nervous system.*
- *More common and severe in African Americans in the U.S.*
- *Diagnosis requires a consistent clinical picture and a biopsy with typical noncaseating granulomas, excluding diseases that can cause similar granulomatous reactions.*

Epidemiology

Sarcoidosis is found worldwide with a prevalence ranging from 10–80 cases per 100,000 in North America and Europe. In the United States, the lifetime risk for developing sarcoidosis is greater in African Americans (2.4%) than in Caucasians (0.85%). Worldwide there is a slight female predominance. Although all ages can be affected, most cases occur between the ages of 20 and 40 years, with a second peak incidence in women over age 50.

Genetics

A genetic predisposition to sarcoidosis is supported by familial clustering in approximately 5–10% of cases of sarcoidosis. A recent multicenter study on the etiology of sarcoidosis in the United States (ACCESS) suggests that the familial relative risk is approximately 5.0 among first-degree relatives, and that this risk is higher in Caucasian families compared with African-American families.

Two recent genome-wide linkage analyses identified an association with the butyrophilin-like 2 gene (*BTNL2*), located within the major histocompatibility locus on chromosome 6, in both Caucasians and African Americans with sarcoidosis.

Etiology

The cause of sarcoidosis is uncertain. The genetic pattern of inheritance suggests that susceptibility to sarcoidosis is polygenic and interacts significantly with environmental factors. Geographic differences in disease prevalence and reports of time-space clustering of cases have also suggested that sarcoidosis may be associated with an environmental, likely microbial exposure. Despite the study's large enrollment, the ACCESS study found no evidence for a single dominant environmental or occupational exposure associated with an increased risk of developing sarcoidosis. Multiple regression analyses found positive associations with modest odds ratios of approximately 1.5 for exposures to molds and mildews, insecticides, or musty odors at work. The ACCESS data supported a negative association of tobacco use or tobacco smoke exposure among sarcoidosis patients. Further studies are necessary to understand the contribution of environmental factors on the development of sarcoidosis.

Since the first description of sarcoidosis, many have speculated that a potential microbial cause of sarcoidosis exists, with mycobacterial and propionibacterial organisms most frequently implicated in laboratory-based studies of sarcoidosis. Recently, a limited proteomic approach identified the mycobacterial catalase-peroxidase protein as a potential pathogenic antigen, supporting a mycobacterial etiology of sarcoidosis.

Pathophysiology

While the etiology of sarcoidosis remains to be elucidated, there is consensus that the pathogenesis of sarcoidosis involves a response to an antigenic stimulus. This antigen-specific T-cell response is polarized towards a T-helper 1 response with expression of interferon-γ and the T-helper 1 immunomodulatory cytokines interleukin-12 and interleukin-18. This response triggers the release of proinflammatory cytokines such as

tumor necrosis factor (TNF), interleukin-1, interleukin-6, and a host of chemokines that orchestrate the granulomatous response. Dysregulated expression of T-helper 1 immunomodulatory cytokines has been hypothesized to contribute to the persistence of the granulomatous inflammation in sarcoidosis.

Clinical Features

The clinical features of sarcoidosis are protean and varied. Initial presentations of sarcoidosis usually have prevailing features of either acute sarcoidosis, pulmonary involvement, or extrapulmonary involvement.

A. SYMPTOMS AND SIGNS

1. Acute sarcoidosis (Löfgren syndrome)—This well-defined syndrome of acute sarcoidosis is characterized by erythema nodosum, bilateral hilar adenopathy, and often polyarthritis and uveitis (Figures 53–1 and 53–2). Löfgren syndrome is common among Scandinavians and Irish women but occurs in fewer than 5% of African-American patients with sarcoidosis. Acute sarcoidosis without erythema nodosum may also occur.

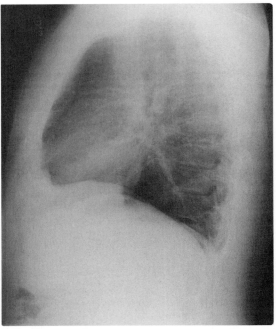

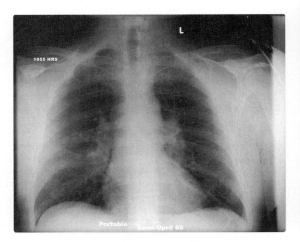

Figure 53–1. Bilateral hilar adenopathy. Posteroanterior and lateral chest x-ray films from a patient experiencing mild dyspnea, dry cough, fevers, and weight loss show bilateral hilar adenopathy and right paratracheal adenopathy. Noncaseating granulomatous inflammation was revealed by bronchoscopy with transbronchial lung biopsy and needle aspiration of the subcarinal adenopathy, providing a diagnosis of sarcoidosis.

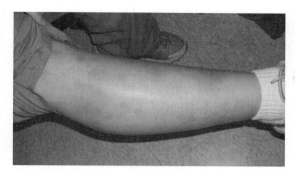

Figure 53–2. Erythema nodosum. These erythematosus plaques are tender and warm to the touch. The constellation of erythema nodosum, bilateral hilar adenopathy, polyarthritis, and often uveitis is a form of acute sarcoidosis called Löfgren syndrome. (Douglas Hoffman, MD, Dermatlas; http://www.dermatlas.org. With permission.)

2. Pulmonary sarcoidosis—The most common symptoms are progressive shortness of breath, nonproductive cough, and chest discomfort (Table 53–1). Chronic sputum production and hemoptysis are more frequent in advanced fibrocystic disease. Typically, there are few physical findings of pulmonary sarcoidosis, with lung crackles heard in fewer than 20% of patients. Clubbing is rare. Airway obstruction is usually fixed (unresponsive to bronchodilators) and observed in a minority of patients, although frank wheezing is an unusual finding.

Pulmonary hypertension or **cor pulmonale** are seen in up to 5% of patients, usually due to severe fibrocystic sarcoidosis, or rarely, a granulomatous pulmonary vasculitis. It is always important to exclude other causes of pulmonary hypertension, such as sleep-disordered breathing or chronic thromboembolic disease, which require different therapeutic approaches. The finding of pulmonary hypertension with sarcoidosis is associated with higher rates of mortality.

3. Ocular manifestations—**Uveitis** is the most common eye lesion in sarcoidosis and may be the initial presenting manifestation. The uveitis is more commonly anterior, may be unilateral or bilateral, and is frequently associated with bilateral hilar adenopathy. Chronic uveitis occurs in as many as 20% of patients with chronic sarcoidosis and is more common in the African-American population. **Granulomatous conjunctivitis** appears as a granular or cobblestonelike appearance of the conjunctivae. Conjunctival nodules are also a common finding. **Optic neuritis** or **retinitis** may present dramatically with blindness. Severe chorioretinitis occurs uncommonly.

4. Chronic cutaneous sarcoidosis—Sarcoidosis commonly involves the skin (20–30%) and may be severe, especially in patients of African descent. Cutaneous

Table 53–1. Clinical Features of Sarcoidosis

Clinically-Evident Organ System Involvement (%)	Major Clinical Features
Pulmonary (70–90%)	Bilateral hilar adenopathy, restrictive and obstructive disease, reticulonodular infiltrates, fibrocystic disease, bronchiectasis, mycetomas
Ocular (20–30%)	Anterior and posterior uveitis, optic neuritis, chorioretinitis, conjunctival nodules, glaucoma, keratoconjunctivitis, lacrimal gland enlargement
Cutaneous (20–30%)	Erythema nodosum, lupus pernio, cutaneous and subcutaneous nodules, plaques, alopecia, dactylitis
Hematologic (20–30%)	Peripheral lymphadenopathy, splenomegaly, hypersplenism, anemia, lymphopenia
Musculoskeletal and joints (10–20%)	Arthralgias, bone cysts, myopathy, heel pain, Achilles tendinitis, sacroiliitis
Hepatic (10–20%)	Hepatomegaly, pruritus, jaundice, cirrhosis
Salivary and parotid gland (10%)	Sicca syndrome, Heerfordt syndrome
Sinuses and upper respiratory tract (SURT) (5–10%)	Chronic sinusitis, nasal congestion, saddle-nose deformity, hoarseness, laryngeal or tracheal obstruction
Cardiac (5–10%)	Arrhythmias, heart block, cardiomyopathy, sudden death
Neurologic (5–10%)	Cranial neuropathy, aseptic meningitis, mass brain lesion, hydrocephalus, myelopathy, polyneuropathy, mononeuritis multiplex
Gastrointestinal (<10%)	Abdominal pain, GI tract dysmotility, pancreatitis
Endocrine (<10%)	Hypercalcemia, hypopituitarism, diabetes insipidus, epididymitis, testicular mass
Renal (<5%)	Hypercalciuria, renal calculi, nephrocalcinosis, interstitial nephritis, renal failure

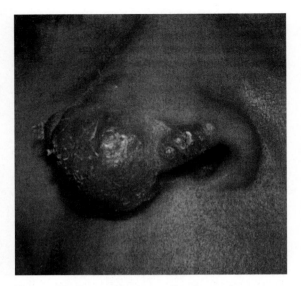

Figure 53–3. Lupus pernio. This form of cutaneous eruption in sarcoidosis is typified by violaceous plaques and nodules that involve the nose, nasal alae, malar areas, nasolabial folds, areas around the eyes, the scalp, and along the hairline. (Bernard Cohen, MD, Dermatlas; http://www.dermatlas.org. With permission.)

nodules, plaques, and subcutaneous nodules, typically located around the hairline, eyelids, ears, nose, mouth, and extensor surfaces of the arms and legs, are common. **Lupus pernio** is a particularly disfiguring form of cutaneous sarcoidosis of the face with violaceous plaques and nodules covering the nose, nasal alae, malar areas, and around the eyes (Figure 53–3).

5. Sarcoidosis of the upper respiratory tract (SURT)—This manifestation occurs in 5–10% of patients, usually in those with long-standing disease. Severe nasal congestion and chronic sinusitis usually are unresponsive to decongestants and topical (intranasal) steroids. Chronic disease or surgical intervention may result in destruction of the nasal septum and a saddle-nose deformity. Laryngeal sarcoidosis may present with severe hoarseness, stridor, and acute respiratory failure secondary to upper airway obstruction. Often, SURT is associated with chronic skin lesions, particularly lupus pernio.

6. Cardiac sarcoidosis—Although myocardial sarcoidosis is diagnosed in fewer than 10% of patients in the United States and Europe, autopsy series suggest that the histologic presence of sarcoidosis in the heart may be as high as 25%. In Japan, cardiac sarcoidosis occurs in nearly 50% of sarcoidosis patients. Arrhythmia, heart block, dilated cardiomyopathy, or sudden death can be the presenting clinical manifestations. Endomyocardial biopsies fail to demonstrate granulomatous inflammation in 80% of cases due to sampling inefficiencies in the setting of patchy inflammatory involvement. A diagnosis of cardiac sarcoidosis can be inferred from a combination of biopsy-proven systemic sarcoidosis and a compatible myocardial imaging study, such as a thallium or sestamibi scan, cardiac magnetic resonance imaging with gadolinium contrast, or positron emission tomography scan.

7. Neurosarcoidosis—This manifestation occurs in 5–10% of patients with sarcoidosis. The most common manifestation is cranial neuropathy with bilateral or unilateral seventh nerve (Bell) palsy or less commonly, glossopharyngeal, auditory, oculomotor, or trigeminal palsies. The palsies may resolve spontaneously or with glucocorticoid therapy but may recur years later. Optic neuritis can result in blurred vision, field defects, and blindness. Other manifestations include mass lesions, aseptic meningitis, obstructive hydrocephalus, and hypothalamic-pituitary dysfunction. Seizures, headache, change in mental status, confusion, and diabetes insipidus can be initial manifestations of sarcoidosis. Spinal cord involvement is rare, but paraparesis, hemiparesis, and back and leg pains may occur. Peripheral neuropathies account for about 15% of cases of neurosarcoidosis, often presenting as mononeuritis multiplex or a primary sensory neuropathy. Recently, small-fiber neuropathy has been implicated as a cause of chronic pain in sarcoidosis.

8. Gastrointestinal sarcoidosis—Although a liver biopsy demonstrates granulomatous inflammation in over 50% of patients, clinically significant liver involvement is documented in only 10–20% of patients and is rarely the sole manifestation of this disease. Active hepatic inflammation may be associated with fever, tender hepatomegaly, and pruritus. Characteristically, the serum alkaline phosphatase and γ-glutamyltransferase are elevated disproportionately higher than the transaminases or bilirubin. This is often part of a constellation of hepatic, spleen, and bone marrow involvement with or without hypercalcemia, sometimes referred to as "abdominal sarcoidosis." Elevated serum liver function tests frequently revert to normal spontaneously or after treatment with glucocorticoids. Progressive cirrhosis may occur if severe, persistent granulomatous hepatitis is not treated.

Symptomatic gastrointestinal involvement in sarcoidosis is rare, and other causes such as Crohn disease or ulcerative colitis must be excluded.

9. Musculoskeletal sarcoidosis—Systemic constitutional symptoms such as fever, malaise, and weight loss are seen in over 20% of patients and may be disabling. **Arthralgias** are common in active multisystem sarcoidosis, although joint radiographs are usually normal. Acute, often incapacitating polyarthritis involving the ankles, feet, knees, and wrists is commonly seen in patients with Löfgren syndrome; usually the polyarthritis regresses within weeks to several months with or without therapy. Persistent joint disease is found in fewer than 5% of patients with chronic sarcoidosis. Pain, swelling, and tenderness of the phalanges (sausage digit) of the hands and feet are most common.

Although random muscle biopsies in autopsy series often demonstrate muscle granulomas in patients with sarcoidosis, symptomatic myopathy with weakness and tenderness is uncommon. Rarely, sarcoidosis can present as a polymyositis with profound weakness and elevated serum creatine kinase and aldolase levels.

Fibromyalgia may be associated with sarcoidosis and causes considerable morbidity in such patients, and does not respond to immunosuppressive therapy. Small-fiber neuropathy may also be a contributor to chronic pain seen in patients with sarcoidosis.

10. Salivary, parotid, and lacrimal gland sarcoidosis—Parotid or lacrimal gland enlargement or sicca syndrome can occasionally be the dominant clinical manifestations of sarcoidosis. Heerfordt syndrome, or uveoparotid fever, is an uncommon acute presentation of sarcoidosis manifesting as fever, parotid and lacrimal gland enlargement, uveitis, bilateral hilar adenopathy, and often cranial neuropathies.

11. Hematologic sarcoidosis—Peripheral lymph node enlargement occurs in 20–30% of patients as an early manifestation of sarcoidosis but then typically undergoes spontaneous remission. Persistent, bulky lymphadenopathy occurs less than 10% of the time. Splenomegaly, occasionally massive, occurs in fewer than 5% of cases and is often associated with hepatomegaly and hypercalcemia. Polyclonal hypergammaglobulinemia is present in 25% or more of patients. Anemia and peripheral lymphopenia are relatively common, while leukopenia and thrombocytopenia are rare. A clinical association exists between sarcoidosis and common variable immunodeficiency; common variable immunodeficiency should be suspected in patients with sarcoidosis who develop increased frequency of infections or hypogammaglobulinemia, both of which are unusual in sarcoidosis.

12. Endocrine abnormalities in sarcoidosis—Hypercalcemia and hypercalciuria are thought to be due to an increased conversion of 1-OH vitamin D_3 to the active $1,25(OH)_2$ vitamin D_3 by macrophages and epithelioid cells from granulomas. In patients with neurosarcoidosis, disturbances to the hypothalamic-pituitary axis may result in diabetes insipidus and other endocrinologic and autonomic problems. Associations have been made between sarcoidosis and autoimmune thyroid disease. Biopsy-confirmed pancreatic involvement is a rare manifestation.

13. Renal involvement in sarcoidosis—Manifestations include direct consequences of hypercalcemia, such as kidney stones or nephrocalcinosis, which can result in significant impairment of renal function. Direct granulomatous involvement of the kidneys causing membranous glomerulonephritis or chronic interstitial nephritis is rare and usually not a cause of renal failure.

14. Psychosocial abnormalities—As many as 30–60% of patients with sarcoidosis report symptoms of depression. One study found this to be associated with female gender, lower socioeconomic status, poor access to health care, and increased disease severity, but not race.

Clinical Assessment & Tests

An initial diagnostic evaluation should consist of tests to evaluate the presence and extent of pulmonary involvement and screen for extrathoracic disease (Table 53–2). Specialized testing is indicated when symptoms or signs suggest extrapulmonary involvement.

A. Imaging Studies

Chest radiographs are abnormal in 90% or more of patients with sarcoidosis and are assigned a category (stage)

Table 53–2. Recommended Tests for an Initial Evaluation of Sarcoidosis

Chest radiograph
Pulmonary function tests
    Spirometry with flow-volume loops (if upper airway obstruction is suspected)
    Diffusion capacity
    Lung volumes
Ophthalmologic examination
Blood work
    Comprehensive metabolic panel
    Renal function
    Liver function
    Serum calcium level
    Complete blood count with differential
Electrocardiogram
Screen for tuberculosis exposure with purified protein derivative skin test
Additional organ-specific tests may be indicated in patients with specific extrapulmonary symptoms. For example:
    Cardiac: echocardiogram, Holter monitor, thallium or sestamibi myocardial scan, cardiac magnetic resonance imaging (MRI), cardiac positron emission tomography scan
    Neurologic: contrast MRI, nerve conduction study, lumbar puncture

based on an internationally acknowledged system devised by Scadding:

0: Normal chest radiograph (extrapulmonary sarcoidosis)

I: Bilateral hilar adenopathy (see Figure 53–1)

II: Bilateral hilar adenopathy plus interstitial infiltrates

III: Interstitial infiltrates only

IV: Fibrocystic lung disease

More unusual findings associated with pulmonary sarcoidosis include large, well-defined nodular infiltrates, miliary disease, a pattern of patchy air space consolidation with air bronchograms (termed "alveolar sarcoidosis"), or the presence of mycetomas. Differential diagnoses often include mycobacterial or fungal infection, malignancy, or Wegener granulomatosis. Pleural effusions and pneumothoraces are unusual in sarcoidosis.

Chest computed tomography typically demonstrates nodular infiltrates that follow central bronchovascular structures, but other patterns including honeycombing may be seen.

Nuclear medicine studies, such as 67-gallium scanning and positron emission tomography using 18-fluorodeoxyglucose, have been used as methods to detect active inflammatory sites in sarcoidosis, potentially aiding in choosing sites for biopsy. 18-Fluorodeoxyglucose positron emission tomography uses less radiation exposure while offering better resolution and has largely replaced gallium scanning. Classic findings using gallium scanning are uptake in the bilateral hilar and right paratracheal lymph node region ("lambda" sign) of the lungs, and uptake in the parotids or lacrimal and salivary glands ("panda" sign). The combination of signs (lambda-panda) is suggestive of sarcoidosis.

Joint radiographs may demonstrate "punched out" lesions with cystic changes and marked loss of trabeculae but without evidence of erosive chondritis (Figure 53–4). Cystic lesions of the long bones, pelvis, sternum, skull, and vertebrae rarely occur.

Magnetic resonance imaging with gadolinium contrast enhancement has an important role in the evaluation of neurosarcoidosis, particularly in cases of suspected brain, cranial nerve, or spinal cord involvement.

B. LABORATORY STUDIES

Recommended initial studies for all patients with presumed or biopsy-proven sarcoidosis include the following:

- A comprehensive metabolic panel is useful to assess renal function, calcium level, and liver function. Abnormalities may reflect additional manifestations of sarcoidosis, but further work-up for other causes is usually warranted.
- The complete blood cell count is usually either normal or demonstrates peripheral lymphopenia.

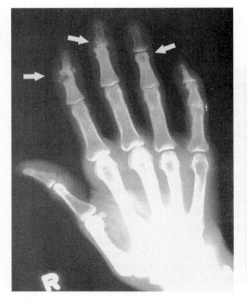

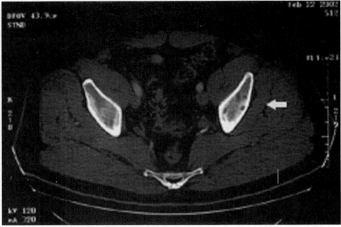

Figure 53–4. Bone involvement in sarcoidosis. Multiple focal "punched-out" lesions (arrows) on a plain x-ray film of the hand (William Herring, MD; http://www.learningradiology.com. With permission.) and from a computed tomography scan of the pelvis (arrow) that are typical for skeletal manifestations of sarcoidosis.

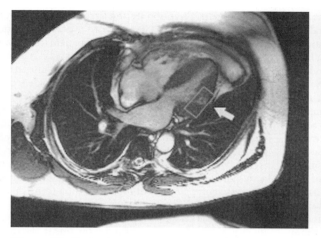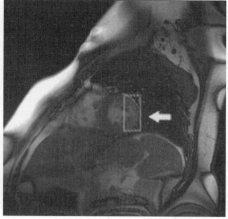

Figure 53–5. Cardiac sarcoidosis. Cardiac magnetic resonance imaging demonstrates gadolinium enhancement in the submyocardial region (arrows) in a patient with cardiac sarcoidosis and non-sustained ventricular tachycardia.

Pancytopenia may be caused by hypersplenism or bone marrow infiltration with granulomas.

C. PULMONARY FUNCTION TESTING

Pulmonary function tests may show restrictive, obstructive, or combined impairment with a parallel reduction in diffusing capacity of carbon monoxide. Gas exchange is usually preserved until extensive fibrocystic changes are evident.

Bronchoalveolar lavage fluid in sarcoidosis is typically characterized by increased proportions and numbers of activated CD4+ alveolar lymphocytes reflective of enhanced cell-mediated immune processes at sites of granuloma formation. These findings are not specific for sarcoidosis and do not predict clinical outcome.

D. OTHER TESTS

A well-recognized feature of sarcoidosis is the impaired cutaneous response to common antigens that elicit delayed-type hypersensitivity reactions, seen in 30–70% of patients. Since anergy to purified protein derivative testing is common in sarcoidosis, active tuberculosis must be strongly considered in any patient in whom a positive tuberculin skin test develops. Purified protein derivative status should be reviewed in all patients prior to beginning immunosuppressive therapy.

An electrocardiogram is routinely performed to screen for conduction abnormalities, which may signal the presence of early cardiac sarcoidosis. When cardiac sarcoidosis is suspected on the basis of symptoms or electrocardiographic abnormalities, Holter monitoring, two-dimensional echocardiography, and radionuclide imaging with gated 201-thallium scanning are indicated to detect myocardial or conduction abnormalities. Electrophysiologic testing may be indicated to exclude arrhythmias undetected by routine studies. If the suspicion for cardiac involvement is high, cardiac magnetic resonance imaging or cardiac positron emission tomography may prove to have greater sensitivity in detecting cardiac sarcoidosis (Figure 53–5).

In patients with suspected neurosarcoidosis, magnetic resonance imaging with gadolinium enhancement of the brain or spine is indicated. The characteristic inflammatory lesions by contrast magnetic resonance imaging have a propensity for periventricular and leptomeningeal areas. These findings are nonspecific and can be produced by infectious (tuberculosis or fungal disease) or malignant (lymphoma or carcinomatosis) disease. A normal scan does not exclude neurosarcoidosis, particularly for cranial neuropathies, peripheral neuropathies, or in the presence of glucocorticoid therapy.

In neurosarcoidosis, the cerebrospinal fluid may demonstrate lymphocytic pleocytosis or elevated protein levels, providing supportive evidence of central nervous system or spinal cord inflammation. A diagnosis of neurosarcoidosis is usually confirmed by biopsy of a non–central nervous system site, generally by bronchoscopic or lymph node biopsy. Rarely, a brain or spinal cord biopsy is needed to exclude infectious or malignant disease. In suspected cases of peripheral neuropathy or myopathy, electromyography or nerve conduction studies are often indicated.

E. DIAGNOSTIC EXAMINATIONS

Identifying the extent of specific organ involvement requires a careful review of localizing symptoms in the setting of biopsy-confirmed granulomatous inflammation. Biopsy of the easiest, most accessible abnormal tissue site is used for confirmation of the diagnosis and to exclude infection, malignancy, or other diseases that have similar clinical manifestations. Biopsy of a skin nodule, superficial lymph node, nasal mucosa, conjunctiva, or salivary gland (lip biopsy) sometimes can establish a diagnosis. Biopsy by fiberoptic bronchoscopy is frequently used to diagnose pulmonary sarcoidosis because of its relative safety and high yield. Endobronchial or transbronchial needle aspiration biopsies may increase the yield further. Biopsy of the liver or bone marrow is nonspecific and should be used to support a diagnosis of sarcoidosis only after malignancy, infectious granulomatous diseases, or other organ-specific diagnoses are excluded. Mediastinoscopy or surgical lung biopsy (open-lung or thoracoscopic) should be considered in cases in whom lymphoma or other intrathoracic malignancy cannot be reasonably excluded. In rare cases, biopsy of critical organs may be necessary to exclude malignancy, such as when sarcoidosis presents as a mass lesion in the brain. Biopsy confirmation of sarcoidosis is usually not necessary in Löfgren syndrome except in regions where histoplasmosis is endemic, and fungal infection must be excluded before initiating glucocorticoid therapy.

Differential Diagnosis

A diagnosis of sarcoidosis is based on a compatible clinical picture, histologic evidence of noncaseating granulomas, and the absence of other known causes of this pathologic response, such as tuberculosis, fungal diseases, and chronic beryllium disease.

Prognosis & Clinical Course

Although sarcoidosis can potentially involve any part of the body, the extent of significant organ system involvement is usually evident within the first 2 years after diagnosis. The recent ACCESS study found that fewer than 25% of the study patients developed *new* evidence for disease in one or more organ systems.

More than 90% of patients with sarcoidosis can be expected to have either a remitting course or a chronic progressive course. It is estimated from various studies that approximately 50–80% of all patients may have a remitting course, which is usually evident within the first 2–3 years following diagnosis. Acute sarcoidosis (Löfgren's syndrome) has the highest remission rate of greater than 70%. Patients with fibrocystic pulmonary sarcoidosis, lupus pernio, nasal or sinus sarcoidosis, neurosarcoidosis, cardiac sarcoidosis, or who have multisystem disease for more than 2–3 years usually will have unremitting, chronic disease.

Such generalizations are not certainties, and careful follow-up for at least several years' (>2–3) duration is necessary to confirm whether a patient has remitting or chronic active sarcoidosis. A waxing and waning course of sarcoidosis is unusual except in patients with ocular, neurologic, peripheral lymph node, or cutaneous involvement. It is important to consider nonsarcoidosis causes of new medical problems that emerge following a long period of clinical stability, either after established disease remission or chronic active disease maintained on a stable regimen. Long-term follow-up is also important to ensure that patients with chronic active disease receive adequate treatment to minimize progressive impairment of organ function from chronic inflammation.

No biomarkers have been found to be useful in predicting outcomes or to assist in treatment decisions. Serum angiotensin-converting enzyme is elevated in 30–80% of patients with clinically active disease. The test has positive and negative predictive values of less than 70–80%, and serum angiotensin-converting enzyme levels do not predict clinical course. Thus, most clinicians agree this test is of limited usefulness in the management of sarcoidosis.

Treatment

A consensus view offers the following indications for treatment:

- Persistent, symptomatic, or progressive pulmonary disease.
- Threatened organ failure, such as severe ocular, central nervous system, or cardiac disease.
- Persistent hypercalcemia or renal or hepatic dysfunction.
- Posterior uveitis or anterior uveitis not responding to localized glucocorticoid therapy.
- Pituitary disease.
- Myopathy.
- Significant splenomegaly or evidence of hypersplenism such as thrombocytopenia.
- Severe fatigue and weight loss.
- Disfiguring skin disease or lymphadenopathy.

A. Medical

1. Glucocorticoids—This class of drugs is the cornerstone of therapy for serious progressive pulmonary or extrapulmonary sarcoidosis (Table 53–3). Guidelines for when to initiate therapy with glucocorticoids and proper dosing have been formulated from extensive clinical experience without being subjected to well-controlled prospective clinical trials. Controversy exists regarding their overall effectiveness in altering the long-term course

Table 53–3. Treatment of Sarcoidosis

Drug	Typical Dose	Major Adverse Effects
Glucocorticoids	Prednisone 20–40 mg/d for 2 wk: decrease by 5 mg every 2 wk until 10–15 mg/d; maintain for 8–12 mo, then taper 2.5 mg/d every 2–4 wk; reinstitute for relapse	Weight gain, hypertension, hyperglycemia, osteoporosis, cataracts, psychosis
Antimalarial drugs Hydroxychloroquine	200 mg once or twice daily	Ocular toxicity. gastrointestinal upset, rashes, hair loss
Chloroquine	250 mg once a day (or 500 mg every other day) for 6 mo followed by 6-mo drug holiday	Ocular toxicity, gastrointestinal upset
Minocycline, doxycycline	100 mg twice daily	Gastrointestinal upset, skin hyperpigmentation, headaches, dizziness, pseudotumor cerebri
Other immunomodulatory drugs Pentoxifylline	400 mg 3 or 4 times a day	Gastrointestinal upset, headaches
Thalidomide	100–200 mg once at bedtime	Teratogenicity, peripheral neuropathy, sedation
Methotrexate	10–20 mg per week PLUS folate 1 mg daily	Hepatic, pulmonary, bone marrow toxicity
Other immunosuppressant drugs Mycophenolate mofetil	1000–2000 mg per day	Bone marrow and hepatic toxicity, gastrointestinal upset, ?Oncogenic potential
Azathioprine	100–200 mg per day	Bone marrow and hepatic toxicity, gastrointestinal upset, ?Oncogenic potential
Anti–tumor necrosis factor agents	Infliximab, adalimumab: dosing varies	Hypersensitivity reaction, severe infection, reactivation tuberculosis, autoimmune phenomena

of the disease. However, clinical experience indicates that glucocorticoids provide prompt symptomatic relief and reverse organ dysfunction in almost all patients with active inflammation. The optimal dose and duration of steroid treatment have not been established by rigorous clinical studies. Topical steroids are usually ineffective except for specific cases of ocular sarcoidosis. Most studies find inhaled steroids for pulmonary sarcoidosis to be ineffective, and only a minority of patients with airway obstruction will demonstrate meaningful responses to bronchodilators.

In general, initial treatment with glucocorticoids should be planned for a period of 8–12 months, except for Löfgren syndrome. In those patients with chronic active disease, a stable maintenance regimen of low-dose glucocorticoids is more effective at preserving lung function than symptomatic use of glucocorticoids followed by repeated aggressive tapering regimens. Existing scarring is not amenable to treatment.

Other medications that are used to treat sarcoidosis have variable efficacy in different individual patients, and may require low doses of glucocorticoids to achieve sufficient suppression of inflammation.

2. Antimalarial drugs—Hydroxychloroquine and chloroquine are used as first-line drugs for dominant skin, nasal mucosal, and sinus sarcoidosis, but have not been consistently effective for pulmonary or systemic disease. Hypercalcemia and laryngeal, bone, and joint involvement have been reported to respond to either hydroxychloroquine or chloroquine. Hydroxychloroquine is usually preferred because of the greater risk for ocular toxicity with chloroquine. Serial ophthalmologic evaluations should be performed during therapy with either drug.

3. Minocycline and doxycycline—These tetracycline derivatives have anti-inflammatory properties. The relatively safe side-effect profile of these medications makes them a reasonable choice for nonthreatening manifestations of sarcoidosis, such as skin lesions, but clinical experience suggests that these drugs usually are not effective in pulmonary or severe multiorgan sarcoidosis.

4. Other immunomodulatory drugs—Pentoxifylline and thalidomide may be effective as glucocorticoid-sparing therapies in only a small subset of patients. Since these medications have significant potential side effects, they are considered second- or third-line drugs for non-threatening manifestations of sarcoidosis.

5. Methotrexate—This drug has been reported to be effective in 50–70% of patients, either as a sole agent or with small doses of glucocorticoids, for the treatment of serious systemic sarcoidosis. In contrast to glucocorticoids that typically induce evident improvement within several days to a few weeks, methotrexate may require up to 6 months or longer to demonstrate clinical effectiveness. The major toxicities of methotrexate may preclude its use in patients with significant liver disease or advanced renal or lung disease.

6. Other immunosuppressive drugs—Azathioprine and more recently mycophenolate mofetil have been commonly used to treat severe extrapulmonary sarcoidosis and pulmonary sarcoidosis that are not well controlled with lower doses of glucocorticoids or when there are unacceptable steroid side effects. Benefits of these drugs have not been established by rigorous clinical trials.

7. Tumor necrosis factor (TNF) inhibitors—There is evidence supporting the effectiveness of anti-TNF therapies in sarcoidosis. Laboratory experiments demonstrate that TNF plays an important role in granuloma formation. A recent large, randomized multicenter Phase II prospective study found that a 24-week course of treatment with infliximab was associated with an improvement in lung function (mean improvement in forced vital capacity of 2.5%). The significant risk for acquiring severe infections, reactivation of indolent infections, and potential risk for malignancy and autoimmune phenomena suggest that anti-TNF agents should be reserved for the most serious cases of sarcoidosis. Further studies are needed to assess their efficacy in different clinical presentations before they can be routinely recommended.

B. SURGICAL

Successful lung, heart-lung, and liver transplantations have been performed in a small number of patients with advanced organ insufficiency. Noncaseating granulomas may develop in the transplanted organs in some lung (and heart) transplant patients but do not seem to have a major impact on overall survival. Heart transplantation for end-stage sarcoidosis cardiomyopathy has also been successful in a small number of patients, although experience remains limited.

Complications

Major causes of death from sarcoidosis include respiratory insufficiency and cor pulmonale, massive hemoptysis, complications from cardiac sarcoidosis, neurosarcoidosis, or uremia from chronic renal failure. Several centers in the United States and Great Britain suggest that race is an important prognostic indicator, with African-American and West Indian patients more likely to have chronic persistent disease and suffer from increased morbidity and mortality. Hospital statistics suggest that sarcoidosis is the direct cause of death in 1–5% of persons admitted with this disease.

When to Refer to a Specialist

A patient should be referred to a specialist in sarcoidosis under the following circumstances:

- Uncertainty of the diagnosis or clinical course.
- Uncertainty whether treatment is indicated.
- Disease that is not responding as expected to therapy.
- Severe extrapulmonary involvement such as cardiac, neurologic, skin, or sinus involvement.
- Unsure about the use of glucocorticoid-sparing or alternative medications.

REFERENCES

Baughman RP, ed. TITLE? Vol. 210. Marcel Dekker, 2005. (A comprehensive and updated reference for many aspects of sarcoidosis ranging from the basic science and pathophysiology of the disease to patient evaluation and treatment.)

Baughman RP, Lynch JP. Difficult treatment issues in sarcoidosis. *J Intern Med.* 2003;253:41. [PMID: 12588537] (A clinical overview of the treatment of sarcoidosis, including a discussion of the role of anti-TNF agents.)

Chapelon-Abric C, de Zuttere D, Duhaut P, et al. Cardiac sarcoidosis: a retrospective study of 41 cases. *Medicine (Baltimore).* 2004;83:315. [PMID: 15525844] (A summary of fifteen years' experience with patients with cardiac sarcoidosis.)

Drent M, Costabel U, eds. *Sarcoidosis.* Vol. 10, Monograph 32. The Charlesworth Group, 2005. (A compendium of the current understanding of sarcoidosis by internationally recognized experts.)

Johns CJ, Michele TM. The clinical management of sarcoidosis. A 50-year experience at the Johns Hopkins Hospital. *Medicine (Baltimore).* 1999;78:65. [PMID: 1019591] (This summary of a 50-year clinical experience offers one of the most comprehensive clinical reviews of this disease.)

Moller DR. Treatment of sarcoidosis—from a basic science point of view. *J Intern Med.* 2003;253:31. [PMID: 12588536] (A review of the scientific foundations for our current treatment strategies in sarcoidosis.)

Newman LS, Rose CS, Bresnitz EA, et al. A case control etiologic study of sarcoidosis: environmental and occupational risk factors. *Am J Respir Crit Care Med.* 2004;170:1324. [PMID: 15347561] (Results from the multicenter ACCESS study regarding the association of environmental and occupational exposures with risk of developing sarcoidosis.)

Rybicki BA, Iannuzzi MC, Frederick MM, et al. Familial aggregation of sarcoidosis. A case-control etiologic study of sarcoidosis (ACCESS). *Am J Respir Crit Care Med.* 2001;164:2085. [PMID: 11734416] (Results from the ACCESS study regarding familial associations in sarcoidosis.)

Statement on Sarcoidosis. Joint Statement of the American Thoracic Society (ATS), the European Respiratory Society (ERS), and the World Association of Sarcoidosis and Other Granulomatous Disorders (WASOG) adopted by the ATS Board of Directors and by the ERS Executive Committee, February 1999. *Am J Respir Crit Care Med.* 1999;160:736. [PMID: 10430755] (Consensus statement of the state of the art of the pathogenesis, diagnosis, and treatment of sarcoidosis from the American Thoracic Society, European Respiratory Society, and the World Association of Sarcoidosis and Other Granulomatous Diseases.)

Stern BJ. Neurological complications of sarcoidosis. *Curr Opin Neurol.* 2004;17:311. [PMID: 15167067] (A comprehensive review of current approaches to patients with neurosarcoidosis.)

Relevant World Wide Web Sites

[National Heart, Lung, and Blood Institute (NHLBI): Sarcoidosis]
http://www.nhlbi.nih.gov/health/dci/Diseases/sarc/sar_whatis.html
[The Foundation for Sarcoidosis Research]
http://www.stopsarcoidosis.org/
[Sarcoid Networking Association]
http://www.sarcoidosisnetwork.org

Endocrine & Metabolic Disorders 54

Jonathan Graf, MD

Endocrine disorders commonly cause musculoskeletal symptoms and may even present with rheumatic syndromes before the nature of the underlying endocrinopathy is apparent (Table 54–1). On occasion, endocrine disorders can mimic rheumatic diseases and be a source of diagnostic error (Table 54–2). Rheumatic manifestations of endocrine diseases are usually a consequence of the hormonal abnormalities, but, in the case of autoimmune thyroid disease, also can be a result of the underlying autoimmune process.

DIABETES MELLITUS

Patients with either type 1 or type 2 diabetes mellitus frequently have musculoskeletal complaints. Although relatively little is understood about the pathophysiologic effects of hyperglycemia on bones, joints, tendons, and muscles, there are well-established associations between diabetes and certain musculoskeletal syndromes (Table 54–3).

Diabetic Cheiropathy (Limited Joint Mobility Syndrome)

Diabetic cheiropathy, or limited joint mobility syndrome, usually develops after 10 or more years of diabetes (type 1 or 2), particularly when glycemic control has been suboptimal. Although most frequently recognized and encountered in the hands, this condition can involve the shoulders, knees, and feet. The limited mobility results from a generalized palmar fasciitis and from progressive thickening and tightening of the skin. In many instances, the skin becomes progressively puffy, shiny, and waxy in appearance, often mimicking the hands of patients with scleroderma and sclerodactyly. In a simple diagnostic maneuver referred to as the prayer sign, the patient places his or her hands together as if in prayer. Patients with limited mobility syndrome are unable to make complete contact between the palmar surfaces of their fingers (Figure 54–1). Improved glycemic control as well as physical and occupational therapy may help slow the progression of diabetic cheiropathy.

Flexor Tenosynovitis of the Hand

Flexor tenosynovitis of the hand may develop in as many as 12–15% of patients with diabetes. Early in its course this condition can present with an isolated nodule on one of the flexor tendons of the hand, most commonly of the long and ring fingers. These nodules become symptomatic when they impede tendon motion, usually locking the finger in flexion or creating a racheting sensation when the finger is flexed and then extended. The nodules can be palpated just distal to the palmar crease of the affected finger. Local glucocorticoid injections into the tendon sheath usually reduce the size of the nodule and alleviate symptoms.

Chronic tenosynovitis of the flexor tendons can progress to Dupuytren contractures. These most commonly involve the fourth finger and can result in significant disability as the affected fingers become locked in flexion. The fibrotic tendon is usually palpable as it courses through the palm proximal to the palmar crease. Glucocorticoid injections provide little benefit.

Adhesive Capsulitis of the Shoulder

Adhesive capsulitis, commonly referred to as "frozen shoulder," occurs in as many as 12% of patients with diabetes. Affected individuals develop relatively rapid and significant loss of the range of motion of the shoulder. Some patients have antecedent calcific tendinitis, peritendinitis, or bursitis of the affected shoulder, conditions that might predispose them to the development of frozen shoulder. Plain radiographs reveal few abnormalities of the glenohumeral joint, despite the degree of immobility. Early and aggressive physical therapy must be used to preserve range of motion and minimize the time that the joint is immobile.

Carpal Tunnel Syndrome

Diabetes and carpal tunnel syndrome are prevalent in Western societies, but the frequent coexistence of these disorders has led many to believe that diabetes predisposes to carpal tunnel syndrome. Patients with carpal tunnel syndrome usually complain of numbness or paresthesias in a distribution consistent with that innervated by the median nerve (see Chapter 6). These symptoms

Table 54–1. Rheumatic Manifestations Associated with Endocrine Disorders

Rheumatic Disorder	Endocrinopathy
Carpal tunnel syndrome	Diabetes
	Hypothyroidism
	Acromegaly
Flexor tenosynovitis	Diabetes
	Hypothyroidism
Chondrocalcinosis/pseudogout	Diabetes
	Hypothyroidism
	Hyperparathyroidism
	Acromegaly
Osteopenia/osteoporosis	Diabetes
	Hyperthyroidism
	Hyperparathyroidism
	Hypoparathyroidism
Destructive arthropathy	Diabetes
	Hypothyroidism
	Hyperparathyroidism
Premature/unusual osteoarthritis	Chondrocalcinosis
	Charcot arthropathy
	Acromegaly
DISH	Diabetes
Myopathy	Diabetes
	Hypothyroidism
	Hyperthyroidism
	Hyperparathyroidism
	Acromegaly

DISH, diffuse idiopathic skeletal hyperostosis.

Table 54–3. Rheumatic Manifestations of Diabetes

Articular
  Charcot arthropathy
  DISH
  Chondrocalcinosis
Bone
  Osteopenia
Soft tissue
  Carpal tunnel syndrome
  Flexor tendon nodule
  Dupuytren contracture
  Cheiropathy
  Adhesive capsulitis

DISH, diffuse idiopathic skeletal hyperostosis.

are often exacerbated at night and may awaken a patient from sleep. Carpal tunnel syndrome can progress from an irritating sensory neuropathy to weakness and wasting of the thenar muscles of the hand. Provocation of paresthesias in a median nerve distribution by either a Phalen maneuver or Tinel sign can help confirm the diagnosis. Nerve conduction studies localize the site of the nerve compression to the wrist and differentiate carpal tunnel syndrome from other types of neuropathy.

Initial treatment focuses on conservative measures. Patients are asked to wear wrist splints, particularly at night, and refrain from various activities that may exacerbate the condition. Local glucocorticoid injection into

Table 54–2. Early Manifestations of Endocrine Disorders that can Mimic Rheumatic Diseases

Manifestation	Endocrine Disorder	Mimics
Myalgias, arthralgias, fatigue	Hyperthyroidism	Fibrositis
	Hypothyroidism	SLE
	Hyperparathyroidism	
Proximal muscle weakness	Hyperthyroidism	Polymyositis
	Hypothyroidism	
	Hyperparathyroidism	
	Acromegaly	
Shoulder girdle pain and stiffness	Hyperthyroidism	Polymyalgia rheumatica
Degenerative arthritis	Acromegaly	Osteoarthritis
	Hypothyroidism	
Distal soft tissue swelling and periosteitis	Graves disease (thyroid acropachy)	Hypertrophic osteoarthropathy
Synovitis with ANA	Hashimoto thyroiditis	SLE, RA
CPPD, pseudogout	Hyperparathyroidism, hypothyroidism, acromegaly	Idiopathic CPPD

ANA, antinuclear antibodies; SLE, systemic lupus erythematosus; RA, rheumatoid arthritis; CPPD, calcium pyrophosphate deposition disease

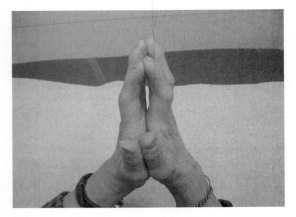

Figure 54–1. Prayer sign in a patient with diabetic cheiropathy.

the carpal tunnel or surgical decompression should be used if symptoms persist or motor signs develop.

Charcot (Neuropathic) Arthropathy

Diabetes mellitus is the leading cause of neuropathic arthropathy, which was first described by Jean Martin Charcot in patients with tabes dorsalis. A common complication of diabetes is a progressive sensory neuropathy that preferentially affects axons with the greatest length—ie, those innervating the extremities. In addition to causing the classic stocking-and-glove distribution of paresthesias and numbness, this sensory neuropa-

thy can impair normal protective mechanisms of the regional joints, particularly those of the foot and ankle. The lack of proprioceptive protection leads to progressive microfractures and subsequent destruction of the joint. The deformities of the affected joints progress with little or no pain or recognition of what is developing.

Patients usually present with a single, painless (or relatively painless), swollen, and deformed joint. Bilateral disease also occurs. The most commonly affected joints are the metatarsophalangeal, tarsal, and talar joints, but the knees, spine, and shoulders may also be involved (Figure 54–2). There are signs of a sensory neuropathy on neurologic examination.

Radiographs confirm the diagnosis. Classic radiographic findings of Charcot arthropathy include subluxations, fractures, bony fragmentation, exuberant sclerosis, and destruction of the joint (see Figure 54–2). Sometimes there is dramatic osteolysis of the bones of the feet, with involvement ranging from areas of patchy osteopenia to marked distal bone resorption. The destruction can be so dramatic as to cause concern for osteomyelitis or a septic joint, especially when there is a contiguous diabetic ulcer. The radiographic appearance sometimes mimics severe osteoarthritis, leading to the admonition to consider Charcot arthropathy when a radiograph reveals "degenerative arthritis times ten." The combination of an unusually destructive degenerative disease in a location not usually affected by osteoarthritis (eg, the tibiotalar, subtalar, and glenohumeral joints) should raise the suspicion of a Charcot joint.

Unfortunately, the treatment of Charcot joints, particularly those below the knee, remains suboptimal once

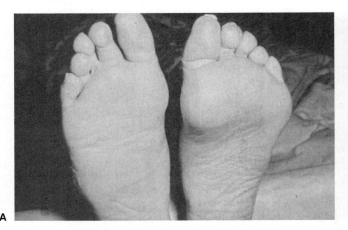
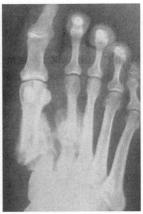

Figure 54–2. Charcot arthropathy. **A:** Deformity of the left foot of a patient with chronic diabetes mellitus and long-standing peripheral neuropathy. **B:** Radiograph of Charcot arthopathy involving the first and second metatarsals. (Courtesy of Dr. Carl Grunfeld, San Francisco Department of Veterans Affairs Medical Center, University of California, San Francisco.)

the destructive process has become advanced. If detected early, the progress of disease can be somewhat slowed by various protective measures, including the limitation of weight bearing on the affected joint and the use of specially crafted orthotic supports for the surrounding joint structures.

Diffuse Idiopathic Skeletal Hyperostosis

Diffuse idiopathic skeletal hyperostosis (DISH) is a disorder of excessive calcification along spinal ligaments and of new bone formation at insertion sites of tendons and ligaments. Although not uncommon in the general population, DISH is found with a higher prevalence among patients with diabetes, particularly those with type 2 diabetes mellitus.

DISH most commonly affects the spine, particularly the midthoracic spine, and causes ossification and calcification of the anterior longitudinal spinous ligament (Figure 54–3). Despite the presence of large, osteophyte-like projections, patients with DISH are rarely symptomatic, and the diagnosis comes to light as an incidental finding on radiographs. In advanced cases, however, the large bony overgrowths can cause spinal rigidity and impingement of nearby structures and nerves; exuberant calcification of the anterior longitudinal ligament in the neck can lead to dysphagia. DISH also can occur in extraspinal sites with prominent bony reactions at ligamentous and tendinous insertions, particularly in the pelvis, greater trochanters, patellae, and calcaneus.

DISH is a radiographic diagnosis, usually based on three general diagnostic criteria: (1) flowing ligamentous calcifications involving at least four contiguous vertebral levels, (2) minimal loss of disk space, and (3) absence of sacroiliitis. DISH can be confused with degenerative

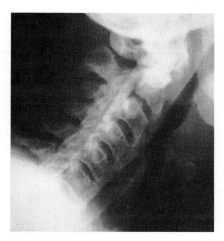

Figure 54–3. Diffuse idiopathic skeletal hyperostosis (DISH).

disk disease and with ankylosing spondylitis. The absence of disc space narrowing, of end-plate sclerosis, and of facet joint degenerative disease helps to distinguish DISH from degenerative spondylitis (although these two entities can coexist). In contrast to ankylosing spondylitis, DISH does not cause inflammatory types of symptoms (eg, morning pain and stiffness in the back) or sacroiliitis.

The treatment of DISH is symptom-based and generally limited to analgesia as needed. Rarely, surgical removal of impinging bone bridges is undertaken when critical functions, such as swallowing, are compromised.

Osteopenia

Type 1 diabetes mellitus appears to predispose to the development of osteopenia. Most often, the degree of osteopenia in diabetic patients is subclinical, and treatment is based on the standard guidelines for managing patients with reduced bone mineral density.

HYPERTHYROIDISM

Myopathy

The spectrum of muscular involvement in hyperthyroidism varies greatly, ranging from minor aches and pains to a profound and usually painless proximal myopathy that can mimic polymyositis (Table 54–4).

With milder muscular involvement, the patient may complain of weakness or easy fatigability, but generally demonstrates minimal findings on physical examination. In its most extreme presentation, the myopathy can cause debilitating proximal muscle weakness with marked muscle wasting. However, hyperthyroid-associated myopathy, unlike inflammatory myopathies, causes minimal elevations of muscle enzymes. Hyperthyroid myopathy usually responds to restoration of the euthyroid state.

Arthralgias and Myalgias

Hyperthyroidism is associated with arthralgias, particularly of the shoulders, that can mimic polymyalgia rheumatica. It also can cause a generalized musculoskeletal pain syndrome that resembles fibrositis and that

Table 54–4. Rheumatic Manifestations of Hyperthyroidism

Articular
Arthralgias
Periarthritis
Thyroid acropachy
Bone
Osteopenia/osteoporosis
Muscular
Proximal myopathy

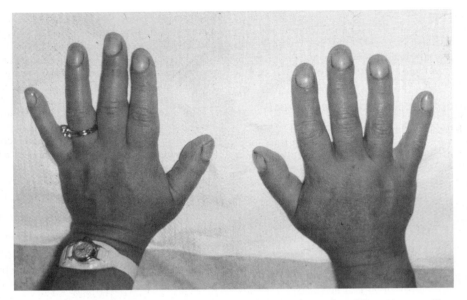

Figure 54–4. Thyroid acropachy in a patient with Graves hyperthyroidism. Note swelling of digits and marked clubbing.

manifests as fatigue, proximal myalgias, and arthralgias. These symptoms usually improve with correction of the hyperthyroidism.

Osteopenia

Both overt and subclinical hyperthyroid states cause increased bone turnover and reductions in bone mineral density that can progress to osteopenia and frank osteoporosis. Subclinical hyperthyroidism is a potentially treatable cause of osteoporosis and should be considered in patients with low bone mineral density.

Thyroid Acropachy

Thyroid acropachy, a complication of Graves disease, is a proliferative dermopathy that tends to occur in patients who also have ophthalmic involvement and pretibial myxedema. It manifests as distal soft-tissue swelling, clubbing, and periostitis, most commonly of the metacarpal bones (Figure 54–4). These abnormalities are thought to be due to effects of circulating thyroid-stimulating autoantibodies rather than of elevated thyroid hormone levels. Indeed, thyroid acropachy may progress, or even begin, after establishment of a euthyroid state due to the persistence of thyroid-stimulating autoantibodies. In some instances, removal of the target antigens via thyroid ablation may diminish the levels of the circulating pathogenic autoantibodies.

HYPOTHYROIDISM
General Considerations

The rheumatic manifestations of hypothyroidism are protean (Table 54–5). Many of these are due to the metabolic abnormalities created by an underfunctioning thyroid. However, autoimmune thyroid disease (Hashimoto thyroiditis) is the most common cause of hypothyroidism, and the autoimmune process, although

Table 54–5. Rheumatic Manifestations of Hypothyroidism

Articular
Inflammatory synovitis associated with thyroiditis
Noninflammatory joint effusions
Arthralgias
Fibromyalgia
Chondrocalcinosis
Erosive osteoarthritis
Charcot-type arthropathy
Bone
Avascular necrosis
Epiphyseal dysplasia
Muscular
Myopathy
Soft tissue
Carpal tunnel syndrome
Flexor tenosynovitis

primarily directed against the thyroid gland, can affect other tissues as well, mimicking several rheumatic diseases. Moreover, rheumatoid arthritis, Sjögren syndrome, mixed connective tissue disease, and systemic lupus erythematosus, can coexist with autoimmune thyroid disease, complicating diagnosis.

Hashimoto Thyroiditis & Immune-Mediated Rheumatic Syndromes

Patients with Hashimoto thyroiditis can develop an overt synovitis that probably is immune-mediated. The synovitis is usually a small-joint, symmetric, polyarthritis that mimics rheumatoid arthritis in its pattern but is nonerosive. Large-joint oligoarthropathies, however, are not rare. Antibodies against thyroid antigens are almost always present. Rarely Hashimoto thyroiditis causes urticarial vasculitis and glomerulonephritis that have been attributed to circulating immune complexes.

Diagnosis often is not straightforward. Depending on the stage of the autoimmune thyroiditis, patients with articular complaints can be euthyroid, hyperthyroid, or hypothyroid. Antibodies against thyroperoxidase and thyroglobulin have specificity for Hashimoto thyroiditis. However, patients also frequently have antinuclear antibodies, and it can be difficult to distinguish autoimmune thyroid disease with rheumatic manifestations from the coexistence of autoimmune thyroid disease and an antinuclear antibody–positive systemic disease. Thyroid replacement alone is often not enough to treat the rheumatic symptoms of these patients, and other medications such as nonsteroidal anti-inflammatory drugs, antimalarials, glucocorticoids, and methotrexate are sometimes used.

Associations Between Hashimoto Thyroiditis & Rheumatic Diseases

Hashimoto thyroiditis also occurs in association with well-defined rheumatic diseases. Ten to fifteen percent of patients with rheumatoid arthritis, for example, suffer from autoimmune thyroid disease, while as many as 15% of patients with Hashimoto thyroiditis may have one or more additional autoimmune diseases such as Sjögren syndrome and systemic lupus erythematosus. There is an association between Hashimoto thyroiditis and specific human leukocyte antigen alleles, particularly HLA-DR3 and HLA-B8.

Articular Manifestations of Hypothyroidism

Hypothyroidism can produce a generalized musculoskeletal pain syndrome and should be included in the differential diagnosis of fibrositis.

Myxedematous arthropathy is a noninflammatory arthritis, classically of the knees and other large, peripheral joints, but now also recognized to frequently involve the hands and wrists. Other patterns of myxedematous arthropathy include involvement of the elbows and metacarpophalangeal joints together with a flexor tenosynovitis of the hands. Joint effusions are common and are characterized by generous quantities of viscous, noninflammatory synovial fluid.

Calcium pyrophosphate crystals and chondrocalcinosis have been identified in the joints of patients with hypothyroidism, but the exact nature of the relationship between calcium pyrophosphate deposition disease, pseudogout, and hypothyroidism is not entirely understood.

Bony Abnormalities & Hypothyroidism

Many studies suggest a link between hypothyroidism and the development of osteonecrosis. There appears to be a peculiar predilection for the tibial plateau, but osteonecrosis has been reported to involve bones ranging in size from the femoral heads to the carpal lunate bones. Other reported bony abnormalities in hypothyroid patients include a Charcotlike destructive process and epiphyseal dysplasia.

Hypothyroid Myopathy

Patients who are hypothyroid frequently have muscle symptoms and can develop a myopathy that varies in severity. Elevations of muscle enzymes, often mild and without associated weakness, are common. However, profound muscle weakness and marked elevations in creatine kinase also occur. Hypothyroidism should always be included in the differential diagnosis of polymyositis and other causes of muscle weakness with an elevated creatine kinase.

Soft Tissue Manifestations of Hypothyroidism

The deposition of mucopolysaccharides in connective tissue may explain many of the soft-tissue manifestations of hypothyroidism. Carpal tunnel syndrome is encountered regularly. In fact, patients with bilateral carpal tunnel syndrome, particularly those with no other known risk factors, should be screened for hypothyroidism. Flexor tenosynovitis of the hand and generalized sensory neuropathy, both associated with hypothyroidism, can mimic this diagnosis as well.

HYPERPARATHYROIDISM

Primary hyperparathyroidism, the most common cause of asymptomatic hypercalcemia, is usually the result of an autonomously functioning parathyroid adenoma.

Chronic renal insufficiency induces secondary and even tertiary parathyroid gland hyperplasia and hormone oversecretion. All forms of hyperparathyroidism can produce rheumatic symptoms.

Chondrocalcinosis & Pseudogout

Primary hyperparathyroidism is a cause of calcium pyrophosphate deposition disease (CPPD). The presence of either chondrocalcinosis or of pseudogout should prompt determination of serum calcium (see Chapter 46).

Effects on Bone

The most common effect of primary hyperparathyroidism on bone is asymptomatic osteopenia and osteoporosis. Because of early detection of primary

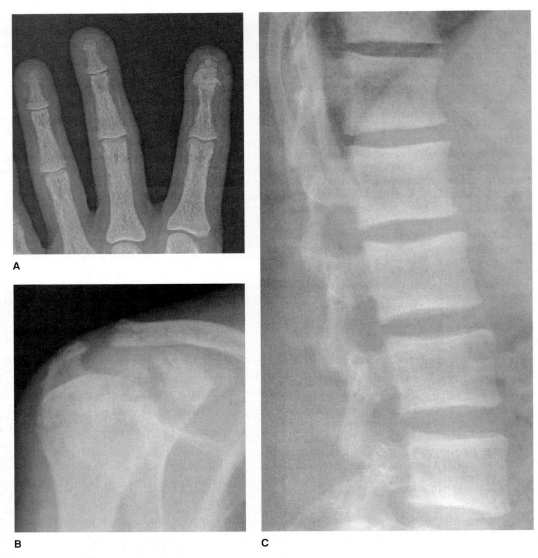

A

B

C

Figure 54–5. Skeletal changes of hyperparathyroidism. **A:** Subperiosteal resorption of the phalanges and calcification of the digital arteries. **B:** Erosion of the distal clavicle and soft-tissue calcification. **C:** "Rugger jersey" spine.

hyperparathyroidism and improved management of chronic renal failure, the classic skeletal effects of long-standing hyperparathyroidism are now uncommon. These include subperiosteal resorption of bone (especially the phalanges and distal clavicle), osteoporosis circumscripta (generalized bone loss of the skull), osteitis fibrosa cystica (cystic lytic lesions of bones), and "rugger jersey" spine (intense sclerosis of the vertebral end-plates alternating with marked osteopenia of the vertebral bodies) (Figure 54–5).

Myalgias

Fatigue and myalgias are frequent complaints in hyperparathyroidism. Patients also may complain of proximal muscle weakness, particularly in the lower extremities; there is little or no elevation of muscle enzymes.

Metastatic Calcification & Calciphylaxis

Advanced renal disease and associated secondary hyperparathyroidism can cause metastatic calcification of soft tissues and muscles, a process which by itself or through the induction of inflammation, can produce various muscle and soft-tissue symptoms. Calciphylaxis, which usually occurs in the setting of end-stage renal failure and severe secondary hyperparathyroidism, results in diffuse calcification of skin and subcutaneous and other soft tissues, leading to painful skin erythema and ulcerations, vascular thromboses, and digital infarctions that can resemble vasculitis.

HYPOPARATHYROIDISM & PSEUDOHYPOPARATHYROIDISM

Hypoparathyroidism is most often the result of surgical damage to, or removal of, the parathyroid glands; autoimmune destruction of the parathyroid glands occurs but is uncommon. Muscle fatigue and weakness usually parallel the degree of hypocalcemia. Neuromuscular irritability and tetany can result from very low levels of ionized calcium. Interestingly, some patients have ectopic soft tissue which rarely can cause calcification of the paraspinous ligaments and result in a restrictive process resembling a spondyloarthropathy.

Pseudohypoparathyroidism, which is due to resistance to parathyroid hormone action, is an inherited disorder that causes low serum calcium levels with elevated levels of parathyroid hormone. Pseudohypoparathyroidism can be associated with distinct skeletal deformities, particularly shortening of the fourth metacarpals bilaterally (Figure 54–6). Examination of the clenched fist reveals a characteristic depression where the knuckle of the fourth metacarpal should be located.

ACROMEGALY

Acromegaly has multiple effects on bone and soft tissues. The anabolic effects of excess growth hormone can cause a marked proliferation of bone, cartilage, synovium, and other soft tissues. Rheumatic symptoms are common in acromegaly and frequently predate recognition of the underlying disorder. The progression of acromegaly is insidious, and therefore attention to the rheumatic manifestations may point to the diagnosis before advanced disease becomes evident.

Degenerative Arthritis

Patients with acromegaly can develop a progressive degenerative arthropathy which can be monarticular or polyarticular and can affect a variety of joints. Initially, cartilage overgrowth leads to joint space widening, but

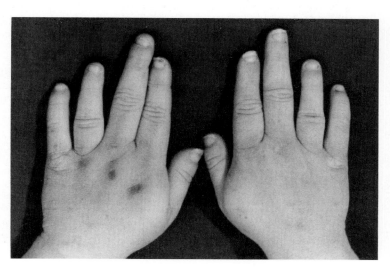

Figure 54–6. Pseudohypoparathyroidism. Shortening of the fourth and fifth metacarpals results in brachydactyly. (Courtesy of Dr. Michael Levine, The Cleveland Clinic.)

Table 54–6. Differential Diagnosis of Bilateral Carpal Tunnel Syndrome

Acromegaly
Amyloidosis
Diabetes mellitus
Rheumatoid arthritis
Hypothyroidism

this overgrowth involves haphazard deposition of matrix, resulting in its fissuring and degeneration. In addition, overgrowth and hypertrophy of joint capsules can cause progressive ligamentous laxity and hypermobility. Premature osteoarthritis ensues, particularly involving the weight-bearing joints, and invariably results in marked joint space narrowing and osteophytosis characteristic of all forms of degenerative joint disease. In addition, acromegaly has been linked to calcium pyrophosphate dihydrate deposition disease, a process that can further exacerbate any ongoing degenerative changes.

Up to 50% of patients with acromegaly have back pain. Patients can have widened disk spaces, large osteophytes, kyphosis and/or loss of lordosis, and ligamentous laxity of the spine. In one series of patients, duration of disease correlated with the height of vertebral bodies and intervertebral spaces, and concomitant DISH was diagnosed in 20% of patients. The degenerative changes in the spine can lead to radiculopathies, and bony overgrowth can impinge on the spinal canal.

Acromegaly should be suspected when precocious degenerative joint disease occurs. Particular attention should be paid to those patients who demonstrate excessive hypermobility or laxity of their joints, a finding that would appear to be in contradiction to the degree of degenerative disease encountered. Early in disease, radiographs of the hands demonstrate increased soft tissue of the hands, joint space widening, and spadelike deformities of the distal phalangeal tufts. Later, the changes observed radiologically resemble those seen in most forms of advanced osteoarthritis.

If treated early enough, most of the rheumatic manifestations of acromegaly will respond to removal of the pituitary adenoma or pharmacologic suppression of growth hormone secretion. However, once advanced degenerative changes have taken place, symptomatic relief is usually provided through conservative measures, including nonsteroidal anti-inflammatory medications. Severe disease may be amenable to surgical correction once the underlying metabolic abnormality has been successfully corrected.

Carpal Tunnel Syndrome

Acromegalic patients often have coarsely enlarged fingers and hands characteristic of the soft tissue, bone, and fibrous proliferation associated with excess growth hormone secretion. As a result of this tissue overgrowth, crowding of the carpal tunnel occurs, leading to carpal tunnel syndrome. This condition is often bilateral and can be the initial clue to the diagnosis of acromegaly (Table 54–6).

Myopathy

A painless, proximal myopathy has been reported in patients with acromegaly. Serum muscle enzyme levels are usually normal in this disorder.

REFERENCES

Biro E, Bako G, et al. Association of systemic and thyroid autoimmune diseases. *Clin Rheumatol.* 2006;25:240. [PMID: 16247581]

Cagliero E, Apruzzese W, Perlmutter GS, Nathan DM. Musculoskeletal disorders of the hand and shoulder in patients with diabetes mellitus. *Am J Med.* 2002;112:487. [PMID: 11959060] (Study of hand and shoulder complications in diabetic patients and controls.)

Kloppenburg M, Dijkmans BA, Rasker JJ. Effect of therapy for thyroid dysfunction on musculoskeletal symptoms. *Clin Rheumatol.* 1993;12:341. [PMID: 8258232]

Lacks S, Jacobs RP. Acromegalic arthropathy: a reversible rheumatic disease. *J Rheumatol.* 1986;13:634. [PMID: 2942687] (Case report and general review.)

Lockshin M. Endocrine origins of rheumatic disease. Diagnostic clues to interrelated syndromes. *Postgrad Med.* 2002;111:87. [PMID: 11985136] (Overview for primary care clinicians.)

McGuire JL. The endocrine system and connective tissue disorders. *Bull Rheum Dis.* 1990;39:1. [PMID: 268759] (A somewhat dated, but more detailed review of the subject published by the Arthritis Foundation.)

McLean RM, Podell DN. Bone and joint manifestations of hypothyroidism. *Semin Arthritis Rheum.* 1995;24:282. [PMID: 7740308] (Case report and good general review.)

Punzi L, Betterle C. Chronic autoimmune thyroiditis and rheumatic manifestations. *Joint Bone Spine* 2004;71:275.

Punzi L, Michelotto M, Pianon M, et al. Clinical, laboratory, and immunogenetic aspects of arthritis associated with chronic lymphocytic thyroiditis. *Clin Exp Rheumatol.* 1997;15:373. [PMID: 9272297]

Ramos-Remus C, Sahagun RM, Perla-Navarro AV. Endocrine disorders and musculoskeletal diseases. *Curr Opin Rheumatol.* 1996;8:77. [PMID: 8867544] (More of an update in selected aspects than a generalized review.)

Scarpa R, De Brasi D, Pivonello R, et al. Acromegalic axial arthropathy: A clinical case-control study. *J Clin Endocrinol Metab.* 2004;89:598.

Rheumatic Manifestations of Malignancy

55

John B. Imboden, MD, & Fiona A. Donald, MD, FRCP(C)

Rarely, tumorlike lesions, benign tumors, and malignancies involve joints directly, producing a monarthritis. More commonly, paraneoplastic syndromes can have rheumatic manifestations. Certain paraneoplastic syndromes have rheumatic presentations that are distinctive, and therefore warrant investigation of an underlying malignancy when recognized. Other paraneoplastic syndromes can mimic idiopathic rheumatic diseases, such as rheumatoid arthritis, and can be a source of diagnostic error.

BENIGN TUMORS & TUMORLIKE LESIONS OF THE SYNOVIUM

 ESSENTIALS OF DIAGNOSIS

- *Insidious onset of pain, swelling, and limited motion of a single joint, usually the knee or other large joint.*
- *Bloody synovial fluid in approximately 75% of cases.*
- *Characteristic histologic findings.*

Pigmented Villonodular Synovitis

Pigmented villonodular synovitis is a rare benign neoplasm of the synovium that typically develops in the knee or other large joint during the third or fourth decade of life, but that can occur in any synovial-lined joint at any age. Involvement of the synovium is usually diffuse, producing boggy swelling that can be massive and disproportionate to the degree of discomfort. Rarely pigmented villonodular synovitis is focal within the joint and presents with locking symptoms. The grossly thickened synovium has friable villi that bleed, leading to diffuse hemosiderin staining of the synovium and bloody or xanthochromic synovial fluid in most, but not all, cases. Plain radiographs do not show specific changes but may reveal

erosions and cystic changes in adjacent bone, usually with preserved joint space. Magnetic resonance imaging is the imaging procedure of choice and may point to the correct diagnosis, but definitive diagnosis requires histologic examination of involved tissue. The treatment of choice for most patients is surgical excision.

Giant Cell Tumors of Tendon Sheaths

Giant cell tumors of tendon sheaths closely resemble pigmented villonodular synovitis histologically. They present as painless finger nodules that can mimic ganglia and foreign-body granulomas. Radiographs show erosion of the underlying bone in a minority of cases. Fine-needle aspiration can be diagnostic; surgical excision is usually curative.

Synovial Chondromatosis

 ESSENTIALS OF DIAGNOSIS

- *Chronic noninflammatory swelling of a single joint.*
- *Multiple calcified loose bodies on radiographs in later stages.*
- *Locking symptoms and secondary osteoarthritis.*

Synovial chondromatosis is a rare tumorlike condition in which metaplastic synovial lesions develop into cartilaginous islands that in turn produce multiple chondroid loose bodies which eventually calcify. The process is monarticular and indolent, with the typical patient presenting with chronic swelling of a knee, hip, or shoulder. In the early phases radiographs may be unremarkable, but in the later stages calcified loose bodies—sometimes numbering in the hundreds—are visible. Synovial chondromatosis is self-limited but can produce painful locking and secondary osteoarthritis. Surgical removal of loose bodies and synovectomy are usually effective.

ARTHRITIS DUE TO DIRECT INVOLVEMENT BY MALIGNANCY

 ESSENTIALS OF DIAGNOSIS

- *Rapidly growing, eccentric mass associated with a joint, tendon, or tendon sheath in an extremity.*
- *Deep radiating pain.*
- *Characteristic histologic and cytogenetic findings.*

Synovial Sarcoma

Synovial sarcoma typically presents as an enlarging mass in an extremity during the third to fifth decades of life. The mass is associated with tendon, tendon sheath, or joint capsule but rarely is truly intra-articular. In 20–40% of cases plain radiographs of the mass reveal amorphous calcification that points to the diagnosis. Magnetic resonance imaging can delineate the extent of the lesion. Treatment consists of wide surgical excision. Five-year survival rates range from 25–60%, and tumor size is an important prognostic factor.

Secondary Tumors

Leukemic and lymphomatous infiltration of synovium can produce an oligoarthritis or a polyarthritis. Metastatic carcinomatous arthritis, arthritis due to direct extension into a joint from a contiguous malignant bone lesion, and synovitis as a reaction to a juxta-articular malignancy are well-recognized but uncommon entities. Metastatic disease to the shoulder and pelvic girdles can produce a syndrome of atypical polymyalgia rheumatica.

RHEUMATIC SYNDROMES THAT SUGGEST A PARANEOPLASTIC PROCESS

These distinctive syndromes have known associations with malignancy. In most cases, their appearance should prompt a search for an underlying cancer.

Hypertrophic Pulmonary Osteoarthropathy

 ESSENTIALS OF DIAGNOSIS

- *Triad of polyarthritis, clubbing, and periostitis.*
- *Rapid progression of symptoms.*
- *Association with intrathoracic malignancies.*

Hypertrophic pulmonary osteoarthropathy may exist in a primary form or in a secondary form associated with infectious diseases (eg, lung abscess) or malignancy. This syndrome is associated most commonly with intrathoracic malignancies (eg, adenocarcinoma of the lung, mesothelioma, and lymphoma) but has also been described in association with other cancers. It may appear several months prior to detection of the associated neoplasm.

Hypertrophic pulmonary osteoarthropathy is characterized by painful polyarthritis, clubbing of the fingers and toes, and periostitis of the long bones. Rapidly progressive symptoms are a feature of paraneoplastic hypertrophic pulmonary osteoarthropathy. The polyarthritis can resemble rheumatoid arthritis in its joint distribution but elicits noninflammatory synovial effusions. The periostitis commonly causes severe pain and tenderness of the long bones of the legs, usually in association with characteristic radiographic and scintigraphic findings. Nonsteroidal anti-inflammatory drugs may improve joint pain. Treatment of the underlying neoplasm often leads to remission of the syndrome.

Palmar Fasciitis-Polyarthritis Syndrome

The development of polyarthritis and rapid progression of palmar fasciitis with flexion contractures of the hands is clearly linked with ovarian cancer but also has been described in patients with gastric, lung, colon, and pancreatic cancer. The syndrome is refractory to treatment, and the prognosis is poor.

Remitting Seronegative Symmetric Synovitis with Pitting Edema

Remitting seronegative symmetric synovitis with pitting edema is characterized by the presence of a symmetric synovitis of the small joints of the hands in association with pitting edema of the hands and feet. Serum rheumatoid factor is negative. Treatment with low-dose systemic glucocorticoids is usually effective. Although there are idiopathic forms of the syndrome, remitting seronegative symmetric synovitis with pitting edema can herald the development of hematologic malignancies or a variety of solid tumors. Treatment of the underlying neoplasm with surgery or chemotherapy can lead to resolution of this disorder.

Panniculitis-Arthritis Syndrome

Patients with pancreatitis or with pancreatic cancer can present with the combination of arthritis and panniculitis. The arthritis is inflammatory and ranges from a monarthritis to a polyarthritis. The panniculitis begins as tender red subcutaneous nodules, usually on the lower extremities, that initially mimic erythema nodosum but that later liquefy and may drain a yellowish material. Release of pancreatic lipase likely plays a role in the pathogenesis of the syndrome.

Erythromelalgia

Erythromelalgia manifests as recurrent attacks of pain and erythema involving the feet, and sometimes the hands. The reversible acral erythema bears a resemblance to Raynaud phenomenon, but the effect of ambient temperature is the converse of that of Raynaud phenomenon: heat exacerbates and cold ameliorates the symptoms of erythromelalgia. Erythromelalgia can be idiopathic but a substantial minority have an underlying myeloproliferative disorder, particularly essential thrombocytosis and polycythemia rubra vera. Approximately 50% of patients with essential thrombocytosis have erythromelalgia.

Dermatomyositis & Polymyositis

Compared with the general population, the incidence ratio of malignancy has been reported to be as high as 6.2 for dermatomyositis and 2.4 for polymyositis at the time of diagnosis (see Chapter 28). Although the incidence of malignancy appears to be highest at the time of diagnosis, an increased risk of malignancy may be present for 2–5 years postdiagnosis. A number of clinical features correlate with the presence of malignancy in association with inflammatory myositis. These include older age, fever, substantial weight loss (>5%), and rapid onset of disease (defined as diagnosis within 2 months of symptoms). Dermatomyositis with cutaneous necrosis of the trunk is also associated with malignancy.

Although the distribution of malignancies seen with the inflammatory myopathies is similar to that of the general population, there are several specific associations with dermatomyositis and polymyositis. Cancer of the

ovaries, lungs, and the gastrointestinal tract is reported most frequently in association with dermatomyositis. Non-Hodgkin lymphoma and cancer of the lung as well as bladder cancer are frequently described in patients with polymyositis. Asian patients with inflammatory myositis have a high incidence of nasopharyngeal cancer.

At a minimum, age-appropriate cancer screening is indicated for patients with dermatomyositis and polymyositis. Although no guidelines exist, some clinicians advocate additional screening, at least in certain circumstances. For example, pelvic ultrasonography and CA-125 are warranted in women with dermatomyositis, given the high incidence of ovarian cancer. Because the risk of ovarian cancer may be elevated for up to 5 years, some experts argue that screening should continue annually during this time.

PARANEOPLASTIC SYNDROMES THAT MIMIC RHEUMATIC DISEASES

Certain paraneoplastic syndromes have manifestations that mimic rheumatic diseases (Table 55–1). When the

Table 55–1. Paraneoplastic Syndromes that Mimic Rheumatic Disease

Syndrome	Malignancy
Cancer-associated polyarthritis	Solid tumors
Jaccoud-like arthropathy	Carcinoma of the lung
Amyloid arthropathy	Myeloma
Secondary gout	Leukemias; lymphomas; myeloma; polycythemia rubra vera; essential thrombocytosis
Lupus-like syndromes	Thymoma; Hodgkin disease; carcinoma of the lung, breast, and ovary
Small-vessel vasculitis	Myeloproliferative and lymphoproliferative disorders
Medium-vessel arteritis	Hairy cell leukemia
Severe Raynaud phenomenon and digital necrosis	Various
Reflex sympathetic dystrophy	Various
Erythema nodosum	Lymphoproliferative disorders
Scleroderma-like skin changes	Carcinoma of the stomach, lung, and breast; melanoma; myeloma; POEMS syndrome
Eosinophilic fasciitis	Myeloproliferative and lymphoproliferative disorders

POEMS, polyneuropathy, organomegaly, endocrinopathy, monoclona protein, and skin changes.

appearance of the paraneoplastic syndrome antedates detection of the associated neoplasm, it may be very difficult to distinguish the paraneoplastic syndrome from its more common rheumatic counterpart. Older age, rapid onset of symptoms, prominent constitutional symptoms, and refractoriness to treatment can be clues to the presence of a paraneoplastic process.

Cancer-Associated Polyarthritis

 ### ESSENTIAL FEATURES

- *May precede or follow the diagnosis of malignancy.*
- *Asymmetric oligoarthritis or polyarthritis, often in the elderly and with abrupt onset.*
- *Frequent sparing of the wrists and hands.*
- *Usually rheumatoid factor negative.*

Cancer-associated polyarthritis is an uncommon paraneoplastic syndrome reported in association with carcinoma of the breast, carcinoma of the lung, and other solid tumors. There is a close temporal relationship between the development of the arthritis and detection of malignancy (usually within 12 months). Characteristic features of cancer-associated polyarthritis include the abrupt onset of an asymmetric arthritis in an elderly patient (age >65). The arthritis often involves the lower extremities with sparing of the small joints of the hands and wrists. Rheumatoid nodules are absent. Less commonly cancer-associated arthritis presents as a symmetric polyarthritis similar in appearance to rheumatoid arthritis. Serum rheumatoid factor is usually absent, and radiographs do not reveal erosions. Typically, cancer-associated polyarthritis responds poorly to nonsteroidal anti-inflammatory drugs. Treatment of the underlying malignancy often results in resolution of the arthritis.

Vasculitis

Small-vessel vasculitis, usually presenting as palpable purpura with biopsy findings of leukocytoclastic vasculitis, can occur in association with myeloproliferative and lymphoproliferative disorders, and less commonly, with various carcinomas. Hairy cell leukemia is associated with a medium-vessel arteritis that resembles polyarteritis nodosa.

REFERENCES

Fam AG. Paraneoplastic rheumatic syndromes. *Baillieres Best Pract Res Clin Rheumatol.* 2000;14:515. [PMID: 10985984]

Naschitz JE, Rosner I, Rozenbaum M, Zuckerman E, Yeshurun D. Rheumatic syndromes: clues to occult neoplasia. *Semin Arthritis Rheum.* 1999;29:43. [PMID: 10468414] (A thorough review of rheumatic associations and malignancy.)

Szendroi M, Deodhar A. Synovial neoformations and tumours. *Best Pract Res Clin Rheumatol.* 2000;14:363. [PMID: 10925750] (An excellent review of tumors that involve joints, tendon sheaths, and bursae.)

Amyloidosis

Paul S. Mueller, MD, MPH

Amyloidosis is not a single disease but a heterogeneous group of diseases that have in common the extracellular deposition of insoluble fibrillar proteins in tissues and organs. These protein deposits derive from diverse and unrelated serum precursor proteins yet have similar β-pleated sheet structural conformations. Furthermore, all forms of amyloid display apple-green birefringence under polarized light when stained with Congo red. Indeed, this observation (in tissue biopsy specimens) remains the primary means of establishing the diagnosis of amyloidosis. Accumulation of amyloid deposits leads to tissue and organ dysfunction, which in turn causes clinical symptoms, and for some patients, death.

Amyloid diseases are classified by the biochemical composition of the serum precursor proteins that form the amyloid fibrils and deposits. Once amyloid deposition has been identified, it is important to identify the precursor protein, because the prognoses and treatments of the various amyloid diseases depend on the underlying cause. To date, more than 20 amyloid fibril precursor proteins and their associated diseases have been identified. Of these, the most common amyloid diseases are (1) primary or immunoglobulin (Ig) light-chain protein–related (AL) amyloidosis; (2) secondary (AA) amyloidosis associated with chronic inflammatory disease; (3) dialysis-associated β_2-microglobulin (β_2-m) amyloidosis; and (4) hereditary amyloidosis. Because the clinical manifestations of these forms of amyloidosis are not identical (Table 56–1), each form is discussed in detail.

AL AMYLOIDOSIS

ESSENTIALS OF DIAGNOSIS

- *AL amyloidosis should be suspected in all patients with unexplained heart failure, nephrotic syndrome, neuropathy, and hepatomegaly.*
- *Approximately 90% of patients with AL amyloidosis have detectable serum or urine monoclonal Ig light-chain protein. However, this finding alone is insufficient to establish the diagnosis of AL amyloidosis.*

- *AL amyloid, like all forms of amyloid, displays apple-green birefringence when viewed under polarized light after staining with Congo red.*
- *Bone marrow examination usually shows a monoclonal population of plasma cells.*
- *Tissue immunohistochemical analysis is necessary to identify the light-chain origin of AL amyloid fibrils. If inconclusive, other diagnostic testing (eg, ultrastructural fibril characterization) should be done.*

General Considerations

AL amyloidosis is a plasma cell dyscrasia associated with multisystem involvement, rapid progression, and short survival. It is a rare disease with an incidence of approximately 8 cases per 1 million persons per year in the United States. It usually affects people older than 40 years of age and men (65%) more than women. Amyloid fibrils derive from the N-terminal region of Ig light chains (λ-more often than κ), produced by a monoclonal population of plasma cells in the bone marrow. Of note, only 10–15% of patients with multiple myeloma, another plasma cell dyscrasia, have AL amyloidosis, and it is unusual for multiple myeloma to develop in patients with AL amyloidosis. AL amyloidosis affects most organs and the vascular system.

Clinical Findings

A. SYMPTOMS AND SIGNS

The symptoms and signs of AL amyloidosis are nonspecific. For example, the most common symptoms are fatigue and involuntary weight loss. Other symptoms and signs of AL amyloidosis reflect the organs and tissues involved. Hence, clinicians should suspect AL amyloidosis in patients with syndromes associated with the disease. The syndromes associated most commonly with AL amyloidosis are nephrotic syndrome, congestive heart failure, idiopathic peripheral neuropathy, hepatomegaly, and carpal tunnel syndrome (CTS).

Table 56–1. Organ Systems Commonly Involved Clinically in Various Forms of Amyloidosis

Organ System	Primary (AL) Amyloidosis	Secondary (AA) Amyloidosis	Dialysis-Associated β_2-Microglobulin (β_2-m) Amyloidosis	Hereditary Amyloidosis[a]
Heart	X			X
Kidney	X	X		X
Vascular	X			
Peripheral nerves	X			X
Autonomic nerves	X			X
Liver	X			
Gastrointestinal tract	X	X		
Joints	X		X	

[a]Organ involvement varies according to the specific amyloid precursor protein mutation.

One-third to one-half of patients with AL amyloidosis have symptoms related to kidney involvement. Nephrotic syndrome (urinary excretion of more than 3 g of protein in 24 hours) with hypoalbuminemia and edema is the most frequent initial manifestation of kidney involvement. Symptomatic cardiac involvement affects up to 40% of patients with AL amyloidosis. Amyloid involvement of the myocardium, intramural coronary arteries, and conduction system may cause congestive heart failure, ischemic syndromes (eg, angina and myocardial infarction), and rhythm disturbances. Nearly 20% of patients with AL amyloidosis have neuropathy. These patients usually present with lower extremity paresthesias. Pain and temperature senses are lost before light touch and vibratory senses. Motor neuropathy is rare. Patients may also have autonomic neuropathy, the manifestations of which include diarrhea, bladder control problems, impotence, and orthostatic hypotension. One-quarter of patients have hepatomegaly. Clinicians should consider AL amyloidosis in all patients who have nephrotic syndrome and unexplained heart disease, peripheral or autonomic neuropathy, or hepatomegaly.

Many patients with AL amyloidosis also have rheumatic manifestations. For example, one-quarter of patients have CTS. Sensory abnormalities caused by amyloid neuropathy may lead to neuropathic joint destruction (Charcot joint). Some patients with AL amyloidosis have joint disease resembling rheumatoid arthritis (RA): bilateral symmetric arthritis of the large and small joints characterized by pain, stiffness, swelling, and palpable nodules. However, unlike patients with RA, those with amyloid arthropathy do not have fevers, joint tenderness on palpation, or evidence of inflammation on synovial fluid analysis. Patients with muscle involvement (amyloid myopathy) present with stiffness, weakness, and enlargement of muscles. Amyloid involvement of joints, muscles, and nerves may also lead to debilitating contractures. Finally, AL amyloidosis may masquerade as giant cell arteritis—patients present with symptoms suggestive of giant cell arteritis (eg, jaw claudication). However, temporal artery biopsy indicates amyloid involvement of the temporal artery rather than giant cell arteritis.

In fact, most patients with AL amyloidosis have vascular involvement, and for some this involvement may be symptomatic (eg, angina pectoris, orthostatic hypotension, and purpura). Less than 20% of patients with AL amyloidosis have pathologic enlargement of the tongue (macroglossia).

Laboratory Findings

No laboratory findings are pathognomonic of AL amyloidosis. Instead, abnormalities in laboratory results reflect the organs and tissues involved. For example, renal insufficiency, hypoalbuminemia, hyperlipidemia, and proteinuria suggest kidney involvement. Hematologic abnormalities are relatively uncommon. However, peripheral blood smear may show Howell-Jolly bodies suggestive of hyposplenism, which is caused by amyloid infiltration of the spleen.

Immunoelectrophoresis of the serum or urine detects a monoclonal Ig light-chain protein in 90% of patients with AL amyloidosis. For those without detectable monoclonal light chain in the serum or urine (nonsecretory AL amyloidosis), bone marrow examination usually indicates a monoclonal population of plasma cells. Patients with AL amyloidosis usually have increased plasma cells (more than 5%) in the bone marrow.

Imaging Studies

In general, imaging studies do not reveal findings specific for AL amyloidosis. Some patients with kidney involvement may have enlarged kidneys when viewed by ultrasonography (most have normal-sized kidneys). Echocardiography usually shows wall thickening (due to amyloid infiltration of the myocardium), evidence of diastolic dysfunction, and a misleadingly normal left ventricular ejection fraction. Reported radiographic findings in patients with AL amyloidosis include osteoporosis, pathologic fractures, osteonecrosis, soft-tissue nodules and swelling, subchondral cysts and erosions, joint contractures, and neuropathic osteoarthropathy.

Quantitative scintigraphy with radiolabeled serum amyloid P (SAP) component is useful in determining the extent and total body burden of amyloid deposits in patients with AL amyloidosis. Serial studies show uptake of the radiolabeled SAP component that correlates with regression or progression of disease. This test, however, is not widely available.

Tissue Biopsy

Tissue biopsy is necessary to establish the diagnosis of amyloidosis. All forms of amyloid display apple-green birefringence when viewed under polarized light after staining with Congo red. The least invasive method of obtaining a biopsy specimen is aspiration of subcutaneous abdominal fat, which indicates amyloid in 70–80% of patients with AL amyloidosis. Bone marrow biopsy (usually performed to evaluate a monoclonal protein) shows amyloid in one-half of patients. Together, fat aspirate and bone marrow biopsy indicate amyloid in 90% of patients. If analyses of aspirated subcutaneous fat and bone marrow do not reveal amyloid, yet suspicion for amyloidosis remains high, other tissue must be obtained. An effective approach is to obtain tissue specimens from organs suspected of having amyloid involvement (eg, kidney, heart, or liver). The presence of a monoclonal light-chain protein in a patient with biopsy-proven amyloidosis strongly suggests, but is not sufficient to establish the diagnosis of, AL amyloidosis. For example, monoclonal gammopathies are not uncommon in the general population, and detecting a monoclonal protein in a patient with a form of amyloidosis other than AL amyloidosis (eg, hereditary amyloidosis) may be misleading. Some patients with AL amyloidosis do not have a detectable monoclonal protein. Hence, tissue immunohistochemical analysis is necessary to identify the light-chain origin of AL amyloid fibrils. If the diagnosis remains inconclusive, other testing (eg, electron microscopy) may be necessary.

Treatment

A major goal in treating AL amyloidosis is the elimination or decrease in the number of monoclonal plasma cells that produce the amyloidogenic proteins. The standard treatment of AL amyloidosis is the combination of melphalan and prednisone. This combination is superior to placebo and to colchicine. Compared with placebo, treatment with melphalan and prednisone increases median survival time from 6 months to 12 months. This treatment, however, is less effective if the disease involves the heart

or kidneys. Although high-dose melphalan followed by autologous stem cell support is a promising treatment for AL amyloidosis, it has high treatment-associated mortality (20–40%) and therefore must be used only in selected patients (eg, those without amyloid cardiomyopathy or without involvement of two or more other major organs). However, in many of the patients who can tolerate this treatment, monoclonal light chains disappear from the serum and urine and the number of bone marrow plasma cells normalizes. Furthermore, the function of organs involved with amyloid may improve (eg, decreased proteinuria). The treatment options for patients with amyloid cardiomyopathy or involvement of two or more other major organs include standard melphalan and prednisone and high-dose dexamethasone (with or without melphalan). Thalidomide is another treatment option but is poorly tolerated. Finally, organ transplantation has been used successfully to treat organ failure in selected patients with AL amyloidosis. Organ transplantation, however, does not prevent amyloid deposition in other organs or in the transplanted organ.

In addition to treatment directed at the specific form of amyloidosis, most patients with amyloidosis, including those with AL amyloidosis, require supportive treatment (Table 56–2). The aims of supportive treatment are to relieve symptoms caused by amyloid involvement of various organ systems and to prolong survival.

When to Refer to a Specialist

Patients with AL amyloidosis should be referred to a hematologist who has experience managing this uncommon disease. Managing organ failure caused by amyloidosis can be challenging and often requires the assistance of a subspecialist (eg, nephrologist or cardiologist). Furthermore, many patients with amyloidosis have daunting psychosocial and spiritual challenges. Under these circumstances, referral to an appropriate allied health colleague (eg, social worker or chaplain) or support group may be helpful.

Prognosis

The prognosis of AL amyloidosis is poor. Overall, the median survival of patients with this disease is 1–2 years. Most deaths are attributable to cardiac involvement (congestive heart failure and sudden death). Indeed, survival depends on which organs and tissues are involved. For example, the median survival of patients with AL amyloidosis who have symptomatic cardiac involvement is only 6 months. However, patients with neuropathy but no involvement of the heart or kidneys have a median survival of nearly 3 years. Patients with nephropathy but no involvement of the heart have a median survival of 21 months. Treatments, including melphalan and

Table 56–2. Supportive Measures for All Forms of Amyloidosis

Organ System	Symptom	Treatment
Heart	Congestive heart failure	Salt restriction
		Diuretics
		ACE inhibitors
		Heart transplantation
		Avoidance of digoxin, calcium channel blockers, and β-blockers
	Heart block	Pacemaker
Kidney	Nephrotic syndrome	Salt restriction
		Elastic stockings
		Adequate dietary protein
		ACE inhibitors
	Kidney failure	Dialysis
		Kidney transplantation
Autonomic neuropathy	Orthostatic hypotension	Salt
		Elastic stockings
		Fludrocortisone
	Gastroparesis	Small, frequent meals low in fat
		Metoclopramide
		Jejunostomy tube
Peripheral neuropathy	Sensory neuropathy	Pain control (eg, amitriptyline or gabapentin)
		Avoidance of trauma
		Proper foot care
	Motor neuropathy	Physical therapy
		Braces, other devices
Gastrointestinal tract	Diarrhea	Psyllium
		Loperamide
		Somatostatin analogues
		Dietary changes
		Total parenteral nutrition
	Macroglossia	Maintenance of airway
Blood	Bruising	Avoidance of trauma
	Factor X deficiency	Factor replacement before surgery and other invasive procedures
	Hyposplenism	Vaccination
		Splenectomy for massive splenomegaly

ACE, angiotensin-converting enzyme.
(Modified from Skinner M. Amyloidosis. In: Lichtenstein LM, Fauci AS, eds. *Current Therapy in Allergy, Immunology, and Rheumatology.* 5th ed. Mosby, 1996. With permission.)

prednisone, and organ transplantation, prolong life in selected patients.

AA AMYLOIDOSIS

 ESSENTIALS OF DIAGNOSIS

- *AA amyloidosis should be suspected in all patients with chronic inflammatory conditions in whom renal insufficiency, nephrotic syndrome, gastrointestinal tract symptoms, or other symptoms and signs of amyloidosis develop.*

- *AA amyloid, like all forms of amyloid, displays apple-green birefringence when viewed under polarized light after staining with Congo red.*

- *Tissue immunohistochemical analysis identifies the serum amyloid A (AA) precursor protein from which AA amyloid fibrils derive.*

General Considerations

AA amyloidosis is an uncommon complication of chronic inflammatory diseases, including rheumatic conditions, infectious diseases, malignancies, and others. Amyloid fibrils derive from the acute-phase reactant serum AA protein. The liver produces serum AA protein in response to inflammation. Serum levels of this protein, which is involved in chemotaxis, cell adhesion, cytokine production, and other immune processes, correlate with disease activity. In fact, serum AA protein levels may increase 1000-fold during an inflammatory response. Chronically elevated serum AA protein levels precede AA amyloid fibril formation. Treating the underlying inflammatory disease suppresses the acute-phase response, normalizes serum AA protein levels, and prevents the development of AA amyloidosis. Indeed, the incidence of AA amyloidosis in the developed world has decreased in recent decades as a result of effective treatment of chronic infections (eg, tuberculosis) and other inflammatory diseases.

Of the cases of AA amyloidosis seen today, about two-thirds are caused by chronic rheumatic diseases, including RA, psoriatic arthritis, ankylosing spondylitis, Reiter syndrome, adult-onset Still disease, juvenile chronic arthritis, systemic lupus erythematosus, Behçet syndrome, Takayasu arteritis, polymyalgia rheumatica, hypersensitivity vasculitis, polymyositis, idiopathic retroperitoneal fibrosis, and the hereditary inflammatory diseases (eg, familial Mediterranean fever [FMF], familial cold urticaria, and Muckle-Wells syndrome). Malignancies associated with AA amyloidosis include Hodgkin disease, renal cell carcinoma, hepatoma, and astrocytoma. Other chronic inflammatory diseases associated with AA amyloidosis include inflammatory bowel disease, primary biliary cirrhosis, bronchiectasis, cystic fibrosis, osteomyelitis, psoriasis, eosinophilic granuloma, and decubitus ulcers. The time from diagnosis of the underlying inflammatory disease to the diagnosis of AA amyloidosis is usually 10–20 years. Because chronic inflammatory illnesses affect persons of all ages, AA amyloidosis may occur at any age.

Two diseases that cause AA amyloidosis, RA and FMF, warrant special attention. RA is the most common rheumatic cause of AA amyloidosis (75% of cases). However, most patients with RA do not have development of AA amyloidosis. The 15-year incidence of AA amyloidosis in RA is about 10%. Patients in whom AA amyloidosis develops have had RA longer than those in whom amyloidosis does not develop. Furthermore, continuously active and inadequately treated RA are risk factors for AA amyloidosis developing. FMF is characterized by recurrent attacks of fever, arthritis, pleuritis, peritonitis, or erysipelaslike erythema lasting 24–48 hours. FMF begins in childhood and usually affects persons of Mediterranean origin. AA amyloidosis develops in one-quarter of patients with FMF. Renal failure due to amyloid deposition usually occurs in the fifth decade of life.

Clinical Findings

A. SYMPTOMS AND SIGNS

The clinical manifestations of AA amyloidosis differ from those of AL amyloidosis in several ways. For example, renal and gastrointestinal tract manifestations are common. More than 90% of people with AA amyloidosis present with renal insufficiency, proteinuria, or both. AA amyloidosis is the most common cause of nephrotic syndrome in people with RA. Gastrointestinal tract involvement affects 20% of patients; the manifestations include nausea, diarrhea, and poor energy intake. Unlike patients with AL amyloidosis, those with AA amyloidosis rarely have cardiac or peripheral nerve involvement. Macroglossia is not a feature of AA amyloidosis.

Laboratory Findings

No laboratory findings are pathognomonic of AA amyloidosis. Abnormalities in laboratory results reflect amyloid involvement of organs and tissues. For example, kidney involvement is common and is suggested by renal insufficiency and proteinuria.

Imaging Studies

Imaging studies usually do not indicate findings specific for AA amyloidosis. Instead, imaging findings usually are associated with the underlying inflammatory condition (eg, RA). As with AL amyloidosis, however, quantitative scintigraphy with radiolabeled SAP component can be used in determining the extent and total body burden of amyloid deposits in patients with AA amyloidosis, as well as regression and progression of disease. However, this test is not widely available.

Tissue Biopsy

Tissue biopsy is required to make the diagnosis of AA amyloidosis. As in other forms of amyloidosis, AA amyloid displays apple-green birefringence when viewed under polarized light after staining with Congo red. Amyloid is found in aspirated subcutaneous abdominal fat samples in 60–70% of patients with AA amyloidosis. If the fat aspirate does not indicate amyloid, yet suspicion remains high, other tissue must be obtained. Because AA amyloidosis commonly involves the kidneys and gastrointestinal tract, kidney and gastric mucosa biopsy specimens almost always show amyloid. Tissue immunohistochemical analysis of the specimens identifies the serum AA precursor protein.

Treatment

The treatment of AA amyloidosis consists of treating the underlying inflammatory disease. This treatment results in decreased levels of serum AA protein and prevents AA amyloid fibril formation and deposition. Treatment may also reverse organ dysfunction caused by amyloid deposits and improve survival. For example, increased use of disease-modifying agents for RA decreases both the need for dialysis and the number of deaths caused by AA amyloidosis. Remissions of nephrotic syndrome caused by AA amyloidosis with the use of azathioprine and the combination of methotrexate and prednisolone also have been reported. Colchicine, the drug of choice for treatment of FMF, prevents inflammatory attacks and the development of AA amyloidosis. Oral chlorambucil has been reported to stabilize amyloid deposits and reverse nephrotic syndrome in a patient with psoriatic arthritis complicated by AA amyloidosis.

Several reports have described the efficacy of tumor necrosis factor-α (TNF-α) antagonists (eg, etanercept and infliximab) in patients with AA amyloidosis due to rheumatic diseases. TNF-α antagonists induce rapid and sustained clinical remission for various rheumatic diseases including RA. In patients with AA amyloidosis due to RA, ankylosing spondylitis, psoriatic arthritis, or other rheumatic conditions, TNF-α antagonists used alone or in combination with other agents (eg, nonsteroidal anti-inflammatory drugs, corticosteroids, and methotrexate) decrease serum acute phase reactants (including serum AA protein), decrease proteinuria, and improve kidney function. TNF induces hepatic production of serum AA protein, whereas TNF-α antagonists inhibit this process, thereby decreasing the potential for AA amyloid deposition.

Depending on the organs and tissues involved, patients with AA amyloidosis may require supportive treatment (see Table 56–2).

Prognosis

Having AA amyloidosis decreases survival. For example, RA patients without AA amyloidosis live nearly 8 years longer than RA patients with AA amyloidosis. Compared with AL amyloidosis, however, AA amyloidosis progresses slowly, and survival is often longer than 10 years.

Treating the underlying inflammatory disease improves survival of patients with AA amyloidosis. In fact, the prognosis of AA amyloidosis is improved if the serum AA level can be kept below 10 mg/L. In addition, treating organ failure caused by amyloid involvement may improve survival. For example, dialysis or kidney transplantation improves survival of patients with AA amyloidosis in whom kidney failure develops.

DIALYSIS-ASSOCIATED β_2-M AMYLOIDOSIS

 ESSENTIALS OF DIAGNOSIS

- β_2-m Amyloidosis should be suspected in all patients treated with long-term dialysis in whom rheumatic symptoms and signs, especially CTS, develop.
- Like all forms of amyloid, β_2-m amyloid displays apple-green birefringence when viewed under polarized light after staining with Congo red.
- Aspiration of subcutaneous abdominal fat is of little value in detecting amyloid in patients with dialysis-associated β_2-m amyloidosis; hence, other tissue (eg, synovium) must be obtained to establish the diagnosis.
- Tissue immunohistochemical analysis identifies β_2-m precursor protein from which β_2-m amyloid fibrils derive.

General Considerations

β_2-m Amyloidosis is a frequent complication of long-term dialysis (hemodialysis or peritoneal dialysis). In fact, β_2-m amyloidosis is a major cause of skeletal morbidity in dialysis-dependent patients. Amyloid fibrils derive from β_2-m, which is part of the class I major histocompatibility complex antigen. Patients with renal failure have chronically elevated serum β_2-m levels because 95% of this protein is eliminated by glomerular filtration. Indeed, β_2-m levels can be elevated 60-fold in anuric patients. Furthermore, β_2-m is only partially cleared during dialysis. Chronically elevated levels of this protein lead to the development of amyloidosis. In fact, β_2-m amyloidosis develops in nearly all patients treated with dialysis for more than 15–20 years. However, this form of amyloidosis may also develop in patients with chronic renal insufficiency not treated with dialysis.

Clinical Findings

A. SYMPTOMS AND SIGNS

β_2-m Amyloidosis has a striking predilection for affecting the joints, especially synovial membranes. Although β_2-m amyloid deposits can be widespread, β_2-m amyloidosis has primarily rheumatic manifestations, including CTS, trigger finger, tendon rupture, arthritis, spondyloarthropathy, and cystic bone lesions.

CTS, caused by deposition of β_2-m amyloid in the synovium of the carpal tunnel, is the most common (and usually the first) manifestation of dialysis-associated β_2-m amyloidosis. Indeed, there is a direct relationship between development of CTS and duration of dialysis. In some patients, CTS develops after only 5 years of dialysis. The prevalence of CTS after 10 years of dialysis is 20%, after 15 years 30–50%, and after 20 years 80–100%.

Roughly one-half of patients treated with dialysis for more than 10 years have persistent joint effusions accompanied by mild discomfort. Joint involvement is bilateral and includes large joints such as the shoulders, knees, wrists, and hips. Spondyloarthropathy is caused by destruction of the intervertebral disks and perivertebral erosions. Juxta-articular bone erosions and cystic defects have been described involving the femoral head, acetabulum, humerus, tibia, vertebral bodies, and carpal bones. These defects are not true cysts but rather eroded cavities. Furthermore, they are prone to pathologic fracture. Although β_2-m amyloid deposits have been found in visceral tissues and organs, this deposition usually does not manifest itself clinically.

Imaging Studies

Imaging studies usually do not indicate findings specific for dialysis-associated β_2-m amyloidosis. The diagnosis is strongly suggested, however, in long-term dialysis patients with rheumatic symptoms and juxta-articular bone erosions or cystic defects on radiography or other imaging studies such as computed tomography.

Tissue Biopsy

Aspiration of subcutaneous abdominal fat is of little value in detecting amyloid in patients with dialysis-associated β_2-m amyloidosis, unlike AL and AA amyloidosis. Hence, other tissue must be obtained to establish the diagnosis (usually from joints and synovial membranes). β_2-m Amyloid displays apple-green birefringence when viewed under polarized light after staining with Congo red. Tissue immunohistochemical analysis identifies the β_2-m precursor protein.

Treatment

The treatment of dialysis-associated β_2-m amyloidosis is largely symptomatic. Rheumatic manifestations are treated with nonsteroidal anti-inflammatory drugs and local glucocorticoids (eg, intra-articular injections). Surgery (eg, carpal tunnel release and stabilization of areas of bone destruction) may be necessary.

Dialysis technology that clears β_2-m is improving. For example, high-flux hemodialysis with bicarbonate-buffered dialysate improves β_2-m clearance, is associated with decreased manifestations of β_2-m amyloidosis, and may improve survival. Kidney transplantation prevents and halts the progression of β_2-m amyloidosis. Serum β_2-m levels normalize and rheumatic symptoms lessen within days after transplantation. It is unclear, however, if kidney transplantation results in mobilization of β_2-m amyloid deposits.

Prognosis

Because β_2-m amyloidosis develops in most patients treated with long-term dialysis, the prognosis of this disease is determined in part by the underlying kidney disease and its cause (eg, diabetes mellitus). Rheumatic manifestations of this disease (eg, destructive spondyloarthropathy) may negatively affect survival.

HEREDITARY AMYLOIDOSIS

 ESSENTIALS OF DIAGNOSIS

- *Hereditary amyloidosis should be suspected in all patients with unexplained neuropathy, cardiomyopathy, or renal insufficiency, especially if there is a family history of these problems.*

- *Hereditary amyloid, like all forms of amyloid, displays apple-green birefringence when viewed under polarized light after staining with Congo red.*

- *DNA analysis of blood and tissue immunohistochemical analysis can be used to identify the mutant precursor protein.*

General Considerations

Hereditary amyloidosis consists of a group of autosomal dominant diseases in which amyloid fibrils derive from mutant serum proteins, including transthyretin, apolipoprotein AI, lysozyme, and fibrinogen A α-chain. Amino acid substitution of these proteins (via gene mutations) render them amyloidogenic. Amyloid fibrils form (with consequent symptoms and signs) in midlife. Not surprisingly, a detailed family history may yield clues to the diagnosis of hereditary amyloidosis.

Many patients with hereditary amyloidosis are mistakenly assumed to have AL amyloidosis. Monoclonal gammopathies are not uncommon in the general population, and detecting a monoclonal protein in a patient with hereditary amyloidosis may be misleading. Hence, it is important for clinicians to be certain of the origin of amyloid precursor protein in all patients with amyloidosis.

Clinical Findings

A. Symptoms and Signs

Peripheral neuropathy is the most common manifestation of the hereditary amyloidoses. Indeed, the term "familial amyloidotic neuropathy" was once used for these diseases. Cardiac involvement is also common, whereas kidney involvement is less common.

Transthyretin is the most commonly involved protein in hereditary amyloidosis. This protein is synthesized by the liver and choroid plexus and transports thyroxine and retinol-binding protein. More than 80 mutations (single amino acid substitutions) of transthyretin have been identified that cause amyloidosis. Peripheral and autonomic neuropathy is the most common manifestation of transthyretin-associated amyloidosis. Cardiac involvement is common but varies among the different transthyretin mutations. However, compared with AL amyloidosis, heart failure is less common and the prognosis is better. In addition, renal involvement is less common and macroglossia does not occur.

Patients with hereditary amyloidosis caused by apolipoprotein AI, lysozyme, and fibrinogen A α-chain mutations usually have kidney disease but not neuropathy.

Laboratory Findings

No laboratory finding is pathognomonic of hereditary amyloidosis. Instead, abnormalities in laboratory results reflect amyloid involvement of organs and tissues.

Imaging Studies

Imaging studies usually do not indicate findings specific for hereditary amyloidosis. As in other forms of amyloidosis, quantitative scintigraphy with radiolabeled SAP component can be used to assess patients with transthyretin-associated amyloidosis. This test is not widely available, however.

Tissue Biopsy

Amyloid deposits caused by the hereditary amyloidoses display apple-green birefringence when viewed under polarized light after staining with Congo red. DNA analysis of blood and tissue immunohistochemical analysis identify the mutant precursor protein.

Treatment

Liver transplantation has been used successfully to treat hereditary amyloidosis caused by mutant proteins synthesized by the liver. For example, liver transplantation to treat hereditary amyloidosis caused by mutations of transthyretin may result in disappearance of the mutant protein from the blood and improvement of neuropathy. Other manifestations of hereditary amyloidosis (eg, kidney failure) are treated with supportive measures (see Table 56–2).

When to Refer to a Specialist

Relatives of patients affected by hereditary amyloidosis should undergo genetic counseling. Because liver transplantation has been used successfully to treat hereditary amyloidosis caused by mutant proteins synthesized by the liver, referral to a liver transplant subspecialist is warranted. Treating other manifestations of hereditary amyloidosis (eg, kidney failure) may also require the assistance of a subspecialist (eg, nephrologist).

Prognosis

Patients with hereditary amyloidosis caused by mutant proteins synthesized by the liver and who undergo liver transplantation have improved symptoms and prolonged survival, especially if transplantation is done before irreversible organ failure has occurred. The rate of progression of hereditary amyloidosis caused by apolipoprotein AI, lysozyme, and fibrinogen A α-chain mutations is usually slow. Patients with these forms of hereditary amyloidosis have kidney involvement and usually respond to supportive measures, and if necessary, kidney transplantation.

REFERENCES

Fernandez-Nebro A, Tomero E, Ortiz-Santamaria V, et al. Treatment of rheumatic inflammatory disease in 25 patients with secondary amyloidosis using tumor necrosis factor alpha antagonists. *Am J Med.* 2005;118:552. [PMID: 15866260] (Case series of patients with AA amyloidosis due to RA, ankylosing spondylitis, and psoriatic arthritis treated with TNF-α antagonists resulting in reduced proteinuria and improved kidney function.)

Floege J, Ketteler M. Beta$_2$-microglobulin-derived amyloidosis: an update. *Kidney Int Suppl.* 2001;78:S164. [PMID: 11169004] (Detailed review of the clinical features, diagnosis, treatment, and prognosis of dialysis-associated β_2-m amyloidosis.)

Lachmann HJ, Booth DR, Booth SE, et al. Misdiagnosis of hereditary amyloidosis as AL (primary) amyloidosis. *N Engl J Med.* 2002;346:1786. [PMID: 12050338] (Amyloidogenic mutations consistent with hereditary amyloidosis in 34 of 350 patients in whom the diagnosis of AL amyloidosis was suggested by clinical and laboratory findings and the absence of a family history.)

Merlini G, Westermark P. The systemic amyloidoses: Clearer understanding of the molecular mechanisms offers hope for more effective therapies. *J Intern Med.* 2004;255:159. [PMID: 14746554] (Detailed review of the clinical features, diagnosis, treatment, and prognosis of the most common systemic amyloidoses.)

Neben-Wittich MA, Wittich CM, Mueller PS, et al. Obstructive intramural coronary amyloidosis and myocardial ischemia are common in primary amyloidosis. *Am J Med.* 2005; 118: 1287.e1. [PMID: 16271914] (Most patients with primary systemic amyloidosis and cardiac involvement have obstructive intramural amyloidosis and associated microscopic changes of myocardial ischemia. Syndromes of myocardial ischemia [eg, angina] may occur in these patients.)

Relevant World Wide Web Sites

[Mayo Foundation for Medical Education and Research: Treatment of Amyloidosis at Mayo Clinic]
http://www.mayoclinic.org/amyloidosis/index.html
[Boston University School of Medicine: Amyloid Treatment & Research Program]
http://www.bu.edu/amyloid/
[Amyloidosis Support Network, Inc.]
http://www.amyloidosis.org

SECTION VIII

Disorders of Bone

Osteoporosis & Glucocorticoid-Induced Osteoporosis

57

Dolores Shoback, MD

Osteoporosis is a systemic skeletal disorder characterized by low bone mass, disruption of the microarchitecture of bone tissue, and compromised bone strength which leads to an increased risk for fracture.

Osteoporosis is common among menopausal women but is often clinically silent until a fragility fracture occurs. Hip fractures are the most devastating of these in terms of medical, psychosocial, and financial consequences. The lifetime probability of sustaining a hip fracture for a 50-year-old white woman is 14%. Osteoporosis is also being recognized with increasing frequency in older men, who account for about one-third of all hip fractures in the United States. The 1-year mortality of men with hip fractures is 30%. Finally, patients receiving long-term glucocorticoid therapy are at increased risk for osteoporosis and should have prevention and treatment approaches implemented.

POSTMENOPAUSAL OSTEOPOROSIS

ESSENTIALS OF DIAGNOSIS

- *Reduced bone mineral density.*
- *Decreased bone strength.*
- *Fragility fractures.*

General Considerations

Bone loss in women begins before the onset of menopause, typically in the late third and early fourth decades, and then accelerates for the 5–10 years after the menopause. Postmenopausal osteoporosis is thought to result from an estrogen-deficiency–induced imbalance between bone formation and resorption such that resorption is favored over formation. Following the increased rate of bone loss immediately surrounding the menopause, a less aggressive phase of bone loss ensues that continues into the eighth and ninth decades. Estrogen deficiency and factors related to aging (reduced osteoprogenitor population, nutritional deficiencies, and malabsorption) play a role in this later phase of bone loss.

Clinically, osteoporosis is diagnosed when **bone mineral density** (BMD) is reduced or when fragility fractures (ie, fractures after little or no trauma) occur. The most common osteoporosis-related fractures involve the thoracic and lumbar spine, the hip, and the distal radius.

Bone densitometry has become widely available as a diagnostic tool in recent years. Several techniques for quantifying BMD have been developed. They include dual-energy x-ray absorptiometry (DXA), single-energy x-ray absorptiometry, quantitative computed tomography, quantitative ultrasound, and radiographic absorptiometry. DXA is by far the best standardized technique and is preferred for diagnosing osteoporosis and monitoring responses to therapy. BMD assessment by DXA has been used by the World Health Organization to define

Table 57–1. WHO Definition of Osteoporosis for Postmenopausal Women Based on DXA Measurements

	Definitions
T-score	Number of SD above or below peak bone mass ("young normal") according to race
Z-score	Number of SD above or below age-matched bone mass according to gender and race
Normal	BMD T-score ≥ -1
Low bone mass (osteopenia)	BMD T-score < -1 and > -2.5
Osteoporosis	BMD T-score ≤ -2.5
Severe osteoporosis	BMD T-score ≤ -2.5 with one or more fragility fractures

WHO, World Health Organization; DXA, dual-energy x-ray absorptiometry; SD, standard deviation; BMD, bone mineral density.

osteopenia and **osteoporosis.** Their criteria are based on a large body of data on postmenopausal white women (Table 57–1).

In addition to age and BMD, there are other risk factors associated with an increased incidence of osteoporotic fractures; the National Osteoporosis Foundation has categorized these as modifiable and nonmodifiable (Table 57–2). As described below, all treatment and prevention strategies for osteoporosis begin with risk factor assessment and modification.

Despite extensive information on risk factors for fracture and low BMD, no single combination—or weighting—of these adequately predicts the prevalent BMD or fracture risk or can substitute for the measurement of BMD at present. Several professional organizations have published guidelines on the use of BMD testing for postmenopausal women and for patients receiving long-term glucocorticoid therapy (Table 57–3). Most of these indications are based on clinical risk factors ascertained during the initial evaluation of the patient.

Clinical & Laboratory Evaluation

The evaluation of perimenopausal or postmenopausal women with osteoporosis or a low BMD begins with the clinical assessment. At least 10–20% of postmenopausal women have an additional secondary cause for their bone loss beyond the estrogen deficiency of menopause. When taking the medical history, the practitioner should pay careful attention to medication use (especially glucocorticoids), smoking, alcohol intake, dietary calcium intake, and family history of osteoporosis and fractures. The physical examination focuses on height loss, the presence of bone pain or deformity, and signs of anemia, hyper-

Table 57–2. Risk Factors for Osteoporotic Fractures in Women Independent of Bone Density

Nonmodifiable
History of fracture as an adult
Presence of fracture (especially of hip) in first-degree relative
White race
Advanced age
Dementia and frailty
Immobilization

Modifiable
Alcohol and tobacco use
Low body weight (<127 lb for white, <100 lb for Asian)
Premature menopause
History of amenorrhea
Low dietary calcium intake
Frequent falls and poor eyesight
Low level of physical activity
Use of glucocorticoids
Vitamin D deficiency

(Modified from National Osteoporosis Foundation, *Physician's Guide to Osteoporosis.* Accessible at http://www.nof.org/physguide/index.htm. 1998; and Kanis JA. Excerpta Medica, Diagnosis of osteoporosis and assessment of fracture risk. *Lancet.* 2002;359:1929. With permission.)

thyroidism, hypercortisolism, malnutrition, and other disorders that cause secondary forms of osteoporosis (Table 57–4).

There is no consensus as to the appropriate and cost-effective laboratory work-up for postmenopausal women with low BMD or osteoporosis. At a minimum, however, laboratory evaluation should include a complete blood cell count, serum chemistry panel, liver function tests, and serum thyroid-stimulating hormone and calcium determinations.

Postmenopausal women as a group are commonly affected by primary hyperparathyroidism (prevalence ~3 per 1000). A serum calcium determination adequately screens for this disorder. In addition, multiple myeloma can be relatively silent clinically and present with osteoporosis, bone pain, pathologic fractures, or anemia. This diagnosis should be considered if BMD is remarkably low for age (ie, a low Z-score) or if low BMD is accompanied by an unexplained anemia or an elevated erythrocyte sedimentation rate. Multiple myeloma can be detected by serum and urine protein electrophoresis.

Measurements of serum 25-hydroxyvitamin D and urinary calcium excretion also can be helpful. Subtle vitamin D deficiency is relatively common in elderly patients and contributes to bone loss because it interferes with the absorption of calcium and phosphorus and thus the mineralization of bone matrix. Low urinary calcium excretion often accompanies vitamin D deficiency but also can be

Table 57–3. Indications for Bone Mineral Density Testing and Medicare Reimbursement

National Osteoporosis Foundation guidelines[a]
- Women ≥65 years regardless of risk factor status
- Younger women after time of menopause with the following risk factors:
  - Positive family history for osteoporosis
  - History of fragility fracture at age 45 or older
  - Smoking
  - Low body weight (<127 lb)

U.S. Preventive Services Task Force[b]
- Women ≥65 years should be screened
- Initiate screening at age 60 if increased risk of fractures is present:
  - Low body weight (<70 kg)
  - Estrogen deficiency
  - Other risk factors

Medicare coverage of bone mineral density testing[c]
- Postmenopausal women at risk for osteoporosis
- Patients with vertebral abnormalities
- Patients receiving glucocorticoids long term (prednisone ≥7.5 mg/d)
- Patients with primary hyperparathyroidism
- Patients receiving approved therapy to monitor response

American College of Rheumatology Ad Hoc Committee on Glucocorticoid-Induced Osteoporosis[d]
- Obtain baseline bone mineral density measurement when initiating long-term (≥6 months) glucocorticoid therapy
- Repeat measurement at 12 months (or 6 months) to ascertain ongoing bone loss
- Monitor patients receiving therapy for osteoporosis annually

[a](Modified from National Osteoporosis Foundation. *Physician's Guide to Osteoporosis.* With permission.)
[b](Modified from data accessible at http://ahcpr.gov/clinic/uspstf/uspsoste.htm. With permission.)
[c](Modified from Health Care Financing Administration. Medicare Program: Medicare coverage of and payment for bone mass measurements. *Fed Reg.* 1998;63:34320. With permission.)
[d](Modified from Recommendations for the prevention and treatment of glucocorticoid-induced osteoporosis: 2001 update. American College of Rheumatology Ad Hoc Committee on Glucocorticoid-Induced Osteoporosis. *Arthritis Rheum.* 2001;44:1496. With permission.)

Table 57–4. Secondary Causes of Osteoporosis in Men and Women

Rheumatologic disorders	Rheumatoid arthritis
	Ankylosing spondylitis
Connective tissue disorders	Marfan syndrome
	Ehlers-Danlos syndrome
	Osteogenesis imperfecta
Endocrine disorders	Primary hyperparathyroidism
	Hyperthyroidism
	Cushing syndrome
	Hypogonadism
	Anorexia nervosa with amenorrhea
	Hyperprolactinemia with amenorrhea or hypogonadism
	Insulin-dependent diabetes
Hematologic disorders	Multiple myeloma
	Systemic mastocytosis
	Lymphoma
	Leukemia
	Disseminated carcinoma
Gastrointestinal disorders	Malabsorption
	Celiac sprue
	Short bowel syndrome
	Crohn disease
	Chronic liver disease (especially cirrhosis)
	Primary biliary cirrhosis
	Postgastrectomy
Other conditions	Chronic obstructive pulmonary disease
	Posttransplantation
	Malnutrition
Drug therapy	Glucocorticoids
	Anticonvulsants
	Excessive thyroxine replacement
	Anticoagulants (heparin)
	Gonadotropin-releasing hormone agonists

Imaging Evaluation

The study of choice to assess BMD in a postmenopausal woman is a DXA measurement of the lumbar spine and hip. DXA reports often include both T- and Z-scores (Figure 57–1). A **T-score** relates the BMD of the patient to peak bone mass for race and gender. A **Z-score** relates the BMD of the patient to persons of the same age, gender, and race. The T-score is the more useful determination clinically. Operationally, the lower of the two T-scores (spine or hip) is used for making the diagnosis. Typically there is concordance between T-scores at both sites. Discordance can be due to artifactual elevation

due to underlying malabsorption or an extremely low calcium intake. Subtle forms of calcium malabsorption (eg, secondary to celiac sprue) are more common than previously thought. High levels of urinary calcium excretion suggest idiopathic hypercalciuria, which can be associated with renal stones and low BMD. Urinary calcium measurements in a patient taking calcium supplements can be informative as to the adequacy of therapy.

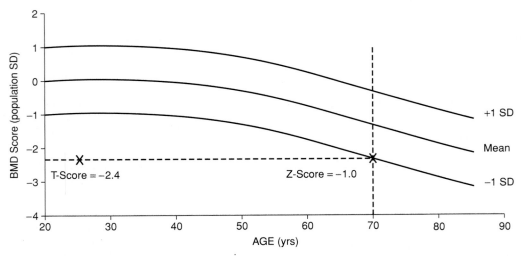

Figure 57–1. This graph shows the mean ± 1 standard deviation for bone mineral density (BMD). For a given femoral neck BMD value in a 70-year-old woman, her Z-score is –1 and her T-score (extrapolated back to the age of 20) is –2.4. (From Orwoll ES, Bliziotes M. *Osteoporosis: Pathophysiology and Clinical Management.* Humana Press, 2003:109. With permission.)

of the spinal measurement as a result of degenerative arthritis, disc disease, or aortic calcification; in such cases, only measurements of the hip and femoral neck should be used.

Obtaining a BMD measurement allows the clinician not only to grade the severity of osteoporosis, but also to predict fracture risk. Several studies have confirmed that the relative risk of fracture approximately doubles with each standard deviation below peak BMD (T-score) that a patient demonstrates.

The combination of BMD measurement and the patient's age is an even more powerful predictor of fracture risk. The 5-year risk of several types of osteoporotic fractures is strongly related to age and BMD T-score (Figure 57–2). Advanced age (over 70 years) dramatically increases the risks of vertebral and hip fractures.

Disease Course & Complications

Postmenopausal osteoporosis can progress silently over years to a dangerously low BMD and to bone strength so markedly reduced that the fracture threshold is reached. At this stage, fragility fractures can occur with minimal impact. Fractures are the dreaded complication of osteoporosis. Fractures of the spine cause pain that is generally self-limited. Multiple vertebral fractures can lead to loss of height, reduced thoracic expansion capacity and difficulty with breathing, progressive thoracic kyphosis, and ultimately increased frailty. Frailty itself is a risk factor for fractures.

Hip fractures have a more dramatic course, and prognosis in the elderly osteoporotic patient is guarded. These fractures require hospitalization and surgery. Because of the underlying frailty of most of these patients, their comorbid conditions and advanced age, and the prolonged immobilization and rehabilitation required, patients who fracture their hips have decreased life expectancy. The overall mortality in the first year after a hip fracture is approximately 20%.

In addition to the medical and financial ramifications of the immediate treatment of the hip fracture, there are substantial long-term human consequences. Hip fractures are life-altering events for elderly people. It is estimated that 50% of patients who sustain a hip fracture do not live independently afterwards. Therefore it is important to recognize osteoporosis early and to intervene with treatment strategies that reduce fracture risk.

MALE OSTEOPOROSIS

 ESSENTIALS OF DIAGNOSIS

- *Usually presents later in life than postmenopausal osteoporosis.*
- *Fragility fractures, height loss.*
- *Most patients have one or more secondary cause of bone loss.*

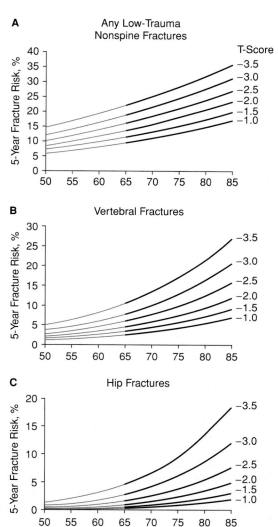

Figure 57–2. These figures show the influence of age and bone mineral density (BMD) on the 5-year fracture risk for any low-trauma non-spinal fracture (**A**), vertebral fractures (**B**), and hip fractures (**C**). At approximately age 65, there is a steep increase in fracture risk at T-scores of –2.0 or –2.5 or greater in panels **B** and **C**. (From Cummings SR, Bates D, Black DM. Clinical uses of bone densitometry: scientific review. *JAMA.* 2002; 288:1889.)

General Considerations

The diagnosis of osteoporosis in men is usually delayed relative to that of postmenopausal osteoporosis and often is made only after the patient presents with fractures, height loss, or obvious stigmata of the secondary causes for bone loss.

In contrast to women, men do not experience a clear-cut, easily defined cessation of gonadal function that raises awareness of risks for bone loss. Testosterone production declines with age, but there is controversy as to what the normal or accepted ranges of testosterone are for elderly men and how age-related declines in testosterone contribute to age-related declines in BMD. It is clear, however, that replacing testosterone does not restore BMD to "normal" even in hypogonadal men and that there are determinants of low BMD and fractures in men beyond hypogonadism.

Differences in the peak bone mass and the rate of bone loss influence the differential clinical expression of osteoporosis in men and women. Men achieve higher peak bone mass than do women, and men lose bone mineral at different rates than do postmenopausal women. In women, once the early rapid phase of postmenopausal bone loss ends, the rate of bone loss slows. Thereafter, the rates of bone loss in men and women are roughly comparable (Figure 57–3). Because of the early rapid phase of menopause-related bone loss and the lower peak bone mass attained by women, women have lower BMDs than men of the same age. This leads to an earlier onset of the typical osteoporotic fractures (hip, vertebral, and Colles fractures) in women compared with men (Figure 57–4). Men with low BMD experience the same fractures, but these fractures occur at later ages—approximately 10 years on average—than they do in women. Osteoporotic fractures therefore tend to occur in men at stages in their lives when they are more likely to be frail and are less able to cope physically and emotionally with the loss of independence and the risks of fracture repair surgery. Hence the morbidity and mortality of hip fractures are much greater in men than in women.

At least 80% of men with osteoporosis have one or more secondary causes of bone loss (Table 57–4 and 57–5). Only 10–20% of men with low BMD have primary osteoporosis. These men are often middle-aged and present with height loss and multiple fractures. Whether they have intrinsic abnormalities in bone remodeling—defects in formation or resorption—is unknown.

Clinical & Laboratory Evaluation

Because of the prominence of secondary forms of osteoporosis, the clinical and laboratory investigation of men with low BMD and fractures must be thorough. The history and physical examination should pay attention

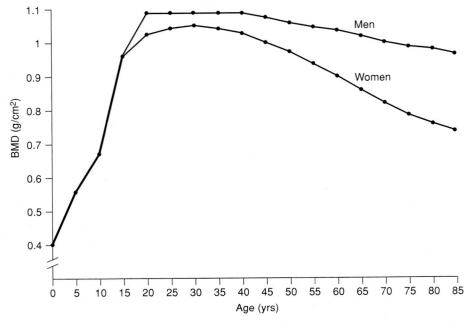

Figure 57–3. Mean bone mineral density (BMD) in men versus women from age 5 to 85 demonstrating the lower peak BMD values for women versus men, the rapid peri-menopausal rates of bone loss in women, and the slow continuous phase of bone loss that continues into the eighth decade. (From Southard RN, Morris JD, Mahan JD, et al. Bone mass in healthy children: measurement with quantitative DXA. *Radiology.* 1991;179:735; and from Kelly TL. Bone mineral reference databases for American men and women. *J Bone Miner Res.* 1990;5(Suppl 2):702. With permission.)

to possible underlying pulmonary, gonadal, adrenal, gastrointestinal, and hematologic disorders. Habits (alcohol and tobacco use) are important risk factors to pursue in men together with the signs and symptoms of the diseases listed in Table 57–4. Men with a history of

prostate cancer should be asked about past (or current) use of long-acting gonadotropin-releasing hormone agonists and androgen blockers. These men lose bone at an accelerated rate and treating them to prevent bone loss is effective.

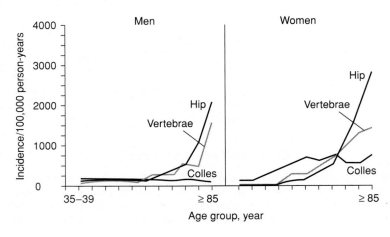

Figure 57–4. The incidence of three common osteoporotic fractures in men and women over decades. (From Cooper C, Melton LJ III. Epidemiology of osteoporosis. *Trends Endocrinol Metab.* 1992;314:224. With permission.)

Table 57–5. Determinants of Low Bone Mineral Density in Men

Advanced age
Frailty
Low body weight
Alcohol intake
Smoking
Caffeine intake
Use of glucocorticoids
History of hyperthyroidism
History of peptic ulcer disease
History of chronic lung disease
History of rheumatoid arthritis
History of fracture after the age of 50
Height loss since age 20

(Adapted from Orwoll ES, Bevan L, Phipps KR. Determinants of bone mineral density in older men. *Osteoporos Int.* 2000;11:815. With permission.)

The complete, cost-effective laboratory evaluation of men with osteoporosis has not been defined. Most would agree that the initial evaluation in men should include a complete blood cell count; liver function tests; determinations of serum chemistries, testosterone, thyroid-stimulating hormone, calcium, and 25-hydroxyvitamin D; and 24-hour urinary calcium excretion.

If anemia is present and no other cause for osteopenia or osteoporosis has been identified, serum and urine protein electrophoresis should be performed to exclude cryptic multiple myeloma. Multiple myeloma should always be considered in older African-American men with unexplained bone loss because of its predilection for that population. Men with low testosterone levels should be referred to an endocrinologist for evaluation for primary or secondary forms of hypogonadism.

While primary hyperparathyroidism is a key consideration in women with low BMD, it is a less prominent cause of accelerated bone loss in men. Nonetheless, because it is a relatively common endocrine disorder, it should be considered if there is a history of renal stones or if the serum calcium value is even marginally elevated.

Hypercortisolism is rare, but bone loss may be the first clinical clue that cortisol excess is present. Cushing syndrome is easily excluded by a 24-hour urinary cortisol determination or overnight dexamethasone suppression testing.

Imaging Evaluation

DXA scanning of the spine of elderly men is often affected by the presence of degenerative arthritis, disc disease, and aortic calcifications. Instant vertebral assessment can be helpful in assessing the presence of vertebral deformities and fractures, although dating such abnormalities is often very difficult. It is important to remember that men experience more traumatic fractures than do women (including fractures of the spine) at young ages.

The most important issue in using bone densitometry in men for the diagnosis of osteoporosis is the lack of sufficiently large databases compared with postmenopausal women. The World Health Organization classification of osteoporosis and osteopenia (see Table 57–1) was developed on the basis of data from postmenopausal white women. It is not rigorously defensible to apply the same DXA T-score cut-points to define osteoporosis and osteopenia in men, but this is widely done. The few randomized trials of drugs to treat osteoporosis in men (summarized below) usually use a T-score of ≤ -2 or -2.5 and/or fractures to enroll patients. Experts in the field are moving toward using absolute BMD measurements and absolute fracture risk to make decisions about treatment in men. Ongoing studies with large cohorts of men should help better define BMD thresholds for treatment in men.

GLUCOCORTICOID-INDUCED OSTEOPOROSIS

General Considerations

Osteoporosis is among the most serious and disabling side effects of glucocorticoid therapy. Adverse skeletal events occur in approximately 50% of patients taking long-term glucocorticoid therapy. These patients are subject to an increased risk of fractures in the spine, hip, and other sites. It has been suggested that glucocorticoid-treated patients fracture at higher BMDs than other groups of patients, but this notion has been challenged.

There is debate about the minimum dose of glucocorticoid required to induce deleterious effects on bone, but the weight of evidence supports the conclusion that chronic therapy with oral doses of ≥ 7.5 mg of prednisone daily (or its equivalent) is associated with an increased risk of both vertebral and hip fractures. The majority of patients receiving glucocorticoids take these drugs orally. Other routes of administration (inhaled, intranasal, or topical) are far less likely to have deleterious skeletal consequences unless particularly high doses of long-acting glucocorticoid preparations are used.

The pathogenesis of glucocorticoid-induced osteoporosis is complex. In the first few weeks of such therapy, there is an increase in bone resorption, and patients can lose considerable bone mass during this initial phase. In addition, glucocorticoids antagonize the actions of vitamin D, especially in the intestine, leading to reduced calcium absorption, and promote calcium excretion by the kidney, producing marked hypercalciuria in some cases. These actions limit the amount of calcium available to form bone matrix properly. Glucocorticoids also act on the pituitary to suppress gonadotropin production, rendering most patients hypogonadal. Chronic glucocorticoid therapy promotes apoptosis (programmed cell death) of osteoblasts, which form new bone, and osteocytes, which are involved in mechanosensing. Therefore ongoing bone resorption is not answered by increased bone formation, and the sensing of normal mechanical forces and physical loading may be impaired. Overall, an imbalance in bone remodeling is favored, and in the end resorption predominates.

When glucocorticoids are discontinued, bone cannot replace the bone mineral that has been lost, and it is impossible to rebuild bone microarchitecture. Hence the prevention of bone loss is the ideal initial strategy.

Not all patients taking high doses of glucocorticoids suffer adverse skeletal consequences. As noted above, only 50% of patients receiving long-term glucocorticoid therapy experience bony complications. What protects the other patients remains unknown. Men and women of all ages and even children can lose bone while taking long-term glucocorticoid therapy. Nonetheless, it is clear that the most vulnerable patients are postmenopausal women. Women who require chronic glucocorticoid therapy often have secondary amenorrhea that contributes to bone loss. Many of the diseases for which they receive glucocorticoids long-term (eg, rheumatoid arthritis) are deleterious to bone.

Clinical, Laboratory, & Imaging Evaluation

Patients who are to receive long-term glucocorticoid therapy should be carefully assessed for relevant skeletal risk factors. The menstrual or menopausal status of women should be recorded. The initial laboratory evaluation should include serum chemistries, serum calcium and 25-hydroxyvitamin D levels, and measurement of 24-hour urinary calcium excretion.

The urinary calcium determination is used in much the same way as described above for postmenopausal women and men with osteoporosis. Because of the propensity of glucocorticoids to interfere with vitamin D action and enhance renal calcium excretion, this is a critical parameter to assess in patients treated with glucocorticoids long term. In addition, a serum testosterone level should be obtained in men due to the effects of glucocorticoids on pituitary release of gonadotropins. Many men taking glucocorticoids long term will often not complain of the typical symptoms of hypogonadism but will have frankly low testosterone levels.

BMD measurements are essential for the evaluation of patients taking glucocorticoids chronically and should inform therapeutic decisions. T-scores that suggest that considerable bone loss has already occurred are usually a signal to treat aggressively.

The American College of Rheumatology published its guidelines for BMD testing among patients taking glucocorticoids long term. Baseline BMD testing and testing patients already receiving treatment were recommended. Depending on the underlying disease, other concomitant risk factors, and the measurement itself, repeat BMD testing is recommended within 12 and sometimes even 6 months. The 6-month interval between repeat testing is appropriate if initial BMD is low, glucocorticoid dose is high, and the patient is not a candidate for the most effective therapies (such as bisphosphonates). Other scenarios could be envisioned in which knowing that bone loss has not progressed rapidly (within 6 months) is helpful in reassuring the patient or in establishing the effectiveness of aggressive therapy.

DIFFERENTIAL DIAGNOSIS OF LOW BONE MINERAL DENSITY

The differential diagnosis of a low BMD measurement is narrow: it is either due to osteoporosis or osteomalacia. Any primary or secondary form of osteoporosis described in this chapter could cause this picture. Osteomalacia causes low bone mass or low BMD because the mineralization of the matrix is defective. Mineral content of the skeleton (not the protein content) is reduced in osteomalacia. A host of different conditions cause osteomalacia. These need to be considered seriously if there is any abnormality in the levels of serum calcium, phosphorus, alkaline phosphatase, or 25-hydroxyvitamin D. Patients with osteomalacia may also have bone pain, pathologic fractures, muscle weakness, and difficulty walking, especially when osteomalacia is moderate or severe and the diagnosis has been delayed. Because the disease is difficult to detect early in its course, the astute clinician must be aware of the manifestations of this less common bone disease and should not ignore subtle clinical and laboratory features that hint at the presence of osteomalacia.

TREATMENT OF OSTEOPOROSIS

The essentials of management for most forms of osteoporosis include the following:

- Lifestyle modifications.
- Nutritional interventions.
- Pharmacologic therapies.

Lifestyle Modifications

Lifestyle modifications should be implemented in all patients in whom the prevention of bone loss is desired and in whom the goals are stopping bone loss and reducing fractures. Initial efforts are directed at increasing the safety of the patient's immediate environment to prevent falls and fractures, eliminating habits that are deleterious to skeletal integrity and that can contribute to falls, and improving the calcium and vitamin D status of the patient. The latter strategy is absolutely essential if the pharmacologic therapies discussed below are to be successful.

The desired lifestyle modifications are straightforward in concept but not always in implementation. Patients should be encouraged to discontinue smoking and alcohol consumption. Both habits are injurious to bone. Patients should be prescribed a weight-bearing exercise program that emphasizes regular participation (five times weekly if possible for at least 30 and preferably 45 or 60 minutes each) and that is suitable for even frail elderly patients. Regular walking can provide benefits to the frail osteoporotic patient beyond positive changes in BMD. Exercise improves well-being and neuromuscular coordination, which can help condition reflexes to respond better to falls. In addition, although there is some controversy as to efficacy, hip protectors are a simple intervention that can help reduce the incidence of hip fractures in the frail elderly patient who is at risk for falls and is ambulatory.

In patients with inflammatory diseases who are receiving long-term glucocorticoid therapy and are at risk for osteoporosis, an exercise and physical therapy program is imperative. Such patients often suffer from glucocorticoid-induced myopathy as well as the disuse and deconditioning attendant to the joint pains, myalgias, and systemic inflammation caused by their underlying disorders (eg, rheumatoid arthritis, systemic lupus erythematosus, ankylosing spondylitis, and so forth).

Nutritional Interventions: Calcium Supplements and Vitamin D

Several studies support the ability of calcium and vitamin D supplements alone to prevent fractures in the elderly. This is especially true for individuals whose calcium intake is below recommended allowances. Every fracture trial done in recent years has included calcium—and usually vitamin D supplementation as well—in both the placebo and treatment groups.

Nutritional interventions for osteoporosis should assure that the diet plus supplements provide at least 1200 mg of elemental calcium per day and up to 1500 mg in high-risk patients over the age of 70 with established disease or with steroid-induced osteoporosis (Table 57–6). Measurements of 24-hour urinary calcium excretion can be used to assure adequate absorption and to avoid hypercalciuria.

There are only two major sources of vitamin D. In the U.S., milk is supplemented with vitamin D and is the main dietary source of this vitamin. The second source of vitamin D is dermal synthesis, which is influenced by latitude and exposure to sunlight. For a variety of reasons, the elderly population and the chronically ill, including those with rheumatologic disorders, are often deficient in dairy intake and sunlight exposure. That vitamin D insufficiency is a substantial problem is

Table 57–6. Management of Postmenopausal and Glucocorticoid-Induced Osteoporosis

• Lifestyle modifications	Discontinue tobacco
	Discontinue alcohol intake
	Wear hip protector
	Exercise regularly
• Nutritional interventions	Increase calcium intake to 1000 mg elemental calcium per day for prevention of osteoporosis in premenopausal women and to 1000–1500 mg elemental calcium per day for postmenopausal women, men, and patients taking glucocorticoids long term; vitamin D intake: 400–800 IU/d for men and postmenopausal women, and for patients taking glucocorticoids long term
• Pharmacologic therapies	• Bisphosphonates
	Alendronate 5 mg/d or 35 mg/wk for prevention of osteoporosis; 10 mg/d or 70 mg/wk for treatment of postmenopausal, male, and glucocorticoid-induced osteoporosis
	Risedronate 5 mg/d or 35 mg/wk for prevention and treatment of postmenopausal and glucocorticoid-induced osteoporosis
	• Parathyroid hormone
	Teriparatide (PTH 1–34) 20 μg subcutaneous per day for postmenopausal and male osteoporosis
	• SERMs
	Raloxifene 60 mg/d
	• Calcitonin
	Nasal spray calcitonin 200 IU intranasally daily

SERMs, selective estrogen response modulators.

strongly supported by a recent survey of 1526 post-menopausal women in North America on prescription drug therapy for osteoporosis. Approximately 50% of these women had 25-hydroxyvitamin D levels below the target of 30 ng/mL.

Vitamin D is universally recommended to preserve bone health. The National Academy of Sciences recommends a daily allowance of 400–600 IU. The National Osteoporosis Foundation recommends slightly more vitamin D per day (800 IU) for individuals at risk for vitamin D insufficiency (eg, the elderly and the housebound).

The definition of vitamin D sufficiency, especially in the elderly, is a controversial issue. 25-Hydroxyvitamin D, which is the metabolite made by the liver and stored in fat, is the best indicator of overall vitamin D status in an individual. However, in a recent publication, experts in the field provided estimates for optimal levels of 25-hydroxyvitamin D that ranged from 50–80 nmol/L (20–32 ng/mL).

Pharmacologic Therapies

Pharmacologic therapies have been intensively researched in recent years. Agents that are effective for treating osteoporosis and approved in the United States are (1) bisphosphonates, (2) selective estrogen response modulators, (3) calcitonin, and (4) teriparatide (parathyroid hormone [PTH] 1-34). Hormone replacement therapy (HRT) remains effective in the prevention of bone loss in postmenopausal women. A summary of the treatment and prevention strategies is outlined in Table 64–6.

Young women of child-bearing age must be treated with circumspection. Bisphosphonates accumulate in the skeleton and may alter fetal skeletal development should pregnancy occur, theoretically even several years after discontinuing bisphosphonate treatment. None of the medications, especially bisphosphonates, are approved for use in pregnant or lactating women.

A. Bisphosphonates

Three drugs in this class are approved for the prevention and treatment of osteoporosis in the United States: alendronate, risedronate, and ibandronate. Alendronate and risedronate are approved for both postmenopausal and glucocorticoid-induced osteoporosis. Alendronate is also approved to treat male osteoporosis. These drugs and the general category of bisphosphonates are discussed in detail in Chapter 67. The BMD changes observed with alendronate therapy in men and women treated with glucocorticoids for 24 months are shown in Table 57–7. Both men and women experience statistically significant increases in BMD by DXA measurements compared with placebo. Overall, drugs of the bisphosphonate class are

Table 57–7. Average BMD Changes (%) Due to Alendronate (ALN) or Placebo in Patients on Glucocorticoids After 24 Months of Therapy

Parameter	Placebo	ALN 5 mg	ALN 10 mg
Lumbar spine BMD	−0.77	2.84	3.85
	(53)	(59)	(51)
Femoral neck BMD	−2.93	0.11	0.61
	(53)	(57)	(51)
Total hip BMD	−1.57	1.64	2.69
	(45)	(47)	(40)
Total body BMD	−0.36	0.77	1.09
	(40)	(44)	(41)
Lumbar spine BMD Men (N=17)	0.65	4.29	6.29
Premenopausal women (N=11)	−0.96	0.75	2.34
Postmenopausal women			
No HRT (N=18)	−0.73	1.95	3.91
HRT (N=7)	−3.98	5.36	1.4

(Adapted from Adachi JD, Saag KG, Delmas PD, et al. Two-year effects of alendronate on bone mineral density and vertebral fracture in patients receiving glucocorticoids: a randomized, double-blind, placebo-controlled extension trial. *Arthritis Rheum.* 2001;44:202. With permission.)

the most frequently prescribed medications for the treatment of osteoporosis.

B. Raloxifene

Raloxifene belongs to a growing class of drugs called selective estrogen response modulators, which differ from estrogen biochemically and structurally but can act as estrogen agonists or antagonists depending on the specific target tissues. Raloxifene was developed with the goal of capitalizing on the benefits of estrogen in bone and eliminating or strongly diminishing the impact of estrogenlike compounds on cardiovascular and breast cancer risks. Results from studies of raloxifene suggest that it may be possible to achieve such outcomes.

The MORE (Multiple Outcomes of Raloxifene Evaluation) study compared the efficacy of raloxifene to placebo in postmenopausal women with osteoporosis. After 3 years of therapy, women treated with raloxifene (60 or 120 mg/d) demonstrated modest (2.1–2.7%) but significant increases in lumbar spine and femoral neck BMD. The occurrence of vertebral fractures was significantly reduced by 30–50% compared with the placebo group. However, the overall incidence of nonvertebral fractures was unchanged by raloxifene, and there was no significant impact on hip fractures (relative risk 1.1; 95% confidence interval [CI] [0.6–1.9]).

Raloxifene was not associated with an increased risk of endometrial carcinoma, vaginal bleeding, or mastalgia. Venous thromboembolic events, however, were increased in women receiving raloxifene compared to women receiving placebo (relative risk 3.1; 95% CI [1.5–6.2]). This incidence of venous thromboembolic events was similar in frequency to that of patients receiving HRT or tamoxifen. Additional adverse events that were increased in women taking raloxifene included hot flashes, leg cramps, edema, and a flulike syndrome.

Interestingly, the incidence of breast cancer was reduced in both groups of women treated for 40 months with either dose of raloxifene (relative risk 0.3; 95% CI [0.2–0.6]) in the initial trial. With continued administration of raloxifene, it appears that the risk of breast cancer is significantly reduced with up to 8 years of treatment. Trials specifically designed to examine breast cancer outcomes are in progress.

In summary, raloxifene has modest positive effects on BMD and reduces vertebral, but not nonvertebral, fractures. It is a useful agent for younger postmenopausal women who have less severe osteoporosis and are at lower risk for hip fracture.

C. NASAL SPRAY CALCITONIN

Calcitonin, a 32-amino-acid peptide hormone, binds to receptors on osteoclasts, and this interaction inhibits osteoclast-mediated bone resorption. Calcitonin in the form of a nasal spray (200 U/d) is approved for the treatment of postmenopausal osteoporosis.

The PROOF (Prevent Recurrence of Osteoporotic Fractures) trial established the efficacy of nasal spray calcitonin by comparing it to placebo in 1255 postmenopausal women. All patients received 1000 mg elemental calcium and 400 IU vitamin D daily. After 5 years of therapy, nasal spray calcitonin (200 IU/d) induced 1.0–1.5% increases in lumbar spine BMD that were accompanied by a 33% reduction in new spinal fractures compared with placebo. Hip BMD and hip fractures were not significantly affected by therapy with calcitonin. Adverse events included nasal irritation (congestion, discharge, or sneezing). Calcitonin therefore has modest effects on spinal BMD and does not reduce hip fractures, but has an excellent tolerability profile.

D. TERIPARATIDE

Teriparatide or parathyroid hormone (PTH) 1-34 was approved by the Food and Drug Administration in 2002 for the treatment of osteoporosis in postmenopausal women and men. This therapy capitalizes on the ability of PTH to produce anabolic effects on the skeleton to stimulate bone formation when it is administered intermittently in low doses. Chronic elevations of PTH, as occurs in primary hyperparathyroidism, are "catabolic" to bone, causing excessive resorption and increased fracture risk. Thus PTH as a therapy for osteoporosis targets the narrow window between the anabolic and catabolic effects of PTH. The studies demonstrating the efficacy of PTH (1-34) in increasing BMD and reducing vertebral and nonvertebral fracture risk in postmenopausal women and the studies in men are described in detail in Chapter 67. Trials are underway to assess the efficacy of teriparatide for glucocorticoid-induced osteoporosis.

1. Indications

a. Postmenopausal osteoporosis—The fracture prevention trial for teriparatide enrolled 1637 postmenopausal women with at least one moderate or two mild nontraumatic vertebral fractures and compared subcutaneous injections of teriparatide (20 μg/d) with placebo. All participants took daily supplements of calcium (1000 mg) and vitamin D (400–1200 IU). After 21 months, teriparatide induced dramatic increases in spinal BMD (+9.7%) and modest but significant increases in femoral neck BMD (+2.8%).

Teriparatide reduced new vertebral fractures by 65% and all nonvertebral fractures combined (ie, hip, wrist, ankle, humerus, rib, and so forth) by 54%, but the number of hip fractures did not significantly differ in teriparatide- versus placebo-treated patients. New moderate or severe vertebral fractures were substantially reduced 78–90% in teriparatide- versus placebo-treated patients. Adverse events due to teriparatide included dizziness and leg cramps (both in <10% of patients). Hypercalcemia (defined as serum calcium >10.6 mg/dL) developed in 11% of patients receiving teriparatide, compared with 2% of patients in the placebo group. Ninety-five percent of these serum calcium values were <11.2 mg/dL and were managed by reducing calcium intake in most patients.

b. Osteoporosis in men—In a study of teriparatide in male osteoporosis, 437 men were enrolled with T-scores <−2 in the lumbar spine or hip. Their average age was 59, and approximately 50% had low serum free testosterone levels. Men were treated for 11 months with teriparatide or with placebo, and all patients received 1000 mg elemental calcium and 400–1200 IU vitamin D per day. This trial was prematurely terminated because ongoing toxicology studies in rats found an increased incidence of osteosarcomas (see below). At study termination, teriparatide (at 20 μg subcutaneously per day) induced significant average increases in spinal BMD of +5.9%, in femoral neck BMD of +1.5%, and in total body BMD of +0.6%. Teriparatide was found to be effective in men regardless of their gonadal status, age, or baseline BMD values. The changes in BMD were impressive, given the short duration of the study, but the short duration of the study and the limited number of subjects rendered it underpowered to assess reduction in fractures.

2. Carcinogenic effect of teriparatide—Both of the above studies were terminated early due to results from standard carcinogenicity studies in rats showing that lifelong daily injections of high-dose teriparatide induced osteosclerosis and a markedly increased incidence of osteosarcomas (48% of rats treated with teriparatide [75 μg/kg for 17 months]). The Food and Drug Administration has concluded that these findings do not preclude the use of teriparatide in humans but requires a black box warning on the package insert to inform practitioners and patients of this result.

3. Guidelines for use—Given the above findings, costs, and inconvenience of daily subcutaneous injections with this hormone, teriparatide is recommended to treat bone loss in the following groups: patients with severe osteoporosis, especially accompanied by fractures; patients intolerant of other therapies for osteoporosis; and patients who have not responded to other drugs for osteoporosis as evidenced by significant losses of BMD by DXA and/or the development of fractures. Treatment is recommended not to exceed 2 years in duration and is approved for use in men and postmenopausal women. Teriparatide is *contraindicated* in growing children (with open epiphyses), patients with bone metastases or those who have had skeletal irradiation, and patients with Paget disease or an unexplained elevation in the alkaline phosphatase value.

Despite the above considerations, teriparatide still holds great promise for both building new bone and increasing the skeleton's biomechanical strength—outcomes that are highly desired to prevent ongoing osteoporotic fractures in high-risk patients. How should teriparatide be best used to treat osteoporosis? It is anticipated that 2 years of therapy with this agent will be followed by long-term therapy with antiresorptive drugs in an effort to maintain the gains in BMD achieved with this anabolic agent. While this idea is at present intuitively sound, the long-term efficacy of such regimens has been evaluated to only a limited extent as described below (see the section on combination and sequential regimens, below).

E. HORMONE REPLACEMENT THERAPY

HRT refers to the combination of estrogen and progestin while estrogen replacement therapy (ERT) involves the use of an estrogen preparation exclusively, typically only in patients who have had a hysterectomy. A variety of estrogen preparations have been used for the prevention and treatment of postmenopausal osteoporosis. Perhaps the most popular and best studied has been the combination of conjugated equine estrogens and medroxyprogesterone acetate in varying dosages. Studies like the PEPI (Postmenopausal Estrogen/Progestin Interventions) trial established the efficacy of various HRT and ERT regi-

mens to prevent postmenopausal bone loss at the spine and hip, based on DXA measurements after 3 years of therapy. This study showed average 3–5% increases in lumbar spine BMD and 1.7% increases in hip BMD after treatment with a variety of ERT and HRT regimens. Placebo-treated patients lost bone mineral (–1.8% and –1.7% changes in BMD values in the lumbar spine and hip, respectively). However, the PEPI trial and other studies of HRT/ERT in postmenopausal osteoporosis did not quantify the antifracture benefit.

Despite the lack of documented fracture protection with HRT/ERT, these treatments were popular preventive strategies for postmenopausal women until recently. HRT/ERT was believed to reduce the risks of coronary heart disease and its complications, based on epidemiologic studies, and to have little or no effect on breast cancer. This view changed dramatically with the publication of findings from the Women's Health Initiative (WHI). The WHI examined the risks and benefits of HRT (0.625 mg conjugated equine estrogens and 2.5 mg medroxyprogesterone acetate per day) in 16,608 women in the primary prevention of several postmenopausal health outcomes. This study found a small but significant increased risk of invasive breast cancer in women receiving HRT compared with those receiving placebo after 5.2 years (HR [hazard ratio] 1.26; 95% CI [1.00–1.59]) and a similarly small increase in coronary heart disease end-points due to HRT (HR 1.29; 95% CI [1.02–1.63]). Ironically, this study did show a reduction in hip fractures (HR 0.66; 95% CI [0.45–0.98]) due to HRT. Despite the salutary effect on fractures, the other negative outcomes from the WHI (increased cardiovascular and breast cancer risks) have strongly discouraged the use of HRT in postmenopausal women.

In 2004, the results of the ERT study in WHI were reported. Of 10,739 postmenopausal women with prior hysterectomies, 5310 were randomized to ERT (0.625 mg conjugated equine estrogens), and 5410 were treated with placebo for 6.8 years. Major clinical outcomes were an increased risk of stroke (HR 1.39; 95% CI [1.10–1.77]) and reduced risk of hip fractures (HR 0.61; 95% CI [0.41–0.91]). There was no increased risk of coronary heart disease, pulmonary embolism, or breast cancer.

The risk of fracture and changes in BMD were further examined in a subset of women in the HRT trial in WHI. Total hip BMD increased by 3.7% after 3 years of therapy compared to 0.14% in the placebo group. The risk of all fractures was significantly reduced in women on HRT (HR 0.76; 95% CI [0.69–0.83]) as were the risks of vertebral and lower arm/wrist fractures.

Despite the positive effects of HRT on reducing fractures, the negative nonskeletal outcomes have made HRT undesirable for treating osteoporosis, given the availability of other options. Present recommendations are that HRT be used for as short a time as possible after menopause, in the lowest possible doses, and mainly for the control of vasomotor symptoms.

F. COMBINATION AND SEQUENTIAL REGIMENS

A small number of trials have combined approved agents for the treatment of osteoporosis, either together or in sequence. In general these studies are smaller than the pivotal trials that established the efficacy of individual therapies in the treatment of osteoporosis and prevention of fractures. The combination of two anti-resorptive therapies typically achieves a small additional increase in BMD beyond that attained with either agent alone. None of the combination or sequential studies has had fracture reduction as an end-point, and therefore a clear role for these approaches to prevent fractures is not yet established. Furthermore, costs and adverse events are potentially additive. There has been the additional concern that excessive blockade of resorption (with two anti-resorptive agents) might produce such marked suppression of turnover as to impair the ability of bone to repair microdamage and microfractures and to respond to the normal forces acting on the remodeling process.

There is theoretical appeal for sequential regimens that first use anabolic agents like teriparatide to promote bone formation and then use potent anti-resorptive drugs to maintain bone. An important trial in this regard, the Parathyroid Hormone and Alendronate Study in postmenopausal women, compared alendronate (10 mg/d) and full-length PTH (PTH [1-84], 100 μg/d) individually or in combination. There was no evidence of synergy when the agents were used concurrently; indeed at 1 year, the concurrent use of alendronate appeared to diminish bone formation. The second year of the study, however, showed that the gains in BMD achieved with PTH (1-84) alone for 12 months were not maintained unless PTH (1-84) was followed by alendronate. Similar conclusions were reached in a study of men using PTH (1-34) and alendronate. It appears that potent anti-resorptive agents such as alendronate tend to blunt the "anabolic" effects of PTH when used concurrently but can maintain PTH-induced increases in BMD when used in a sequential regimen.

Currently there are insufficient data to firmly establish how best to use combinations of currently available therapies for osteoporosis. In the near future, however, the therapy of osteoporosis likely will combine the unique features of the available drugs with a better understanding of how to manipulate the bone remodeling cycle to the best advantage.

TREATMENT FAILURES

An ominous clinical development in a patient already on treatment for osteoporosis is the occurrence of multiple fractures. Loss of BMD during therapy is also a cause for concern if the decrement in BMD exceeds the precision errors of DXA measurements.

Noncompliance is a common explanation for treatment failure. Although the therapies discussed above (especially the bisphosphonates and teriparatide) are highly efficacious, no treatment strategy completely prevents all fractures. If noncompliance is not the explanation, then the clinician must decide whether the fracture was expected or unexpected in the context of the individual patient. The clinician must consider the length of therapy, underlying risk factors contributing to the patient's bone loss, baseline BMD values, the degree of trauma if any, and other medications and conditions that might exacerbate the fracture risk or bone loss. The clinician must also decide whether the initial work-up was sufficient and whether possible secondary causes were considered and properly eliminated. On many occasions, especially in postmenopausal women, treatment failures prompt the first thorough investigation to exclude secondary causes of low BMD (eg, primary hyperparathyroidism, multiple myeloma, vitamin D deficiency, or celiac sprue). If the clinician is inexperienced with the evaluation of secondary osteoporosis or deciding whether BMD determinations indicate adequate responses to treatment, then this is an excellent time to refer a patient with fractures or ongoing bone loss while receiving therapy to a specialist (rheumatologist or endocrinologist) experienced in the care of patients with osteoporosis.

REFERENCES

Dawson-Hughes B, Heaney RP, Holick MF, et al. Estimates of optimal vitamin D status. *Osteoporos Int.* 2005;16:713. [PMID: 15776217]

Health Care Financing Administration. Medicare program; Medicare coverage of and payment for bone mass measurement. Interim final rule with comment period. *Fed Reg.* 1998;63:34320. [PMID: 10180295]

Hodsman AB, Bauer DC, Dempster DW, et al. Parathyroid hormone and teriparatide for the treatment of osteoporosis: a review of the evidence and suggested guidelines for its use. *Endocr Rev.* 2005;26:688. [PMID: 15769903]

Holick MF, Siris ES, Binkley N, et al. Prevalence of Vitamin D inadequacy among postmenopausal North American women receiving osteoporosis therapy. *J Clin Endocrinol Metab.* 2005;90:3215. [PMID: 15797954]

Kanis JA. Diagnosis of osteoporosis and assessment of fracture risk. *Lancet.* 2002;359:1929. [PMID: 12057569]

Maricic M. Glucocorticoid-induced osteoporosis: treatment options and guidelines. *Curr Osteoporos Rep.* 2005;3:25. [PMID: 16036098]

Mosekilde L. Vitamin D and the elderly. *Clin Endocrinol.* 2005;62:265. [PMID: 15730407]

National Osteoporosis Foundation. *Physician's Guide to Prevention and Treatment of Osteoporosis.* Excerpta Medica, 1998.

Nelson HD, Helfand M, Woolf SH, Allan JD. Screening for postmenopausal osteoporosis: a review of evidence for the U.S.

Preventive Services Task Force. *Ann Intern Med.* 2002;137:529. [PMID: 12230356]

National Institutes of Health Consensus Statement. Osteoporosis Prevention, Diagnosis, and Therapy, Office of the Director, 2000;17:5.

Orwoll ES, Bevan L, Phioos KR. Determinants of bone mineral density in older men. *Osteoporos Int.* 2000;11:815. [PMID: 11199184]

Orwoll ES, Bliziotes M. *Osteoporosis: Pathophysiology and Clinical Management.* Humana Press, 2003.

Recommendations for the prevention and treatment of glucocorticoid-induced osteoporosis: 2001 update. American College of Rheumatology Ad Hoc Committee on Glucocorticoid-Induced Osteoporosis. *Arthritis Rheum.* 2001;44:1496. [PMID: 11465699]

Rosen CJ. Postmenopausal osteoporosis. *N Engl J Med.* 2005;353:6. [PMID: 16093468]

U.S. Preventive Services Task Force. Screening for osteoporosis in postmenopausal women: recommendation and rationale. *Ann Intern Med.* 2002;137:526. [PMID: 12230355]

Relevant World Wide Web Sites

[The American Society for Bone and Mineral Research]
http://www.asbmr.org
[National Osteoporosis Foundation]
http://www.nof.org

Osteonecrosis

Carol M. Ziminski, MD

ESSENTIALS OF DIAGNOSIS

- *Pain is the most frequent symptom of osteonecrosis (ON).*
- *The most commonly affected sites are the proximal and distal femoral heads, resulting in hip or knee pain. The ankles, shoulders, or elbows may also be affected.*
- *Groin pain is most common in patients with femoral head disease; thigh and buttock pain occur less often.*
- *Most patients have pain with weight bearing and joint motion.*
- *Pain at rest occurs in two-thirds of patients. One-third report night pain.*
- *A small proportion of patients are asymptomatic, in which case the diagnosis is generally incidental.*

General Considerations

Osteonecrosis is a generic term that refers to cell death in the two components of bone, both hematopoietic fat marrow and osteocytes. Other terms frequently used for this condition are "ischemic necrosis," "avascular necrosis," "aseptic necrosis," and "osteochondritis dissecans."

ON, which represents an inability to supply adequate oxygen to underlying bone, is extremely uncommon in healthy individuals. The condition typically occurs only in the fatty marrow, which contains a sparse vascular supply. In contrast, hematopoietic marrow has a rich blood supply. The femoral head is the most vulnerable site for the development of ON. The site of necrosis is typically just below the weight-bearing articular surface of the bone, the anterolateral aspect of the femoral head. This is the site of greatest mechanical stress.

Osteonecrosis is characterized by areas of dead trabecular bone and marrow extending to the subchondral plate. The anterolateral aspect of the femoral head, the principal weight-bearing region, is involved most often. In the adult, the involved segment never fully revascular-izes. Once radiographic detection is possible, collapse of the femoral head is usually inevitable, at intervals ranging from weeks to years.

Elderly persons seem to be at decreased risk for developing ON. In this age group, fat cells become smaller. The space between fat cells fills with a loose reticulum and mucoid fluid that is resistant to ischemic necrosis. This is termed gelatinous marrow, and even in the presence of increased intramedullary pressure, interstitial fluid is able to escape into the blood vessels, leaving the spaces free to absorb additional fluid.

Osteonecrosis is not a discrete disease but represents the final common pathway of several conditions, most of which result in impairment of the blood supply to the bone. ON may occur in a variety of clinical settings, in association with defined diseases (eg, an infiltrative process such as Gaucher disease), medications (eg, glucocorticoids), physiologic or pathologic conditions (eg, pregnancy, thromboembolism, or trauma), or without identifiable predisposing factors (idiopathic).

The true prevalence of ON is unknown, but it is estimated that there are approximately 10,000–20,000 new cases annually in the United States, and ON is the underlying diagnosis in approximately 10% of all total hip replacements. For the most part, ON affects the epiphyses of the long bones, such as the femoral and humeral heads, but other bones (eg, carpal and tarsal) can also be affected. The disease occurs more frequently in males than females, with the overall male:female ratio in the range of 8:1. The age distribution is wide, although most patients are younger than age 50 at the time of diagnosis. The average age of female cases exceeds that of males by almost 10 years.

Pathogenesis

Osteonecrosis may be seen in association with a number of different conditions (Table 58–1). A definitive etiologic role has been established for some of these factors but most are probable relationships. Glucocorticoid use and excessive alcohol intake reportedly account for more than 90% of cases.

A variety of pathways are believed to contribute to the pathogenesis of ON. Some pathways figure more prominently in certain cases than in others. One pathway

Table 58–1. Etiologic Factors Associated with Osteonecrosis

Osteonecrosis of known etiology
  Traumatic
    Femoral neck fracture
    Dislocation or fracture dislocation of the hip
  Nontraumatic
    Sickle cell disease
    Gaucher disease
    Caisson disease (decompression sickness or diver's disease)
    Radiotherapy
Osteonecrosis with probably etiologic relationships
  Traumatic
    Minor trauma
  Nontraumatic
    Glucocorticoids (exogenous and endogenous)
      Enteral, intra-articular, pulse intravenous
      Organ transplantation
      Cushing disease
    Alcohol use
    Connective tissue diseases (may occur independent of glucocorticoid use)
    Systemic lupus erythematosus
    Rheumatoid arthritis
    Systemic vasculitis
    Antiphospholipid antibody syndrome
    Other connective tissue diseases
    Metabolic disorders
      Hyperuricemia/gout
      Hyperlipidemia
      Chronic renal failure or hemodialysis
    Disorders associated with fat necrosis
      Pancreatitis
      Pancreatic cancer
    Hematologic disorders
      Intravascular coagulation
      Thrombophlebitis
    Pregnancy
    Cigarette smoking
    Tumors (infiltrative)
    Idiopathic

is thrombosis or embolization of smaller arteries of the femoral head by lipid droplets (potentially an important contributor in glucocorticoid-associated ON), abnormal red blood cells (as in sickle cell disease), or nitrogen bubbles from caisson disease (ON associated with decompression illness or deep sea diving). In other cases, vasculopathy may result from structural damage to the arterial or venous walls from vasculitis, radiation necrosis, or release of vasoactive substances (as in Gaucher disease). In others, increased intraosseous pressure from enlargement of intramedullary fat cells or osteocytes may play a role.

Through one or more of these pathways, ON begins with interruption of the blood supply to bone; subsequently, the adjacent area becomes hyperemic, leading to demineralization, trabecular thinning, and if stressed, bony collapse. The process is usually progressive, resulting in joint destruction within 3–5 years if left untreated.

Trauma with fracture of the femoral neck, especially in the subcapital region, interrupts the major part of the blood supply to the femoral head and may lead to ischemia and ON. ON can occur within 8 hours of traumatic disruption of the blood supply. The superior retinacular vessels and the nutrient artery can be damaged as they enter the femur. The artery of the ligamentum teres also may be damaged. Intracapsular hematoma increases intracapsular pressure, which can cause tamponade of the joint capsule. The incidence of ON in such cases, at least 30%, increases for badly displaced fractures, particularly in young adults. Intertrochanteric and extracapsular fractures of the femur rarely develop ON. Following hip dislocation, circulation is interrupted because of tears of the ligamentum teres, tearing the artery of the ligamentum teres. Tearing of the joint capsule compromises the vessels within the capsular reflections. ON following subcapital fractures of the femur may develop as late as 10 years following the fracture. Dislocation and fracture-dislocation are much less common than hip fracture, but the incidence of ON may be quite high if reduction is accomplished more than 6 hours after dislocation.

Many studies have related **glucocorticoid** use to the development of ON. A possible mechanism for steroid-induced ON involves alterations in circulating lipids, with resultant microemboli in the arteries supplying bone. A more recent theory proposes that steroids induce changes in venous endothelial cells, leading to stasis, increased intraosseous pressure, and eventual necrosis.

The overall incidence of developing ON as a result of glucocorticoid therapy is small but significant, and appears to be dose-related. Patients treated with prolonged high doses of glucocorticoids are at greatest risk for the development of ON. ON may develop in patients treated with physiologic glucocorticoid replacement for adrenal insufficiency. In comparison, ON is a rare complication of short-term glucocorticoid use, including pulse therapy and intra-articular glucocorticoid injections.

Most studies have found that the risk is low (less than 3%) in patients treated with doses of prednisone less than 15–20 mg/d. In one series, the prednisone dose in the highest month of therapy exceeded 40 mg/d in 93%, and 20 mg/d in 100% of patients with ON. The only clinical finding that distinguished patients with ON from those without this complication was a cushingoid appearance (86% versus 15%). ON is a rare complication of primary **Cushing disease.** This probably reflects the lower glucocorticoid exposure than that seen with high-dose exogenous glucocorticoid therapy.

ON has been reported in 3–30% of patients with **systemic lupus erythematosus.** This range reflects the use of different techniques in defining the disorder (from the less sensitive radiography to the very sensitive magnetic resonance imaging [MRI]), variations in glucocorticoid doses, and variable periods of follow-up. At greatest risk are patients with systemic lupus erythematosus who have taken glucocorticoids, although occasional cases have occurred in the absence of glucocorticoid treatment.

ON often develops in patients with systemic lupus erythematosus a relatively short time after the initiation of glucocorticoid therapy. The strongest risk factors appear to be doses of prednisone consistently greater than 20 mg/d and evidence of glucocorticoid-associated end-organ effects. Other potential contributors in systemic lupus erythematosus are Raynaud phenomenon, antiphospholipid antibodies, and hyperlipidemia, but none of this is proven.

ON is probably the most debilitating of the musculoskeletal complications following **renal transplantation.** In this setting, it is usually multifocal, with 50–70% of affected persons having more than one joint involved. The risk has decreased since the introduction of cyclosporine, with resultant decrease in glucocorticoid dose. Osteopenia and preexisting hyperparathyroidism have been proposed as independent risk factors in this population, but these are not proven.

Excessive alcohol use and the development of ON have been linked for decades: fat emboli, venous stasis, and increased cortisol levels have all been implicated as etiologic factors. An elevated risk for regular drinkers and a clear dose-response relationship has been noted.

ON is common in patients with homozygous **sickle cell disease** because of red blood cell sickling and bone marrow hyperplasia. ON develops in about 50% of affected patients by age 35.

Gaucher disease is an autosomal recessive disorder of glucocerebroside metabolism that leads to the accumulation of cerebroside-filled cells within the bone marrow. This may result in compression of the vasculature and subsequent ON. ON has been reported in 60% of patients with Gaucher disease.

The increased pressure associated with **caisson disease (diver's disease)** can lead to the formation of nitrogen bubbles, which may occlude arterioles and cause ON. This may develop years after the exposure. The number of exposures and the magnitude of depth or pressure to which the diver is exposed are important risk factors.

Another potential cause of ON is **inherited thrombophilia.** There are conflicting data from small retrospective series regarding the role of mutations in genes for proteins in the coagulation cascade and fibrinolytic pathways in the pathogenesis of ON. Four reports suggested an increased prevalence of the factor V Leiden mutation in patients with ON of the hip or knee compared with healthy controls, a finding that was not seen in another study.

Infection with the **human immunodeficiency virus** may confer an increased risk of developing ON of the femoral head. Additional risk factors in this population may be use of glucocorticoids, lipid-lowering drugs, testosterone, and weight training. Use of highly active antiretroviral therapy does not appear to be an independent risk factor.

Clinical Findings

A. Symptoms and Signs

Many patients with ON have had the disease for some time before symptoms are present. Initial symptoms are often felt during activity and include pain or aching in the affected joint. In some instances, the pain may begin quite suddenly. Many patients have bilateral involvement at the time of diagnosis, including disease of the hips, knees, and shoulders.

Physical findings are largely nonspecific. In early stages of hip ON, for example, decreased range of motion is related primarily to pain, particularly with forced internal rotation and abduction. Bone remodeling allows some patients to remain functional for years, despite limited range of motion. As the disease progresses, the pain increases, associated with stiffness and restricted range of motion of the involved joint. Limping becomes common late in the course of lower extremity disease. With hip involvement, the pain is usually felt in the groin. The time from onset of symptoms to development of end-stage joint disease varies widely, from months to years.

MRI studies comparing symptomatic and asymptomatic joints in people at high risk for development of ON have demonstrated a preclinical stage. Abnormalities in asymptomatic joints may predate clinical symptoms by weeks to months.

B. Imaging Studies

1. Radiography—The diagnosis of ON has been based on plain radiographs, which may identify advanced disease but are less helpful in early stages. The evaluation for suspected ON of the femoral head should begin with anteroposterior and frog-leg lateral radiographs. Lateral views are necessary to evaluate the superior portion of the femoral head, where subchondral abnormalities may be seen. The plain radiograph may remain normal for months after onset of symptoms; the earliest findings are mild density changes followed by sclerosis and cysts as the disease progresses (Figures 58–1 and 58–2). The pathognomonic crescent sign (subchondral radiolucency) is evidence of subchondral collapse. Later stages show loss of sphericity or collapse of the femoral head. Eventually,

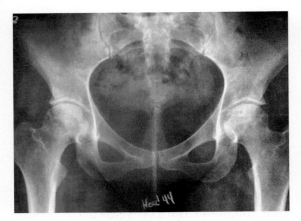

Figure 58–1. Plain anteroposterior radiograph demonstrating features consistent with osteonecrosis of the femoral head. There is bilateral cystic change and sclerosis at the margins. There is a mottled increased density because of destruction of the bony trabecula. There is some evidence of collapse of the femoral head, as the joint space is not a smooth hemisphere.

joint space narrowing and degenerative changes in the acetabulum are apparent (Figure 58–3).

2. Radionuclide bone scan—Technetium-99m bone scanning is useful for patients with suspected disease who have normal radiographs, unilateral symptoms, and no risk factors. Increased uptake, either because of new bone formation or simply as a result of metabolic activ-

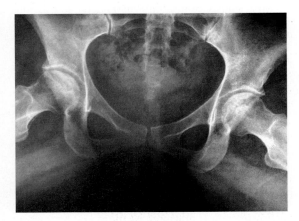

Figure 58–2. Lateral/frog-leg radiography of the same patient shown in Figure 58–1, again demonstrating bilateral cystic change and sclerosis. There is some evidence of collapse of the femoral head, as the joint space is not a smooth hemisphere.

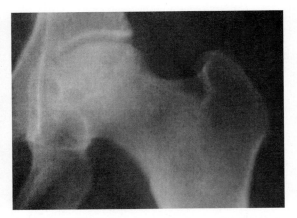

Figure 58–3. Osteonecrosis of the femoral head. There is cystic change and sclerosis of the femoral head. There is evidence of collapse with irregular joint space narrowing and loss of sphericity of the joint space.

ity around the necrotic area, can be demonstrated. This technique has limitations, however:

- Bone scan findings are nonspecific, except when a characteristic (but unusual) sign is observed: the donut sign or "cold in hot" image. This scintigraphic finding consists of decreased uptake observed within the center of an area of increased uptake.
- Potential bone scan abnormalities in one joint are usually judged by comparison to the contralateral joint. In the setting of bilateral disease, the interpretation of bone scan findings may be challenging.

3. Computed tomography—Computed tomography images can display early sclerosis in the central part of the femoral head ("asterisk sign") and give an evaluation of the size of the sequestrum. Computed tomography also demonstrates well the anterior part that is preferentially involved in ON of the femoral head, and slight anterior collapse is in some cases visible only on computed tomographic images.

4. Magnetic resonance imaging—In the early stages of ON, before collapse of the femoral head, MRI is the most sensitive test. The reported overall sensitivity of MRI for ON is 91%. Changes can be seen early in the course of disease when other studies are negative. In early ON, there is an area of low-intensity signal in the medial aspect of the femoral head, particularly in the subchondral zone. The focal defect involving the anterosuperior aspect of the femoral head, but occasionally extending to the metaphysis, is the most common abnormality observed (96% of cases).

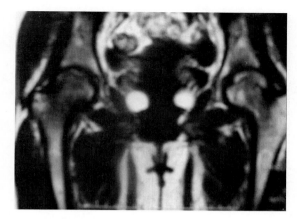

Figure 58–4. Coronal magnetic resonance image demonstrates osteonecrosis bilaterally, with irregular shape of the femoral head, suggesting early collapse.

The most characteristic image, seen in 60–80% of cases, is a margin of low signal on T1- and T2-weighted images (Figure 58–4). An inner border of high signal associated with this low-signal line on T2-weighted images, the "double-line sign," is considered pathognomonic for ON and has been described in 50–80% of cases. This high signal intensity on T2-weighted images is thought to result from an increased water content in either the intravascular or interstitial spaces. The high signal intensity may also reflect the presence of mesenchymal tissue in the marrow surrounding the interface.

In some cases, caution must be exercised in interpreting MRI findings, particularly in asymptomatic patients. Treatment based on abnormal MRI findings alone in the absence of symptoms may result in overtreatment of some patients.

C. STAGING

Staging of ON is usually based on radiologic and histologic features. Several proposed systems of staging, based on the sequence of changes seen by radiography and by other investigative techniques, have been proposed since the initial description by Arlet and Ficat, which was based primarily on radiographic findings. Newer imaging modalities and the need for quantification of involvement have led to these revisions. Recently, the Subcommittee of Nomenclature of the International Association on Bone Circulation and Bone Necrosis (ARCO: Association of Research Circulation Osseous) has reassembled the various staging systems to establish an internationally accepted system of classification of the various stages of ON (Table 58–2). This standardized system is designed to enhance uniformity among comparative epidemiologic studies and to facilitate clinical trials of treatment strategies.

Table 58–2. Stages of Osteonecrosis

Stage 0
All diagnostic studies normal; diagnosis by histology, necrosis on biopsy. Thus, osteonecrosis can exist histologically without any associated clinical signs or symptoms.

Stage 1
Plain radiographs and computed tomography (CT) normal; radionuclide scan or magnetic resonance imaging (MRI) abnormal and biopsy positive, extent of involvement A, B, or C (less than 15%, 15–30%, and > 30%, respectively). The patient may or may not be symptomatic at this Stage.

Stage 2
A variety of radiographic abnormalities that are signs of eventual bone death are evident within the femoral head. These may include areas of linear sclerosis, focal mineralization, or cysts in the femoral head or neck. The femoral head, however, is still spherical, as evidenced on both anteroposterior and lateral radiographs and on the CT scan. There is no subchondral lucency or collapse; extent of involvement A, B, or C.

Stage 3
The femoral head has begun to fail mechanically. The radiolucent "crescent sign" appearing just beneath the subchondral end-plate is the hallmark of this Stage; it indicates collapse of the subchondral cancellous trabeculae. The spherical configuration of the articular surface remains intact. The crescent sign does not always develop as the femoral head progresses from earlier to later Stages of involvement. Because the femoral head remains spherical, it should theoretically be possible to preserve its integrity by surgical measures that allow the necrotic and collapsed bone to be replaced by viable tissue. Extent of involvement A, B, or C.

Stage 4
The first sign of Stage 4 is any evidence of flattening of the femoral head with joint space narrowing. This has important therapeutic implications because the hip has now progressed to the point at which the changes are irreversible. The collapse usually occurs in the anterolateral or superior weight-bearing region. The distinction between Stage 2 and Stage 4 is best demonstrated by CT scan, which is more sensitive than plain radiographs. Extent of involvement is quantitated A, B, or C as above, with further characterization by amount of depression (in millimeters).

Stage 5
Any or all of the preceding radiographic changes may be seen, and in addition there is a decrease in the joint space. In this situation, there is osteoarthritis secondary to the mechanical collapse of the femoral head, with sclerosis, cysts of the acetabulum, and occasionally marginal osteophytes.

Stage 6
Extensive destruction of the femoral head following the degenerative process.

(From the Subcommittee on Nomenclature of the International Association on Bone Circulation and Bone Necrosis [ARCO: Association of Research Circulation Osseous. With permission.])

Differential Diagnosis

At stages 3 and 4, radiographic findings are specific for ON. If stage 5 or 6 is present at diagnosis, however, it is impossible to diagnose ON as the cause of destruction of the hip, as virtually any cause of end-stage hip disease will lead to the same appearance. The challenging differential diagnoses relate to stages 1 and 2. In stage 1, all diseases that may affect bone, cartilage, or synovial tissue must be considered as possible explanations for the joint pain. In stage 2, nonspecific bone lesions on radiographs should prompt radionuclide scan or MRI in patients at risk for ON. One entity in the differential diagnosis that can be difficult to distinguish from ON clinically is transient osteoporosis of the hip (see references), which commonly occurs during pregnancy.

Treatment

The management of ON remains one of the most controversial topics in the orthopedic literature. The goal of treatment is to preserve the native joint for as long as possible. There are four main therapeutic options:

- Conservative management
- Joint replacement (eg, total hip arthroplasty)
- Core decompression with or without bone grafting
- Osteotomy

Conservative measures may be the only treatment needed for patients with stages 0 and 1 disease, although core decompression may provide some advantages in these cases. Total joint replacement in later-stage disease should be performed before total collapse of the femoral head occurs.

A. Conservative Therapy

Stages 0, 1, and 2 may be treated by conservative measures or by core decompression (see below). Conservative treatment includes bed rest, partial weight bearing with crutches, and weight bearing as tolerated, in addition to nonsteroidal anti-inflammatory drugs or other analgesics, physical therapy to maintain muscle strength and prevent contractures, and assistive devices to facilitate ambulation. This approach is generally ineffective in halting the progression of disease.

Patients with ON of non–weight-bearing joints may not require any intervention because they may have only mild to moderate pain, and minimal, tolerable functional limitation. Results of conservative therapy in non–weight-bearing joints may be more successful.

There is no consensus on the appropriate management of patients with asymptomatic ON. Some have suggested that patients with lesions affecting less than 15% of the volume of the femoral head should be managed conservatively; those with lesions greater than 30% by elective total hip arthroplasty; and those with lesions of intermediate size (ie, between 15% and 30%) by either core decompression or osteotomy. Opinions on the optimal approach to certain ON lesions, particularly those of intermediate severity and extent, vary from center to center. In ON of the shoulder, results with conservative treatment (eg, analgesia, avoidance of overhead use of the arm, gentle stretching, and strengthening exercises) may be more efficacious.

B. Joint Replacement

Patients with persistent, intractable pain and progressive functional loss should be considered for arthroplasty. Ideally, this should be accomplished before total collapse of the femoral head occurs in patients with hip involvement. The usual treatment for late stage 3 or stage 4 disease has been total hip arthroplasty, but results have been inconsistent. Most studies suggest a worse prognosis in this disease than for others, with a higher rate of early failures compared with age-matched patients with other diagnoses. Possible reasons for the higher failure rate in patients with ON include poor bone quality (size of necrotic area and degree of bone collapse), bilateral disease, and presence of an underlying condition.

C. Core Decompression

The failure of conservative management and the poor long-term survival of prosthetic devices in the early days of joint arthroplasty necessitated the development of other interventions aimed at preserving the femoral head and slowing or stopping the progression of ON. The technique of core decompression was initially used as a diagnostic tool to measure bone marrow pressure and obtain biopsy specimens. It evolved into a treatment mode when it was observed that some patients had pain relief following the procedure. In the core decompression procedure, the orthopedist drills a hole through the femoral neck into the head of the femur.

The rationale for core decompression is to reduce intraosseous pressure, re-establish blood supply, and allow living bone adjacent to dead bone to contribute to the reparative process. Good to excellent results have been obtained in most patients with stages 1 and 2 ON, and in a significant proportion of patients with stage 3 disease. The results of this technique are still controversial, and the best results vary from 34–95% in early stages, but they are always better than simply discontinuing weight bearing.

D. Osteotomy

Osteotomy has also been used as a joint-sparing technique. The stated goal of this procedure is to remove the diseased section of the femoral head from the region of major weight bearing, and to redistribute the weight-bearing forces to articular cartilage that is supported by healthy bone.

There are many reports in the European and Japanese literature concerning the use of osteotomies for salvage of hips with stage 2 and 3 disease, with variable results. All of these osteotomies require a period of restricted weight bearing of 3 months to 1 year, and usually until there is radiographic evidence of healing of the osteotomy. One potential problem with the use of an osteotomy is that it may complicate the performance of total hip arthroplasty if that procedure is required in the future.

E. OTHER

In theory, bisphosphonates may be used to slow the resorption of necrotic bone and prolong the time to femoral head collapse. This approach has not yet been subjected to prospective, randomized studies.

Complications

The optimal treatment for ON has not yet been determined. Early diagnosis of ON may lead to better outcomes. Unfortunately, the natural history of ON is usually progressive disease with cortical collapse and joint dysfunction. The outcome is influenced by many factors, particularly the size and localization of the bone necrosis. ON is not a life-threatening process, but it can be a debilitating condition that frequently leads to destruction of the hip joint in patients in their third, fourth, or fifth decades of life. Early intervention, both surgical and nonsurgical, has improved the outcome, but still nearly 50% of cases of femoral head ON require arthroplasty.

Based on available data, the following recommendations can be made concerning ON of the femoral head:

- Asymptomatic lesions that involve less than 15% of the femoral head may resolve without surgical intervention and may therefore be treated conservatively.
- Asymptomatic lesions that involve more than 30% of the femoral head are likely to progress to collapse despite core decompression or osteotomy. Thus, these patients should be managed conservatively, in anticipation of the eventual need for total hip arthroplasty.

- In early stage 0–2 lesions in young, active patients, core decompression provides the best chance at preserving the femoral head.
- In later stage 2 lesions with cyst formation and stage 3 disease, osteotomy may be the best option.
- In stage 4 disease and in older sedentary patients with less severe disease, total hip replacement is the treatment of choice.

Acknowledgments

The author wishes to express her thanks to Harpal S. Khanuja, M.D. (Department of Orthopedics, Johns Hopkins University) for providing the radiographic and magnetic resonance images.

REFERENCES

Arlet J, Ficat RP. Diagnosis of primary femur head osteonecrosis at stage I (preradiologic stage). *Rev Chir Orthop Reparatrice Appar Mot.* 1968;54:637. [PMID: 4236312] (Early description of stages of osteonecrosis based on radiographs.)

Balakrishnan A, Schemitsch EH, Pearce D, McKee MD. Distinguishing transient osteoporosis of the hip from avascular necrosis. *Can J Surg.* 2003;46:187.

Ficat RP. Idiopathic bone necrosis of the femoral head. Early diagnosis and treatment. *J Bone Joint Surg Br.* 1985;67:3. [PMID: 3155746] (Review and discussion of osteonecrosis.)

Mont MA, Hungerford DS. Non-traumatic avascular necrosis of the femoral head. *J Bone Joint Surg Am.* 1995;77:459. [PMID: 7890797] (Current concepts, extensive review of etiology, pathogenesis, staging, and treatment options, from a group with decades of interest and experience.)

Pavelka K. Osteonecrosis. *Ballieres Best Pract Res Clin Rheumatol.* 2000;14:399. [PMID: 10925752] (Thoughtful discussion of evidence-based diagnosis and treatment.)

Stulberg BN, Bauer TW, Belhobek GH. Making core decompression work. *Clin Orthop.* 1990;261:186. [PMID: 2245544] (Randomized, controlled study with compelling evidence for efficacy of core decompression.)

Relevant World Wide Web Site

[Center for Osteonecrosis Research & Education]
http://www.osteonecrosis.org
[National Osteonecrosis Foundation]
http://www.nonf.org
[The Osteonecrosis/Avascular Necrosis Support Group International Association]
http://osteonecrosisavnsupport.org/index.html

SECTION IX

Special Topics

Common Rheumatologic Problems Encountered by the Hospitalist: Pearls & Myths

59

John Stone, MD, MPH, John Imboden, MD, & David Hellmann, MD

Clinical Problem: The Patient with an Active Rheumatic Disease

Pearl: Make sure the "punishment" fits the "crime."

Comment: One of the fundamental principles of rheumatology is to make certain that the intensity of treatment matches the severity of the disease. Pleuritis, arthralgia, and low-grade fever with systemic lupus erythematosus (SLE) will respond to 60 mg of prednisone given daily. But these manifestations will also respond generally to far less prednisone, eg, 10–20 mg daily, doses associated with a much lower risk of infection or other complications. In contrast, severe hemolytic anemia and glomerulonephritis in SLE may not respond to low dose prednisone and often must be treated not only with high doses of prednisone but also additional agents.

Clinical Problem: Supplemental Therapy for the Glucocorticoid-Treated Patient Who Is Stressed by Serious Illness or Major Surgery

Myth: A normal cosyntropin stimulation test excludes adrenal insufficiency induced by glucocorticoid therapy.

Comment: The cosyntropin stimulation test determines the ability of the adrenal gland to produce cortisol in response to an exogenous corticotropin (adrenocorticotropic hormone, ACTH). However, the endogenous response to stress requires that all components of the hypothalamic-pituitary-adrenal axis be intact. Individuals treated currently with glucocorticoids and for many months after such therapy can have insufficiency of the central components of this axis (ie, normal adrenal response to exogenous ACTH but subnormal ability to produce ACTH endogenously).

Because tests of the central components of the axis are complex, most authorities recommend empiric hydrocortisone supplementation (100 mg tid) when these patients face major surgery or the stress of serious medical illness. Once the patient is beyond the perioperative period, the baseline prednisone dose can be resumed.

Clinical Problem: Fever in the Patient with Rheumatic Disease: Underlying Disease or Superimposed Infection

Pearl: Rheumatoid arthritis rarely causes high-grade fever.

Comment: Although low-grade fevers in the range of 37.5°C often accompany active rheumatoid arthritis (RA), high-grade fevers are rare. Only 5% of cases manifest fever >38°C, and less than 1% have temperatures >38.3°C. Therefore, high-grade fever in a patient with well-established RA should prompt an investigation for an underlying cause (eg, infection) other than RA. In a patient with the new onset of inflammatory arthritis, the presence of high-grade fever is an argument against the diagnosis of RA or even a complication of RA, such as rheumatoid vasculitis (Chapter 43). (See Chapter 4 for a discussion of the differential diagnosis of fever and arthritis).

Pearl: Flare of a single joint in an RA patient signals serious concern about septic arthritis.

Comment: Most flares of RA are polyarticular. When signs of new, increased inflammation affect only one joint, infection should be strongly considered. The most common cause of septic arthritis in RA is *Staphylococcus aureus*. Absence of fever does not exclude infection because only 50% of patients with septic arthritis present with fever. In the RA patient with only one "active" joint, arthrocentesis should be performed to exclude infection before intensifying anti-inflammantory therapy.

Pearl: Always consider tuberculosis when a febrile illness develops in a patient treated with an anti–tumor necrosis factor agent.

Comment: Because tumor necrosis factor-α (TNF-α) is required for an intact host immune response to *Mycobacterium tuberculosis,* treatment with anti–TNF-α agents greatly increases the risk of TB. Although infliximab has been most closely associated with the greatest risk of TB in studies, the risk is likely a class effect shared by all anti–TNF-α agents. Most cases, caused by reactivation of infection, have developed within weeks of starting anti–TNF-α therapy. There is almost certainly an increased risk of disease from primary exposure as well, however.

In the setting of anti–TNF-α therapy, tuberculosis can be acute, is often disseminated or extrapulmonary, and has an atypical histopathology (TNF-α is required for granuloma formation). Anti–TNF-α therapy also carries an increased risk of infection with other intracellular pathogens, including *Listeria monocytogenes,* and fungi, such as *Histoplasma capsulatum* and *Coccidioides immitis.*

Pearl: When trying to distinguish between infection and active disease in a patient with SLE, the presence of rigors favors infection.

Comment: One of the great quandaries of hospital medicine for patients with SLE is determining whether an acute change is caused by infection or a flare of the disease. The presence of rigors *clearly* favors infection. Other clues may come from the complete blood count: many SLE patients have a baseline tendency toward neutrope-nia (particularly lymphopenia) and thrombocytopenia. Elevations in either of these two blood counts raises the likelihood of infection.

Pearl: Fever that develops in a patient with SLE treated with high-dose glucocorticoids is due to infection until proven otherwise.

Comment: Infection is a leading cause of morbidity and mortality in SLE, particularly in the setting of immunosuppression with high-dose glucocorticoids. Although SLE itself can cause fever >39°C, fever due to SLE most often occurs in the setting of clinically active disease (particularly serositis) and usually responds to glucocorticoid therapy. Fever that develops *after* high-dose glucocorticoids have been started should be attributed to SLE only after a vigorous search for infectious causes, including opportunistic infections.

Pearl: When a patient with SLE remembers the precise hour that the disease "flared," the patient more likely has an acute infection.

Comment: Most flares of SLE develop over days or weeks. Infections tend to present more abruptly. Therefore, a patient who says, "my disease flared at 10 o'clock" probably has an infection.

Pearl: Apparent "flares" of rheumatic disease that occur while the patient is taking cyclophosphamide are almost always caused by a superimposed opportunistic infection rather than by activation of the underlying disease.

Comment: Over the last 25 years at one large medical center, not one patient transferred to that center because of "refractory vasculitis" has had active vasculitis: every one of the transferred patients has had an opportunistic infection.

Clinical Problem: The Patient with Acute Monarthritis

Pearl: Acute monarthritis has three major causes: trauma, infection, and microcrystalline disease.

Comment: In the absence of trauma, acute monarthritis usually means that the patient has an infection or has gout or pseudogout. Although crystal-induced arthritis is more common, it is critical not to overlook septic arthritis. Delay in its treatment of joint infections increases morbidity and mortality substantially.

Pearl: The wrist and knee are to pseudogout what the great toe and foot are to gout.

Comment: The most commonly affected joints in gout are the great toe and other sites of the foot. Pseudogout in contrast most commonly affects the wrist and the knee.

Pearl: Monarthritis of the knee is the most common articular manifestation of chronic Lyme arthritis.

Comment: In regions where *Ixodes* complex ticks and *Borrelia burgdorferi* are endemic, an individual with chronic, unexplained inflammation of the knee (synovial fluid negative for crystals and organisms) may well have Lyme disease. Knee effusions due to Lyme disease can be intermittent.

Pearl: Arthrocentesis is the diagnostic procedure of choice for the patient with unexplained, acute monarthritis.

Comment: Analysis of synovial fluid allows the physician to answer three questions: Is the joint inflamed? Is infection present? Is crystal disease present? The synovial fluid WBC count is the best single discriminator between inflammatory (>2000 WBC/mm^3) and non-inflammatory (<2000 WBC/mm^3) arthritis. In cases of nongonococcal septic arthritis, examination of synovial fluid by Gram staining has limited sensitivity (approximately 50%), but culture of the synovial fluid is positive in $>90\%$. Polarized light microscopy is a sensitive and specific test for the presence of urate and calcium pyrophosphate dihydrate crystals in synovial fluid.

Myth: Synovial fluid should be tested for glucose level.

Comment: Synovial fluid glucose levels tend to be low when there is intense inflammation, especially when the joint is infected. The synovial fluid WBC count, however, is a far better measure of the severity of joint inflammation. The synovial fluid glucose level adds nothing to what is learned from the synovial fluid WBC count and should not be ordered. When the diagnosis is in question, synovial fluid should always be sent for the three Cs: cell count, culture, and crystals.

Myth: The serum uric acid is a reliable test for the presence or absence of gout in the patient with acute monarthritis.

Comment: The serum uric acid level neither establishes nor refutes the diagnosis of acute gout. Most patients develop gout after years of hyperuricemia, but it is not uncommon for the serum uric acid level to fall to within the normal range at the time of an acute attack. Determining the serum uric acid has some value in that a low level makes gout quite unlikely. A high serum uric acid level increases the probability of gout but is not definitive; asymptomatic hyperuricemia is common and can be present in patients with acute arthritis unrelated to gout. The definitive test for the diagnosis of acute gout is demonstration of intracellular urate crystals in synovial fluid from the affected joint.

Clinical Problem: The Patient with Acute Gout

Pearl: Gout has never killed a single patient. Not so its treatment.

Comment: Imprudent or improper use of gout therapies can be associated with a host of serious and even fatal complications. Gout should be treated, but treated wisely by informed clinicians mindful of the patient's entire clinical status. See the comments below on the potential dangers of specific gout treatments.

Myth: Intravenous colchicine is a first-line therapy for acute gout.

Comment: There is almost always a better option than intravenous colchicine for the treatment of gout. Intravenous colchicine can cause fatal bone marrow and multiorgan failure, particularly in patients who have renal insufficiency or liver disease or who have been taking oral colchicine. Because of its toxicity and the availability of safer alternatives (ie, NSAIDs and glucocorticoids), intravenous colchicine should be administered very rarely (if ever), and only by clinicians who are very familiar with its use.

Myth: Allopurinol is useful for the treatment of acute gout.

Comment: A common mistake in the treatment of acute gout is the failure to separate therapy of the acute arthritis from management of the chronically elevated serum uric acid. During a flare of gout, attention should focus on treating the acute arthritis with NSAIDs or glucocorticoids (see Chapter 45). In fact, the use of allopurinol in this setting may have a counterintuitive—and counterproductive—effect: by lowering serum uric acid abruptly, allopurinol may exacerbate the acute gout flare. Thus, initiation of allopurinol should be deferred until several weeks after resolution of the acute attack.

Pearl: Glucocorticoids are an effective treatment for acute gout in the patient with a contraindication to nonsteroidal anti-inflammatory drugs.

Comment: Glucocorticoids are an excellent therapeutic option for the gout patient who has a contraindication to NSAIDs (eg, renal insufficiency). When gout involves a readily accessible joint, an intraarticular glucocorticoid injection is a safe, rapidly effective treatment. For cases of polyarticular gout in which the injection of all involved joints is not possible, the efficacy of oral glucocorticoids (eg, prednisone 20–40 mg daily, tapered over 1–2 weeks) is comparable to or greater than that of NSAIDs (and may have fewer side effects).

Because of the multiple co-morbidities found in many hospitalized patients today, a short course of glucocorticoids (with close attention to the risk of hyperglycemia) is often the best approach to treating acute gout on the in-patient service.

Myth: Acute gout does not cause high fever.

Comment: Acute gout can present in myriad ways on the inpatient service. Polyarticular gout, which may develop after years of recurrent podagra, can mimic RA. Acute gout affecting many joints of one limb can mimic a stroke. Not infrequently, polyarticular gout can be associated with high fevers (ie, $>39°C$.) Septic arthritis or another infection should always be excluded in this setting, but in the end the explanation is often gout.

Clinical Problem: Gout Prophylaxis

Pearl: Avoid using a dose of colchicine higher than one tablet (0.6 mg) per day in patients over the age of 65, especially if the serum creatinine is above 1.5 mg/dL.

Comment: Daily oral colchicine can rarely cause proximal muscle weakness (a neuromyopathy) that mimics polymyositis. Almost all the patients with this drug complication are older than the age of 60 and have decreased renal function. The dose of colchicine must be decreased in patients with kidney dysfunction.

Pearl: Avoid starting allopurinol in any patient taking azathioprine.

Comment: Allopurinol blocks the catabolism of azathioprine by xanthine oxidase, greatly augmenting the effect of this immunosuppressive agent. Failure to stop azathioprine or to reduce the daily dose dramatically (by at least 50%) can result in life-threatening cytopenia.

Clinical Problem: The Patient with Nongonococcal Septic Arthritis

Pearl: Carefully examine all joints, particularly shoulders and hips, in a patient with suspected septic arthritis.

Comment: Nongonococcal septic arthritis is oligoarticular in approximately 15% of cases. Focus on an obviously inflamed joint (eg, a septic knee) can lead to the failure to appreciate infection of less visible joints, such as the shoulders and hips.

Pearl: Nongonococcal septic arthritis requires drainage.

Comment: Many physicians are surprised to learn that viable organisms can be obtained from a previously untapped septic joint despite two or more days of antibiotics. "Pus under pressure" prevents antibiotics from working effectively. Drainage is as important as antibiotics in the treatment of septic arthritis.

Clinical Problem: Hypertension in a Patient with Scleroderma

Pearl: Elevated blood pressure in a patient with scleroderma may be an indication of incipient scleroderma renal crisis.

Comment: Prior to the availability of angiotensin-converting enzyme inhibitors, the most common cause of death in patients with diffuse systemic sclerosis was scleroderma renal crisis. Scleroderma renal crisis occurs characteristically in diffuse (as opposed to limited) disease. Asymptomatic hypertension, particularly if documented to be new, may be a primary clue. Failure to recognize scleroderma renal crisis may lead to malignant hypertension with all of its attendant complications, renal failure, and a microangiopathic picture in the peripheral blood smear. On renal histopathology, scleroderma renal crisis is indistinguishable from thrombotic thrombocytopenic purpura. The cornerstone of therapy for scleroderma renal crisis is aggressive angiotensin-converting enzyme inhibition.

Clinical Problem: The Patient with Giant Cell Arteritis

Pearl: Consider giant cell arteritis (GCA) in any adult over the age of 60 who has "above-the-neck" pain that cannot otherwise be explained.

Comment: Headache, scalp tenderness, and jaw claudication are among the most common symptoms in patients with GCA. But GCA can also produce pain in other locations, including the tongue, the ear, the back of the neck, over the carotids, and along the jaw line. Thus, any pain above the neck that is not explained readily by trauma or some other cause should prompt consideration of GCA.

Pearl: Consider GCA in the differential diagnosis of the elderly patient with fever of unknown origin.

Comment: GCA usually presents with symptoms referable to involvement of the cranial circulation (eg, headache, scalp tenderness, visual symptoms, and jaw claudication) but can cause fever without localizing signs or symptoms. Fever can be the sole clinical manifestation of the disease for weeks or months. Even in the absence of temporal artery abnormalities on physical examination, the diagnostic test of choice is temporal artery biopsy. If large-vessel disease (eg, subclavian or aortic involvement) is suspected on the basis of arm claudication or a diastolic murmur, magnetic resonance imaging/angiography of the great vessels may also be helpful.

Pearl: Among all GCA symptoms, jaw claudication is the most specific for that disease.

Comment: Jaw claudication has a likelihood ratio of greater than 4 for the diagnosis of GCA, making it more likely than any other symptom to be associated with a temporal artery biopsy. The problem is that patients do not complain flagrantly about "jaw claudication". Further, unless prompted, they will not mention that they have pain in their jaw when they chew unless you specifically ask. The symptom of jaw claudication, which may present as facial pain or pressure felt soon after the initiation of chewing, must be actively elicited when taking the patient's history. In short, the clinician must be attuned to patients' describing synonyms for use of this phenomenon.

Myth: Glucocorticoid therapy for suspected GCA should be administered only after temporal artery biopsies have been obtained.

Comment: Glucocorticoid therapy, which can prevent irreversible blindness and other feared complications of GCA, and should be administered promptly when the diagnosis is considered. Glucocorticoid therapy does not interfere with histopathologic findings in the temporal arteries for at least 2 weeks. Start treatment, then get the biopsy (but don't fail to get the biopsy).

Pearl: GCA does not occur among individuals under the age of 50.

Comment: This is a remarkably true statement. Among 1435 patients with biopsy-proven temporal arteritis, only two cases occurred in individuals younger than 50 years of age. It is possible that even those two patients did not have GCA but rather some other form of systemic vasculitis involving the temporal arteries (microscopic polyangiitis, Wegener granulomatosis, and polyarteritis nodosa, for example, are known to do this).

Pearl: The addition of low-dose aspirin to glucocorticoid therapy may reduce the risk of blindness or stroke in patients with GCA.

Comment: A retrospective review of patients with GCA revealed that those receiving concomitant low-dose aspirin had a fivefold lower incidence of intracranial ischemic events compared to patients treated with glucocorticoids alone.

Clinical Problem: The Patient with Suspected Primary Vasculitis

Pearl: Subacute bacterial endocarditis can cause palpable purpura, glomerulonephritis, and hypocomplementemia.

Comment: Chronic bacterial infections such as subacute bacterial endocarditis and chronic osteomyelitis can cause an immune-complex–mediated vasculitis. These diagnoses should always be considered in the differential diagnosis of a patient with small-vessel vasculitis.

Pearl: Consider cholesterol emboli syndrome when an elderly man with atherosclerotic disease develops "vasculitis."

Comment: Cholesterol emboli syndrome can be a remarkable mimic of vasculitis. Its diverse manifestations include peripheral emboli (often producing "blue toes"), livedo reticularis, cutaneous ulcers, acute renal failure, elevated erythrocyte sedimentation rate, and eosinophilia. The syndrome, which typically develops days to weeks after an intravascular procedure (eg, cardiac catheterization) or the institution of anticoagulation therapy and is due to shedding of cholesterol emboli from destabilized atherosclerotic plaques.

Myth: Cold-induced symptoms dominate the clinical presentation of hepatitis C–associated cryoglobulinemia.

Comment: The cryoglobulins associated with hepatitis C (types II and III) are immune complexes that precipitate in the cold eg, several days at 4°C—not conditions

that occur physiologically. Immune-complex–mediated disease accounts for the major clinical manifestations, such as palpable purpura and glomerulonephritis. In contrast, type I cryoglobulins (cryoprecipitating monoclonal gammopathies) can precipitate at temperatures achieved in the distal extremities, nose, ears, and elsewhere. Type I cryoglobulins often present with cold-induced symptoms.

Pearl: Suspect mixed cryoglobulinemia in a patient with a very low serum level of C4 and normal or near-normal level of C3.

Comment: Immune complexes in types II and III cryoglobulinemia activate the classical complement pathway leading to depletion of C4 and other early pathway components. In mixed cryoglobulinemia, the C4 level is usually disproportionately low compared to other complement components, even C3.

Myth: Patients with diffuse alveolar hemorrhage always have hemoptysis.

Comment: Diffuse alveolar hemorrhage is a life-threatening complication of vasculitis associated with antineutrophil cytoplasmic antibodies (ANCA), anti–glomerular basement membrane disease, SLE, and other conditions. Classically, diffuse alveolar hemorrhage presents with hemoptysis, dyspnea, a fall in hematocrit, and the abrupt appearance of new infiltrates on chest radiography. Unfortunately, the presentation is highly variable, and hemoptysis, the clinical finding most suggestive of diffuse alveolar hemorrhage, is absent in up to one-third of cases.

Myth: In a patient whose serum tests positively for antibodies that produce either a perinuclear or cytoplasmic P- or C-ANCA pattern on indirect immunofluorescence, primary systemic vasculitis is likely.

Comment: ANCA assays are enormously helpful in making the diagnosis of certain forms of vasculitis, specifically Wegener granulomatosis, microscopic polyangiitis, and the Churg-Strauss syndrome. However, positive perinuclear and circulating ANCA test results are actually quite nonspecific (perinuclear ANCA results particularly so). A host of nonvasculitic inflammatory disorders—inflammatory bowel disease, SLE, RA, and infections—may be associated with a positive perinuclear ANCA IIF result. The ANCA-associated vasculitis patients comprise only a minority of patients with positive perinuclear ANCA results. Similarly, in one study, 50% of patients with C-ANCA immunofluorescence—a pattern considered more specific for vasculitis—had nonvasculitic conditions.

The key to using ANCA assays appropriately in the diagnosis of vasculitis is confirming all positive immunofluorescence results (P- or C-ANCA) with enzyme immunoassays to detect antibodies directed against either myeloperoxidase (MPO-ANCA) or proteinase 3

(PR3-ANCA). The combination of a positive immunofluorescence assay (a P- or C-ANCA pattern) and either MPO-ANCA or PR3-ANCA has a high positive predictive value for vasculitis.

Clinical Problem: Gauging Disease Activity in Patients with ANCA-Associated Vasculitis

Myth: ANCA assays are useful in predicting disease flares in Wegener granulomatosis.

Comment: Used properly, ANCA serologies may be invaluable in making the diagnosis of ANCA-associated vasculitis. Even so, significant numbers of patients with "ANCA-associated" vasculitis are ANCA negative. This is true for approximately 15% of patients with Wegener granulomatosis (and an even higher percentage of Wegener patients with limited disease), approximately 30% of those with microscopic polyangiitis, and 50% or more of those with the Churg-Strauss syndrome. Moreover, a number of studies have demonstrated that elevations in ANCA titers bear only a poor temporal correlation with disease activity. Specifically, given a significant rise in ANCA titer (either two- or fourfold, depending on the study), a disease flare may not present itself (if it presents at all) until 1 year or more after the ANCA elevation. Consequently, treatment decisions should never be predicated on ANCA titers.

Pearl: Arthritis is a common presentation of a flare in ANCA-associated vasculitis.

Comment: Perhaps because it improves so quickly after the institution of therapy, arthritis is a frequently overlooked sign of ANCA-associated vasculitis and a very common tip-off to disease flare. The arthritis commonly involves large joints in a migratory, asymmetric, oligoarticular pattern, one day involving a knee and an ankle, the next day a shoulder. Small joints may also be involved.

Pearl: Once renal involvement by Wegener granulomatosis begins, organ- or life-threatening disease may ensue swiftly.

Comment: Cases of Wegener granulomatosis "smoldering" in the upper respiratory tract for years (undiagnosed) are well documented in the literature. In many cases, the explanation for the chronic sinus dysfunction, nasal pain and bleeding, and other symptoms is understood only in retrospect, upon the occurrence of disease manifestations that threaten vital organs. Few diseases can cause renal deterioration as rapidly as Wegener granulomatosis. Once the serum creatinine begins to rise in Wegener granulomatosis, the disease often appears to accelerate substantially, with rapidly progressive glomerulonephritis, swift progression to renal failure, and the appearance of "disseminated" involvement (alveolar hemorrhage, mesenteric vasculitis, and so on).

Thus, once the diagnosis of Wegener granulomatosis is considered, the evaluation must occur swiftly, especially if the patient has hematuria or an elevated serum creatinine.

Clinical Problem: Evaluating Shortness of Breath in the Patient with ANCA-Associated Vasculitis

Pearl: Patients with Wegener granulomatosis are at substantially increased risk of deep venous thrombosis and pulmonary emboli.

Comment: In the Wegener Granulomatosis Etanercept Trial (WGET), 13 of the 180 patients had had venous thrombotic events prior to enrollment. During 228 person-years of prospective follow-up, venous thrombotic events occurred in 16 of the remaining 167 patients with no prior history of such events. The incidence rate of venous thrombotic events in Wegener granulomatosis was more than seven times higher than that of a comparable group of patients with SLE—a group known to have an increased thrombotic risk.

The etiology of venous thrombotic events in Wegener granulomatosis, which is likely multifactorial, remains unclear. One possibility in addition to the debility, proteinuria, and other predisposing factors that may be associated with this disease is the fact that Wegener granulomatosis involves veins as well as arteries. It is conceivable that venous inflammation contributes in a major way to the elevated risk of venous thrombotic events in Wegener granulomatosis. Vasculitic conditions related to Wegener granulomatosis such as microscopic polyangiitis and the Churg-Strauss syndrome are probably also associated with an increased risk of venous thrombotic events, although this has never been studied formally.

Pearl: Patients with either Wegener granulomatosis or relapsing polychondritis may have difficult airways.

Comment: The potential presence of subglottic stenosis is important to keep in mind among patients with Wegener granulomatosis or relapsing polychondritis, particularly those who may be undergoing bronchoscopy or elective intubation. Subglottic stenosis, a vasculitis complication that is peculiar to these two conditions, may lead to life-threatening narrowing of the airway just below the vocal cords. Passage of a bronchoscope or endotracheal tube may be difficult or impossible.

Pearl: The patient with inspiratory sounds most likely has subglottic stenosis and not asthma.

Comment: Asthma produces expiratory sounds; loud inspiratory sounds audible without the stethoscope are a sign of stridor, which in patients with Wegener granulomatosis, is commonly caused by subglottic stenosis.

Subglottic stenosis can usually be detected by observing patients as they talk: because of their upper airway narrowing, they must often pause slightly to suck in air before beginning a sentence.

Clinical Problem: Treating Cryoglobulinemic Vasculitis Associated with Hepatitis C

Myth: The optimal therapy for hepatitis C–associated cryoglobulinemic vasculitis is always antiviral treatment.

Comment: Under ideal conditions, the treatment of vasculitis is directed against the underlying cause—in this case, hepatitis C. Currently, this means the combination of pegylated interferon and ribavirin. In the setting of severe, multiorgan system vasculitis, however, control of the underlying inflammation initially with anti-inflammatory therapies—glucocorticoids, cyclophosphamide, and even plasmapheresis—is recommended. In such situations, initial treatment with antiviral therapies alone may trigger a paradoxical worsening of the vasculitis through an unfavorable alteration of the antigen:antibody ratio. Initial treatment aimed at controlling the inflammatory response may prevent this complication. Following a couple of weeks of treatment with immunosuppressive agents, antiviral therapy may begin. Glucocorticoids and other therapies may be discontinued swiftly.

Clinical Problem: Diagnosing Small-Vessel Cutaneous Vasculitis

Pearl: Direct immunofluorescence (DIF) should be performed on all skin biopsies performed to diagnose small-vessel vasculitis.

Comment: Hospitalists may have the opportunity to diagnose vasculitis by ordering skin biopsies. Full pathologic assessment of cutaneous vasculitis involves examination of a skin biopsy specimen by both light microscopy and DIF. DIF involves the testing of the skin biopsy sample for immunoglobulin, complement, and other immunoreactants. The presence of immunoreactants in the skin as well as their precise location (along the dermal epidermal border, around blood vessels, etc.) and pattern of deposition, reveals important characteristics about the underlying disease process. This information cannot be gleaned from the usual hematoxylin and eosin (H & E) stains examined by light microscopy; it requires DIF. The omission of DIF—an unfortunately common occurrence—wastes an opportunity to observe potentially valuable information and often leads to misdiagnoses (eg, the failure to distinguish Henoch-Schönlein purpura from a drug-induced vasculitis). DIF can only be performed on fresh skin biopsy samples, cannot be added on later, and therefore must be planned at the time of the biopsy. Insist that the dermatologist send skin biopsies for both H & E and DIF.

Approach to the Patient with a Painful Prosthetic Joint

60

Steven A. Lietman, MD

ESSENTIALS OF DIAGNOSIS

- *Revision arthroplasty is indicated for a painful prosthetic joint in three major circumstances: prosthetic failure, loosening, and infection.*
- *Prosthetic joints that are infected are generally not as painful as native septic joints with range of motion.*
- *Infection is always in the differential diagnosis of a painful prosthetic joint.*
- *Wound drainage beyond the third postoperative week is usually related to infection.*
- *Prosthetic loosening usually occurs more than 10 years after the procedure.*
- *Radiographs are insensitive for early osteolysis.*
- *The spine is the most common cause of referred pain when the prosthetic joint itself is not the cause of the pain.*

Total joint arthroplasty represents one of the most successful operations performed in the United States, with excellent results for more than 90% of patients. There is a small subset of patients, however, who have chronic pain after total joint replacement.

Prevention

The life of a prosthetic joint can be extended by the following preventive measures:

- *Prophylaxis against infection.* The risk of infection after joint replacement can be decreased with antibiotic prophylaxis with amoxicillin for dental visits or a cephalosporin for surgical procedures.
- *Avoidance of high-impact exercise.* Patients with prosthetic joints should avoid high-impact activities such as running, aerobics, and playing tennis on hard courts.

- *Body positioning.* In order to decrease the risk of dislocation, patients should avoid crossing their legs and sitting in low chairs for at least 6 weeks after surgery.
- *Moderation in physical therapy.* Overly aggressive physical therapy may lead to periarticular muscle damage in tissues already compromised by the operation. Gentle passive and active assisted range-of-motion exercises are preferred to extreme range-of-motion maneuvers, particularly in the hip and shoulder.

Clinical Findings

A. HISTORY

There are several critical questions to ask in taking the history of a patient with prosthetic joint pain:

- Is pain present at the time of the visit?
  If the patient has no pain that can be elicited with use of the extremity at the time of the visit, major problems with the prosthesis are unlikely unless the patient is immunosuppressed (in which case infection remains a possibility).
- Where is the pain?
  Many patients say they have hip pain, but when they are asked to show the clinician the specific location, they point to the sacrum or lumbar spine, indicating a possible lumbar strain, disc herniation, or spinal stenosis as the potential cause; or to the trochanteric bursa, suggesting the possibility of trochanteric bursitis.
- When did the pain start?
  If the patient's pain is unchanged from before the initial prosthetic implantation, then the pain for which the joint replacement was performed may not have been related to the joint at all. With the exception of Charcot joints, pain relief obtained from a joint replacement correlates well with the severity of joint disease before surgery.
- What triggers the pain?
  Except in infection and fracture, pain without use of the extremity is rarely related to a prosthetic problem.
- Could the pain be referred and due to other medical problems?

Spinal stenosis, disc herniation, and arthritis of the lumbar and cervical spine are the most common causes of referred extremity pain.

B. Physical Examination

A general physical examination can delineate other potentially relevant issues, such as hernias or spinal disease. The area around the prosthetic joint must be examined systematically by inspection, palpation, evaluation of range of motion, and special tests.

For patients with lower extremity joint prostheses, observation of their gait is extremely important and can help define the cause of the pain. Patients with pain from their prostheses generally walk with limps, and frequently have worse pain with the use of the extremity. Specific tenderness in the area of the prosthesis is generally present. Range of motion is generally decreased.

C. Radiographs

A set of radiographs should always be taken of the entire painful prosthesis. The standard radiographic approach to painful prosthetic joints according to the joint involved is shown in Table 60–1.

Aspiration of the joint should be performed if infection is suspected. Aspiration is urgent if the problem has been present for less than 2–3 weeks, because irrigation and débridement may salvage the prosthesis.

Differential Diagnosis

A. Infection

Infection is always in the differential diagnosis of the painful prosthetic joint. Prosthetic joint infections can cause myriad symptoms and signs, including constitutional symptoms such as fever, chills, and night sweats, and pain at rest. An infected prosthesis generally is less painful with range-of-motion exercises than a native septic joint. A history of difficulty with healing of the wound postoperatively and/or what was termed a "superficial infection" should be noted. In addition, a history of infections in other areas and particularly a history of recent dental procedures should be obtained.

On physical examination, the wound and area around the involved joint should always be examined for evidence of drainage. Wound drainage beyond the third postoperative week is usually related to infection. Laboratory tests such as white blood cell count, C-reactive protein, and erythrocyte sedimentation rate are frequently, but not always, elevated. In one study, among 23 patients with deep hip arthroplasty infections, only one patient had a C-reactive protein <20 mg/dL and an erythrocyte sedimentation rate <30 mm/h.

Aspiration of the joint (under fluoroscopy in the case of the hip and sometimes shoulder) is the gold standard for diagnosis and should be repeated at least 2 weeks after the patient has discontinued antibiotic therapy. At the time of all revision surgery for hip pain or loosening, Gram stains and cultures for aerobic and anaerobic organisms, as well as acid-fast bacilli and fungal organisms, are essential.

B. Prosthetic Loosening

The patient with prosthetic loosening generally has pain of the involved joint with the use of the extremity. The pain is particularly severe with weight bearing in the lower extremity and with lifting objects or simply raising the involved upper extremity. This pain can be present even immediately after the surgery (if the implant was improperly fixed), but more commonly occurs more than 10 years after implantation. The average longevity of a prosthetic implant depends on many factors including the patient's age, but is generally 10–20 years.

Patients with prosthetic loosening in a lower extremity joint nearly always have an antalgic gait or limp, and the pain is generally demonstrable with lifting or use of that extremity. They may have pain with palpation or range of motion of the involved joint. Some patients have more pain in the area of loosening with an active straight leg raise (raising the leg off the examination table with the knee straight) than with a passive straight leg raise. This pain is presumably due to the increased joint reaction force created by the contraction of the hip flexor muscles.

Radiographs nearly always demonstrate at least a 2-mm lucency around the entire prosthesis. Radiographic techniques should be standardized so that accurate serial radiographs can reveal progressive loosening. Standardization of radiographic technique is particularly important in the evaluation of knee arthroplasties. In loosening of knee prostheses, the lucency may not be seen if the x-ray beam is not tangential to the interface between the cement and bone.

Table 60–1. Radiographic Evaluation of the Painful Prosthetic Joint

Joint	Radiographic Studies
Hip	AP pelvis and AP and lateral of the entire femur
Knee	AP weight-bearing, sunrise view, and lateral knee (consider hip films if the patient also has groin pain or decreased hip ROM)
Shoulder	Axillary view (Y view can be substituted if the patient cannot raise the arm high enough for the cassette to be placed properly) and AP and lateral of the entire humerus
Elbow	AP and lateral of the elbow

AP, anteroposterior; ROM, range of motion.

C. OSTEOLYSIS

Osteolysis manifests itself as a lucent area around the prosthesis and is the most common cause for eventual prosthetic loosening. It is generally the result of polyethylene wear debris that stimulates a foreign-body inflammatory response, resulting in bone resorption and manifested as radiographic lucency. Osteolysis can, but does not always, cause pain in the absence of loosening; it is a progressive process in which there is probably a release of polyethylene particles with every motion of the prosthetic joint. However, the rate of bone resorption can be variable and can be quite slow. Osteolysis may cause pain with the provocative maneuvers described above for prosthetic loosening, and the patient may limp. Radiographs frequently do not demonstrate osteolysis until the bone mass in the area of lucency has been decreased by 30–50%.

D. PERIPROSTHETIC FRACTURE

Fracture around the prosthesis is relatively uncommon, but it is usually related to osteolysis and implant loosening. The history may relate relatively minor trauma, particularly in areas of significant osteolysis. Physical examination should be limited based on the significant discomfort generally present with motion of the involved extremity. Standard radiographs will nearly always reveal the fracture.

E. COMPONENT FRACTURE OR FAILURE

The metal of modern prostheses rarely fractures, but the polyethylene, particularly as it wears in a joint arthroplasty, can suddenly break. This will usually—but not always—present with a change in pain and instability, and the use of the extremity will be less effective. Radiographs demonstrate joint asymmetry.

F. PROSTHETIC DISLOCATION OR SUBLUXATION

Prosthetic dislocation is most common in the hip, less common in the shoulder, and rare in the knee and elbow. In general, the patient describes an unusual or extreme motion of the joint and pain afterwards. The dislocated joint is not functional and the problem can be seen on standard radiographs; however, it can be missed if only one radiographic view is used.

G. REFERRED PAIN

Pain at a site remote from the joint is particularly important to try to identify. The most common cause of pain referred to the hip or knee is a spinal disorder. Nerve impingement in the lumbar spine can cause pain similar to that of a loose hip or knee prosthesis. Abdominal and pelvic abnormalities can also cause pain in the hip, and thoracic tumors can cause shoulder pain. Nerve root impingement in the neck can cause pain very similar to that of a loose shoulder implant. In general, the symptoms and signs of nerve root impingement from either spinal stenosis or a herniated disc are numbness and weakness. In addition, the pain will not generally increase with an active straight leg raise compared with a passive straight leg raise. The classic presentation of nerve root impingement at the neck is reproducible pain with neck range of motion or rotation. The classic manifestation of spinal stenosis is a stooped posture; leaning forward (as when pushing a grocery cart) relieves the pain. Radiographs, computed tomography scans, and magnetic resonance imaging all may be helpful in the evaluation of potential spinal disorders.

H. BURSITIS

Bursae around prosthetic joints are potential sites of inflammation and sources of pain after joint arthroplasty. Patients with subacromial, olecranon, trochanteric, pes, patellar, or anserine bursitis describe pain in the bursal region and tenderness to touch. In 14% of human cadavers, the iliopsoas bursa communicates with the hip joint, explaining the common finding of an iliopsoas mass in patients with inflamed or infected hip arthroplasties.

I. SCAR NEUROMATA

Any cutaneous nerve transected at surgery may (in theory) cause pain after the incision for joint arthroplasty. The infrapatellar branch of the saphenous nerve, cut at knee arthroplasty, is a particular problem. Patients with painful neuromata generally have pain out of proportion to physical examination results and cutaneous hypersensitivity.

J. REFLEX SYMPATHETIC DYSTROPHY

Compared to patients with scar neuromata, those with reflex sympathetic dystrophy generally have pain that is less focal in nature. Patients with reflex sympathetic dystrophy generally have joint stiffness, as well as hyperhidrosis and discoloration over the involved area (see Chapter 63). Limbs affected by reflex sympathetic dystrophy demonstrate local osteopenia on radiography.

K. PROSTHETIC STEM PAIN

Pain in the area of long uncemented stems can be present even with well-fixed implants and is primarily believed to be due to a mismatch in the modulus between a stiff implant and the less stiff bone. In most cases, this condition is believed to improve within 2 years of implantation and is uncommon with newer uncemented prostheses with lower moduli of elasticity.

Treatment

A. INFECTION

If treatment is begun within 3 weeks of the onset of the infection (to the extent to which this can be determined), therapy of the infected total joint involves careful irrigation and débridement and change of the polyethylene liner. In most cases, however, the infection is not detected within 3 weeks of onset and all foreign bodies in the joint (prosthetic components, methyl methacrylate, cement restrictors, cables and plate and screws) should be removed. At this point, multiple culture specimens should be obtained and at least 6 weeks of antibiotics should be given. Following this initial treatment, antibiotic therapy should be discontinued for at least 2 weeks and re-aspiration of the joint should be performed. If there is no evidence of infection at this point, a revision arthroplasty can be performed. If infection persists, then another course of antibiotics for at least 3 months is given before reimplantation. Reimplantation is not recommended if the aspirate or a Gram stain at the time of surgery reveals evidence of continued infection.

B. Osteolysis

The treatment of osteolysis in the patient with minimal symptoms and bone loss is somewhat controversial. Antiresorptive agents such as alendronate (70 mg orally every week) may be considered. In the patient with severe pain or dysfunction, joint revision or (occasionally) bone grafting of the defect without implant revision may be recommended.

C. Periprosthetic Fracture

Usually fracture of the bone around the prosthesis does not heal with immobilization and requires surgery, except in the severely debilitated or ill patient. Component loosening often accompanies these fractures. At the time of fixation, the components should be examined for signs of loosening. The revision surgery in these situations generally requires implant change to a long-stem model, which will in essence bypass the fracture or defect.

D. Component Fracture or Failure

The failure of a component requires exchange of at least that component, except in the most severely ill or debilitated patients.

E. Prosthetic Dislocation or Subluxation

Prosthetic subluxation can generally be treated with avoidance of the activity that causes the subluxation. Progressively increasing prosthetic subluxation, however, can be a harbinger of polyethylene wear and failure.

F. Bursitis

The approach to the patient with bursitis following joint arthroplasty is different than that in the patient with bursitis around a native joint. Postsurgical joints are less likely to have capsules or boundaries between the bursae and the joint spaces. Contamination of the bursa is associated with a greater risk of joint infection. Consequently, bursal injections are discouraged.

G. Scar Neuromata and Reflex Sympathetic Dystrophy

Cutaneous nerve resection may be useful in patients who have pain for at least 6 months after a joint replacement in the absence of other causes. Sympathetic nerve block has relieved pain in selected patients with reflex sympathetic dystrophy.

H. Prosthetic Stem Pain

This condition is usually self-limited, resolving within 2 years. Revision of uncemented to cemented components in this situation has not yielded consistently favorable results.

REFERENCES

Chandler SB. The iliopsoas bursa in man. *Anat Rec.* 1934;58:235.

Gusenoff JA, Hungerford DS, Orlando JC, Nahabedian MY. Outcome and management of infected wounds after total hip arthroplasty. *Ann Plast Surg.* 2002;49:587. [PMID: 12461440] (Salvage of the infected hip prosthesis is accomplished best via early recognition, irrigation, and débridement. In the setting of complex wounds, plastic surgery consultation may be important for muscle flap coverage.)

Sanzen L, Carlsson AS. The diagnostic value of C-reactive protein in infected total hip arthroplasties. *J Bone Joint Surg Br.* 1989;71:638.

Tsukayama DT, Goldberg VM, Kyle R. Diagnosis and management of infection after total knee arthroplasty. *J Bone Joint Surg Am.* 2003;(Suppl 1):S75. [PMID: 12540674]

Relevant World Wide Web Site

[The Cleveland Clinic]
http://www.clevelandclinic.org/quality/leaders/orthopaedics.htm

The Patient with a Red Eye

61

James T. Rosenbaum, MD, & Lyndell L. Lim, MD

Ocular or peri-ocular inflammation is a frequent accompaniment of joint disease in rheumatic syndromes. Rheumatologists should be familiar with the differential diagnosis of a red eye, know when to refer a patient for specialized eye care, and recognize the implications of ocular inflammatory disease for patients who may have an associated rheumatologic condition.

Differential Diagnosis

The differential diagnosis of a red eye is given in Table 61–1. Put simply, the causes of a red eye can be subdivided into unilateral or bilateral involvement (Table 61–2). Other distinguishing features of each diagnosis are outlined in Table 61–3. Some conditions such as conjunctivitis are common, while others such as scleritis are rare. A patient with a red eye should be referred to an ophthalmologist if (1) the redness lasts more than a few days; (2) pain, as opposed to mild discomfort, is present; or (3) visual acuity is affected.

Conjunctivitis is by far the most common cause for ocular redness. Patients with conjunctivitis will experience discomfort but not frank pain. Conjunctivitis has multiple causes including viral infection, allergy, toxins, trauma, or rarely immunologic disease. Conjunctivitis, for example, is seen in conditions such as classic reactive arthritis. In general, however, patients with conjunctivitis are unlikely to have an associated diagnosis related to systemic inflammation and the disease is typically self-limiting, resolving within 1–2 weeks.

Blepharitis is inflammation or infection of the lid margins. Although this common condition does not typically cause a red eye, it does result in symptoms similar to those of conjunctivitis, notably ocular irritation and tearing. It especially affects the elderly, and responds to lid soaks and improved ocular hygiene such as scrubs with a non-irritating shampoo. Blepharitis is not associated with autoimmunity.

Pinguecula and pterygia are also common ocular conditions that are both benign and are not associated with autoimmune disease. They are degenerative, raised, conjunctival growths that are typically found on either the temporal or nasal portions of the eye. A pterygium is a growth that extends onto the cornea, while a pingueculum is confined to the scleral portion of the globe. They are not premalignant and usually do not require surgical treatment unless a pterygium extends across the pupil. Occasionally they may become inflamed, resulting in mild ocular discomfort and localized injection; however, this is usually self-limiting and responds well to topical artificial tears or a short course of weak topical steroid eye drops.

Episcleritis is another cause of redness that is generally not related to rheumatic disease. The episcleral vessels are more superficial than scleral vessels. The clinical distinction between scleritis and episcleritis is given in Table 61–4. Patients with episcleritis may have diffuse redness or the condition could be limited to just a sector of the eye. Episcleritis does occur in association with relapsing polychondritis, inflammatory bowel disease, and rheumatoid arthritis, but the majority of patients with episcleritis do not have an identifiable systemic immunologic disease.

In contrast to episcleritis, approximately 50% of patients with scleritis do have an associated systemic illness. Scleritis is a vasculitis of scleral vessels. As is true for episcleritis, the redness can be diffuse or limited to a sector of the eye. A rare form of scleritis involves only the sclera in the posterior portion of the eye such that no redness is visible on examination. These patients may have choroidal or retinal changes that are visible on a dilated examination. Ultrasound or some other imaging study is required to verify the diagnosis. Patients with scleritis usually have intense pain and the disease tends to be very persistent with a mean duration of 7 years. Intraocular complications such as uveitis, choroidal effusions, glaucoma, optic nerve edema, and corneal melt can be associated with scleritis.

Rheumatologic Disease and Medication Related Associations

Diseases most frequently associated with scleritis are listed in Table 61–5. By far the most common systemic disease is rheumatoid arthritis. In general, the subset of patients with RA who develop scleritis is distinct. These patients have a high titer of rheumatoid factor, rheumatoid nodules, and evidence for vasculitis or pleuropericarditis. Scleritis in the setting of rheumatoid arthritis is associated with a shortened life expectancy. Rheumatoid

Table 61–1. The Differential Diagnosis of a Red Eye

Conjunctivitis
Ocular cicatricial pemphigoid
Episcleritis
Scleritis
Anterior uveitis
Acute closed-angle glaucoma
Dryness
Keratitis
Exophthalmos

Table 61–2. Predominant Patterns of Disease: Unilateral Versus Bilateral Red Eyes

Unilateral	Bilateral	Either Unilateral or Bilateral
Acute closed-angle glaucoma	Conjunctivitis	Uveitis
Keratitis	Ocular cicatricial pemphigoid	Episcleritis
Noninfective orbital inflammation	Thyroid eye disease Sjögren syndrome	Scleritis

Table 61–3. Characteristic Features of Specific Causes of a Red Eye

Diagnosis	Defining Features
Conjunctivitis	Grittiness, ocular discharge, normal vision
Ocular cicatricial pemphigoid	Chronic ocular discomfort and injection followed by the development of conjunctival keratinization, symblepharon, ankyloblepharon, corneal ulceration and scarring, eyelid scarring (entropion)
Uveitis	Photophobia, periocular ache, floaters, decreased vision
Acute closed-angle glaucoma	Severe, sudden onset, periocular ache; middilated fixed pupil; decreased vision; corneal edema
Keratitis	Pain, photophobia, corneal opacity, decreased vision
Orbital inflammation	Proptosis, diplopia, restricted eye movements
Scleritis and episcleritis	See Table 61–4

Table 61–4. Distinguishing Scleritis from Episcleritis

Scleritis	Episcleritis
Painful	Irritation without pain
Persistent	Transient
Frequently associated with a systemic disease	Rarely associated with systemic disease
Associated with ophthalmic complications	No ophthalmic complications
Vessels do not blanch with a topical vasoconstrictor	Vessels blanch with a topical vasoconstrictor
Vessel color: deep red to blue	Vessel color: pink to light red

nodules can also occur in the sclera. This condition is known as scleromalacia perforans (Figure 61–1). This form of scleritis can be associated with minimal pain.

Systemic forms of vasculitis, especially Wegener granulomatosis, are also associated with scleritis. Several authorities recommend obtaining a test for antineutrophil cytoplasmic antibodies in evaluating patients with scleritis, although it is currently not proven that a patient with a positive antineutrophil cytoplasmic antibody test, scleritis, and no other evidence of Wegener has a distinct prognosis or a risk for developing a more complete form of Wegener.

Bisphosphonates, especially intravenous bisphosphonates, can cause a scleritis and this cause is often overlooked. The disease is usually unilateral and the onset is typically soon after the initiation of the treatment. An adverse effect from a bisphosphonate should especially be considered in an older patient who develops the new onset of scleritis.

Diseases Causing Red Eye

Ocular cicatricial pemphigoid is an autoimmune cicatrizing conjunctivitis. Although the early stages of the disease may mimic simple conjunctivitis with symptoms of ocular irritation, redness, and tearing, the onset is more insidious and the course is chronic and progressive, with the eventual development of severe conjunctival, corneal,

Table 61–5. Systemic Diseases Most Often Associated with Scleritis

Rheumatoid arthritis
Vasculitis, especially Wegener
Inflammatory bowel disease
Ankylosing spondylitis
Relapsing polychondritis
Behçet disease

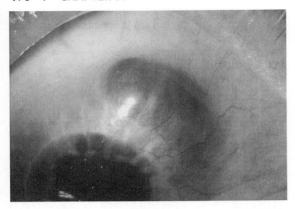

Figure 61–1. Rheumatoid scleromalacia perforans characterized by the prolapse of (dark) uveal tissue.

and lid scarring that results in permanent visual loss if left untreated (Figure 61–2). Ocular cicatricial pemphigoid should therefore be suspected in patients who present with chronic, persistent symptoms that fail to resolve within 1–2 weeks and are associated with the development of conjunctival keratinization and shortened fornices due to conjunctival symblepharon and ankyloblepharon. These cases require an ophthalmic examination to confirm the diagnosis (usually with a conjunctival biopsy) to enable the institution of treatment, which typically consists of aggressive systemic immune suppression in combination with local/surgical therapies.

The most common cause of a red eye that is causally related to a rheumatic disease is dryness or Sjögren's syn-

drome. Although disease of the lacrimal gland does not cause redness directly, a dry eye is often red secondary to irritation and injected conjunctival vessels. Sjögren's syndrome is discussed separately in Chapter 27.

Orbital disease resulting in proptosis and often diplopia can be a manifestation of a rheumatic disease, especially Wegener granulomatosis; however, the most common cause of orbital disease is thyroid eye disease. Redness results indirectly either from corneal exposure secondary to exophthalmos, and/or increased intraorbital pressure from the inflammatory mass that results in raised venous pressure and vascular engorgement. Visual loss due to optic nerve compression may also occur.

Acute closed-angle glaucoma, which is extremely painful and a medical emergency, is associated with eye redness, but this condition is not typically associated with rheumatic disease.

Keratitis is inflammation or infection of the cornea that is characterized by a red eye and a corneal infiltrate (Figure 61–3). There are many causes of keratitis including infections, toxins, trauma, and immunologic disease. One of the most common causes of keratitis is marginal keratitis, which is associated with acne rosacea and blepharitis. Unlike infective keratitis, marginal keratitis has a benign course and responds well to treatment of the acne rosacea with oral tetracyclines in combination with local measures such as lid scrubs and a short course of topical steroid eye drops. However, patients with any form of suspected keratitis require an ophthalmic assessment to distinguish between infective keratitis (which can progress rapidly to permanent visual impairment) and other more benign forms.

Thinning of the corneal periphery is sometimes known as corneal melt or marginal keratolysis and can also occur in the setting of a systemic autoimmune

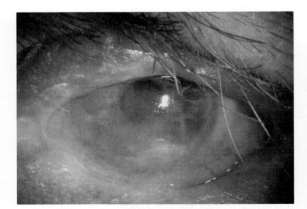

Figure 61–2. End-stage ocular cicatricial pemphigoid with obliteration of the conjunctival fornices due to symblepharon and ankyloblepharon, deformed lower eyelid (entropion), and extensive scarring of the cornea with pannus ingrowth.

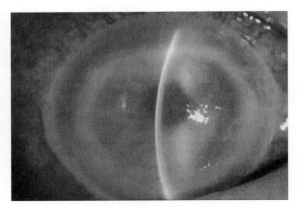

Figure 61–3. Severe infective keratitis as evidenced by marked ocular injection, corneal edema, and a ring infiltrate involving the mid-periphery of the cornea.

Table 61–6. Causes of Uveitis

Infections such as herpes simplex, herpes zoster, or toxoplasmosis

Syndromes confined to the eye such as pars planitis, sympathetic ophthalmia, or birdshot retinochoroidopathy

Masquerade syndromes such as lymphoma, leukemia, or retinal degeneration

Systemic immunologic disease as listed in Table 61–7

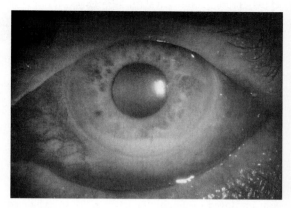

Figure 61–4. Acute anterior uveitis with a hypopyon.

disease. This condition is usually but not always found in association with scleritis. It can be associated with severe rheumatoid arthritis or vasculitis. Cataract surgery in a patient with a very dry eye and severe rheumatoid arthritis can sometimes trigger a corneal melt. The treatment usually consists of oral glucocorticoids and medications that control the underlying rheumatic condition.

Uveitis describes inflammation of the uvea, which consists of the iris, ciliary body, and choroid. A simplified differential diagnosis of anterior uveitis is given in Table 61–6. Table 61–7 lists the most common systemic diseases associated with uveitis. Patients with uveitis often have associated inflammation of adjacent structures such as the retina or the vitreous humor. Anterior uveitis is synonymous with iritis or iridocyclitis. Anterior uveitis, especially if it begins suddenly, is associated with a red eye (Figure 61–4). In contrast, patients with juvenile idiopathic arthritis whose anterior uveitis has begun insidiously usually do not experience prominent redness. Similarly uveitis which is mainly posterior to the lens may not display redness. Approximately 50% of patients with anterior uveitis are human leukocyte antigen (HLA)-B27 positive and the majority of B27-positive patients with iritis have joint symptoms such as inflammatory low back pain consistent with a spondyloarthropathy.

Table 61–7. Systemic Immunologic Diseases Commonly Associated with Uveitis

Ankylosing spondylitis
Behçet disease
Drug reactions (eg, rifabutin)
Familial granulomatous synovitis with uveitis
Inflammatory bowel disease
Interstitial nephritis
Juvenile idiopathic arthritis
Multiple sclerosis
Neonatal-onset multisystem inflammatory disease
Psoriatic arthritis
Reactive arthritis
Relapsing polychondritis
Sarcoidosis
Systemic lupus erythematosus
Vasculitis, especially Kawasaki syndrome and Cogan syndrome
Vogt-Koyanagi-Harada syndrome

The cause of ocular redness is best evaluated with a slitlamp examination, a biomicroscope that is designed specifically to examine the eye.

Treatment

The treatment for ocular redness depends greatly on the underlying disease and ranges from no treatment for a minor irritation to an oral alkylating agent for some forms of scleritis.

It should also be emphasized that many rheumatic diseases that involve the eye do so without causing any redness. The optic nerve ischemia that characterizes temporal arteritis is a classic example of this.

REFERENCES

Ahmed M, Zein G, Khawaja F, Foster CS. Ocular cicatricial pemphigoid: pathogenesis, diagnosis and treatment. *Prog Retin Eye Res.* 2004;23:579. (This extensive review of a relatively rare but blinding disease covers current concepts of pathogenesis, clinical features, histology, and treatment modalities.)

Gordon LK. Diagnostic dilemmas in orbital inflammatory disease. *Ocul Immunol Inflamm.* 2003;11:3. (This article gives a step-by-step approach to the patient presenting with orbital inflammatory disease and covers both infective and autoimmune causes of this presentation.)

Okhravi N, Odufuwa B, McCluskey P, Lightman S. Scleritis. *Surv Ophthalmol.* 2005;50:351. (This thorough review covers the clinical features of scleritis and its differentiation from episcleritis, as well as its classification, complications, systemic disease associations, and current treatments.)

Suhler EB, Martin TM, Rosenbaum JT. HLA-B27-associated uveitis: overview and current perspectives. *Curr Opin Ophthalmol.* 2003;14:378. (This comprehensive and easily readable review covers current concepts of HLA-B27–related uveitis, including the current understanding of disease pathogenesis, clinical patterns of presentation, common systemic disease associations, and new treatment developments.)

Common Injuries from Running

62

Calvin R. Brown JR, MD

Approximately 11 million people in the United States run more than 100 days per year. Recreational exercise is attractive because it improves the quality of life and increases longevity. Runners note a range of salutary effects, from improved cardiopulmonary capacity to enhanced mental health, less depression and anxiety, and a greater sense of tranquility.

Regular exercise enhances sleep patterns; promotes a stronger and more stable musculoskeletal system; and results in decreases in disability, hypertension, diabetes, cancer, stroke, and osteoporosis. Runners report increased appetite and healthier weight, a desirable combination. Except for walking, running may be the most easily accessible and least expensive form of regular exercise.

However, there are important health concerns that develop as a consequence of running as well. These include the risk of sudden death, musculoskeletal injuries, and potentially deleterious effects on joints. Approximately 45–70% of runners will experience musculoskeletal injuries each year.

RISK FACTORS

Repetitive use, rather than a single traumatic event, causes the majority of running injuries. Table 62–1 lists the 10 most common injuries seen in one clinic and is representative of reports from other large series. Risk factors for running injuries include history of a previous injury, competitive running, high weekly mileage (>25 miles per week), and abrupt increases in the intensity or duration of training. Injuries are more likely to occur when the runner's shoes are worn down, leading to the recommendation that shoes be replaced every 6 months or 400 miles of use.

Stretching is of particular interest because runners frequently report performing better and feeling better after stretching. However, a large controlled trial of stretching as taught by an Olympic marathon coach showed no difference in injury type or frequency between the intervention and control groups. Thus, the well-entrenched lore of stretching and running does not have evidence-based support. Similarly, there is little or no evidence to support proposed links between running injuries and

age, gender, body mass, hill running, running on hard surfaces, time of year, and time of day.

CLINICAL FINDINGS

Physical Examination

The physical examination of an injured runner should not only focus on the area of pain, but should also include an examination of adjacent joints, alignment, and flexibility. Approximately 20–40% of running injuries can be related to structural abnormalities. The foot must dissipate 110 tons of force for every mile run, and alignment abnormalities of the foot are associated with increased frequency of injury. A high-arched foot (pes cavus) is rigid and tends to transmit impact up the leg. A flat foot (pes planus) leads to excessive pronation of the foot during running, which in turn increases stress on the medial structures of the ankle, shin, and knee. Orthotics may be helpful for either type of structural abnormality.

Hamstring and calf flexibility can be assessed with the runner in the supine position on the examining table, the femur at 90 degrees to the table, and the foot at 90 degrees to the tibia. The physician should be able to passively extend the knee to within 15 degrees of full extension. Although there is little evidence that stretching prevents running injuries, stretching may be of therapeutic value for the injured runner with limited flexibility.

Shoe Evaluation

The athletic shoe industry is a $13-billion-per-year industry that sells more than 350 million pairs of shoes annually. Sports shoes, particularly running shoes, have penetrated into every facet of mainstream America. They have become a fashion statement, and some of us even wear them to work. Consequently the use of athletic shoes for casual and fashion wear has had a large influence on their appearance and features. Fortunately, podiatric biomechanical thought and technology have penetrated deeply into the psyche of the industry and buying public. Terms such as pronation, stability, and motion control are now widely used in the description and rankings of running shoes.

Today's running shoes are designed with an eye toward accommodating various types and shapes of feet. Shoes

Table 62–1. The 10 Most Common Running Injuries

Medical Diagnosis	Percentage	N
Patellar pain syndrome	25.8	468
Stress fractures	13.2	239
Achilles tendinitis	6.0	109
Plantar fasciitis	4.7	85
Patellar tendinitis	4.5	81
Iliotibial band syndrome	4.3	78
Metatarsalgia	3.2	58
Tibial stress syndrome	2.6	47
Tibialis posterior tendinitis	2.5	45
Peroneus tendinitis	1.9	34
Total	68.7	1224

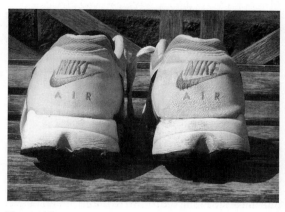

Figure 62–1. Shoe wear. The upper of the left shoe tilts toward the inside, a finding indicative of overpronation.

are made that allow for differences between men and women, light- and heavyweight runners, pronated and supinated (underpronated) feet, and narrow and wide feet. Increasingly sport-specific shoes meet the diverse needs of different sports, and even different running conditions such as trail running and racing on various surfaces.

Evaluation of an injured runner should always include examination of a well-used pair of running shoes, so patients coming in for the first visit should be advised to bring a pair with them as part of the evaluation. The most important aspect is to examine shoe tilt by looking at the shoes from the rear at eye level. Do not pay attention to the heel or outsole wear, but rather look at the angle of the upper (the top part of the shoe that the foot fits into) relative to perpendicular. If the upper is tilting, bent, or smashed toward the inside of the foot, overpronation is occurring (Figure 62–1). If the upper has no tilt, the biomechanics are normal or neutral. Finally, if the upper is tilting or bent toward the outside of the foot, the biomechanics are those of supination, also known as underpronation.

Current thinking is that runners with excessive pronation need a shoe that has more rearfoot control but can have a bit less shock absorption. These shoes are described as "motion control" shoes, and employ dual-density midsoles and medial posts to control excessive pronation. Neutral runners can use a shoe without this technology, saving both cost and weight. These are referred to, somewhat confusingly, as "stability" shoes. People with a high-arched (cavus) foot need more cushioning because of the rigid nature of their feet. These are more obviously referred to as "cushioned" shoes. Some general principles

of shoe fitting for all running athletes are outlined in Table 62–2.

PATELLOFEMORAL PAIN SYNDROME

By far the most common injury in runners, and probably the most common cause of knee pain in all active individuals, is the patellofemoral or anterior knee pain

Table 62–2. Athletic Shoe Fitting: Advice for Patients

1. Buy shoes for the specific sport for which you intend to use them.
2. Shop at a reputable store with a knowledgeable staff.
3. Bring the socks you plan to wear with the new athletic shoes.
4. Bring your orthotic or other inserts with you to try on shoes.
5. Allow one finger's width (about $3/8$ inch) space at the front of the shoe in front of the big toe.
6. Running shoes should fit bigger than casual shoes.
7. Make certain that the shoe flexes only where the toes bend, which should also be the widest part of the shoe.
8. Check the inside and outside of the shoe for defects. The shoe should sit level when checked on a flat surface.
9. Check your shoes often for wear such as (1) the outsole worn to the midsole, (2) the heel counter tilted inward (valgus) or outward (varus), and (3) the forefoot upper shifted medially or laterally. Replace shoes every 400 miles, even in the absence of noticeable wear.
10. For a listing of shoes that have been evaluated, visit the website of the American Academy of Podiatric Sports Medicine at www.aapsm.org.

syndrome. Persons seek medical attention complaining of the insidious onset of poorly localized pain on the anterior surface of the knee. Pain is worse when arising from a seated position, particularly after sitting for several minutes (the "theater sign") and when walking up, or more commonly, down stairs.

On physical examination, the Q angle between the femur and tibia should be measured (see Chapter 12). An angle greater than 16 degrees is associated with a higher incidence of patellofemoral pain syndrome. Compression of the patella will cause pain, particularly when the quadriceps muscle is contracted simultaneously. The "patellar inhibition sign" can be assessed by compressing the patella against the femur with the leg extended, and simultaneously asking the patient to isometrically contract the quadriceps, causing loading of the patellofemoral joint. This maneuver should reproduce the patient's knee pain.

STRESS FRACTURES

A stress fracture is an incomplete fracture that results from repetitive strain on the bone rather than a single traumatic episode. Stress fractures occur in all sports that require repetitive running and jumping, but are far more common in long-distance runners than in any other athletes. The vast majority occur in people who are running more than 20 miles per week. Continued, repetitive stress on the bone leads to a normal remodeling response that is gradually overcome, and trabecular microfractures occur. The tibia and fibula are most commonly involved (Figure 62–2). Displacement of stress fractures is rare

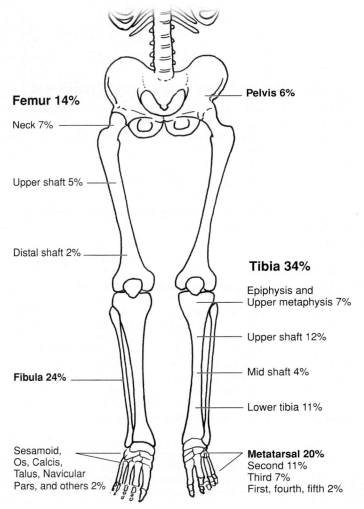

Femur 14%
Pelvis 6%
Neck 7%
Upper shaft 5%
Distal shaft 2%

Tibia 34%
Epiphysis and Upper metaphysis 7%
Upper shaft 12%
Mid shaft 4%
Lower tibia 11%

Fibula 24%

Sesamoid, Os, Calcis, Talus, Navicular Pars, and others 2%

Metatarsal 20%
Second 11%
Third 7%
First, fourth, fifth 2%

Figure 62–2. Stress fractures resulting from failure of bone remodeling.

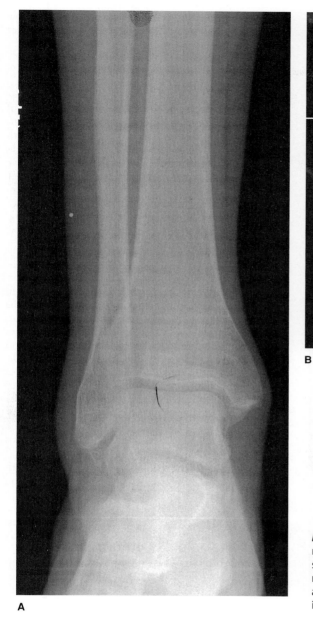

A

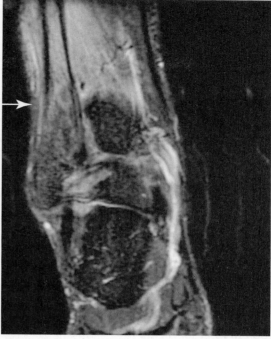

B

Figure 62-3. Detection of early stress fracture using magnetic resonance imaging. **A:** The initial radiograph shows no abnormality. **B:** The fat suppression magnetic resonance image shows increased signal in the fibula at the area indicated by the arrow, indicative of bone injury.

except for femoral neck fractures, which also carry the risk of avascular necrosis.

In most patients, the diagnosis of a stress fracture should be made on the clinical history. Any running athlete who complains of pain localized to a bone in the lower extremity should be considered to have a stress fracture. If local tenderness over the bone is found, further work-up should include radiographs or bone scan. Magnetic resonance imaging is expensive but can be used in rare in-

stances when the lesion is indistinct on bone scan (Figure 62–3).

Some general rules can be applied to treatment of stress fractures regardless of their location. Pain can usually be controlled with nonsteroidal anti-inflammatory drugs. The patient must significantly decrease or stop running to reduce the excess strain that is causing the stress fracture. During this rest phase of treatment, alternative exercise possibilities include swimming, biking,

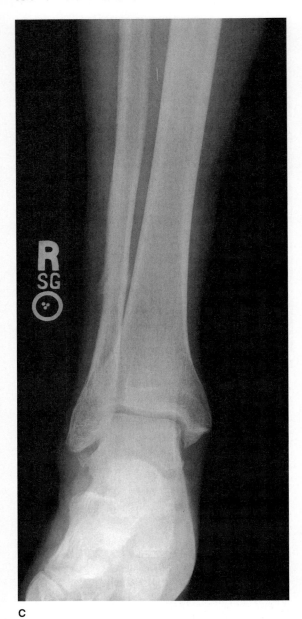

C

Figure 62–3. (***Continued***) **C:** The follow-up radiograph 1 month later confirms periosteal bone reaction indicative of stress fracture.

and the use of a stair-climber or elliptical trainer. This hiatus offers an excellent chance to increase muscle mass and strength and thereby avoid further stress fractures. When local tenderness has disappeared, a final radiograph can be obtained, and running activities can be gradually reintroduced. At this point one has to know the previous running history and must be certain that the return to running is gradual.

MEDIAL TIBIAL STRESS SYNDROME (SHIN SPLINTS)

Persons with medial tibial stress syndrome complain of diffuse, nagging pain over the tibia that worsens with running. If the pain persists after running and is noted with routine ambulation, the diagnosis of a tibial stress fracture should be suspected. Medial tibial stress syndrome is common in beginning runners. The pathophysiology is thought to be inflammation of the anterior and posterior calf musculature and periostitis of the tibia. Treatment consists of a break from full or vigorous training, correction of any misalignment, and substituted aerobic activities to prevent deconditioning.

ACHILLES TENDINITIS

Runners and jumping athletes may complain of pain in the substance of the Achilles tendon, which connects the soleus and the gastrocnemius muscles to the calcaneus. A relatively avascular or "watershed" area in the Achilles tendon approximately 4–5 cm proximal to its insertion is a factor in its vulnerability to injury and rupture. Diverse factors are thought to incite overuse injuries of the Achilles tendon, including running on hard surfaces, abrupt increases in mileage or training intensity, and shoe design. Fortunately, the latter has been addressed in contemporary running shoes. A person with a high-arched foot may also be at increased risk for Achilles tendinitis and rupture.

Clinically, fusiform swelling with or without warmth may be evident along the Achilles tendon. Crepitation may be present with motion. Palpation along the tendon will elicit pain. The calf should be squeezed with the foot held in dorsiflexion; this should result in a modest amount of plantar flexion if the Achilles tendon is intact (the Thompson squeeze test).

Treatment of Achilles tendinitis consists of reduction of activities, anti-inflammatory medication, heel lifts or orthotics, and gentle stretching. Once the Achilles tendon is no longer tender to palpation and the athlete has restored his or her flexibility, slow progressive return to activity is permitted. There have been reports of iatrogenic Achilles tendon rupture secondary to inadvertent intratendinous glucocorticoid injection, and thus injection should be avoided.

PLANTAR FASCIITIS

Plantar fasciitis typically occurs over the midportion of the plantar fascia and is usually exacerbated by dorsiflexion of the toes and direct pressure over the fascia. Lateral squeeze of the heel also precipitates pain. Individuals with chronic plantar fascial pain have microtears and partial rupture of the plantar fascia near its origin. In the case of rupture, a gap in the tendon is often palpable.

Treatment consists of ice, anti-inflammatory drugs, and physical therapy to increase heel and Achilles flexibility in order to relieve stress and tension on the plantar fascia. Orthotics may be useful.

PATELLAR TENDINITIS

Patellar tendinitis is often referred to as "jumper's knee" because of its common association with jumping sports such as basketball. However, it can occur in any running sport, which can be thought of as a series of onelegged jumps. Abnormal foot biomechanics and running up hills are cited as aggravating factors.

Pain is localized to the inferior pole of the patella, and swelling is generally not present. Knee range of motion is within normal limits. Affected persons feel a sensation of the knee giving way with hard jumping. On examination, tenderness is felt directly on the lower tip of the patella. Radiographs are normal, but bone scans may be positive at the inferior pole of the patella, and magnetic resonance imaging may show chronic tendinopathy.

Unfortunately, patellar tendinitis is often chronic, taking many months to a year for complete healing. Nonsteroidal anti-inflammatory drugs are helpful, as are exercises to stretch and strengthen leg muscles. In some cases, surgery is needed to remove scarred portions of the tendon. Long-term restriction of jumping may be required for 1 or 2 years. Patellar tendinitis can affect the long-term playing ability of jumping athletes, such as volleyball or basketball players and long-distance runners.

ILIOTIBIAL BAND SYNDROME

Iliotibial band syndrome is an overuse condition that is common in runners and cyclists and is characterized by an ache or burning sensation of the lateral aspect of the knee during or after activity. Iliotibial band syndrome is thought to be due to local friction of the tendon band as it rubs over the lateral femoral condyle. Clinically, pain symptoms are localized to the lateral aspect of the femoral condyle and may radiate up the side of the thigh to the hip. Motion of the knee is normal, but tightness and snapping may be perceived. Apart from well-localized tenderness, the knee examination is normal. Radiographs generally are normal, and magnetic resonance imaging is not indicated.

Progressive healing is the rule with iliotibial band syndrome. The athlete can continue moderate activities during this condition. Treatment consists of local icing both before and after activities, and frequent regular stretching of the lateral hip muscles and iliotibial band.

METATARSALGIA

Metatarsalgia, which is more a description than a diagnosis, refers to a syndrome of pain in one or more metatarsophalangeal (MTP) joints due to a variety of causes, including capsulitis and synovitis, degenerative arthritis, neuroma, synovial cyst, and stress fracture. Synovitis and capsulitis are probably the most common causes. Although any of the MTP joints can be affected, the second MTP joint is the most commonly involved.

Biomechanical factors such as a hypermobile first MTP joint accompanied by a long second metatarsal can result in second MTP synovitis. Anterior ankle impingement may cause diffuse forefoot pain. Plantar fat pad atrophy and plantar flexion of the metatarsal may also cause MTP joint synovitis.

Physical findings associated with MTP joint synovitis include swelling and pain with manipulation of the joint. Vertical subluxation of the toe places pressure on the plantar capsule, eliciting pain.

Treatment is almost always conservative and is generally successful. Ice massage and anti-inflammatory medications reduce swelling and pain. Orthotics with metatarsal relief padding reduce stress on the joint and can be of great help. In resistant cases, an intra-articular injection is indicated. This should be done judiciously because repeated injections may be destructive to the ligamentous capsular support of the joint. Surgery, in the form of synovectomy and metatarsal osteotomy, is rarely necessary.

REFERENCES

Akuthota V, Harrast MA. Running injuries. *Phys Med Rehabil Clin N Am.* 2005;16:623 [PMID: 16324969].

Browning KH, Donley BG. Evaluation and management of common running injuries. *Clev Clin J Med.* 2000;67:511. [PMID: 10902242]. (A concise review of rapid diagnosis and conservative management techniques.)

World Wide Web Sites

[The U.S. National Library of Medicine/National Institutes of Health homepage for sports injury information]

http://www.nlm.nih.gov/medlineplus/sportsinjuries.html

[The American Academy of Podiatric Sports Medicine website that contains up-to-date running shoe evaluations]

www.aapsm.org

Complex Regional Pain Syndromes: Reflex Sympathetic Dystrophy & Causalgia

63

Ralf Baron, MD, Janne Ludwig, MD, & Jon D. Levine, MD, PhD

ESSENTIALS OF DIAGNOSIS

- *Disabling neuropathic pain affecting a limb.*
- *Develops after trauma or minor tissue injury.*
- *Spontaneous pain, hyperalgesia, swelling, autonomic abnormalities, and impaired motor function of the affected limb.*
- *Trophic changes and restricted passive range of motion in the chronic stages.*

General Considerations

Complex regional pain syndromes (CRPS) are painful disorders that develop as a disproportionate consequence of trauma to a limb. Sensory abnormalities, autonomic abnormalities, trophic changes, and motor weakness are the dominant clinical manifestations and form the basis for diagnostic criteria (Table 63–1). These abnormalities have a distal distribution, are not confined to the innervation territories of peripheral nerves or nerve roots, and tend to spread. Two types of CRPS can be distinguished. There is no overt nerve lesion in CRPS 1 (also called reflex sympathetic dystrophy). In contrast, the diagnosis of CRPS 2 (also known as causalgia) is confirmed by the identification of a partial peripheral nerve lesion.

The pathophysiology of CRPS is not well understood. Inflammatory reactions due to neurally-released substances—"neurogenic inflammation"—appear to be involved in the edema, vasodilatation, skin warming, heat hyperalgesia, and increased sweating observed in the acute phase of CRPS; immune-mediated inflammation may contribute as well.

The spontaneous pain and various forms of stimulus-evoked pain that characterize CRPS are thought to be generated by peripheral and central sensitization of the nociceptive system. Altered somatosensory perceptions are probably the result of changes in the central representation of somatosensory maps in the thalamus and cortex. For example, somatosensory evoked potential mapping demonstrates smaller cortical representation of the CRPS-affected hand than that of the contralateral healthy hand. Cortical reorganization correlates with the amount of CRPS pain, consistent with the possibility that mechanical hyperalgesia is associated with cortical plastic changes.

CRPS 1 is associated with alterations in sympathetic reflex patterns that cause unilateral abnormalities in skin blood flow, temperature, and sweating. Pathologic interactions of sympathetic and afferent neurons may stimulate nociceptors, leading to sympathetically maintained pain in some cases. About half of patients with CRPS 1 show evidence of motor abnormalities, possibly as a result of abnormal central programming and processing of motor tasks.

Clinical Findings

A. SYMPTOMS AND SIGNS

1. CRPS type 1 (reflex sympathetic dystrophy)— Bone fracture, surgery (eg, for carpal tunnel syndrome), minor soft tissue trauma, and rarely stroke or myocardial infarction can precipitate CRPS type 1. Typically pain and swelling of a distal extremity develops after trauma (Figure 63–1). There is no overt nerve lesion. The swelling and pain often occur at a site removed from the inciting injury, and obvious local tissue-damaging processes are absent.

Patients with CRPS 1 often report a burning spontaneous pain in the distal part of the affected extremity. The intensity of the pain is disproportionate to the inciting event and usually increases when the extremity is in a dependent position. Pain evoked by mechanical and thermal stimuli is a striking clinical feature. These sensory abnormalities often appear early, are most pronounced

Table 63–1. Revised Diagnostic Criteria for Complex Regional Pain Syndrome (CRPS)

Clinical Signs and Symptoms
1. Positive sensory abnormalities:
   - Spontaneous pain
   - Mechanical hyperalgesia
   - Thermal hyperalgesia
   - Deep somatic hyperalgesia
2. Vascular abnormalities
   - Vasodilatation
   - Vasoconstriction
   - Skin temperature asymmetries
   - Skin color changes
3. Edema and sweating abnormalities
   - Swelling
   - Hyper- or hypohidrosis
4. Motor and trophic changes
   - Motor weakness
   - Tremor
   - Dystonia
   - Coordination deficits
   - Nail and hair changes
   - Skin atrophy
   - Joint stiffness
   - Soft tissue changes

Diagnosis of CRPS:
Clinical use: At least one symptom from three or more categories AND at least one sign from two or more categories ; sensitivity 85%, specificity 60%
Research use: At least one symptom in EACH category AND at least one sign in two or more categories; sensitivity 70%, specificity 96%

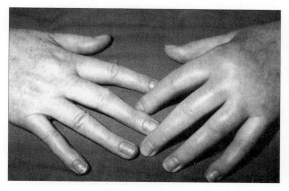

Figure 63–1. Complex regional pain syndrome developed in this patient after a radial fracture in the left hand. The marked swelling seen in the left hand started 2 weeks after the initial trauma. (From Baron R, Levine JD, Fields HL. Causalgia and reflex sympathetic dystrophy: does the sympathetic nervous system contribute to the generation of pain? *Muscle Nerve.* 1999;22:678. With permission.)

distally, and have no consistent spatial relationship to individual nerve territories or to the site of the inciting lesion. Pain also is elicited by movement and by pressure at the joints in the affected region, even though these joints are not directly affected by the inciting lesion. In many cases, symptoms are also present in more proximal joints (eg, the ipsilateral shoulder).

Autonomic abnormalities include swelling and changes in sweating and blood flow in the skin. In the acute stages of CRPS 1, the affected limb is often warmer than the contralateral limb. Sweating abnormalities (hypohidrosis, or more frequently, hyperhidrosis) are present in nearly all CRPS 1 patients.

Trophic changes, such as abnormal nail growth, increased or decreased hair growth, fibrosis, thin glossy skin, and osteoporosis, may develop, particularly in the chronic stages. Restriction of passive movement is often seen in long-standing cases and may be related to functional motor disturbances and to trophic changes of joints and tendons.

Muscles of the affected distal extremity are often weak. Small, accurate movements are impaired. Nerve conduction and electromyography studies are within normal ranges, except among patients in whom CRPS 1 is chronic or advanced. About half of patients have postural or action tremors that represent exaggerated physiologic tremors. In about 10% of cases, dystonia of the affected hand or foot develops.

It is not possible to identify those who are at risk for CRPS 1 following a potential precipitating event. During the normal course of fracture healing, pain is felt predominantly within the traumatized area. If CRPS 1 develops, the pain changes in quality (often described as burning), becomes more intense, spreads to the entire affected distal extremity, and is located deep within the bone or joints. Movement of all distal joints elicits discomfort, and the patient experiences disproportionate muscle weakness.

2. CRPS type 2 (causalgia)—CRPS 2 presents as a burning pain that develops in a distal extremity after a traumatic partial injury of a peripheral nerve. In addition to spontaneous pain, patients report hypersensitivity of the skin to light mechanical stimulation. Movement, loud noise, or strong emotion can trigger the pain. There is swelling of the distal extremity and smoothness and mottling of the skin. The affected limb is usually cold and sweaty. In some cases, acute arthritis is present. Sensory and trophic abnormalities spread beyond the innervation territory of the injured peripheral nerve and often develop at a site remote from the original injury. CRPS 2 occurs in approximately 1–5% of partial nerve lesions.

There are no known predictors for the development of CRPS 2.

3. Sympathetically maintained pain—Some patients with either CRPS 1 or CRPS 2 have pain that is sympathetically maintained and that responds to selective sympathetic blockade or to antagonism of α adrenoceptors. The presence of sympathetically maintained pain defines a subset of patients with CRPS, not a separate clinical entity.

B. LABORATORY STUDIES, IMAGING, AND SPECIAL TESTS

The results of routine blood studies, including erythrocyte sedimentation rate and C-reactive protein, are usually normal.

Certain tests provide supportive evidence for the diagnosis of CRPS. Bone scintigraphy can show significant changes during the subacute period (up to 1 year) (Figure 63–2). Plain radiographs can demonstrate demineralization in the chronic stages (Figure 63–3). Skin temperature measurements using infrared thermometry assess vascular function and are particularly helpful in the diagnosis of CRPS. Under normal conditions, only minor skin temperature asymmetries are present between both limbs. Prominent asymmetries of skin temperature distinguish CRPS from other extremity pain syndromes with high sensitivity and specificity.

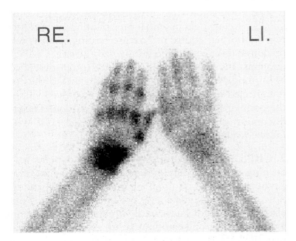

Figure 63–2. Three-phase bone scintigraphy of a patient presenting with a complex regional pain syndrome after distal radius fracture of the right hand. The scintigram shows increased bone metabolism in the traumatic wrist area as well as in the metacarpophalangeal and interphalangeal joints, typical findings for CRPS.

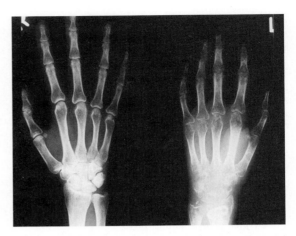

Figure 63–3. Radiograph of both hands in a patient with chronic complex regional pain syndrome of the left hand. The radiograph shows a soft-tissue swelling of the dorsum of the hand and around the metacarpophalangeal joints as well as a generalized demineralization, particularly in the distal metacarpal bones.

Differential Diagnosis

A. OTHER DISORDERS WITH UNILATERAL VASCULAR DISTURBANCES

Inflammatory arthritis and soft-tissue infections can cause unilateral skin warming and a vascular regulation pattern that mimics CRPS. Arterial or venous occlusive diseases can present with marked temperature differences between the affected and healthy limbs. Repetitive artificial occlusion of the blood supply to a limb (as in the psychiatric factitious syndrome) can induce secondary structural changes of the blood vessels with consecutive abnormalities in perfusion.

B. POSTTRAUMATIC NEURALGIA AND TERRITORIAL NEUROPATHIC PAIN SYNDROMES

Neuralgia (eg, trigeminal neuralgia) is a type of neuropathic pain located within the innervation territory of the affected nerve. Some patients with focal painful neuropathies are more complex than neuralgia patients, but do not have the full clinical picture of CRPS 2. Patients with territorial neuropathic pain syndromes, which can follow traumatic or postherpetic nerve damage, have spontaneous burning pain and pain that can be evoked by mechanical or cold stimuli. In contrast to CRPS 2, these sensory symptoms are confined to the territory of the affected peripheral nerve, although the mechanically evoked pain may extend somewhat beyond the border of nerve territories. Patients with territorial neuropathic pain syndromes do not have marked swelling and do not exhibit a progressive spread of symptoms.

C. METABOLIC AND TOXIC NEUROPATHIES

Polyneuropathies induced by metabolic disorders (eg, diabetes mellitus) or toxins (eg, alcohol) characteristically demonstrate a diffuse symmetric distribution of symptoms and therefore can be distinguished clearly from CRPS, which in most cases is confined to one extremity.

Treatment of Complex Regional Pain Syndrome

Only a few evidence-based treatment regimens for CRPS are available. Therefore, the clinician must rely on studies of other neuropathic pain syndromes, on treatments based on hypothetical mechanisms, and on expert opinion.

Treatment should be individualized. In mild cases of CRPS (defined by pain present only under load and with only mild joint symptoms), conventional pain therapy and carefully increasing physiotherapy may lead to resolution within weeks. If symptoms are severe, however, pain therapy should be immediate, aggressive, and most importantly, directed toward restoration of full function of the extremity. This objective is best attained in a comprehensive multidisciplinary setting with emphasis on conventional and interventional pain management and functional restoration. Pain specialists should include neurologists, anesthesiologists, orthopedists, physiotherapists, and psychologists.

In rare cases, treatment of an underlying disorder is associated with complete resolution of CRPS. In patients with carpal tunnel syndrome, for example, continuous nociceptive input from the nerve compression site can initiate and maintain CRPS 2. Adequate decompression of the nerve will rapidly relieve CRPS symptoms in these patients.

Destructive surgery on the peripheral or central afferent nervous system in patients with CRPS always generates further deafferentation and provides an increased risk for the persistent pain associated with destruction of afferent pathways.

A. PHARMACOLOGIC THERAPY

The general principles of pharmacologic treatment are the individualization of therapy and the titration of a specific pharmacologic agent to maximize effect and minimize negative side effects. "No response" should not be accepted as a result until enough time (2–4 weeks) has passed to accurately judge the efficacy of the drug.

1. Analgesics—Nonsteroidal anti-inflammatory drugs can provide relief of mild to moderate pain. Opioids have been shown in short-term studies to be efficacious in other neuropathic pain syndromes but have not been rigorously studied in CRPS; however, expert opinion supports the use of opioids in a comprehensive pain treatment program for CRPS. Antidepressants have analgesic effects in several neuropathic pain states and should be tested as part of the treatment regimen. Lidocaine and the anticonvulsant carbamazepine relieve neuropathic pain. Intravenous lidocaine is effective in CRPS. Gabapentin and pregabalin modulate central calcium channels that presynaptically inhibit the distribution of pain-inducing neurotransmitters. In one study, gabapentin had a promising effect on CRPS.

2. Anti-inflammatory agents—Oral glucocorticoids have demonstrated efficacy in controlled trials of acute CRPS. There are also reports of sustained relief of pain and an improvement of symptoms in CRPS patients in response to anti–tumor necrosis factor agents, lenalidomide (a thalidomide analogue that inhibits the secretion of proinflammatory cytokines), and intravenous gamma globulin.

3. Other pharmacologic modalities—There is clinical evidence for efficacy of radical scavengers such as topical dimethylsulfoxide and N-acetylcysteine. Transdermal application of the α_2-adrenoceptor agonist clonidine, which is thought to prevent the release of catecholamines by a presynaptic action, may be helpful when small areas of hyperalgesia are present. The administration of intravenous bisphosphonates (alendronate and clodronate) has been shown to provide significant relief from pain and swelling and improve movement. Studies of calcitonin in CRPS have yielded contradictory results.

B. INTERVENTIONAL THERAPY IN THE SYMPATHETIC NERVOUS SYSTEM

Sympatholytic therapy can result in substantial or even complete pain relief in some patients and can improve other symptoms of CRPS. Approximately 85% of patients in the acute stage report a positive short-term effect, but far fewer experience long-term relief. Two therapeutic techniques to block sympathetic nerves are currently used: (1) injections of a local anesthetic around sympathetic paravertebral ganglia that project to the affected body part (sympathetic ganglion blocks), and (2) regional intravenous application of guanethidine, bretylium, or reserpine (which deplete noradrenaline in the postganglionic axon) to an isolated extremity blocked with a tourniquet (intravenous regional sympatholysis).

C. STIMULATION TECHNIQUES AND SPINAL DRUG APPLICATION

Transcutaneous electrical nerve stimulation may be effective in some cases and produces minimal side effects. Epidural spinal cord stimulation was effective in one randomized study in selected patients with chronic CRPS and may be a promising treatment for such individuals.

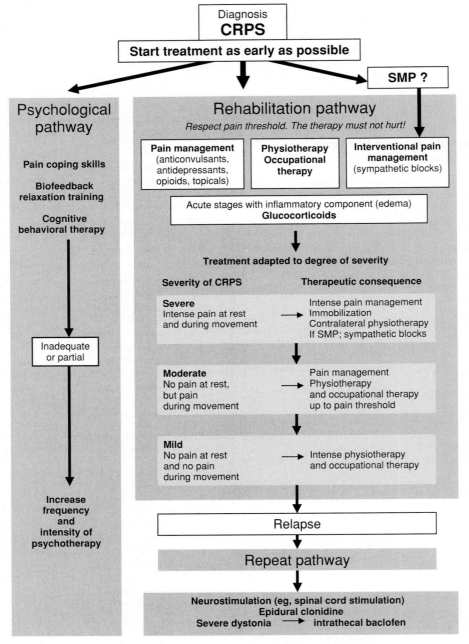

Figure 63–4. Treatment algorithm. CRPS, complex regional pain syndrome; SMP, sympathetically maintained pain. (Modified from Stanton-Hicks M, Burton AW, Bruehl SP, et al. An updated interdisciplinary clinical pathway for CRPS: Report of an Expert Panel. *Pain Practice.* 2002;2:1. With permission; modified from Baron R, Binder A, Ulrich W, Maier C. [Complex regional pain syndrome. Reflex sympathetic dystrophy and causalgia.] *Nervenarzt.* 2002;73:305. With permission; and from McMahon S, Koltzenberg M, eds. *Wall & Melzack's Textbook of Pain.* 5th ed. Churchill Livingstone, 2005:1011. With permission.)

Other stimulation techniques, such as peripheral nerve stimulation with implanted electrodes and deep brain stimulation (sensory thalamus and medial lemniscus), have been reported to be effective in selected cases of CRPS.

In selected patients with severe refractory CRPS, epidural administration of the N-methyl-D-aspartate antagonist ketamine or the adrenoceptor agonist clonidine induced analgesia, but was associated with marked side effects such as sedation and hypotension. Intrathecal baclofen resulted in positive outcomes for CRPS patients with severe dystonia.

D. PHYSICAL THERAPY

Aggressive physical therapy is not feasible and may be harmful in the acute stage of CRPS, when patients still suffer from severe pain. Short periods of immobilization and careful contralateral physical therapy should be the treatment of choice in the acute stages. Later, when pain subsides, passive physical therapy followed by active isometric and later active isotonic training should be combined with sensory desensitization programs. Clinical experience strongly suggests that physiotherapy and occupational therapy are of utmost importance in achieving recovery of function and in rehabilitation. Recent studies have shown that special motor imagery techniques can improve symptoms of CRPS.

E. TREATMENT ALGORITHM

There are no treatment guidelines for CRPS. Nonetheless an algorithm for the treatment of CRPS has been developed on the basis of expert opinion, empiric observations, those few clinical trials that have been conducted, and the authors' personal preferences (Figure 63–4).

Anticonvulsants, antidepressants, and opioids are used for pain relief; it is often preferable to start with a combination of these drugs rather than to use monotherapy. Therapy of the acute phase of the CRPS should also include anti-inflammatory agents, usually oral glucocorticoids, and application of free radical scavengers. Other drugs such as clonidine, nifedipine, and bisphosphonates can be added as well, but their use should be determined by the presence of vasomotor disturbances or demineralization. It is useful to try a series of sympathetic blocks at least once for each patient with CRPS, because these can reduce pain and provide additional benefit beyond that achieved with conventional pharmacologic therapy.

Physiotherapy, occupational therapy, and psychotherapy should be part of the therapeutic regimen in every CRPS patient. Transcutaneous electrical nerve stimulation and topical therapy can be used as well at every stage of the disease as an add-on therapy. Invasive stimulation techniques should be used only if conservative therapy strategies failed over a prolonged time period.

Prognosis

In patients with mild CRPS who experience pain only under physical load and have few articular symptoms, conventional pain therapy and carefully increased physiotherapy may relieve the disorder within weeks. In patients with moderate CRPS, a multidisciplinary approach with interventional treatment options and frequent occupational and physiotherapy often leads to successful relief of symptoms within 1 year. In most patients with severe CRPS, however, the prognosis is poor despite aggressive therapy. Improvement followed by relapse of symptoms is common. More than 60% of patients with severe CRPS continue to suffer from many of the primary symptoms for years after the initiating trauma. Spontaneous remissions of associated shoulder symptoms occur more often than remissions of hand symptoms, which may progress to severe dystonia. Complete loss of function is the final stage in severe CRPS cases.

REFERENCES

Baron R. Complex regional pain syndromes. In: McMahon S, Koltzenberg M, eds. *Wall & Melzack's Textbook of Pain.* 5th ed. Churchill Livingstone, 2005:1011.

Harden N, Bruehl S. Diagnostic criteria: The statistical derivation of the four criterion factors. In: Wilson P, Stanton-Hicks M, Harden N, eds. *CRPS: Current Diagnosis and Therapy,* IASP Press, 2005.

Jänig W, Baron R. Complex regional pain syndrome: mystery explained? *Lancet Neurology.* 2003;2:687. [PMID: 14572737].

Ludwig J, Baron R. Complex regional pain syndrome: an inflammatory pain condition? *Drug Discov Today.* 2004;1:449.

Perez RS, Kwakkei G, Zuurmond WW, de Lange JJ. Treatment of reflex sympathetic dystrophy (CRPS type 1): a research synthesis of 21 randomized clinical trials. *J Pain Symptom Manage.* 2001;21:511. [PMID: 11397610]

Relevant World Wide Web Site

[International Research Foundation for RSD/CRPS]
www.rsdfoundation.org

Sensorineural Hearing Loss (Immune-Mediated Inner Ear Disease)

64

John H. Stone, MD, MPH, & Howard W. Francis, MD

ESSENTIALS OF DIAGNOSIS

- *When sensorineural hearing loss occurs in the context of an inflammatory condition, it is referred to most appropriately as immune-mediated inner ear disease (IMIED).*
- *May be associated with disturbances of balance as well as hearing loss, because the inner ear mediates vestibular function as well as hearing.*
- *May occur as a primary inner ear problem, or as a complication of a recognized inflammatory condition such as Cogan syndrome, Wegener granulomatosis, Sjögren syndrome, and others.*
- *Symptoms include tinnitus, vertigo, nausea, and difficulties with two issues related to hearing: acuity and speech discrimination.*

General Considerations

This chapter focuses on sensorineural hearing loss (SNHL) as an idiopathic inflammatory disorder, either secondary to a known autoimmune disease or occurring as a primary form of disease limited to the ear. The anatomy of the inner ear is shown in Figure 64–1. SNHL is a common feature of some primary forms of vasculitis (eg, Cogan syndrome, Wegener granulomatosis, and giant cell arteritis). SNHL also occasionally occurs in association with systemic autoimmune disorders such as systemic lupus erythematosus and Sjögren syndrome. Finally, SNHL may represent an organ-specific inflammatory process confined to the inner ear. Because hearing loss is often not the sole feature of this syndrome—vertigo, tinnitus, and a sense of aural fullness often occur as well—and because the symptoms respond frequently to immunosuppression, *immune-mediated inner ear dis-*

ease (IMIED) is presently the preferred term for this disorder when symptoms and signs are confined entirely to the ear. Devastating disabilities such as profound deafness and severe vestibular dysfunction are potential sequelae of IMIED. Yet if diagnosed promptly, IMIED is amenable to treatment.

Several characteristics distinguish IMIED from other syndromes of inner ear dysfunction. First, its time course is relatively rapid. IMIED is analogous to rapidly progressive glomerulonephritis in that inner ear inflammation progresses to severe, irreversible damage within 3 months of onset (and often much more quickly). With IMIED, in fact, the complete loss of hearing within a week or two of symptom onset is not unusual. Second, IMIED is usually bilateral to some degree, albeit the left and right sides may be affected asymmetrically and asynchronously. Typically, weeks or months separate involvement of the two sides, but the interval may be as long as a year or more. Finally, although some cases of IMIED are marked by precipitous, unrecoverable losses of inner ear function, others demonstrate fluctuating symptom patterns over a period of several months. Recurrent bouts of SNHL often lead to consistent decrements in hearing capabilities, causing profound hearing deficits in many patients over time.

Although IMIED usually occurs in middle-aged individuals, the syndrome has been described in young children and also in the elderly. Two-thirds of the patients with IMIED are women.

Clinical Findings

A. SYMPTOMS AND SIGNS

1. Hearing—Hearing loss in IMIED may take two forms. First, patients may complain primarily of diminished hearing *acuity* (the ability to perceive sound). Crude assessments of hearing sensitivity using the mechanical sounds of a watch, the dial tone of a telephone, or the rubbing of fingers, are inadequate to detect

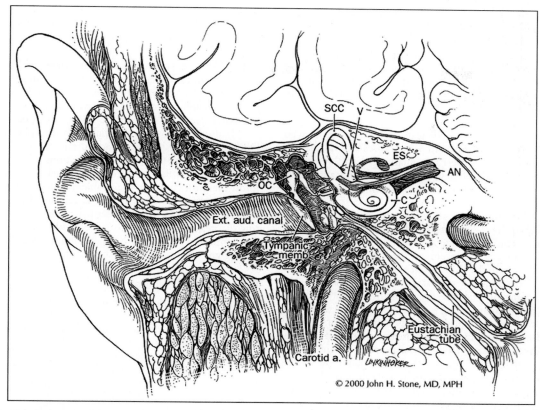

Figure 64–1. Anatomy of the temporal bone and audiovestibular apparatus. AN, auditory nerve; C, cochlea; ES, endolymphatic sac; OC, ossicular chain; SCC, semicircular canals; V, vestibule.

subtle but clinically significant deficits in hearing acuity or speech discrimination. Second, patients may also note decreased *discrimination* (the ability to distinguish individual words). Communication problems arising from poor word discrimination often constitute the chief complaint. Patients with significant deficits in word discrimination are able to hear voices on the telephone, but fail to understand what is being said. They also have difficulty participating in conversations conducted amid background noise. Understanding conversations in crowded rooms or restaurants is particularly problematic.

Otoscopy is usually normal in IMIED, even among patients with profound SNHL. In patients with SNHL secondary to Wegener granulomatosis, otoscopy may reveal findings consistent with otitis media (caused by granulomatous inflammation within the middle ear cavity), tympanic membrane clouding or even rupture.

In Wegener granulomatosis, conductive hearing loss caused by middle ear disease is more common than SNHL, but SNHL occurs with a frequency that is prob-

ably underrecognized because of failure to obtain audiologic testing in all patients. Conductive hearing loss in Wegener results from a variety of mechanisms, including opacification of the middle ear cleft with fluid or discontinuity of the ossicular ear chain. In contrast, the ischemic sequelae of vasculitis are believed to be responsible for SNHL. Both vasculitis of the vasa nervorum and compressive granulomatous inflammation of the seventh cranial nerve (as it courses through the middle ear) may cause peripheral facial nerve paralysis.

Two simple physical examination tests are useful in distinguishing SNHL from conductive hearing loss:

- *Weber test:* A vibrating 512-Hz tuning fork is placed on an upper incisor tooth or mid-forehead. The tone will sound louder in the ipsilateral ear if conductive hearing loss is present, and in the contralateral ear if SNHL is present. The test can be repeated for higher frequencies.
- *Rinne test:* A vibrating 512-Hz tuning fork is first placed 3 cm from the opening of the ear and then

in contact with the mastoid bone. A comparison is made between the loudness of the tone generated in air and that on the bone. When bone conduction exceeds air conduction in loudness, a conductive hearing loss of over 30 dB is suggested. A normal Rinne test (air conduction is greater than bone conduction) in an ear to which the Weber has lateralized, suggests SNHL in that ear.

2. Balance—Otolaryngologists and neurologists, who should become involved in patient cases if SNHL is suspected, should be expert at evaluating patients' vestibulo-ocular reflexes (VORs). Other tests, including audiometric testing and electronystagmography, are also essential components of the work-up.

Evaluations of the VORs consist of assessments for nystagmus in response to rapid repetitive head shaking, and gaze stability during rapid lateral rotation of the head. By detecting head movement, the inner ear provides afferent input to the VOR upon which the central nervous system depends for accuracy in the compensatory saccadic movements of the eyes. Disturbance of the inner ear's role in maintaining a stable image on the retina will lead to a perception of dizziness which is worsened by head movement and relieved at rest. The rapid changes in afferent input to the central nervous system associated with IMIED lead to the decompensation of the VOR, an inability to maintain a stable retinal image, and a persistent illusion of movement known as vertigo. The acute phase of vertigo will resolve to motion-induced dizziness after central compensation has occurred in days to weeks. In the acute phase of vestibular decompensation, spontaneous nystagmus may be seen when visual fixation is suppressed (eg, in the dark or behind Frensel lenses). The VOR can be assessed for each ear separately at the bedside by asking the patient to fix her eyes on the examiner's nose while the examiner quickly turns the patient's head 30 degrees towards the ear in question. Normal VORs generate smooth, accurate compensatory ocular saccades. In contrast, an abnormal VOR will cause the eyes to under- or overshoot followed by a corrective saccade.

A feeling of perpetual motion known as oscillopsia is a disabling consequence of bilateral loss of the VOR. The presence of oscillopsia and bilateral vestibular hypofunction can be detected by comparing visual acuity with a Snellen chart while the head is at rest versus acuity during head shaking. A difference in visual acuity of three or more lines is an indication of peripheral vestibular dysfunction, with larger decrements expected in bilateral disease.

Electronystagmography provides objective measure and comparison between ears of peripheral vestibular function, more specifically the lateral semicircular canal. The vestibular electromyographic potential measured in the sternocleidomastoid muscle in response to stimulation of the saccule by low-frequency sound assesses another component of peripheral vestibular function.

3. Eyes—Cogan syndrome can be associated with virtually any form of ocular inflammation, including orbital pseudotumor, scleritis, and uveitis. The most characteristic ocular manifestation of Cogan syndrome, however, is interstitial keratitis. Wegener granulomatosis (see Chapter 33) also has a host of potential ocular complications. Diplopia, amaurosis fugax, and anterior ischemic optic neuropathy are common manifestations of giant cell (temporal) arteritis. Aside from secondary sicca symptoms, the most common eye problem in systemic lupus erythematosus (see Chapter 22) is retinopathy, which may be associated with either retinal vasculitis or a clotting diathesis, such as that associated with antiphospholipid antibody syndrome. Xerophthalmia is a hallmark of Sjögren's syndrome see (Chapter 27).

B. LABORATORY FINDINGS

The results of routine laboratory tests in IMIED are usually unremarkable. There is typically no indication, for example, of a systemic inflammatory response; acute phase reactants are usually normal. The measurement of several types of autoantibodies is highly appropriate, however, in the search for an underlying cause of SNHL that might have alternative treatment indications. As discussed below (see the section on special tests), the optimal use of testing for antibodies against HSP-70, a 68-kDa antigen, remains unclear. Autoantibody testing relevant to the assessment of a patient with SNHL are shown in Table 64–1.

Table 64–1. Autoantibodies and Other Assays Appropriate in the Evaluation of Sensorineural Hearing Loss

Test
Antinuclear antibody
Anti-Ro antibody
Anti-La antibody
dsDNA antibody
Serum C3 and C4
Antineutrophil cytoplasmic antibody (ANCA)
FTA-Abs
Lyme serology
Antibodies to HSP-70 (68-kDa antigen)
Routine blood and urine tests to exclude signs of systemic disease: Complete blood count, serum chemistries, urinalysis with microscopy

FTA-Abs, fluorescent treponemal antibody, absorption test.

C. IMAGING STUDIES

Magnetic resonance imaging studies are essential to exclude tumors of the cerebellopontine angle.

D. SPECIAL TESTS

1. Audiogram and electronystagmogram—Formal hearing tests should be performed on any patient with a complaint of hearing loss. The audiogram (Figure 64–2A) is a graphical representation of the lowest volume at which individual tones ranging from 250–8000 Hz can be distinguished. An audiogram from a patient with classic SNHL is depicted in Figure 64–2B. The *reception threshold* measures the lowest volume at which speech is heard. The *discrimination score* measures the ability to discriminate words. Electronystagmography measures ocular movement in response to various stimuli, including warm and cold caloric stimulation of the ears. This test assesses the functional strength and symmetry of the vestibulo-ocular reflexes in response to input from both ears. Audiometry and electronystagmographic testing may confirm clinical impressions of inner ear dysfunction and quantify the degree of organ involvement.

2. Serologic testing for antibodies to the 68-kDa antigen—The impact of early diagnosis and treatment on long-term hearing prognosis in patients with IMIED has prompted the search for specific markers of inner ear inflammation. The serum of patients with rapidly progressive bilateral SNHL contains antibodies that react with a variety of antigens from human and bovine inner ears. However, antibodies to cochlear-specific antigens have low specificities for rapidly progressive SNHL. In contrast, antibodies to a non–organ specific protein, a 68-kDa antigen found in the inner ear, kidney, brain, and other organs of nonhuman species (eg, cows), appear to have relatively high specificity for IMIED in humans. In a group of 72 patients with rapidly progressive bilateral SNHL, one group found that 58% possessed antibodies to the 68-kDa antigen, compared to only 2% of normal subjects and none of the subjects with otosclerosis or Cogan syndrome (p <0.01). This test may therefore be useful in making the diagnosis of IMIED, but its true-positive and negative predictive values as well as its role (if any) in following disease activity and guiding therapy remain undefined.

Differential Diagnosis

Because the treatments for various inner ear disorders vary dramatically according to cause, precise distinction between etiologies is critical. Table 64–2 depicts the major disease categories that require exclusion in the workup of patients with possible IMIED. The etiologies of inner ear dysfunction may differ in several respects: (1) their rates of progression; (2) their degrees of symmetry; and (3) their relative effects on hearing and balance. The

etiologies may be divided into six major categories: aging, trauma, tumors, infections, ototoxic drugs, and finally, cases presumed to be immunologic in nature.

Slowly progressive, symmetric loss of high-frequency hearing without vestibular symptoms distinguishes hearing loss due to aging and chronic noise exposure from IMIED. In addition, rapidly progressive hearing loss and dysequilibrium due to ototoxic drugs, sudden acoustic trauma, or barotrauma can be excluded by taking a careful history. Meniérè syndrome, a symptom complex of gradual, fluctuating hearing loss punctuated by episodes of vertigo, tinnitus, and aural fullness, is a common sequela to many causes of inner ear inflammation, including IMIED. In the absence of identifiable causes, the syndrome is termed Meniérè *disease.*

Time course is the principal criterion for distinguishing Meniérè disease from IMIED. In Meniérè disease, hearing loss occurs over a period of several years, rather than the weeks or months characteristic of IMIED. Meniérè disease is also usually limited to one ear, but delayed involvement of the contralateral ear occurs in approximately one-third of cases. Because IMIED is more likely to respond to the early institution of aggressive immunosuppression, distinguishing between these two disorders is critical.

Other causes of rapid changes in auditory and balance function are difficult to distinguish from IMIED by history alone. For example, tumors that compress the eighth cranial nerve (eg, schwannomas at the cerebellopontine angle) cause asymmetric hearing loss with variable rates of progression, ranging from days to years. Magnetic resonance imaging with gadolinium is essential to rule out such tumors. Rapid increases in intracranial or middle ear pressures (eg, as induced by trauma or a forceful Valsalva maneuver) may lead to a breach in the bony capsule of the inner ear. This condition, known as a perilymph fistula, produces rapid unilateral hearing loss accompanied by vertigo. Patients with perilymph fistulas are candidates for prompt surgical repair.

Bacterial and viral causes of inner ear dysfunction, including meningitis, may lead to swift, dramatic, irreversible hearing loss. These must be excluded quickly with appropriate cultures and serologies. Table 64–2 includes a partial list of infections associated with inner ear disease. Syphilis deserves special emphasis because of the many similarities between otosyphilis and IMIED. Syphilitic complications span the entire spectrum of inner ear disease, ranging from the sudden onset of hearing loss and vertigo associated with secondary syphilis to the gradual hearing loss associated with latent and tertiary stages of disease (sometimes accompanied by Meniérè syndrome). Specific treponemal tests (eg, the fluorescent treponemal antibody, absorbed assay) are indicated in all patients with unexplained hearing loss. Nontreponemal tests such as the rapid plasma reagin have unacceptably

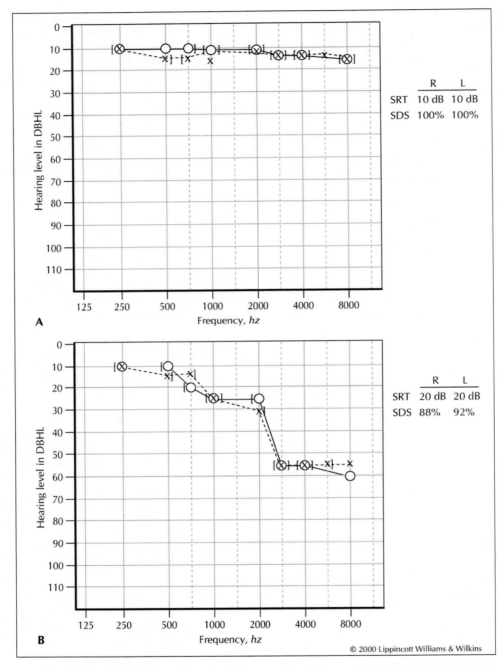

Figure 64–2. Audiogram. **A:** Normal bilateral hearing. **B:** Symmetrical high-frequency hearing loss in a patient with IMIED. Bone conduction thresholds (R = [and L =]) are measures of auditory function of the cochlea and proximal neural pathway, whereas air conduction thresholds (R = circle and L = X) measure function of the entire auditory system. SRT, speech reception threshold; SDS, speech discrimination score.

Table 64–2. Differential Diagnosis of Sensorineural Hearing Loss

Time Course	Associated Disorders	Vestibular Symptoms	Distinguishing Features
Slowly-progressive (>3 months-years)	Meniérè syndrome	+	Episodic vertigo, unilateral hearing loss, tinnitus, aural fullness
	Presbyacusis	−	Symmetric high-frequency hearing loss
	Latent or tertiary syphilis	+/−	+ FTA-Abs, +/− RPR
	Acoustic neuroma	+/−	Unilateral hearing loss, tinnitus; enhancing lesion on MRI
Intermediate (days-3 months)	IMIED	+/−	
	• Primary		See text
	• Secondary (vasculitis, connective tissue disorder)		Signs and symptoms of systemic inflammatory disorders
	Drugs		
	• Aminoglycosides	+	Chronic dysequilibrium; signs of bilateral vestibular hypofunction (eg, oscillopsia)
	• Antimalarials		
	• Loop diuretics		
	• NSAIDs		
	Lyme disease	+/−	Exposure risk; + *Borrelia burgdorferi* serology
	Latent or tertiary syphilis	+/−	+ FTA-Abs, +/− RPR
	Acoustic neuroma	+/−	Unilateral hearing loss, tinnitus; enhancing lesion on MRI
Sudden (hours to days)	Acoustic trauma	−	Recent intense noise exposure
	Barotrauma	+/−	Recent deep sea diving, barotrauma
	Perilymph fistula	+	Otolaryngology evaluation
	Viral/bacterial labyrinthitis	+	Acute vertigo and/or hearing loss
	Early or secondary syphilis	+	+ FTA-Abs, + RPR
	Acoustic neuroma	+/−	Unilateral hearing loss, tinnitus; enhancing lesion on MRI

FTA-Abs, fluorescent treponemal antibody, absorption test; IMIED, immune-mediated inner ear disease; MRI, magnetic resonance imaging; NSAID, nonsteroidal anti-inflammatory drug; RPR, rapid plasma reagin.

high false-negative rates in latent and tertiary infection. Susac syndrome is a poorly-understood disease entity, marked by encephalopathy, branch retinal artery occlusion, and sensorineural hearing loss.

Treatment

In the absence of significant numbers of rigorous, controlled studies, the treatment approach for IMIED is based largely upon anecdotal experience, case series, and inference from the treatment of related conditions. Because of the devastating nature of severely impaired hearing and vestibular function, IMIED should be regarded in the same fashion as any other threat to vital organs mediated by an immunologic injury. In such conditions, aggressive immunosuppression—glucocorticoids, and in most cases a cytotoxic agent—may halt the inflammatory response and prevent permanent organ damage. In contrast, failure to treat these disorders promptly leads to substantial, irreversible organ dysfunction within a brief time.

Numerous case reports and small case series demonstrate the responsiveness of IMIED to immunosuppression in its early stages, including recovery of vestibular function. The authors' approach to the treatment of IMIED is guided by the concept that if IMIED is worth treating (ie, if significant inner ear function appears recoverable), it is worth treating aggressively. Thus in the setting of rapidly progressive SNHL, we institute treatment with at least 1 mg/kg/d of prednisone. If there is significant improvement in auditory and vestibular function within 2 weeks, prednisone is continued at this dosage for a total of 1 month, and then slowly tapered over 2 additional months. In patients with recurrent disease, some maintenance prednisone (eg, 5–10 mg/d) may be prudent.

If hearing and balance deteriorate despite prednisone or do not improve significantly within the 2 weeks of treatment, we add cyclophosphamide (2 mg/kg/d) to the regimen. We also consider cyclophosphamide if patients do not maintain audiovestibular gains during their prednisone tapers. For patients with other types of organ-threatening disease (eg, pulmonary or renal involvement), we sometimes employ intravenous pulses of glucocorticoids at the start of treatment (1 g of methylprednisolone per day for 3 days), but we do not routinely use pulse glucocorticoids in IMIED.

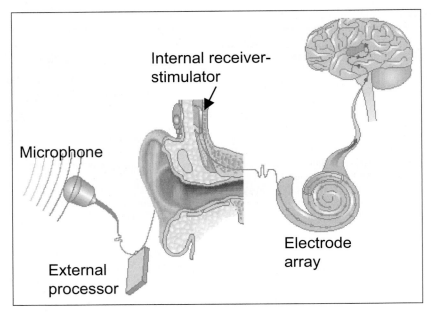

Figure 64–3. Cochlear implant. (From Niparko JK, Kirk KI, Mellon NK, et al. *Cochlear Implants: Principles and Practices.* Lippincott Williams & Wilkins, 2000. With permission.)

Unless active disease in other organ systems justifies continuation of significant immunosuppression, the maintenance of such therapy after irreversible organ damage (ie, profound hearing loss) has occurred places patients at risk for treatment complications with little potential benefit. In the setting of profound hearing disturbances despite aggressive immunosuppression, the hearing that a patient may derive from a cochlear implant (Figure 64–3) may render this the most appropriate course of action. Consequently, if patients have not demonstrated a response by the end of 3 months of therapy, the medications should be discontinued.

The treatment of SNHL associated with Wegener granulomatosis, Cogan syndrome, and other primary disorders are discussed in their appropriate chapters.

Prognosis

Seropositivity for antibodies to the 68-kDa antigen may correlate with both active disease and the likelihood of a treatment response. One group of researchers found that antibodies against the 68-kDa antigen were significantly more prevalent in patients with rapidly progressive SNHL of less than 3 months' duration (89%) compared with patients whose hearing loss had been present for more than 3 months (0%; p <0.001). Compared to seronegative patients, seropositive patients were also more likely to respond to glucocorticoid therapy (75% versus 18%; p <0.001). These observations support an association between antibodies to the 68-kDa antigen and the early stages of IMIED. Other studies of antibodies directed against this antigen, however, have been significantly less conclusive about its relevance to IMIED.

Hearing & Vestibular Rehabilitation

All patients with functionally significant bilateral hearing loss should be supplied with appropriate hearing aids. When speech discrimination remains poor in both ears despite maximal medical therapy and the use of powerful hearing aids, the patient may be a candidate for cochlear implantation. Cochlear implants process and deliver sound to the auditory nerve in the form of encoded electrical signals, increasing both hearing acuity and speech understanding. For patients with dizziness due to a significant loss of peripheral vestibular function, compensation by the central nervous system is effectively enhanced through a program of vestibular rehabilitation. Such programs, administered by appropriately trained physical therapists, promote a variety of strategies to maintain balance and minimize fall risk. In the treatment of dizziness, chronic use of vestibular suppressant drugs (eg, meclizine) should be avoided, because they impede the development of central compensation mechanisms.

REFERENCES

Bhat V, Naseeruddin K. Combined tuning fork tests in hearing loss: explorative clinical study of the patterns. *J Otolaryngol.* 2004;33:227.

Broughton SS, Meyerhoft WE, Cohen SB. Immune-mediated inner ear disease: Ten-year experience. *Semin Arthritis Rheum.* 2004;34:544.

Brown KE, Whitney SL, Wrisley DM, Furman JM. Physical therapy outcomes for persons with bilateral vestibular loss. *Laryngoscope.* 2001;111:1812.

Deutschlander A, Glaser M, Strupp M, et al. Immunosuppressive treatment in bilateral vestibulopathy with inner ear antibodies. *Acta Otolaryngol.* 2005;125:848.

Harris JP, Weisman MH, Derebery JM, et al. Treatment of corticosteroid-responsive autoimmune inner ear disease with methotrexate: a randomized, controlled trial. *JAMA.* 2003;290:1875.

Koch DB, Staller S, Jaax K, et al. Bioengineering solutions for hearing loss and related disorders. *Otolaryngol Clin North Am.* 2005;38:255.

Loveman DM, de Comarand C, Cepero R, Baldwin DM. Autoimmune sensorineural hearing loss: Clinical course and treatment outcome. *Semin Arthritis Rheum.* 2004;34:538.

Moscicki RA, San Martin JE, Quintero CH, et al. Serum antibody to inner ear proteins in patients with progressive hearing loss. Correlation with disease activity and response to corticosteroid treatment. *JAMA.* 1994;272:611.

Relevant World Wide Web Site

[The Johns Hopkins Vasculitis Center]
http://vasculitis.med.jhu.edu

SECTION X

Special Topics

Legal Issues

65

Victor R. Cotton, MD, JD, & Joanne E. Pollak

The practice of medicine is an increasingly complex endeavor in which errors, omissions, and miscommunications are not entirely preventable. In addition, a variety of societal changes have combined to make it easier to sue a physician for malpractice. Practicing "good medicine" is no longer a guarantee that one will not be sued, and an understanding of the origins of lawsuits, along with how to manage them once they occur, is essential.

Although the field of rheumatology is not particularly laden with malpractice concerns, the potential for difficulty in diagnosis and the complex and potentially debilitating nature of the disease processes combine to create a legitimate level of risk.

FACTORS IN MALPRACTICE LAWSUITS

The medical malpractice problem is multifactorial in nature. The increasing incidence and financial impact of this problem can be linked to a variety of medical, societal, and legal phenomena. The exact contribution of each factor is the subject of some debate and probably varies by location and situation.

Medical

Although scientific advancement has greatly enhanced the ability to care for patients, the practice of medicine is more difficult than it has ever been. The number of diseases, tests, and treatments that must be managed can be overwhelming. The challenge is made greater by the financial pressure to see more patients in less time, and the

barriers that are often created by formulary and managed care requirements.

The increased mobility of physicians and greater role that large corporations have taken in the practice of medicine have attenuated the interpersonal aspects of medicine. Unfortunately, the impact on the doctor-patient dynamic hurts not only the diagnostic and treatment capabilities but also the patient's tolerance of mistakes.

Finally, medical training has traditionally provided little instruction on the legal process and how risk can be reduced. Although physicians are well trained in science, they receive little guidance when it comes to cultivating the doctor-patient relationship and avoiding situations that increase the risk of malpractice litigation.

Societal

A generation ago, the advice that physicians gave was referred to as "doctor's orders," and given a degree of respect that was almost never questioned. Today, patients are more willing to question the accuracy of their physician's decisions and often second-guess what has been done. In addition, most of the stigma associated with bringing a lawsuit has disappeared, eliminating a barrier that previously provided a reasonable amount of physician protection.

Relying on what they have heard in the lay press or read on the Internet, many patients enter the medical system with enormous, unrealistic expectations. When these expectations are not met, disappointment occurs, and blame sometimes follows. There is often little tolerance for what are unpreventable side effects and unavoidable consequences.

Finally, there is no question that the possibility of financial enrichment leads many patients to bring a medical malpractice lawsuit. The regularity with which enormous sums of money are awarded for intangible damages like pain and suffering leads many patients to seek compensation through litigation.

Legal

The increased number of attorneys drawn to the field by the potential for lucrative reward has certainly contributed to the medical malpractice risk. In conjunction with this, advertising by attorneys, a phenomenon that was prohibited until the late 1980s, has made some plaintiff attorneys into household names and undoubtedly has led more patients to seek their services.

The widespread availability of physicians who are willing to serve as expert witnesses against other physicians has increased the legal risk for all physicians. The law contains few penalties for physicians who testify in a manner that may skew the facts, and the financial reward for doing so often makes this an irresistible temptation.

Geography

Physicians who practice in large metropolitan areas are much more likely to be sued than physicians who practice in smaller towns. There are more law firms in larger towns, patient expectations are often higher, and the anonymity of living in a city helps the plaintiff avoid any stigma that might otherwise be associated with bringing a lawsuit. In addition, juries in metropolitan areas are more willing to find physicians liable for malpractice and generally award larger amounts of money when they do so.

Patient Age

Younger patients are associated with a greater medicolegal risk. Although most debilitating and fatal illnesses generally spare young people, rheumatologic disease does not, and it can have devastating consequences. When this occurs, patients and their families can suffer enormous physical, emotional, and financial burdens. These burdens are often accompanied by a strong urge to look for answers and an explanation. In the end, what started as a search for answers often becomes a means of blaming someone, and this occasionally is the physician.

Type of Illness

Every lawsuit begins with an accident or illness that results in injury to a patient. The injury is usually physical in nature but can be psychological or financial. Although any patient who suffers an injury may choose to sue for medical malpractice, injuries that are severe, occur with suddenness, or are unexpected are more likely to result in a lawsuit.

Nearly 40% of all medical malpractice lawsuits arise because of errors or perceived errors that occur in the course of a procedure. Many rheumatologic patients undergo procedures to alleviate the functional and cosmetic impact of their disease. Because it is not possible to guarantee a perfect result, time should be taken to ensure that patient expectations are not unrealistically high.

Approximately one-third of medical malpractice lawsuits arise as a result of a "failure to make a timely diagnosis." Although cancer and heart disease are the usual culprits, any disease state that presents a challenging diagnosis contributes to this phenomenon. Because rheumatologic disease can present with vague, seemingly unrelated complaints accompanied by nonspecific laboratory abnormalities, any patient situation that eludes diagnosis should be considered for referral. This is especially true for patients who repeatedly seek medical attention for the same complaint or who become progressively ill despite treatment.

A large number of lawsuits are directly or indirectly related to the treating physician's level of recent experience with the disease process and its treatment. The threshold for referral should be lower when the patient has an uncommon disease or requires an unusual treatment. Although many rheumatologic diseases can be managed by nonrheumatologists, the medicolegal risks associated with the potential for the sudden onset of blindness from giant cell arteritis or severe joint deformity caused by progressive rheumatoid arthritis should not be underestimated. It is worth noting that no physician has ever been sued for making a referral to a specialist, while many have been sued for not doing so. The medical and medicolegal value of a properly timed second opinion should not be underestimated.

Patient Motive

Some patients see medical malpractice lawsuits as a way to obtain a monetary windfall. Driven primarily by a desire to "get rich," these persons can be best viewed as plaintiffs looking for defendants. In the worst cases, no amount of due care, communication, and documentation will be sufficient to insulate the physician from an allegation of medical malpractice. The only lawsuit avoidance strategy that works in such a case is termination of the doctor-patient relationship prior to occurrence of an adverse outcome.

On occasion, physicians encounter patients with whom it is not possible to develop the proper relationship of trust and open communication. These patients may be confrontational, manipulative, dishonest, accusatory, or argumentative. To some degree, this type of behavior can be accepted, but it occasionally reaches the point of undermining the ability to properly care for the patient.

Physicians should be attentive to patients who are not approaching the doctor-patient relationship in an appropriate manner. If these relationships cannot be re-habilitated, they should be terminated. As a general rule, physicians have the right to unilaterally terminate vir-tually any doctor-patient relationship at any time. The only requirements are that the patient must be given no-tice of the physician's choice to end the relationship, and afforded sufficient time to establish a relationship with a new physician. The exact amount of time is not written in any law or regulation but is generally regarded to be 30 days.

Degree of Empathy

A perception that the physician did not "care" is the most common reason cited by patients who sue for medical malpractice. Despite all of the changes that have occurred in the medical field, the majority of patients are still look-ing for a physician who "cares." As has been taught for many years, a strong doctor-patient relationship remains the most valuable lawsuit prevention technique.

Patients are generally more willing to forgive mistakes when they perceive that their physician put his heart into the case and tried his best. On the other hand, patients are often led to suspicion and open dissatisfaction when they believe that their physician approached the situation with anything less than a caring, fully committed attitude. Answering questions, explaining the disease process, and clarifying the goals of treatment are all valuable in this regard. In a sense, being sued has more to do with what the physician says than what the physician actually does.

Family Discord

Serious illness can bring out both the best and the worst in the patient's family. Although a patient may be fully satisfied with the care that he or she is receiving, a member of the family will occasionally express dissatisfaction. The family member is generally not directly involved in the patient's care and is often driven by factors that are totally unrelated to the care at hand. Nonetheless, physicians can be caught in the middle of what is primarily family discord and are occasionally blamed as a result.

In dealing with family discord, it is important to make clear that the physician's obligation is to the wishes of the patient, and that disagreement with these wishes is between the patient and his or her family. In addition, the family should be asked to designate one person as the point of contact with the physician, so as to improve efficiency and decrease confusion. In those unfortunate cases in which the family is unmanageable, consideration

to termination of the doctor-patient relationship should be given. Although the circumstances may not be the patient's "fault," the consequences of an unmanageable clinical and medicolegal situation are the same.

Miscommunication

Errors in communication are at the root of many, if not the majority, of medical malpractice cases. Effec-tive patient care requires the coordination of respon-sibilities among treating physicians, other health care providers, and the patient. Although physicians regu-larly co-manage patients, it is generally undesirable to co-manage a given aspect of a patient's disease process. Because the risk of miscommunication and error is greatly multiplied when two or more persons are responsible for the same issue, clear delineation of roles should exist.

Anytime that a new physician becomes involved in a patient's care, everyone who is also involved, includ-ing the patient, should have a working understanding of their respective roles. This is especially important in the outpatient setting, where there are less opportunities to review one another's progress notes and treatment plans.

Proper communication with the patient is also es-sential. Many patients suffer adverse consequences as a result of not understanding or remembering their physi-cian's instructions. What may seem routine and simple to a physician is often new and complex to the patient, and patients regularly make mistakes with medications and other treatments. Although this is often the patient's own "fault," some patients use the legal system to try to hold their physician responsible.

In order to provide the best possible patient care and also prevent the possibility of legal entanglement, it is im-perative that every reasonable effort be made to ensure that the patient knows what he or she is to do. When feasible, verbal instructions should be accompanied by a written summary. Although written instructions are not legally required, they make sense when the patient is be-ing asked to undertake a new or complex endeavor. If the patient receives both verbal and written instructions, the chance of error is reduced and the likelihood of a fa-vorable outcome is increased. In addition, the probability that the treating physician can be held responsible should the patient choose to do otherwise is virtually eliminated.

PRIVACY ISSUES

Although historically patients seldom bring a malpractice claim based on privacy issues, privacy issues can become part of the claim if physicians do not approach patients' requests and rights with sensitivity.

Privacy regulations adopted under the Health Insur-ance Portability and Accountability Act (HIPAA) apply in all states. Under these regulations, a patient has the right to see the medical record, to have a copy of the record, to request an amendment to the record, and except for certain exceptions, to request a limit on who may see the record. In addition, many states have privacy protections which are stronger than those under the HIPAA privacy regulations. And even though a plaintiff has no direct claim against a provider under the HIPAA privacy regulations, if the plaintiff is able to assert state law privacy rights, a judge may use HIPAA as the standard of care for the provider under the state law claim.

One common claim is that a plaintiff's health information has been provided to someone without the patient's authorization. This may be part of a claim for emotional distress. Again, the claim may arise under state law, but the federal HIPAA regulations will be used as the standard of care under the state law claim.

In connection with a privacy claim, physicians should promptly produce the plaintiff's medical record and be sure they have handled any requests for amendments to the record. The manner in which requests are handled is very important. Timeliness and completeness avoid motions to the judge or mediator that the defense is obstructing the proceeding, or worse, hiding evidence.

PREVENTION

Like most problems in medicine, the best approach to a medicolegal problem is prevention. Recognizing cases in which the patient's condition is worsening, eludes diagnosis, or is not responding to treatment and making a timely referral are paramount. Drawing limits in terms of the type of patient and family conduct that will be permitted, and rehabilitating or ending those relationships that fall outside these boundaries are things that most physicians are not accustomed to doing but are necessary nonetheless. When co-managing a patient with another physician, time should be dedicated to the communication of the scope of one another's responsibilities.

Most importantly, it is not possible to spend too much time answering patients' questions, addressing their concerns, and ensuring that they understand what their role will be in the diagnostic or treatment plan. In the event that the patient is unwilling to go along with the physician's recommendation, the risks of making this choice should be discussed in terms that the patient can understand. Although physicians are not required to persuade the patient to submit to the recommended treatment, clinicians should be sure that patients understand the potential consequences of any decision.

In cases in which the patient chooses an option other than the physician's suggestion, an entry noting the physician's recommendation, the resulting discussion, and the patient's choice should be made in the medical record. In making this entry, it is not necessary or desirable to note every word that was said. However, some notation should be made. It is also helpful to have the patient sign the medical record entry. Although it is not legally required, the patient's act of signing reinforces the seriousness of the decision and also decreases the viability of a later claim of misunderstanding or miscommunication.

MANAGEMENT OF ADVERSE OUTCOMES

The majority of adverse outcomes are not caused by medical malpractice. They arise because medical science is not perfect and the human body is mortal. Physicians cannot control these variables and are not legally expected to do so. Other adverse outcomes are the result of medical malpractice, medical care that falls below recognized standards. These events are within the control of physicians.

Regardless of their cause, adverse outcomes are the reason that patients sue doctors. Put another way, all lawsuits begin with a "bad" outcome. Sometimes the adverse event is caused by a physician's mistake. In others, physicians are sued despite the fact that the adverse event was not their fault. Although many of these latter cases will be dismissed or otherwise successfully defended, the experience is unpleasant and something that most physicians want to avoid. Moreover, after viewing a person's devastating injuries, juries sometimes award damages to help the injured party—regardless of fault. Because adverse outcomes of any cause are inherently linked to the risk of litigation, they must be effectively managed.

Patient Care

The most important aspect of managing an adverse outcome is taking care of the patient's medical needs. This alleviates the patient's suffering, demonstrates attentiveness, and reduces any ongoing medicolegal injury that the patient has suffered. The sooner that a patient can regain function and return to normal activities, the less likely it is that he or she will have a viable lawsuit. Plaintiff attorneys work on a contingency basis, receiving a percentage of any verdict or settlement. Adverse events that have minimal injury and quick recovery are unappealing to a plaintiff attorney, and most will never result in a lawsuit.

Communication

Communication with the patient is the next most important function. When an unexpected outcome, adverse event, or treatment error occurs, malpractice literature suggests that aggrieved patients want three things: to learn what happened, to receive acknowledgement of their suffering, and to know that lessons have been learned and corrective steps taken. These discussions are an important part of the practice of medicine and a valuable medicolegal strategy. They require a measured, well-timed, and empathic approach that avoids both self-criticism and blame of others.

Documentation

Documentation is the final consideration in the management of an adverse outcome. The medical record is a powerful legal document. It is entirely admissible as evidence and almost uniformly believed by judges and juries. Most physicians understand the need for documentation, but many are unfamiliar with the manner in which adverse outcomes should be handled in the medical record.

No amount of documentation can change a bad outcome, undo a mistake, or alter a test result. Whatever happened is over and done. It is a mistake to attempt to use documentation to recharacterize or change events that have already occurred. Efforts to do so invariably create inconsistency and might even be interpreted as attempting to hide the truth. At best, the additional documentation draws attention to the matter. This, too, is undesirable.

Physicians must also resist the urge to make "heat of the moment" entries in the medical record. Efforts to document the physician's thought process and explain why a certain choice was made are among the most harmful entries that are ever made. Once these items are recorded in the patient's chart, the physician is legally bound to them. The problem is that the pressure of the situation may result in a poorly worded explanation that omits critical facts. This creates a compromised medicolegal situation that is best avoided. Explanations and thought processes should be saved for a time when they can be carefully measured.

Self-criticism should never be present in a medical record. Physicians, as a group, are very self-critical. To an extent, this criticism is a necessary part of molding one's skills to the highest possible level. However, when self-criticism becomes a part of the medical record, it becomes an unmanageable liability. The appearance in a medical record of self-criticism of any type or degree is inappropriate. It does not advance the care of the patient in any way, and renders the physician indefensible in any subsequent legal action. When a physician openly blames himself for the plaintiff's condition, there is little likelihood of convincing a judge and jury otherwise.

The legal tragedy of self-criticism is deepened by the fact that much of it results from physicians holding themselves to an inappropriately high and unachievable standard.

Physicians can raise their awareness of self-criticism by exercising care when using the pronoun "I" in the medical record. As a general rule, the word "I" should appear very infrequently in the medical record. Because self-criticism can be subtle with statements like "I did not have a chance to look at the lab report," one must always be careful when using the word "I."

The only thing worse in a medical record than self-criticism is criticism of other health care providers. Unfortunately, there exists a potentially devastating misperception that it is possible to cover oneself by documenting the shortcomings of others. The extent to which this occurs between physicians, nurses, pharmacists, and other hospital staff is sometimes alarming.

There is no question that pointing the finger at another health care provider is likely to bring his or her conduct under scrutiny. However, if a lawsuit arises, the plaintiff usually looks for as many potential defendants as he can find. The conduct of everyone who was involved with the case will eventually be brought under scrutiny. This will usually include the person who did the original finger-pointing along with the person against whom the criticism was levied. Regardless of the facts, this type of case is inherently compromised from a defense perspective and most can never be won.

Unless there is a desire to express appreciation or agreement, references to the conduct of another provider should not be made in the medical record. Any concern for the care that has been delivered by someone else should be expressed directly and in person. Once the matter is resolved, the medical record can reflect that an agreement has been reached.

Exclamation points or big, block letters should generally not be used in the medical record. The presence of these notations in a patient's chart suggests frustration or dissatisfaction. This draws attention to the events and can serve as a nidus for additional scrutiny. Although these feelings can be normal, it is better if they are left out of the medical record.

When an adverse outcome occurs, the patient should be treated and apprised of the situation. An entry should be made in the medical record that objectively describes the patient's condition and the treatment plan. Explanations, second-guessing, and any type of criticism should be avoided. From both a patient care and a liability perspective, it is better to spend any extra time with the patient rather than with the chart.

It is worth noting that physicians are not sued over documentation. Patients do not care about documentation. Patients want proper care, communication, and empathy.

MANAGEMENT OF LITIGATION

Litigation is a difficult and unrewarding experience for most physicians. There is limited satisfaction even when the case has been successfully defended. There are virtually no means by which physicians can obtain compensation for the loss of their practice time and financial expenditures. The litigation process should be viewed as something that must be avoided if possible and endured when necessary. There is simply no way for a physician defendant to truly "win" a medical malpractice case.

Lawsuits begin with service of the court-related documents. This is done in person at the physician's office or residence by a sheriff, deputy, or officer of the court. A physician who is served with a lawsuit should immediately contact his malpractice insurance carrier. Most carriers require immediate notification as a condition of coverage. Any instructions that the carrier gives should be followed.

The relevant medical records should be located and secured. From a litigation perspective, the only way to deal with a lost record is to find it. Lost records create the appearance of sloppiness or concealment, neither of which is desirable. Cases that involve lost records are generally considered to be severely compromised from a defensive perspective.

Nothing should be added to or subtracted from the record. This includes modifications, addendums, and clarifications. The patient and his attorney probably obtained a copy of the record months earlier, and any type of modification creates suspicion. At the least, modifications draw attention to an area of concern of which the plaintiff may not have been aware. Nothing should be written in any other log, diary, or journal about the case. The discovery process that accompanies litigation generally gives the parties access to any documents or records relating to the case. The fact that notes are not in the patient's "official" medical record will not protect them from discovery, nor will it prevent the plaintiff from using those notes against the physician.

The only writings and communications that are protected from the plaintiff's discovery are those that occur between the physician and his attorney and those made as part of a peer review proceeding or process protected under many state laws.

With rare exception, communication between attorney and client is protected from discovery. Physicians can record their thoughts, recollections, or strategy insights on paper, but the writing must be part of a confidential communication between attorney and client. Any such document should be addressed to one's attorney, and as an added measure, be prefaced with the words "Confidential, Attorney-Client Privilege."

The protection from discovery of writings and communications made as part of a hospital's or other health care facility's peer review process varies based on each state's laws and regulations governing these proceedings. The physician's attorney should advise regarding these protections, if any, and the legend that should be noted on any documents submitted to or produced in the process.

Nothing should be said about the case to anyone other than the physician's attorney or the physician's spouse, or if applicable, those involved in the peer review process. Although spouses are not part of the attorney-client privilege, spousal immunity generally limits the ability of spouses to testify against one another. Physicians who are facing litigation have an understandable desire to seek reassurance from colleagues, but this must be avoided. Other physicians may also be involved as defendants or be serving as witnesses for the plaintiff. Even when they are not involved, any conversation that takes place is not protected from discovery, unless the conversation is part of the peer review process.

The patient should not be contacted. Once litigation has been initiated, there is no longer an opportunity to clarify a misunderstanding or miscommunication. Apologies should be strictly avoided, and hostility must be contained. Sometimes the patient will want to continue to see a physician whom he has sued for malpractice. Physicians should not see such an individual. The purpose is not to punish the person, but simply to avoid the possibility of further conflict. The patient should be asked to find another physician and should be assisted in doing so if the need is acute or emergent.

Most lawsuits involve depositions as part of the discovery process. These generally occur even in cases that are eventually dropped or settled before trial. A deposition is a question and answer session that is conducted under oath. For the defendant physician, most of the questions will come from the plaintiff's attorney. Depositions are not conducted in front of a judge or jury. There are no scorekeepers at a deposition, and it is impossible to win a deposition. For a physician defendant, the only goal is to keep from losing. Depositions are lost when major discrepancies about the patient's care are uncovered, when the physician repeatedly contradicts himself or herself, and when the physician loses his or her composure.

Demeanor and candor are everything. It is imperative that the physician be himself or herself. Jurors are ordinary people who function at the level of most patients. They are asked to solve a complex problem and are generally not permitted to take notes. They are much better at assessing credibility and candor than they are at engaging in a complex analysis of the therapeutic options. If the defendant physician's testimony is logical and the delivery is respectful, then the story is credible. Malpractice cases are not about technical minutia. They are about whether a witness is believable. Personable, patient, and respectful witnesses are the most believable. The ability to demonstrate these characteristics at a deposition and at trial are as important as the facts of the case.

Tennenhouse DJ, Kasher MP. *Risk Prevention Skills.* PMSLIC Press, 1996.

Complementary & Alternative Therapies

66

Sharon L. Kolasinski, MD

The majority of patients with chronic rheumatic diseases seek adjunctive care outside the medical mainstream. Although patients usually maintain relationships with medical physicians and take prescription medications, most will add some form of complementary and alternative therapy at some point during the course of their illness. Patient choices reflect their cultural and ethnic background, financial resources, and the availability of alternative providers. Not all interventions have yet been studied in a scientifically rigorous manner, but well-designed clinical trials continue to be published in a wide range of areas relevant to patients with rheumatic diseases.

GENERAL CONSIDERATIONS

Definition

Complementary and alternative medicine (CAM) has been defined as that which is not traditionally taught in U.S. medical schools and not traditionally available in U.S. hospitals. With the recognition of its widespread use and the provision of services like acupuncture within academic medical centers, however, defining the limits of alternative medicine has become more difficult. The National Center for Complementary and Alternative Medicine, established by Congress in 1998 as one of the centers within the National Institutes of Health, has divided CAM therapies into (1) alternative medical systems (eg, traditional Chinese medicine, Ayurvedic medicine, naturopathy, and homeopathy); (2) mind-body interventions (eg, meditation and spiritual healing); (3) biologic-based therapies (eg, herbal medicines, dietary supplements, and special diets); (4) manipulative and body-based therapies (eg, chiropractic, massage and osteopathy); and (5) energy therapies (eg, reiki, therapeutic touch, and magnets). Furthermore, with the increasing number of randomized controlled trials examining these therapies, practitioners have a growing body of resources with which to evaluate the usefulness of CAM therapies, provide advice to patients, and consider incorporating CAM into standard treatment plans.

Epidemiology

Initial epidemiologic work suggested that overall about 35% of the general public seeks alternative care in a given year. Demographic data showed that these patients were more likely to be between the ages of 25 and 49, have some college education, be in higher income brackets, and live in the western United States, and were less likely to be African American. More recent epidemiologic data show that almost half of Americans surveyed use alternative therapies for medical conditions. Patients with rheumatic disease who seek alternative care, however, use CAM more frequently and are demographically diverse. Use correlates with pain and over 90% of patients with diagnoses such as fibromyalgia may seek alternative care. Similarly, a variety of ethnic and racial groups and the elderly with musculoskeletal complaints have higher rates of CAM use than average American populations. However, patients with rheumatic diseases are unlikely to discuss their CAM use with their physician, similarly to patients in general, unless the physician specifically asks.

Quality & Safety Issues

Practitioners have a responsibility to help inform patients regarding their choices of alternative therapies, particularly where medical data exist. However, in this developing field, data may be lacking and patients often hold strong beliefs that alternative products are effective and safe. Despite this, only about 10% believe that CAM therapies will cure arthritis.

Efforts to study aspects of traditional Chinese and Ayurvedic medicine and many herbal therapies have been hampered by the passage of the Dietary Supplement and Health Education Act (DSHEA) by the U.S. Congress in 1994. This legislation permitted the classification of numerous over-the-counter products with pharmacologic activity as dietary supplements. Dietary supplements are regulated like food. As such, they are exempted from the safety and efficacy requirements that must be met by prescription drugs. In fact, this legislation mandated that the U.S. Food and Drug Administration (USFDA)

Table 66–1. Potential Adverse Effects of Herbal Remedies and Their Major Constituents

Cardiotoxicity	*Alocasia macrorrhiza* root tuber
Aconite root tuber	*Artemisia* spp. rich in santonin
Herbs rich in cardioactive glycosides	Essential oils rich in ascaridole
Herbs rich in colchicine	Essential oils rich in thujone
Leigongteng	Gingko seed or leaf
Licorice root	Herbs rich in colchicine
Ma huang	Herbs rich in podophyllotoxin
Pokeweed leaf or root	Indian tobacco herb
Scotch broom	Kava rhizome
Squirting cucumber	Ma huang
Hepatotoxicity	Nux vomica
Certain herbs rich in anthranoids	Pennyroyal oil
Certain herbs rich in protoberberine alkaloids	Star fruit
Chaparral leaf or stem	Yellow jessamine rhizome
Germander spp.	**Renal toxicity**
Green tea leaf	β-Aescin (saponin mixture from horse chestnut leaf)
Herbs rich in coumarin	Cape aloes
Herbs rich in podophyllotoxin	Cat's claw
Herbs rich in toxic pyrrolizidine alkaloids	Certain essential oils
Impila root	Chaparral leaf or stem
Kava rhizome	Chinese yew
Kombucha	Herbs rich in aristolochic acid
Ma huang	Impila root
Pennyroyal oil	Jering fruit
Skullcap	Squirting cucumber
Soy phytoestrogens	Star fruit
Neurotoxicity, convulsions	
Aconite root tuber	

(From De Smet PA. Herbal remedies. *N Engl J Med.* 2003;347:2046. With permission.)

assume the burden of proof when a product is considered for removal from the market as unsafe. Furthermore, consumers may make certain assumptions about testing, quality, and efficacy since the DSHEA permits labeling claims regarding "structure and function" that may suggest to the consumer that the products being sold have been proved to have health benefits.

Recently, a number of safety considerations concerning herbal remedies were reviewed. A variety of herbs may themselves have toxic side effects (Table 66–1). They may also have important interactions with prescription medications. Garlic and gingko may increase bleeding risk in patients on warfarin, whereas ginseng may reduce the ability of warfarin to lead to appropriate anticoagulation. St. John's wort may reduce the plasma levels of numerous medications, including antidepressants, antiretroviral agents, and immunosuppressive drugs. Thus, even if a patient is not taking an herbal product to address arthritis symptoms, he or she should be questioned about all over-the-counter product use since medication interactions may be significant.

Adulterants and contaminants in herbal preparations have been reported, including heavy metals, microor-ganisms and their toxins, and pesticides. Unsuspected botanicals other than those identified on the label may be present. One such case involved contamination of a weight loss preparation with the root of *Aristolochia fangchi,* resulting in interstitial renal fibrosis, renal failure and in some, urothelial carcinoma. Pharmaceuticals may be present as well. A number of reports have detailed the presence of glucocorticoids and nonsteroidal anti-inflammatory drugs (NSAIDs) in herbal arthritis preparations, with resultant side effects including gastrointestinal bleeding and hepatotoxicity. Contamination of other herbal products with warfarin, estrogen, fenfluramine and glyburide has been reported.

To date, the USFDA has issued specific warnings about a number of alternative products (Table 66–2) but has only banned those containing ephedrine alkaloids (21 CFR Part 119), effective April 2004. Ephedrine alkaloids were found to present an unreasonable risk under ordinary conditions of use, including myocardial infarction, cerebrovascular accident, seizure and death, after numerous reports of toxicity and an extensive review of the literature, as well as congressional hearings on these agents. In November 2004, the USFDA announced three

Table 66–2. U.S. FDA Warnings and Safety Information on Dietary Supplements

Year	Dietary Supplement	Action	Area of Concern
1999	Triax Metabolic Accelerator	Consumer warning	Thyroid hormone leading to myocardial infarction and cerebrovascular accidents
2000	St John's wort	Public health advisory	Interaction with indinavir, others
2001	Weight loss preparation contaminated by *Aristolochia fangchi*	Statement issued	Interstitial renal fibrosis, renal failure, urothelial carcinoma
2001	Comfrey	Advisory to industry to remove from market	Hepatotoxicity
2001	LipoKinetix	Consumer advisory, letter to health care professionals, letter to distributors	Hepatotoxicity
2002	Chaso (Jianfei) diet capsules, Chaso Genpi	Consumer warning	Contamination with fenfluramine
2002	Kava	Consumer advisory, letter to health care professionals	Hepatotoxicity
2002	PC SPES	Consumer warning	Contamination with warfarin, estrogen
2004	Androstenedione	Industry warning	Altered secondary sexual characteristics, carcinogenesis
2004	Ephedrine alkaloids	Declared by federal rule to be adulterated under the Federal Food, Drug and Cosmetic Act	Myocardial infarction, cerebrovascular accidents, seizure, psychosis, death

initiatives to further implement DSHEA: formulating a regulatory strategy that will improve the evidenciary basis for USFDA actions with regard to dietary supplements by working collaboratively with the National Institutes of Health and federal regulatory bodies; holding a public meeting for discussion of issues arising from the regulation of dietary supplements; and formulating a draft document detailing the amount and type of evidence that should be used to substantiate "structure function claims." The USFDA encourages the reporting of adverse events by consumers, physicians, and manufacturers via their web site (www.fda.gov/medwatch) or telephone (consumers: 1-800-MEDWATCH; physicians: 1-800-FDA-1088).

There has been a long-standing interest in systematic investigation and regulation of herbal medications in Germany. The Federal Health Agency Commission E was formed in 1978 and has amassed over 400 monographs on herbal medicines that provide a resource for practitioners attempting to inform themselves and advise patients. An additional up-to-date guide with references regarding herbal and other alternative therapies has recently been published.

The American College of Rheumatology has issued a position paper on the use of CAM therapies. The College acknowledges that CAM use is widespread among patients with rheumatic diseases. It notes that all therapies must meet the same rigorous standards of scientific scrutiny using scientific methods and that those proven safe and effective can be integrated into the therapeutic armamentarium. It further suggests that rheumatologists should be informed about CAM therapies and be able to knowledgeably discuss them with their patients. Many studies show that little discussion about CAM occurs in the office visit setting, however. Several authors have offered advice to physicians on what information should be discussed in order to facilitate the dialogue, particularly when patients are using herbal products (Table 66–3).

Barnes P, et al. Complementary and Alternative Medicine Use Among Adults: United States, 2002. *Advance Data form Vital and Health Statistics. No. 343*, May 27, 2004. (Report of a survey by the Division of Health Statistics of the Centers for Disease Control National Center for Health Statistics and the National Center for Complementary and Alternative Medicine on computer-assisted personal interviews of 31,044 adults regarding CAM use, examining frequency of use and types of therapies used.)

Table 66–3. Obtaining and Providing Information about CAM Therapies

Questions for patients

1. Are you taking any vitamins, supplements, or herbal remedies? If so, which ones?
2. How much are you taking of each? How often do you take each? How long have you been taking each?
3. What are the symptoms you want to treat?
4. Do you have a prescription medication for the same symptoms? If so, are you still taking it?
5. Have you noticed any improvement or worsening of symptoms since taking the remedy?

Information for patients

1. Natural does not always mean safe.
2. Commercial availability does not guarantee safety and efficacy. Manufacturers are not legally required to back their claims with scientific studies.
3. The quantity and quality of active ingredients may vary from product to product and from time to time in the same product.
4. Herbal products are not regulated like prescription drugs, and contamination can occur.
5. Supplements or remedies may interact with prescribed medication or with each other with possible serious consequences.
6. Some products are safe for short-term use but long-term studies with appropriate controls are generally lacking.
7. Infants, children, pregnant women, women trying to conceive, and the elderly should not use any CAM therapy without medical supervision.

CAM, complementary and alternative medicine.
(From Kolasinski SL. Complementary and alternative therapies for rheumatic disease. *Hosp Pract.* 2001;36:31. With permission.)

Blumenthal M, et al, eds. The complete German Commission E monographs: therapeutic guide to herbal medicine. Integrative Medicine Communications, 1998. (This compendium has been the standard source of information on herbal medicine for many years and reflects an accumulation of data from studies and anecdotal experience, analysis, and recommendations.)

De Smet PA. Herbal remedies. *N Engl J Med.* 2003;347:2046. [PMID: 12490687] (This review article summarizes the current state of knowledge on quality and safety issues regarding herbal products.)

Ernst E, ed. *The Desktop Guide to Complementary and Alternative Medicine. An Evidence-Based Approach.* Mosby, 2001. (This up-to-date encyclopedia of alternative therapies is edited by one of the foremost authorities on evidence-based analysis of CAM. The format includes listings of herbal medicines, physical interventions, and other therapeutic methods and beliefs with cross-references by diagnosis or condition.)

Peng CC, Glassman PA, Trilli LE, Hayes-Hunter J, Good CB. Incidence and severity of potential drug-dietary supplement interactions in primary care patients: an exploratory study of 2 outpatient practices. *Arch Intern Med.* 2004;164:630–636.

[PMID: 15037491] (Survey of 458 outpatients at two Veterans Affairs medical centers showed that 43% of those surveyed were taking prescription medications and dietary supplements at the same time and that 45% had the potential to have adverse effects as a result, 6% of which were serious.)

HERBAL MEDICINES

Avocado/Soybean Unsaponifiables

A very popular treatment for osteoarthritis (OA) in western Europe, avocado/soybean unsaponifiables is an extract of oils in a one-third avocado to two-thirds soybean mixture. A large body of in vitro and animal data suggests that this mixture possesses anti-inflammatory actions. A prospective, randomized, double-blind, placebo-controlled multicenter clinical trial of patients with knee and hip OA showed promising results. After 6 months of treatment with 300 mg of the extract, patients experienced significant reductions in pain and functional disability. Many required less NSAIDs. No significant side effects were reported. Patients with hip OA seemed to benefit more than those with knee OA. Avocado/soybean unsaponifiables may achieve these benefits through structural effects on cartilage, as suggested by a subsequent study. This 2-year trial showed that avocado/soybean unsaponifiables may reduce cartilage loss in patients with hip OA and advanced joint space narrowing at baseline. This product has just become available in the U.S. but the utility of the product to alter the course of OA has yet to be confirmed.

Capsaicin

The American College of Rheumatology Subcommittee on Osteoarthritis identifies topical capsaicin cream as an option for treatment of OA symptoms. It may be used as an adjunct to systemic therapy or as monotherapy in those who wish to avoid oral medications. The cream should be applied four times daily. It initially results in a burning sensation but judicious and repeated use lessens the severity of the burning, which rarely results in discontinuation of therapy.

Capsaicin is one of a number of pharmacologically active substances found in the *Capsicum* red pepper. It is known to initially induce the release of the neurotransmitter substance P from skin sensory C fibers when applied topically. Repeated application leads to specific blockade of transport and de novo synthesis of substance P, resulting in desensitization to pain by raising the pain threshold. A number of randomized trials have suggested that capsaicin is useful in the treatment of neurogenic pain, including the pain of diabetic neuropathy, as well as low back pain and pain due to OA.

Ginger

Extracts of members of the Zingiberaceae family have been used in Chinese traditional medicine and Ayurvedic tradition for millennia. Over a hundred species have been tested and a number have been found to have anti-inflammatory effects, including inhibition of the actions of cyclooxygenase and lipoxygenase, synthesis of leukotrienes, and rat paw edema in an animal model of inflammation. As with other herbal products, ginger is pharmacologically complex and may contain salicylate (though in amounts that are not thought to account for all of its anti-inflammatory effect), gingeroles, β-carotene, capsaicin, caffeic acid, and curcumin.

Fifty-six patients in Copenhagen with radiographically verified OA of the knee participated in a study in which they received either a ginger extract (Eurovita Extract 33, 170 mg orally three times a day), ibuprofen 400 mg orally three times a day, or placebo in each of three treatment periods of 3 weeks each. Overall, the investigators could demonstrate no differences between ginger and placebo. A larger, more recent multicenter study included 247 patients with radiographically confirmed knee OA. Participants were required to have visual analog scores between 40 mm and 70 mm on a 100-mm scale for pain on standing during the 24 hours preceding the baseline visit. They received either placebo or ginger extract (Eurovita Extract 77, 255 mg orally twice daily) for 6 weeks in this double-blind, randomized trial. Patients in both placebo- and ginger-treated groups had improvement in pain on standing, but the ginger group had a higher percentage of responders (63% versus 50%), a greater degree of response on average (8.1 mm more in the ginger group), and a greater percentage of participants with large responses. Pain after walking and overall functioning measured by the Western Ontario and McMaster Universities OA composite index (WOMAC) were also significantly improved in the ginger group. Gastrointestinal side effects (eructation, dyspepsia, and nausea) were more common in the ginger group (45% versus 16%), but none were serious. The investigators concluded that ginger has efficacy for pain management in knee OA, but that a future dose-finding study would be of benefit as would long-term investigation of side effects.

Thundergod Vine

Extracts of *Tripterygium wilfordii* Hook F, or thundergod vine, have been used in traditional Chinese medicine to treat a variety of autoimmune and inflammatory disorders, including rheumatoid arthritis, systemic lupus erythematosus (SLE), ankylosing spondylitis, psoriasis, and idiopathic IgA nephropathy. Traditional use dates back centuries, and while the Chinese literature has been uncontrolled, it does represent observations made on thousands of patients for time periods as long as a decade. In addition, several preliminary controlled trials have suggested that use of thundergod vine may represent a promising herbal therapy for a number of rheumatic diseases. Laboratory data suggest that active ingredients include triptolide and tripdiolide and that these substances inhibit in vitro inflammation, delayed-type hypersensitivity reactions, and primary antibody responses.

Uncontrolled reports from China on a total of about 250 patients have shown that thundergod vine can be of benefit in treating SLE. Subjects have experienced improvements in fatigue, arthralgias, fever, skin rash, lymphadenopathy, hepatomegaly, and laboratory abnormalities including proteinuria, renal function, thrombocytopenia, and the presence of antinuclear antibodies. Reports have suggested that glucocorticoid doses can be reduced, and sometimes eliminated.

The Chinese experience with thundergod vine has also been considerable with rheumatoid arthritis patients. An early placebo-controlled trial of 70 patients with rheumatoid arthritis had a crossover design. The majority of subjects improved in parameters of disease activity and laboratory abnormalities. Peripheral blood mononuclear cells from those receiving active treatment produced less IgM rheumatoid factor than cells from placebo-treated persons. Adverse effects gleaned from the Chinese experience include dry mouth, loss of appetite, nausea or vomiting, abdominal pain, diarrhea, leukopenia, thrombocytopenia, rash, skin pigmentation changes, and amenorrhea.

The safety and efficacy of the herb have been most recently examined in a small, double-blind, placebo-controlled trial of patients with rheumatoid arthritis seen at the National Institutes of Health and at the University of Texas Southwestern Medical Center. Twenty-one participants completed the 20-week study. They received either placebo or an oral dose of thundergod vine of 180 mg/d or 360 mg/d. Eighty percent of those receiving the higher dose, 40% of those receiving the lower dose, and none of those receiving placebo had at least a 20% improvement in the criteria for a clinical response (as established by the American College of Rheumatology). In this trial, the most common side effect was diarrhea and no person withdrew due to an adverse event. Investigations into the role of thundergod vine extract in the treatment of rheumatoid arthritis are continuing.

Altman RD, Marcussen KC. Effects of a ginger extract on knee pain in patients with osteoarthritis. *Arthritis Rheum.* 2001;44:2531. [PMID: 11710709] (Two hundred forty-seven participants were evaluated in a double-blind, randomized, placebo-controlled trial over 6 weeks. There were statistically significant differences between the ginger extract used and placebo for pain on standing and WOMAC scores, with more gastrointestinal side effects in the ginger group.)

American College of Rheumatology Subcommittee on Osteoarthritis Guidelines. Recommendations for the medical management of osteoarthritis of the hip and knee; 2000 update. *Arthritis Rheum.* 2000;43:1905. [PMID: 11014340] (This position statement outlines current best practices in the management of symptoms due to osteoarthritis of the hip and knee.)

Bliddal H, Rosetzsky A, Schlichting P, et al. A randomized, placebo-controlled, crossover study of ginger extracts and ibuprofen in osteoarthritis. *Osteoarthritis Cartilage.* 2000;8:9. [PMID: 10607493] (Fifty-six participants were evaluated in a double-blind, randomized, placebo-, and NSAID-controlled trial. Participants sequentially received placebo, ibuprofen, or a ginger extract for 3 weeks each in random sequence and the effects of ginger could not be distinguished from those of placebo.)

Lequesne M, Maheu E, Cadet C, Dreiser RL. Structural effect of avocado/soybean unsaponifiables on joint space loss in osteoarthritis of the hip. *Arthritis Rheum.* 2002;47:50. [PMID: 11932878] (This prospective, multicenter, randomized, parallel group, double-blind, placebo-controlled trial of 2 years' duration included 108 patients with hip OA. In those most severely affected, there was a significant reduction in joint space loss in those who received avocado/soybean unsaponifiables compared with those who received placebo.)

Maheu E, et al. Symptomatic efficacy of avocado/soybean unsaponifiables in the treatment of osteoarthritis of the knee and hip: a prospective, randomized, double-blind, placebo-controlled, multicenter clinical trial with a six-month treatment period and a two-month followup demonstrating a persistent effect. *Arthritis Rheum.* 1998;41:81. [PMID: 9433873] (This clinical trial treated 85 OA patients with avocado/soybean unsaponifiables for 6 months and compared them to 79 patients receiving placebo. Participants in the treatment group experienced reductions in pain, functional disability, and NSAID use.)

Setty AR, Sigal LH. Herbal medications commonly used in the practice of rheumatology: mechanisms of action, efficacy, and side effects. *Semin Arthritis Rheum.* 2005;34:773. [PMID 15942912] (This comprehensive literature review discusses a variety of herbal preparations used in rheumatologic conditions in the U.S. and elsewhere with an emphasis on potential anti-inflammatory and immunomodulatory mechanisms of action.)

Tao X, Younger J, Fan FZ, Wang B, Lipsky PE. Benefit of an extract of *Tripterygium wilfordii* hook F in patients with rheumatoid arthritis: a double-blind, placebo-controlled study. *Arthritis Rheum.* 2002;46:1735. [PMID: 12124856] (This is the most recent clinical publication addressing the specific effects of thundergod vine extract in subjects with rheumatoid arthritis. Patients with treatment-refractory rheumatoid arthritis benefited and tolerated the preparation well.)

DIETARY SUPPLEMENTS

Dehydroepiandrosterone

The wild Mexican yam is a natural source of diosgenin, an inactive prohormone of dehydroepiandrosterone (DHEA). However, wild yam products do not contain DHEA and require chemical treatment to yield usable hormone. DHEA is widely available without prescription in pharmacies and health food stores. However, before passage of the Dietary Supplement and Health Education Act, DHEA was considered a drug and was banned from over-the-counter sales since the 1980s. DHEA is a weak androgen and increases testosterone and estrogen levels as well as altering cytokine production.

The observations that there is a striking female predominance among SLE patients, that there are low circulating levels of DHEA in lupus patients, and that DHEA is beneficial in a mouse model of lupus have fueled interest in DHEA as a treatment for SLE. Several human trials have now been published and offer intriguing findings.

A double-blind, randomized trial monitored 191 patients with SLE for 7–9 months. The investigators found that a significantly greater proportion of persons who took oral DHEA (at the 200-mg/d dose but not at the 100-mg/d dose) were able to reduce their prednisone dose to ≤ 7.5 mg/d orally and sustain disease quiescence for 2 months than were those persons receiving placebo. However, differences between groups were small. Forty-one percent of the placebo-treated group responded, compared with 44% of the low-dose DHEA group and 51% of the higher-dose group. Furthermore, 65% of those with SLE disease activity index scores of 0 or 1 were responders and the percentage of responders decreased progressively and rapidly as baseline scores increased. The most common side effect was acne, occurring in twice as many DHEA-treated patients as those receiving placebo. High-density lipoprotein cholesterol and C3 levels were reduced, and serum levels of testosterone and estrogen were increased.

A second multicenter, randomized, double-blind, placebo-controlled trial was published later in 2002 that monitored 120 female patients with SLE in Taiwan. Participants took either placebo or 200 mg/d of oral DHEA for 6 months. These investigators found no difference between the clinical status of patients in the two groups as measured by the systemic lupus activity measure or SLE disease activity index. However, the number of disease flares were significantly lower in the DHEA group, and this group had a significant improvement in the patient global assessment. Serious adverse events were mostly characterized as disease flares and were increased in the placebo group. Increased levels of testosterone and increased incidence of acne were noted in the DHEA group. C3 and C4 levels declined in the DHEA group in this study as well.

A subsequent follow-up report of 293 patients receiving prasterone 200 mg/d or placebo for up to 12 months showed a small but statistically significant difference between groups. Those who took prasterone more frequently demonstrated improvement or stabilization of symptoms of lupus without clinical deterioration. A third of prasterone-treated patients developed acne and 16% developed hirsutism, but most did not withdraw from the trial as a result.

None of the trials published to date, however, is large enough to answer questions about the possible contribution of this hormone to risk of myocardial infarction or cerebrovascular accidents due to accelerated atherogenesis, altered cholesterol profile, or increased insulin resistance. In addition, concern has been raised because consequent elevations in sex hormones levels could result in increases in breast, ovarian, uterine, and prostate cancer risk.

Glucosamine Sulfate & Chondroitin Sulfate

Glucosamine sulfate and chondroitin sulfate are the most commonly used over-the-counter alternative therapy for arthritis. Their tremendous popularity in the United States results in part from the best selling book, *The Arthritis Cure,* by Jason Theodosakis, MD, who drew on decades of use and study in Europe in making his recommendations. While not a cure, glucosamine and chondroitin are of interest because they occur naturally in connective tissue, and are therefore intrinsically appealing as "nutraceuticals" for OA. In vitro work suggests a multitude of potential mechanisms, including inhibitory effects on cartilage-damaging agents like lysosomal enzymes, oxygen free radicals, matrix metalloproteinases, and aggrecanase, as well as dose-dependent increases in proteoglycan synthesis.

Glucosamine is available in a sulfate and a hydrochloride form, but studies have been carried out most often with the sulfate form. Most studies have been small and short in duration. Meta-analyses suggest that an analgesic benefit can be obtained from an oral dose of 1500 mg/d in a majority of those who take it. The effect is similar in magnitude to that of NSAIDs but is delayed in onset. The duration of the analgesic benefit is not known.

Controversy remains concerning the interpretation of two long-term studies of glucosamine because they suggested that glucosamine could halt radiographic progression of OA. In a 3-year Belgian trial, 212 patients received either 500 mg of oral glucosamine sulfate three times daily or placebo. Radiographs obtained at baseline and at 1 and 3 years of follow-up suggested that no radiographic progression occurred in those taking glucosamine while those receiving placebo had 0.34 mm joint space narrowing detectable after 3 years. However, the radiographic technique used and its ability to detect the very small differences noted have been questioned. Nonetheless, a 3-year study of 202 OA patients seen at the Prague Institute of Rheumatology had similar results: those who took glucosamine had no radiographic progression while those on placebo lost 0.35 mm of joint space after 3 years. Both studies have reported a reduction in the rate of joint replacement surgery needed for those who took glucosamine at 5-year follow-up. Trials suggest that chondroitin has analgesic benefit in OA as well. An oral dose of 1200 mg/d has generally been used. Studies of chondroitin are subject to the same criticisms as those of glucosamine; namely, they involve small numbers of participants and are of short duration, in addition to often being industry-sponsored.

The side-effect profiles of glucosamine and chondroitin have been indistinguishable from those of placebo in many of the short-term studies that have been carried out. Occasionally, gastrointestinal intolerance leads to discontinued use.

Methylsulfonylmethane

Methylsulfonylmethane (MSM) is a commonly used ingredient in over-the-counter topical and oral preparations for the treatment of a wide variety of conditions, including musculoskeletal pain, inflammation, asthma, allergies, headaches, cancer prevention, gastrointestinal complaints, and parasitic infections. Despite considerable popularity and millions of dollars in sales annually, few data support its use as an arthritis treatment. MSM is naturally present in a variety of foods including grains, meat, eggs, and fish, as well as raw broccoli, peppers, brussels sprouts, onions, and cabbage. When taken as a dietary supplement, doses of 1000–6000 mg/d are generally recommended.

MSM is a metabolite of dimethyl sulfoxide, which was itself popular as a topical arthritis treatment throughout the last century. However, the pungent odor and occasional skin irritation associated with use of dimethyl sulfoxide have likely contributed to its decline and the increase in popularity of MSM. Until recently, few toxicologic data were available on MSM. A study in rats showed no toxicity from a dose 5–7 times higher than the recommended human dose when given as a single gavage dose nor from long-term use of a 1.5-g/kg dose over 90 days.

Evidence that MSM is of benefit in arthritis treatment is largely anecdotal and published in the lay press. Celebrity endorsements and a best-selling volume by two physician proponents have enhanced public awareness of this substance, but rigorous trials and convincing evidence that it might have a specific role in thwarting pathophysiologic processes in arthritis are lacking.

Omega-3 Fatty Acids

Omega-3 fatty acids have been well documented to have a range of in vitro and in vivo effects of relevance to the treatment of rheumatic diseases, including antagonism of the production of proinflammatory and prothrombotic eicosanoids, suppression of production of proinflammatory cytokines, and reduction of cartilage-degrading enzymes. Omega-3 fatty acids are most readily available via the consumption of fish oil which contains both eicosapentaenoic acid and docosahexaenoic acid. Eicosapentaenoic acid competitively inhibits utilization of arachidonic acid and becomes a substrate for the production of alternative products of the cyclooxygenase and 5-lipoxygenase pathways. Thromboxane A_3 and prostacyclin I_3 are increased, resulting in decreased platelet aggregation, and leukotriene B_4 is decreased, presumably an important mechanism in reducing inflammation. A considerable number of short-term clinical trials performed over the last two decades have suggested efficacy in the treatment of rheumatoid arthritis. When given a daily dose of 3 g of omega-3 fatty acids, investigators have confirmed a reduction in morning stiffness, in the number of tender joints, and in the dose of NSAIDs required. Concomitant reduction in the level of interleukin-1 has been reported but fish oil has not been demonstrated to act as a disease-modifying agent in rheumatoid arthritis.

The clinical status of patients with systemic lupus erythematosus may also be affected by ingestion of fish oil. Murine models have suggested that consumption of an omega-3 fatty acid–rich diet could reduce autoantibody and inflammatory cytokine production and result in a prolonged lifespan in lupus-prone mice. A number of small, short-term trials in humans suggested improvements might occur but rigorous outcome measures were not generally used. A recent 6-month trial compared the status of lupus patients who received fish oil or placebo olive oil with or without copper supplements using the systemic lupus activity measure. Significant improvements of systemic lupus activity measure scores were noted at 6 months, as was an overall sense of well-being, but no detectable difference was found in weight, blood pressure measurements, blood counts, blood chemistry, erythrocyte sedimentation rate, complement levels, or levels of antibodies to double-stranded DNA or anticardiolipin.

Vitamins

Vitamins are among the most popular and readily accessible supplements that patients might choose to treat their arthritis symptoms. There are a number of possible mechanisms through which vitamins could be of benefit, particularly in the pathogenesis of OA. It is thought, for example, that oxidative stress is a major contributor to the progression of OA and antioxidant vitamins like C and E might, therefore, have a role in slowing progression. The current concept of OA is that it is a disease of not only the articular cartilage, but also of the subchondral bone and that the nature of the bone response to OA determines outcome. Vitamin D appears to play an important role in bone mineralization, in proteoglycan synthesis by chondrocytes, and in reduction of degradative matrix metalloproteinases, all of which could be protective from OA progression. Epidemiologic surveys have suggested that

there may be a role for optimizing vitamin intake, but prospective intervention trials have not yet emerged.

A 1996 study analyzing Framingham data was the first to suggest that vitamin D intake could have an impact on OA progression. Participants had been followed for more than 40 years and had had radiographs performed in the early 1980s and again in the early 1990s. Serum 25-hydroxyvitamin D levels had been obtained in the late 1980s, along with a dietary questionnaire. The investigators analyzed 788 normal and 126 osteoarthritic knees and found that the risk of progression of prevalent OA at baseline was markedly increased in those in the middle and lower tertiles for both intake and serum levels of vitamin D.

The importance of dietary vitamin D was again addressed in a more recent study of hip OA. A subset of participants in the Study of Osteoporotic Fractures was randomly selected for further investigation of the biochemical antecedents of fractures. Serum 1,25-dihydroxyvitamin D and 25-hydroxyvitamin D levels were measured and radiographs of the hip were obtained. Participants were women with a mean age of 71 years. The investigators found that in those with low serum 25-hydroxyvitamin D—but not 1,25-dihydroxyvitamin D—levels there was a threefold increase in the incidence of hip OA characterized by joint space narrowing rather than osteophyte formation. This result supported the hypothesis that the action of vitamin D was likely to be through effects on cartilage metabolism.

Data have also appeared regarding the role of dietary antioxidant vitamins and the risk of OA. Framingham data were analyzed for a relationship between knee OA and intake of vitamins B_1, B_6, C, E, β-carotene, niacin, and folate as assessed by food frequency questionnaire. Six hundred forty participants were available for analysis and incident and progressive OA developed in 81 and 68 knees, respectively. The investigators found a threefold reduction in risk of OA progression for the middle and highest tertiles of vitamin C intake. This finding correlated predominantly with a reduced risk of cartilage loss. Interestingly, those with high vitamin C intake also had a reduced risk of developing knee pain. A less consistent reduction in risk of OA progression was also seen for β-carotene and vitamin E. However, a more recent long-term prospective trial of vitamin E supplementation in patients with osteoarthritis of the knee has failed to demonstrate efficacy.

Duffy EM, Meenagh GK, McMillan SA, et al. The clinical effect of dietary supplementation with omega-3 fish oils and/or copper in systemic lupus erythematosus. *J Rheumatol.* 2004;31:1551. [PMID: 15290734] (Lupus patients were found to have improvements in validated clinical outcomes measures of overall status, but no changes in laboratory values as a result of ingestion of fish oil supplements.)

Horvath K, Noker PE, Somfai-Relle S, et al. Toxicity of methyl-sulfonylmethane in rats. *Food Chem Toxicol.* 2002;40:1459. [PMID: 12387309] (This report details the only public information on the toxicology of MSM.)

Kolasinski SL. Dimethylsulfoxide (DMSO) and methylsulfonylmethane (MSM) for the treatment of arthritis. *Altern Med Alert.* 2000;3:115. (This review article summarizes the history and current use of MSM for musculoskeletal complaints.)

Kremer JM, Lawrence DA, Jubiz W, et al. Dietary fish oil and olive oil supplementation in patients with rheumatoid arthritis. Clinical and immunologic effects. *Arthritis Rheum.* 1990;33:810. [PMID: 2363736] (This classic article documented a significant clinical response of rheumatoid arthritis patients to supplementation with fish oil that correlated with a shift to production of less inflammatory cytokines.)

Lane NE, Gore LR, Cummings SR, et al. Serum vitamin D levels and incident changes of radiographic hip osteoatoid arthritis: A longitudinal study. Study of Osteoporotic Fractures Research Group. *Arthritis Rheum.* 1999;42:854. [PMID: 10323440] (This subset analysis of participants in a trial examining osteoporosis quantified the risk of incident hip OA as threefold greater in those with low serum 25-hydroxyvitamin D levels.)

McAlindon TE, LaValley MP, Gulin JO, Felson DT. Glucosamine and chondroitin for treatment of osteoarthritis: a systematic quality assessment and meta-analysis. *JAMA.* 2000;283:1469. [PMID: 10732937] (This report is the most authoritative meta-analysis of data on glucosamine and chondroitin for osteoarthritis symptom reduction. Careful selection of trials for analysis and assessment of their design and findings result in the conclusion that these substances are likely to be modestly effective and safe.)

Petri MA, Mease PJ, Merrill JT, et al. Effects of prasterone on disease activity and symptoms in women with active systemic lupus erythematosus. *Arthritis Rheum.* 2004;50:2858. [PMID 15452837] (The most recent of a series of publications detailing the effects of DHEA in lupus patients.)

Reginster JY, Deroisy R, Rovati LC, et al. Long-term effect of glucosamine sulphate on osteoarthritis progression: a randomised, placebo-controlled clinical trial. *Lancet.* 2001;357: 251. [PMID: 11214126] (This is the longest study to date to assess the benefit of glucosamine in knee OA. It remains controversial because of the type of radiographic assessment that was performed.)

PHYSICAL INTERVENTIONS

Acupuncture

Acupuncture is a centuries-old practice of inserting needles into predetermined locations. In the traditional Chinese explanation for the efficacy of acupuncture, the movement of chi, or vital energy, along channels called meridians is influenced by the placement of the needles. An imbalance in the flow of chi can be redressed by certain needle placements, depending on the ailment being treated, and may improve health and well-being. In the Western medical tradition, it is recognized that one explanation, although incomplete, of the efficacy of acupuncture may be that needle placement stimulates the production of endogenous opioids. Inadequate understanding of the mechanism of action of acupuncture, however, is not as much of an impediment to systematic study as is the very nature of the intervention. Deciding what an appropriate control is (Can an intervention that does not use needles provide adequate control? Where should the control needles be placed? How many? For how long?) has an important bearing on interpretation and comparison of trials. Regardless of the availability of scientific appraisal of acupuncture, about 1 million consumers in the United States seek treatment each year.

No individual trials have been adequately designed to address the efficacy of acupuncture in pain control in rheumatic diseases. The National Institutes of Health compiled a consensus statement in 1998 on the use and efficacy of acupuncture in a variety of medical conditions. The statement concluded that acupuncture might be useful for analgesia in tennis elbow, fibromyalgia, myofascial pain, OA, low back pain, and carpal tunnel syndrome, but that there was a paucity of high-quality research from which to draw conclusions.

The largest and most definitive study of acupuncture for treatment of osteoarthritis of the knee has suggested that acupuncture may offer modest benefit in patients who have had inadequate analgesia from other therapies. Five hundred seventy patients were randomly assigned to receive true or sham acupuncture over a 26-week period. Both groups received about 23 hours of contact during the study. The sham procedure used insertion of acupuncture needles at sham points, as well as the application of sham needles at true acupuncture points with adhesive tape. The investigators showed that WOMAC function scores improved significantly in the true acupuncture–treated group at 8 weeks and that this persisted and improved further at the 26-week time point. Also, at the study's conclusion, participants receiving true acupuncture had significantly greater improvements in pain scores and patient global assessment scores. No adverse effects due to acupuncture were noted.

Acupuncture has been used in several trials as a therapy for the pain of fibromyalgia. No single trial definitively establishes the place of acupuncture in the treatment regimen for fibromyalgia. However, the systematic review of one high-quality and six lower-quality studies provides some guidance. This clinical review concluded that the high-quality study suggested that acupuncture was more effective than sham acupuncture for relieving pain, increasing pain thresholds, improving global ratings, and reducing morning stiffness. It was unclear how long-lasting the benefits were. Some patients received no benefit, and others had an exacerbation of pain. The lower-quality studies were in agreement with these results.

Few trials have addressed the use of acupuncture in rheumatoid arthritis. However, available evidence suggests no improvement in parameters of inflammation. Methodologic limitations need to be taken into account in the interpretation of the data.

Despite the fact that trials in patients with rheumatic diseases have affirmed the safety of acupuncture, adverse events due to acupuncture have been documented and include serious consequences such as pneumothorax, cardiac tamponade, spinal injuries, and septic complications. However, considerable additional evidence supports the safety of acupuncture. A survey was conducted of preceptors and interns at a Japanese national medical facility at which about 60% of the patients undergo acupuncture. Results were compiled on over 55,000 acupuncture treatments and 64 adverse events were identified. The most frequent was failure to remove the needle after the procedure was completed. Almost as common were dizziness, discomfort, and perspiration thought to be associated with a transient vasovagal episode. Less common side effects were burn injuries due to moxibustion, ecchymoses, and needling site reactions. A systematic review of the literature revealed a similar safety record. Nine prospective surveys encompassing over 250,000 acupuncture treatments were reviewed. Minor side effects were common. These included pain at the site of needling and pain due to aggravation of the presenting condition that occurred in up to half of those undergoing acupuncture. Postprocedure fatigue was noted in up to about 40%; an unusual feeling of relaxation (characterized by some as necessary for efficacy) was seen in over 80%. Minor bleeding was seen in up to about 40% as well. Fainting was reported in less than 0.2%. Serious side effects reported included two cases of pneumothorax and two cases in which needles needed to be retrieved surgically after they fractured.

Tai Chi

Tai chi is a centuries-old Chinese form of conditioning exercise based in martial arts traditions and consisting of slow, flowing movements, relaxation, and deep breathing. The aim of the practice is balance of mind and body by stimulating chi. Tai chi involves cognitive, cardiovascular, and musculoskeletal responses that evoke physiologic and psychological changes including maximum oxygen consumption, muscular strength, and flexibility. Early studies encouraged enthusiasm for tai chi as an intervention for geriatric patients since these small trials suggested that improvements in balance and fall prevention could follow training in tai chi. A more recent study of 72 patients with OA showed that a 12-week program held three times weekly improved WOMAC scores for pain and function. Participants reported significantly less pain at the completion of the study, as well as reduced stiffness, reduced perception of difficulty in activities of daily living, and improved physical functioning. It was particularly noteworthy that on physical fitness testing, subjects demonstrated enhanced balance and abdominal muscle strength. No serious side effects of tai chi have been reported.

Yoga

Yoga derives from a more than 2000-year-old Indian tradition based on eight branches of practice, including postures (asanas), breathing, and meditation. The aim of hatha yoga, or the practice of asanas, is to prepare the practitioner for the spiritual experience of purifying the body. The ultimate goal of this practice is the achievement of harmony in body, mind, and spirit. A number of studies have attempted to quantify physiologic effects of yoga and found reductions in oxygen consumption, minute ventilation, and heart rate after exercise in persons participating in regular yoga practice.

Small studies have suggested that yoga may be efficacious for a variety of musculoskeletal conditions, but all studies to date have methodologic limitations that reduce their generalizability. Nonetheless, the trials that have been carried out support a role for yoga in reducing pain and increasing function. Persons with carpal tunnel syndrome participated in an 8-week yoga program and had significant improvements in grip strength and pain. A study of the effects of a 10-week course of yoga for symptoms of OA of the hands showed reductions in finger joint tenderness and range of motion and hand pain during activity. A more recent trial has suggested that yoga represents an exercise alternative for even obese patients with OA of the knee who are not regular exercisers. Reductions in pain and functional disability using WOMAC scores were demonstrated in a group who completed an 8-week yoga program.

No serious side effects have been reported in the trials assessing yoga for musculoskeletal complaints. There have been rare reports of reversible compression neuropathy after 6 hours of kneeling and very rare instances of vertebral and basilar artery occlusion after neck standing and prolonged flexion of the cervical spine.

Berman BM, Lao L, Langenberg P, et al. Effectiveness of acupuncture as adjunctive therapy in osteoarthritis of the knee: a randomized, controlled trial. *Ann Intern Med.* 2004;141:901. [PMID: 15611487] (This large, carefully designed trial showed adjunctive analgesic benefit from acupuncture in OA patients who had previously been maximally medically treated.)

Berman BM, Swyers JP, Ezzo J. The evidence for acupuncture as a treatment for rheumatologic conditions. *Rheum Dis Clin North Am.* 2000;26:103. [PMID: 10680198] (This is a very readable overview that provides a wealth of references and analysis of the use of acupuncture for a broad range of rheumatologic conditions.)

Ernst E, White AR. Prospective studies of the safety of acupuncture. A systematic review. *Am J Med.* 2001;110:481. [PMID: 11331060] (A review of nine surveys from the literature detailing acupuncture side effects in an attempt to get a more realistic assessment of acupuncture safety than is available from the anecdotal, case report literature. It concludes that serious adverse events are rare.)

Kaptchuk TJ. Acupuncture: theory, efficacy and practice. *Ann Intern Med.* 2002;136:374. [PMID: 11874310] (A scholarly discussion of the traditional concepts and theoretical underpinning of acupuncture in the context of current practice.)

Kolasinski SL. Acupuncture for arthritis. *Altern Med Alert.* 2002;5:37. (This review article provides an overview of methodologic considerations, mechanism of action, and trials in OA and rheumatoid arthritis. Side effects of acupuncture are reviewed.)

Kolasinki SL, Garfinkel M, Tsai AG, et al. Iyengar yoga for the treatment of symptoms of osteoarthritis of the knees: a pilot study. *J Altern Complement Med.* 2005;11:689. [PMID: 16131293] (This pilot study suggests that significant reductions in pain and improvements in physical functioning can result from an 8-week yoga program even in obese, sedentary subjects who have not previously practiced yoga.)

Song R, Lee EO, Lam P, Bae SC. Effects of tai chi exercise on pain, balance, muscle strength, and perceived difficulties in physical functioning in older women with osteoarthritis: a randomized clinical trial. *J Rheumatol.* 2003;30:2039. [PMID 12966613] (Seventy-two patients with OA were assigned to either Sun-style tai chi or control. Those participating in tai chi had improvements in pain, stiffness, balance and abdominal muscle strength.)

SECTION XI

Therapies

Medications

■ NONSTEROIDAL ANTI-INFLAMMATORY DRUGS

John B. Imboden, MD

MECHANISM OF ACTION

- Inhibition of prostaglandin synthesis: Nonsteroidal anti-inflammatory drugs (NSAIDs) inhibit cyclooxygenase (COX), which converts arachidonic acid to prostaglandins. NSAIDs are competitive antagonists and reversible inhibitors of COX. Aspirin, on the other hand, inhibits COX through the acetylation of the enzyme, a process that is irreversible. There are two isoforms of COX: COX-1, whose expression is constitutive and ubiquitous, and COX-2, which is not constitutively expressed by most tissues but can be induced by inflammatory stimuli. In general, it is thought that inhibition of COX-2 accounts for the anti-inflammatory, antipyretic, and analgesic effects of NSAIDs, while inhibition of COX-1 explains much of the gastrointestinal toxicity of NSAIDs. Inhibition of COX-1 accounts for the inhibitory effect of NSAIDs on platelets, which do not express COX-2. COX-2 appears to be the major source for the production of prostacyclin, which has antiplatelet and vasodilatory effects. COX-2 is constitutively expressed in the kidney and contributes to the production of prostaglandins that regulate renal blood flow.

- Inhibition of COX may not explain all the effects of NSAIDs, but there is no consensus as to other pharmacologically relevant targets.

PHARMACOKINETICS

- Bioavailability: Very high.
- NSAIDs circulate tightly bound to plasma proteins (>99% protein-bound for most; approximately 70% for aspirin).
- Metabolism: The liver converts NSAIDs to inactive metabolites. Some NSAIDs undergo extensive enterohepatic circulation.
- Half-life: Varies greatly among individual NSAIDs (Table 67–1). Longer half-lives permit once-daily dosing but lead to substantial delays in reaching steady-state levels of drug (eg, 7–12 days in the case of piroxicam).
- Aspirin and diflunisal exhibit concentration-dependent elimination kinetics with the result that small increases in doses can produce disproportionately large increases in plasma drug levels.
- Clearance: Renal excretion is the major means of elimination of metabolites. Usually only a small percentage of the parent drug is renally cleared.

USES IN RHEUMATIC DISEASE

NSAIDs are used in a wide range of rheumatic conditions. The Food and Drug Administration has approved most for use in osteoarthritis and many for rheumatoid arthritis as well. NSAIDs are used for treatment of the spondyloarthropathies, are effective in the management of acute flares of gout and pseudogout, and are prescribed

Table 67–1. Selected Nonsteroidal Anti-Inflammatory Drugs

Drug (Trade Name)	Half–Life (h)	Dosing	Comments
Arylcarboxylic acids			
Diflunisal (Dolobid)	8–12	250–500 mg bid	Concentration-dependent elimination kinetics
Arylalkanoic acids			
Diclofenac (Voltaren, Cataflam)	2	50–75 mg bid	
Ibuprofen (Motrin, Advil, Rufen)	2–2.5	200–800 mg qid	Available over the counter
Fenoprofen (Nalfon)	2–3	300–600 mg qid	
Naproxen (Naprosyn, Aleve, Anaprox, Naprelin)	12–17	250–500 bid	Available over the counter
Indomethacin (Indocin)	4.5	25–50 mg tid	
Sulindac (Clinoril)	16	150–200 mg bid	Converted by liver to an active metabolite
Enolic acids			
Piroxicam (Feldene)	50	10–20 mg daily	
Meloxicam (Mobic)	15–20	7.5–15 mg daily	
Nonacidic			
Nabumetome (Relafen)	24	1000 mg daily	Prodrug rapidly converted to an active metabolite by the liver
Coxibs (selective COX-2 inhibitors)			
Celecoxib (Celebrex)	11	100-200 mg bid	Coxibs have an increased risk of adverse cardiovascular events, particularly at higher doses and with prolonged use; sulfonamide hypersensitivity is a contraindication for celecoxib

COX, cyclooxygenase.

widely for bursitis, tendinitis, and other soft-tissue complaints.

CHOICE OF NSAID

- A large number of NSAIDs are available in the United States. As a general rule, the NSAIDs are comparable in efficacy, but individual patients may exhibit different responses to particular NSAIDs. Physician and patient preferences, concerns regarding toxicity, and cost usually determine the choice of NSAID. See Table 67–1 for typical dosing ranges of selected NSAIDs in common use in the U.S.
- Traditional NSAIDs inhibit both COX-1 and COX-2. Although considered "nonselective," these nonetheless vary in their relative selectivity for COX-1 and COX-2 in vitro (*N Engl J Med.* 2001;345:433; *J Clin Invest.* 2006;116:4). Indeed, the in vitro selectivity of diclofenac, meloxicam, and nabumetone for COX-2 is comparable to that of celecoxib. On the other hand, indomethacin, ibuprofen, and naproxen display modest in vitro selectivity for COX-1. The clinical significance of differential selectivity for COX-1 and COX-2 by traditional NSAIDs remains to be determined.
- Selective COX-2 inhibitors (the "coxibs") were developed in an effort to reduce gastrointestinal toxicity, but an increase in adverse cardiovascular events (myocar-

dial infarction and stroke) led to the withdrawal of two of these: rofecoxib and valdecoxib. Longer duration of therapy, higher dose, and the presence of cardiac risk factors appear to increase the risk of coxib-associated adverse cardiovascular events. The major underlying mechanism is thought to be inhibition of COX-2-mediated production of prostacyclin; loss of prostacyclin removes a vascular protective mechanism, thereby predisposing to thrombosis and accelerating atherogenesis (*J Clin Invest.* 2006;116:4). The inability of coxibs to inhibit platelets (which only express COX-1) also likely contributes to the increase in thromboembolism (*Nat Rev Drug Discov.* 2003;2:879). Celecoxib is the only coxib currently available in the United States. Low doses of celecoxib (total dose <200 mg per day) do not appear to be associated with increased cardiovascular risk in short-term studies, but safety data for long-term use are limited. The evidence that celecoxib has a favorable gastrointestinal-toxicity profile relative to traditional NSAIDs has been questioned (*BMJ.* 2002;324:1287).

INITIATING THERAPY

Complete blood cell (CBC) count, serum electrolytes and creatinine, and liver function tests should be obtained prior to initiating long-term therapy with NSAIDs.

Table 67–2. Risk Factors for NSAID-Induced Hemodynamically Mediated Renal Failure

Intrinsic renal disease
Volume depletion
Diuretic use
Use of an angiotensin-converting enzyme inhibitor
Cirrhosis
Heart failure
Advanced age

NSAID, nonsteroidal anti-inflammatory drug.

MONITORING THERAPY

Serum electrolytes and creatinine should be monitored closely (eg, weekly for several weeks) if NSAIDs are started in a patient at risk for renal toxicity (Table 67–2). Many clinicians check liver function tests 6–12 weeks after initiating NSAID therapy and periodically monitor the CBC count and liver function tests thereafter (guidelines from the American College of Rheumatology call for yearly testing of patients with rheumatoid arthritis; *Arthritis Rheum.* 2002;46:328).

SPECIAL PRECAUTIONS

- The presence of one or more of the risk factors for gastrointestinal toxicity listed in Table 67–3 should prompt consideration of an alternative to NSAIDs (eg, acetaminophen) or the concomitant use of a proton pump inhibitor. Celecoxib has not been shown to have a clearly favorable gastrointestinal side-effect profile relative to traditional NSAIDs (*BMJ.* 2002;324:1287; *J Clin Invest.* 2006;116:4).
- Patients with known cardiovascular disease or with cardiac risk factors are likely at greater risk for adverse car-

Table 67–3. Risk Factors Associated with NSAID-Induced Gastrointestinal Toxicity

Age >60 years
Previous history of peptic ulcer or gastrointestinal bleeding
Concomitant glucocorticoid therapy
Anticoagulation
Prolonged use of maximum doses of NSAID
Comorbid conditions (cardiovascular disease, renal insufficiency, hepatic impairment, diabetes, hypertension)

NSAID, nonsteroidal anti-inflammatory drug.
(Adapted from Wolfe MM, Lichtenstein DR, Singh G. Gastrointestinal toxicity of nonsteroidal antiinflammatory drugs. *N Engl J Med.* 1999;340:188. With permission.)

diovascular events associated with COX-2 inhibitors. Whether traditional NSAIDs also carry an increased cardiovascular risk is not known. Early work in this area suggests that naproxen may be neutral or slightly protective and that diclofenac may carry risk with prolonged use (*J Clin Invest.* 2006;116:4).

- Patients on low-dose aspirin for primary or secondary cardiac protection present a complex problem. Traditional NSAIDs are reversible inhibitors of platelet COX-1 and may not mimic the sustained inhibition that occurs with aspirin. Indeed, concomitant treatment with certain traditional NSAIDs such as ibuprofen (and possibly indomethacin and naproxen as well) diminishes the protective effect of aspirin, probably by limiting access of aspirin to the acetylation site of platelet COX-1 (*N Engl J Med.* 2001;345:1809; *J Clin Invest.* 2006;116:4). Clopidogrel has been suggested as a rational alternative to low-dose aspirin for the patient who requires chronic NSAID therapy and has significant cardiovascular risk factors (*J Clin Invest.* 2006;116:4). The coxibs do not interfere with the inhibitory effects of low-dose aspirin on platelets, but there is no evidence that low-dose aspirin provides consistent protection against the increased cardiovascular risk associated with coxibs.
- NSAIDs (including the coxibs) should be used cautiously, if at all, when one or more of the risk factors for NSAID-induced hemodynamically mediated renal failure is present (see Table 67–2) and should not be used when the creatinine clearance is less than 30 ml/min.
- Severe anemia places a patient at greater risk in the event of NSAID-induced gastrointestinal blood loss.
- NSAIDs can induce a modest elevation in blood pressure and can blunt the antihypertensive effects of β-blockers, angiotensin-converting enzyme inhibitors, and diuretics. NSAIDs can worsen heart failure.
- NSAIDs can displace drugs from binding sites on plasma proteins, can alter their metabolism or excretion, and can interfere with their actions. The physician should determine whether there are any known interactions with coadministered medications (for example, by using the drug interaction search available at www.PDR.net).
- Patients should be cautioned that combining over-the-counter drugs (eg, aspirin, naproxen, ibuprofen, and ketoprofen) with prescription NSAIDs can increase toxicity.
- Aspirin should be discontinued 1–2 weeks before surgery because its effect on platelets is irreversible. Other NSAIDs should be discontinued for a period equal to five times their half-life prior to surgery.
- Aspirin and other NSAIDs can trigger attacks of severe asthma and marked nasal congestion, particularly

in persons with a history of asthma and nasal polyposis. Up to 10% of asthmatic patients display aspirin sensitivity, which usually develops in the third or fourth decade. This reaction is due to inhibition of COX and is a class effect, not an immune response to a specific drug. NSAIDs are absolutely contraindicated for patients with known aspirin sensitivity.

- NSAIDs should be avoided during pregnancy if possible. Concerns regarding bleeding and premature closure of the ductus arteriosus preclude the use of NSAIDs in the final months of pregnancy.

COMPLICATIONS

Common

- Upper gastrointestinal toxicity: Dyspepsia, gastritis, peptic ulceration, hemorrhage, and perforation (*N Engl J Med.* 1999;340:1888; *Gut.* 2003;52:600). Dyspepsia is not a reliable indicator of patients at risk for ulceration, hemorrhage, or perforation; the majority of patients with serious gastrointestinal complications do not have antecedent dyspepsia. Proton pump inhibitors reduce NSAID-induced dyspepsia, are an effective treatment for NSAID-induced ulcers, and protect against ulcers detected endoscopically. Coadministration of misoprostol prevents ulcerations and reduces the rate of complications due to ulcers. However, side effects such as diarrhea and abdominal pain are common and limit the usefulness of misoprostol. Coadministration of H_2-receptor antagonists is not recommended for the routine prevention or treatment of NSAID-induced dyspepsia. Although these agents reduce dyspepsia, they do not protect against, and may even increase, serious gastrointestinal complications.
- Renal: Retention of sodium and fluid is common. Hemodynamically mediated acute renal failure is reversible and generally occurs when NSAIDs are administered to patients with risk factors for this complication (see Table 67–2).
- Hepatic: Transient, modest (< two- to threefold) elevations of serum aminotransferases are common and do not predict severe liver damage.
- Tinnitus and hearing loss: This frequent complication of high doses of aspirin also occurs with other NSAIDs.

Uncommon or Rare

- Renal: Interstitial nephritis, nephrotic syndrome, papillary necrosis.
- Acute liver injury.
- Lower gastrointestinal: Small bowel ulcers; strictures of the small or large bowel.
- Neutropenia.

- Central nervous system: aseptic meningitis, headaches, dysphoria, cognitive impairment.
- Hypersensitivity reactions.

■ SYSTEMIC GLUCOCORTICOID THERAPY: PREDNISONE, PREDNISOLONE, & METHYLPREDNISOLONE

John B. Imboden, MD

MECHANISM OF ACTION

- Glucocorticoids bind to cytoplasmic receptors that translocate to the nucleus and affect the transcription of target genes, thereby inducing the production of anti-inflammatory proteins and repressing the production of proinflammatory proteins. Glucocorticoids also inhibit inflammation through mechanisms that are independent of transcriptional effects (*N Engl J Med.* 2005;353:1711).
- Anti-inflammatory effects: The direct and indirect effects on inflammation are diverse and include reduction of arachidonic acid release, inhibition of production of proinflammatory cytokines, decreased migration of neutrophils to sites of inflammation, impaired T-cell function, and decreased numbers of eosinophils.

PHARMACOKINETICS

- Bioavailability: 50–90%.
- Metabolism: Prednisone is biologically inactive until reduced to prednisolone in the liver. Prednisone, prednisolone, and methylprednisolone are converted to inactive metabolites by the liver.
- Half-life: 2–3 hours for prednisolone and methylprednisolone; 3–4 hours for prednisone
- Clearance: Metabolites are excreted in the urine.

USES IN RHEUMATIC DISEASE

Glucocorticoids are used for a wide variety of rheumatic diseases, but controlled studies documenting their efficacy in these conditions are few.

Rheumatoid Arthritis

Low-dose glucocorticoids (eg, prednisone or prednisolone ≤10 mg/d) are frequently used as "bridge therapy" to suppress disease activity while introducing slower acting disease-modifying antirheumatic drugs (see

Chapter 16). The addition of low-dose prednisolone (5–7.5 mg/d) for 2 years to standard care with disease-modifying antirheumatic drugs slows radiographic progression in patients with recent-onset rheumatoid arthritis (*N Engl J Med.* 1995;333:142; *Arthritis Rheum.* 2005;52:3360, 3371). There is debate as to whether the benefits of therapy outweigh the risks of prolonged glucocorticoid therapy for chronic rheumatoid arthritis.

Systemic Lupus Erythematosus & Mixed Connective Tissue Disease

Despite a paucity of controlled trials, the efficacy of glucocorticoids is accepted. Glucocorticoids are a mainstay of regimens to treat acute flares of systemic lupus erythematosus (SLE) and to maintain remissions (see Chapter 23).

Vasculitis

High-dose glucocorticoids are often used in conjunction with cytotoxic drugs in the initial management of Wegener granulomatosis, microscopic polyangiitis, Churg-Strauss syndrome, and polyarteritis nodosa. Giant cell arteritis and Takayasu arteritis are often treated with glucocorticoids alone (see Chapters 31–36).

Polymyositis & Dermatomyositis

High-dose glucocorticoids are standard first-line therapy (see Chapter 28).

DOSAGE

- Methylprednisolone is slightly more potent than prednisone or prednisolone. Equivalent doses of these and other commonly used exogenous glucocorticoids are: prednisone 5 mg; prednisolone 5 mg; methylprednisolone 4 mg; hydrocortisone 20 mg; dexamethasone 0.7 mg (*Medicine [Baltimore]*. 1976;55:39).
- High-dose oral glucocorticoids (eg, prednisone or prednisolone 1 mg/kg/d or 60 mg/d) are used in an attempt to control severe disease activity rapidly in cases of SLE, vasculitis, inflammatory myopathies, and the like. Because substantial toxicity is likely if high doses are maintained, the dose should be tapered as permitted by the activity of the disease or the use of glucocorticoid-sparing agents, or both.
- Intravenous "pulses" of methylprednisolone (eg, 500–1000 mg/d for 3 days) are sometimes used for severe complications of SLE, vasculitis, and the inflammatory myopathies. Pulses are infused over 1–2 hours (there are rare reports of sudden death and ventricular arrhythmias with rapid infusions).
- Generally only low-dose glucocorticoids (eg, prednisone or prednisolone ≤10 mg/d) are used in the treatment of RA. Maintenance doses in SLE are often somewhat higher (prednisone or prednisolone 10–15 mg/d).

INITIATING THERAPY

If prolonged therapy is contemplated, bone density should be determined, particularly for patients with risk factors for osteoporosis. Chapter 57 reviews the prophylaxis of glucocorticoid-induced osteoporosis.

MONITORING THERAPY

Serum glucose should be monitored closely when patients with diabetes are treated with systemic glucocorticoids. Routine laboratory studies otherwise are not necessary to monitor therapy but may be indicated to assess the underlying disease.

SPECIAL PRECAUTIONS

In the setting of active infection, diabetes, or osteoporosis, systemic glucocorticoids should be used only after very careful consideration of the indications for treatment, the risks of treatment, and the alternatives to glucocorticoids.

Renal failure does not affect dosing. Some clinicians argue that prednisone should not be used in the setting of severe liver disease, but delayed conjugation to inactive metabolites may offset impaired conversion of prednisone to prednisolone.

SUPPRESSION OF THE HYPOTHALAMIC-PITUITARY-ADRENAL AXIS

Glucocorticoid therapy can suppress the hypothalamic-pituitary-adrenal (HPA) axis. The dose and duration of therapy influence the onset and magnitude of this effect, but individual variation is substantial and prevents accurate identification of adrenally-suppressed patients in the absence of endocrine testing. As a rough guide, treatment with prednisone 7.5 mg daily for 3 weeks can be sufficient to induce suppression.

The evaluation for adrenal insufficiency includes measurements of serum cortisol and stimulatory tests of the HPA axis. Basal plasma cortisol levels, however, correlate poorly with HPA suppression and are helpful only when very low or very high (*N Engl J Med.* 1992;326:226). Thus, a serum cortisol level <3 μg/dL indicates glucocorticoid-induced adrenal insufficiency if the sample is drawn at 8 AM (the time of peak endogenous production). Conversely, a serum cortisol level >20 μg/dL at any time renders adrenal insufficiency unlikely. Serum cortisol should be measured at least 24 hours after the last dose of prednisone, prednisolone, or methylprednisolone, because these exogenous glucocorticoids interfere with measurements of serum cortisol.

The short 250-μg corticotropin stimulation test is the most widely used stimulatory test of the HPA axis and is easily performed. An important limitation of the corticotropin stimulation test is its failure to detect patients with isolated suppression of the hypothalamic-pituitary component of the axis (25% of glucocorticoid-treated patients in one series). The corticotropin-releasing hormone stimulation test reliably assesses all components of the HPA axis but is very expensive.

SUPPLEMENTAL THERAPY FOR PATIENTS STRESSED BY SURGERY OR INTERCURRENT ILLNESS

Patients who are receiving glucocorticoid therapy, or who were treated with glucocorticoids within the previous 12 months, are at risk for adrenal insufficiency when stressed by surgery or intercurrent illness. Most clinicians recommend empiric supplementation for adrenal insufficiency in these patients. Although this approach undoubtedly results in overtreatment, it is well tolerated, eliminates all risk of adrenal insufficiency, and is more feasible, and perhaps more cost-effective, than performing tests of the HPA axis (*JAMA.* 1999;282:671).

Supplemental doses of glucocorticoids are usually not necessary for mild, nonfebrile illnesses (eg, a "cold"). Prednisone doses should be increased to 15 mg/d for patients undergoing minor surgical procedures or with uncomplicated febrile illnesses; the dose can be returned promptly to baseline with resolution of the event. Patients with severe medical illness or major trauma or facing major surgery should be treated with hydrocortisone 50 mg intravenously or intramuscularly every 6 hours for several days; the dose can be tapered by 50% per day as the intercurrent event resolves. Patients with septic shock generally require a week of therapy before taper and may require supplementation with fludrocortisone as well (*N Engl J Med.* 1997;337:1285; *N Engl J Med.* 2003;348:727).

COMPLICATIONS

Virtually all complications of glucocorticoids are dose-dependent and increase with the duration of therapy.

- The risk of infection is substantial with prolonged high-dose therapy. The anti-inflammatory effects of systemic glucocorticoids can mask the signs and symptoms of infection, making diagnosis difficult. Systemic glucocorticoids cause the demargination of neutrophils, producing a peripheral leukocytosis in the absence of infection.

- Fat redistribution commonly produces a cushingoid appearance (truncal obesity, "buffalo hump," and "moon facies") in patients treated with moderate to high doses for prolonged periods but is unusual with low-dose therapy.
- The complex effects of glucocorticoids on carbohydrate metabolism can exacerbate hyperglycemia in known diabetics or induce clinically apparent diabetes.
- Proximal muscle weakness without elevations of muscle enzymes is a common, reversible side effect of high-dose glucocorticoids (eg, prednisone ≥30 mg/d for several weeks).
- Osteoporosis: See Chapter 57.
- Osteonecrosis: See Chapter 58.
- The risk of peptic ulcer disease is increased in patients receiving systemic glucocorticoids and concomitant nonsteroidal anti-inflammatory drugs.
- Striae, acne, and ecchymoses.
- Hypertension.
- Cataracts.
- Insomnia and mood disturbances are common. Severe side effects (eg, psychosis) can occur with high doses of glucocorticoids.
- Pseudotumor cerebri and pancreatitis are rare side effects.

DISCONTINUING THERAPY

The nature of the underlying disease, the activity of that disease, the use of glucocorticoid-sparing agents, the presence of comorbidities, and practice styles influence the rate at which glucocorticoid therapy is tapered; guidelines for tapering, therefore, are only approximate. For SLE and other diseases that require prolonged treatment with glucocorticoids, high doses (eg, 60–80 mg of prednisone daily) should be continued no longer than necessary and in general should be reduced to moderate levels (eg, 30 mg/d) after 6–10 weeks. Tapering from moderate levels to low doses (10–15 mg/d) can occur at a rate of 2.5 mg every week or 5 mg every other week. Most clinicians taper very slowly (1 mg per month) when the daily dose is 10 mg or less.

Tapering glucocorticoids can lead to flares of the underlying disease. In addition, when glucocorticoid doses are reduced to physiologic replacement levels (5–7.5 mg prednisone daily) or below, patients can develop symptoms from adrenal insufficiency or from the "steroid withdrawal syndrome." The latter, which manifests as myalgias, arthralgias, fatigue, and malaise, can mimic adrenal insufficiency or even a flare of the underlying disease; the HPA axis is intact, and the basis for the syndrome is not understood.

Following discontinuation of glucocorticoids, the time to recovery of the HPA axis varies widely (from days to 1 year).

KEY POINTS

- Glucocorticoids are widely used in the treatment of rheumatic disease.
- Toxicity is substantial and increases with dose and duration of treatment.

■ METHOTREXATE (MTX)

John B. Imboden, MD

MECHANISM OF ACTION

- Inhibits dihydrofolate reductase and other folate-dependent enzymes. Inhibition of dihydrofolate reductase accounts for its antineoplastic effects (fully reduced folate is required for DNA synthesis) and much of its toxicity (eg, mucositis and cytopenias).
- The mechanism of action in rheumatoid arthritis (RA) is unclear but may relate to the ability of polyglutamates of MTX to cause the release of extracellular adenosine, which has anti-inflammatory and immunomodulatory properties.

PHARMACOKINETICS

- Bioavailability of low-dose oral MTX: Generally high (mean 70%) but there is considerable individual variability (40–100%).
- 50–60% of MTX is bound to plasma proteins and can be displaced by aspirin and nonsteroidal anti-inflammatory drugs—not clinically significant for low-dose regimens used in rheumatology, but very important in high-dose chemotherapy.
- Metabolism: Can be metabolized to polyglutamated derivatives that are active and are retained intracellularly longer than MTX.
- Half-life: 3–10 hours for low-dose MTX.
- Clearance: MTX and metabolites are renally cleared (filtered and secreted).

USES IN RHEUMATIC DISEASES

Rheumatoid Arthritis

MTX reduces the signs and symptoms of RA and slows the rate of radiographic changes. It is the most commonly prescribed disease-modifying antirheumatic drug (DMARD) in the United States and is used as monotherapy or as the "anchor drug" in combinations with other conventional DMARDs or with anti–tumor necrosis factor agents.

Psoriasis

Although widely used for the treatment of psoriatic arthritis, low-dose weekly MTX has been studied in only one randomized controlled study (*Arthritis Rheum.* 1984;27:376), which showed a trend in favor of MTX compared with placebo. High-dose MTX is efficacious in psoriatic arthritis (Jones G, Crotty M, Brooks P. Interventions for treating psoriatic arthritis [Cochrane Review]. In: *The Cochrane Library,* Issue 1, 2003. Oxford: Update Software). MTX has been used to treat the skin disease of psoriasis since the 1950s.

Other Spondyloarthropathies

Although sometimes used in the treatment of reactive arthritis and ankylosing spondylitis, MTX has not been rigorously studied in these diseases.

Juvenile Chronic Arthritis

MTX is the most widely used DMARD for juvenile chronic arthritis, but data from controlled trials are limited (Takken T, Van der Net J, Helders PJM. Methotrexate for treating juvenile idiopathic arthritis [Cochrane Review]. In: *The Cochrane Library,* Issue 1, 2003. Oxford: Update Software).

Polymyositis & Dermatomyositis

MTX, sometimes in doses higher than those generally used in the treatment of RA, appears to be effective as an adjunct to glucocorticoid therapy and as a glucocorticoid-sparing agent. The combination of MTX and azathioprine probably has efficacy in refractory disease (*Arthritis Rheum.* 1998,41:392).

Systemic Lupus Erythematosus

MTX is superior to placebo in the management of articular and cutaneous manifestations of the disease and may have glucocorticoid-sparing effects (*J Rheumatol.* 1999;26:1275; *Lupus.* 2001;10:162).

Vasculitis

In an effort to minimize toxicity due to prolonged exposure to cyclophosphamide, MTX has been used to maintain remissions induced in antineutrophil cytoplasmic antibody (ANCA)-associated vasculitis by cyclophosphamide (*Arthritis Rheum.* 2002;47:326).

DOSING

- Given *weekly* as a single dose (can split dose over 24 hours if gastrointestinal symptoms occur).
- Usual starting dose is 7.5 mg orally every week.

- Dose can be increased by increments of 2.5–5 mg every 4–8 weeks until (1) there is a therapeutic effect, (2) the maximal dose is attained (generally 15–20 mg/wk in RA; higher doses are sometimes used in inflammatory diseases of muscle and psoriasis), or (3) toxicity develops. Some clinicians increase the dose to 15 mg/wk at week 4, and if there is no response, then to 20 mg/wk at week 8. Clinical responses generally occur after a lag of 3–6 weeks in RA.
- Because there is individual variability in bioavailability, many clinicians switch to parenteral administration (usually subcutaneous injection) of MTX before discontinuing for lack of efficacy.
- Use oral folate concomitantly (1 mg/d) to reduce side effects.

INITIATING THERAPY

- Before initiating therapy, the following laboratory tests should be obtained: CBC with platelets; serum electrolytes and creatinine; liver function tests (LFTs), including serum albumin; and tests for hepatitis B and C.
- Chest radiograph (particularly important for patients with underlying pulmonary disease).
- MTX is a hepatotoxin and should be used cautiously, and only after careful consideration of the alternatives to MTX and the risks of MTX, if the patient has a prior history of excessive alcohol consumption, persistently abnormal levels of transaminases, or chronic hepatitis B or C infection. Under these circumstances, a liver biopsy should be performed prior to starting MTX (*Arthritis Rheum.* 1994;37:316).
- Document the mode of contraception, if applicable.

MONITORING THERAPY (ADAPTED FROM *ARTHRITIS RHEUM.* 2002;46:328)

- CBC, creatinine, and LFTs monthly for the first 6 months and then every 1–2 months *as long as the patient is taking MTX.*
- For minor elevations in aspartate aminotransferase (AST) or alanine aminotransferase (ALT) (< twofold the upper limit of normal): repeat LFTs in 2 weeks.
- For moderate elevations in AST or ALT (> twofold but < threefold the upper limit of normal): closely monitor with LFTs every 2 weeks and reduce MTX dosage as necessary.
- For persistent elevations of AST or ALT (> two- or threefold the upper limit of normal): discontinue MTX and perform liver biopsy as necessary.

SPECIAL PRECAUTIONS

- Pregnancy is an absolute contraindication because MTX is an abortifacient and teratogenic. Adequate contraception (for male as well as female patients) is absolutely necessary while taking MTX. Women should not breastfeed while taking MTX.
- Cytopenias (except due to Felty syndrome), active liver disease, alcoholism, and active infections are contraindications to the use of MTX.
- Renal insufficiency reduces the clearance of MTX and its active metabolites and substantially increases the risk of toxicity. Other factors that predispose patients to MTX toxicity include dosing errors, advanced age, untreated folate deficiency, and the use of drugs that block tubular secretion (eg, probenecid and salicylates). Major surgery often leads to transient decreases in renal function and may predispose patients to toxicity.
- MTX should not be given to anyone with a history of "MTX lung" or any other allergic reaction to MTX.
- MTX therapy requires ongoing monitoring and should be used cautiously, if at all, in patients with records of poor compliance.
- Patients taking MTX should not receive live virus vaccines.

COMPLICATIONS

- Common toxicities (likely due to inhibition of dihydrofolate reductase) include gastrointestinal disturbances (nausea, vomiting, diarrhea, and anorexia), stomatitis, and cytopenias (especially leukopenia). An elevated mean corpuscular volume may presage hematologic toxicity. The incidence of these common toxicities is reduced by daily folate therapy.
- MTX lung is a hypersensitivity reaction that can develop at any time during therapy but occurs most often within the first year (50% within 32 weeks; *Arthritis Rheum.* 1998;42:1327). The onset is usually subacute (weeks) but can be acute (days) or chronic (months). Dyspnea, cough, fever, headache, and malaise are common complaints. Bilateral interstitial infiltrates are the classic radiographic findings, but alveolar infiltrates are not rare. The major diagnostic issues are (1) recognition of MTX as the cause of the symptoms and (2) ruling out infectious causes. MTX should be discontinued; most patients receive glucocorticoids.
- Hepatotoxicity correlates with total cumulative dose and manifests as fibrosis of increasing severity, culminating in cirrhosis. The mechanism is unknown. Clinically significant MTX-induced liver disease in appropriately selected patients with RA is very rare in the absence of abnormalities of either transaminases or albumin *when monitoring is performed regularly* (every 4–8 weeks).
- Other toxicities include reversible oligospermia, rash (including urticaria and cutaneous vasculitis), alopecia, accelerated nodulosis, dysphoria and headache,

infections (localized and disseminated zoster and opportunistic infections), and low-grade lymphomas.
- Overdoses should be treated as quickly as possible with leucovorin.

KEY POINTS

- MTX has established efficacy in RA and is commonly used in the treatment of other rheumatic diseases.
- MTX should only be administered in the form of weekly pulses; regular monitoring of CBC and LFTs is mandatory during therapy.

■ LEFLUNOMIDE (ARAVA)

John B. Imboden, MD

MECHANISM OF ACTION

- Activity requires conversion to the active metabolite, M1.
- M1 inhibits dihydro-orotate dehydrogenase, the rate-limiting enzyme for de novo pyrimidine synthesis, and thereby inhibits B and T lymphocytes, whose proliferation depends on the de novo pathway of pyrimidine synthesis.

PHARMACOKINETICS

- Bioavailability: 80%.
- Metabolism: Rapid metabolism to M1 following oral administration.
- Half-life: The half-life of M1 is approximately 2 weeks.
- Clearance: M1 is eliminated by biliary excretion (about 40%) and further metabolism and renal excretion (about 40%).

USES IN RHEUMATIC DISEASE

Rheumatoid Arthritis

In its ability to improve clinical outcomes and to delay radiographic progression, leflunomide is superior to placebo and comparable to sulfasalazine and to moderate doses of methotrexate (*Lancet.* 199;353:259; *Arch Intern Med.* 199;159:2542; *Rheumatology (Oxford).* 2000;39:655).

DOSING REGIMEN

- Because steady-state levels are not reached for 2 months, a loading dose of 100 mg/d for 3 days has been recommended. However, many patients experience gastrointestinal toxicity during loading, and most rheumatologists now forego loading and begin therapy with 20 mg/d.
- Maintenance dose: 20 mg/d (may be reduced to 10 mg/d if not tolerated).

INITIATING THERAPY

- Laboratory evaluation prior to initiating leflunomide should include CBC, serum creatinine, LFTs, tests for hepatitis B and C, and urinalysis.
- The possibility of pregnancy must be excluded prior to starting leflunomide.

MONITORING THERAPY (ADAPTED FROM *ARTHRITIS RHEUM.* 2002;46:328)

- CBC, creatinine, and LFTs monthly for the first 6 months and then every 1–2 months *as long as the patient is taking leflunomide.*
- For minor elevations in AST or ALT (< twofold the upper limit of normal): repeat LFTs in 2–4 weeks.
- For moderate elevations in AST or ALT (> twofold but < threefold the upper limit of normal): closely monitor with LFTs every 2–4 weeks and reduce dose of leflunomide.
- For persistent elevations of AST or ALT (> two- or threefold the upper limit of normal): discontinue leflunomide, eliminate leflunomide with cholestyramine, and perform a liver biopsy as necessary.

SPECIAL PRECAUTIONS

- Pregnancy is an absolute contraindication. Mothers should not breastfeed. Adequate contraception is required for female and male patients.
- Preexisting liver disease, obstructive biliary disease, excessive consumption of alcohol, and infection with hepatitis B or C viruses are contraindications.
- Because renal excretion is an important mechanism of drug elimination, leflunomide should be used cautiously, if at all, in patients with renal insufficiency.
- Leflunomide should not be used in the setting of severe immunodeficiency, active infection, or bone marrow dysplasia.
- Patients taking leflunomide should not receive live virus vaccines.
- Concomitant rifampin therapy, which increases leflunomide levels, is contraindicated.

COMPLICATIONS

- Gastrointestinal toxicity is common, especially within the first 2 weeks of therapy and may manifest as nausea and vomiting, abdominal pain, and diarrhea.

- Mild elevations (< twofold) in serum transaminases are common and often resolve on therapy. Elevations > threefold occurred in 2–4% of patients in initial clinical trials and reversed with discontinuation of leflunomide. There are post-marketing reports of severe liver disease temporally associated with leflunomide (see www.fda.gov).
- Rash and allergic reactions (including, rarely, Stevens-Johnson syndrome and toxic epidermal necrolysis).
- Reversible alopecia.
- Headache.
- Cytopenias appear to be rare.

DISCONTINUING THERAPY

Because of the unusually long half-life of leflunomide, drug elimination therapy with cholestyramine is recommended for (1) serious toxicity (eg, hypersensitivity reactions or liver toxicity) and (2) women of childbearing age who have stopped taking leflunomide. Serum levels of M1 should be documented to be <0.02 mg/L prior to attempts to become pregnant; unless cholestyramine elimination therapy is used, it can take up to 2 years for M1 levels to reach this level after the drug has been discontinued.

LONG-TERM CONCERNS

The risk of developing malignancy with long-term treatment is unknown but is increased with several other immunosuppressive therapies.

KEY POINTS

- Leflunomide is effective for the treatment of rheumatoid arthritis.
- Most physicians reserve leflunomide for patients with rheumatoid arthritis who have not responded to methotrexate.

■ SULFASALAZINE (SSA)

John B. Imboden, MD

MECHANISM OF ACTION

- SSA consists of salicylic acid joined to sulfapyridine (SP) by an azo bond.
- The mechanism of action is not certain; SSA may affect inflammatory mediators and may have immunomodulatory activity.

PHARMACOKINETICS

- Bioavailability: <15% of SSA is absorbed as intact drug. SSA undergoes cleavage by intestinal bacteria, releasing 5-aminosalicylic acid, which is poorly absorbed (bioavailability 10–30%), and SP, which is well absorbed (bioavailability 60%).
- Half-life: Serum levels of SP peak 10 hours after ingestion of SSA. SP, which is metabolized by acetylation, has a half-life of 10–15 hours depending on acetylation status.
- Clearance: SP and its metabolites are excreted in the urine.

USES IN RHEUMATIC DISEASE
Rheumatoid Arthritis

SSA is superior to placebo in control of disease activity (*J Rheumatol.* 1992;19:1672; *Arthritis Rheum.* 1993;36:1501) and slows radiographic progression (*Arthritis Rheum.* 2000;43:495). In short-term studies, SSA appears comparable to leflunomide and moderate doses of methotrexate. In long-term studies, leflunomide is superior to SSA in terms of clinical responses (*J Rheumatol.* 2001;28:1983), and the drop-out rate is higher for SSA than for methotrexate. The combination of SSA, hydroxychloroquine, and methotrexate is superior to methotrexate alone in patients with suboptimal responses to methotrexate (*N Engl J Med.* 1996; 334:1287).

Spondyloarthropathies

The superiority of SSA over placebo in the management of psoriatic arthritis and reactive arthritis has been demonstrated in controlled studies (*Br J Rheumatol.* 1996;35:664; *Arthritis Rheum.* 1996;39:2013; *Arthritis Rheum.* 1996;39:2021). In ankylosing spondylitis, SSA does not have efficacy in the treatment of disease of the axial skeleton but is superior to placebo in controlling the activity of peripheral arthritis (*Arthritis Rheum.* 1996;39:2004). SSA is widely used in the treatment of inflammatory bowel disease.

DOSING REGIMEN

- Start with a low dose (0.5 g/d or 0.5 g twice daily) and increase by 0.5-g increments at intervals of a week or more in order to reduce gastrointestinal side effects.
- Maintenance dose: 1 g twice daily.

INITIATING THERAPY

- Prior to initiating therapy: CBC, electrolytes, and creatinine; LFTs should be obtained.
- Determine glucose-6-phosphate dehydrogenase levels in persons at risk for glucose-6-phosphate

dehydrogenase deficiency (eg, males of African or Mediterranean descent).
- Advise patient that treatment for 4–12 weeks is required before benefit is observed.

MONITORING THERAPY

- CBC and LFTs every 2 weeks for the first 3 months of therapy; monthly for the next 3 months of therapy; and then every third month. Periodic urinalyses and determinations of serum creatinine.

SPECIAL PRECAUTIONS

- Contraindicated for patients with a history of allergies to sulfonamides, aspirin sensitivity, or hypersensitivity to SSA.
- Should be used cautiously, if at all, in patients with blood dyscrasias, liver disease, renal insufficiency, or severe asthma.
- Patients with glucose-6-phosphate dehydrogenase deficiency are at risk for hemolytic anemia.

COMPLICATIONS

- Gastrointestinal side effects (nausea, vomiting, dyspepsia, anorexia, and abdominal discomfort), headache and dizziness, and reversible oligospermia are common.
- Rash, pruritus, photosensitivity.
- Leukopenia (usually in the first few months but can occur at any time), thrombocytopenia, and hemolytic anemia.
- Hepatitis.
- Rare toxicities include aplastic anemia, agranulocytosis, and Stevens-Johnson syndrome.

KEY POINTS

- SSA has proved effective in the treatment of rheumatoid arthritis and the spondyloarthropathies.

ANTIMALARIAL DRUGS: HYDROXYCHLOROQUINE (PLAQUENIL) & CHLOROQUINE

John B. Imboden, MD

MECHANISM OF ACTION

- Raise the pH of acidic intracellular compartments such as endosomes and lysosomes.

- The mechanism of action of antimalarial drugs in treating rheumatic disease, however, is not clear.

PHARMACOKINETICS

- Bioavailability: Both drugs are well absorbed.
- Half-life: The drugs concentrate in tissues, and as a result have a long terminal half-life (50 days).
- Clearance: Approximately 50% of drug is excreted unchanged in the urine; another 25–30% is metabolized prior to renal clearance.

USES IN RHEUMATIC DISEASE

Discoid Lupus

Hydroxychloroquine and chloroquine have been used for decades in the treatment of discoid lupus and are considered effective.

Systemic Lupus Erythematosus

Hydroxychloroquine is widely used for the treatment of SLE. A controlled, double-blinded study demonstrated that withdrawal of hydroxychloroquine led to flares of disease (*N Engl J Med.* 1991;324:150).

Rheumatoid Arthritis

Hydroxychloroquine is superior to placebo for the treatment of relatively mild rheumatoid arthritis (*Am J Med.* 1995;98:156; *Arthritis Rheum.* 1995;38:1447) but is generally considered to be less effective than other commonly used DMARDs, such as methotrexate. The onset of action may be slow (up to 6 months). Hydroxychloroquine may be useful in combination with other DMARDs. For example, the combination of hydroxychloroquine, sulfasalazine, and methotrexate is superior to methotrexate alone in patients with suboptimal responses to methotrexate (*N Engl J Med.* 1996;334:1287).

DOSING REGIMEN

- Hydroxychloroquine: Initial therapy 400 mg/d; maintenance therapy 200–400 mg/d.
- Chloroquine: Initial therapy 500 mg/d; maintenance therapy 500 mg every other day.

INITIATING THERAPY

- Baseline ophthalmologic examination should be performed.

MONITORING THERAPY

- Ophthalmologic examination for retinal toxicity every 12 months.

SPECIAL PRECAUTIONS

- Hydroxychloroquine and chloroquine are contraindicated in persons with retinopathy due to any cause.

COMPLICATIONS

- In general, antimalarials are well tolerated and have the lowest incidence of side effects of DMARDs.
- Rash.
- Gastrointestinal side effects (dyspepsia, nausea, and vomiting).
- Headache, insomnia.
- Neuromuscular syndrome (uncommon) presents with proximal lower extremity weakness and can mimic steroid myopathy.

Ocular Toxicity

- Retinal toxicity: Irreversible retinal damage has occurred with long-term therapy and has been reported more with chloroquine than hydroxychloroquine. With regular ophthalmologic examinations and appropriate dosing, irreversible retinal damage should be rare.
- Extraocular muscle palsy producing diplopia.
- Corneal deposits.

KEY POINTS

- Antimalarial drugs are commonly used to treat discoid lupus and appear to be useful adjunctive therapy for SLE. In rheumatoid arthritis, they are generally reserved for mild disease or used in combination with other DMARDs.
- Although antimalarials are well tolerated relative to other DMARDs, regular monitoring for retinal toxicity is required. There are fewer reports of retinopathy associated with hydroxychloroquine, which as a result is preferred by many clinicians over chloroquine.

■ INTRAVENOUS IMMUNE GLOBULIN (IVIG)

Fiona A. Donald, MD

DEFINITION

- Pooled immune globulin from human plasma, 3000–10,000 donors per batch.
- Contains 95% IgG, <2.5% IgA, and trace IgM.
- IgG antibodies are directed against a wide variety of antigens.

- Contains trace amounts of soluble CD4, CD8, and human leukocyte antigen molecules.

MECHANISMS OF ACTION

Multiple mechanisms are likely, including the following:

- Modulation of Fc receptor function.
- Suppression of antibody synthesis.
- Direct inhibition of cytokines by naturally occurring anticytokine antibodies.
- Inhibition of superantigen-mediated T-cell activation.
- Inhibition of complement component binding and activation.

PHARMACOKINETICS

- Serum levels of IgG increase immediately postinfusion (fivefold increase with a dose of 2 g/kg) and then decrease by 50% after 72 hours due largely to equilibration between the intravascular and extravascular spaces.
- In-vivo half-life: Approximately 3 weeks.

USES IN RHEUMATIC DISEASE

Kawasaki Disease

Administration of IVIG within 10 days of onset reduces coronary artery involvement according to well-controlled trials (*N Engl J Med.* 1991;324:1633; *N Engl J Med.* 1986;315:341).

Inflammatory Myopathy

IVIG has demonstrated benefit in refractory adult dermatomyositis (DM). Uncontrolled trials suggest benefit in refractory adult polymyositis and juvenile DM. A double-blind, placebo-controlled trial of 15 patients with refractory adult DM demonstrated improvement in neuromuscular symptoms, muscle power, and rash in treated patients after one or two infusions. No patients in the placebo group showed improvement (*N Engl J Med.* 1993;329:1993). Ten patients with polymyositis and five with DM demonstrated improvement in muscle strength and creatinine kinase in an open trial of IVIG in 14 patients with polymyositis and 6 with DM. Improvement occurred after two infusions, with maximum benefit after four infusions (*Am J Med.* 1991;91:162). Due to cost considerations, it is unlikely that IVIG will become a first-line therapy for inflammatory myositis.

Systemic Lupus Erythematosus

The addition of IVIG to a standard treatment regimen for class III or IV lupus nephritis did not result in improvement in creatinine clearance or protein-uria according to a small randomized trial (*Lancet.* 1999;354:569). An uncontrolled trial of IVIG in 20 patients with SLE reported clinical benefit in 17 of 20 patients. Improvements were seen in arthritis, thrombocytopenia, fever, and neuropsychiatric manifestations (*Semin Arthritis Rheum.* 2000;29:321). Many case reports suggest that thrombocytopenia, psychosis, pleural effusions, carditis, and vasculitis due to SLE may respond to IVIG.

Other Vasculitides

Beneficial effects of IVIG in Wegener granulomatosis, Churg-Strauss syndrome, and microscopic polyangiitis have been suggested by case reports and small open studies. However, the only prospective randomized controlled trial of IVIG in Wegener granulomatosis and microscopic polyangiitis failed to show benefit in terms of reduced disease activity at 3 months versus placebo (*Q J Med.* 2000;93:433).

Rheumatoid Arthritis

IVIG is ineffective in adult rheumatoid arthritis. Two randomized controlled trials (*Arthritis Rheum.* 1996;39:1027; *Arthritis Rheum.* 1993;36[Suppl]:S57) failed to show benefit of IVIG over the placebo arm.

Antiphospholipid Antibody Syndrome

For recurrent fetal loss, the addition of IVIG to a standard regimen of aspirin plus heparin did not achieve statistical benefit compared with placebo in a randomized double-blind controlled trial of 16 patients (*Am J Obstet Gynecol.* 2000;182:122).

Other Uses

Efficacy of IVIG in managing idiopathic thrombocytopenic purpura, Guillain-Barré syndrome, and chronic inflammatory demyelinating polyneuropathies has been demonstrated in controlled clinical trials.

COMPLICATIONS

- Nonanaphylactic reactions (5–10%): Fever, chills, dyspnea, back pain, and modest hypotension. Treatment includes nonsteroidal anti-inflammatory drugs, antihistamines, and glucocorticoids.
- Aseptic meningitis: Occurs in up to 10% of patients 48–72 hours postinfusion; unrelated to underlying disease.
- Acute renal failure: Due to acute tubular necrosis; diabetes, preexisting renal disease, and advanced age are risk factors.

- Other (rare): Thromboembolic events due to increased serum viscosity.

SPECIAL PRECAUTIONS

- Contraindicated in patients with selective IgA deficiency due to the risk of anaphylaxis.

KEY POINTS

- IVIG is effective in the treatment of Kawasaki disease and refractory dermatomyositis and may have efficacy in polymyositis.
- IVIG has been used in a wide variety of rheumatic diseases. While its use may be warranted in patients with SLE and severe thrombocytopenia, the evidence to date does not support routine use of IVIG for SLE, rheumatoid arthritis, vasculitis other than Kawasaki disease, or the antiphospholipid antibody syndrome.

ABATACEPT (ORENCIA)

John B. Imboden, MD

STRUCTURE

- Abatacept is a recombinant receptor-IgG Fc fusion protein consisting of the extracellular domain of human cytotoxic T-cell–associated antigen-4 linked to the hinge, CH2, and CH3 domains of human IgG1.

MECHANISM OF ACTION

- Inhibition of T-cell co-stimulation: During the T-cell response to antigen, the T-cell molecule CD28 engages CD80 and CD86 molecules on antigen-presenting cells, and as a result of these interactions, delivers a co-stimulatory signal necessary for full T-cell activation. Abatacept binds CD80 and CD86, blocking their interactions with CD28 and preventing delivery of the CD28 co-stimulus.

PHARMACOKINETICS

- Bioavailability: Abatacept is administered intravenously.
- Average half-life: 13 days
- Clearance: The mechanism of clearance has not been determined. Methotrexate, nonsteroidal anti-inflammatory drugs, and glucocorticoids do not alter clearance. There have been no formal studies of the impact of liver disease or renal insufficiency.

USES IN RHEUMATIC DISEASE

The Food and Drug Administration has approved abatacept for the treatment of moderate to severe rheumatoid arthritis refractory to one or more DMARDs or to a tumor necrosis factor (TNF) inhibitor. The combination of abatacept plus methotrexate was superior to placebo plus methotrexate in a randomized, double-blind study of patients with rheumatoid arthritis and inadequate responses to methotrexate alone (*N Engl J Med.* 2003;349:1907). In a second randomized, double-blind study, the combination of abatacept plus a DMARD was superior to placebo plus DMARD for patients with rheumatoid arthritis unresponsive to TNF inhibitors (*N Engl J Med.* 2005;353:1114).

DOSING

Abatacept is given as an intravenous infusion over 30 minutes. Initial doses should be administered at 0, 2, and 4 weeks; thereafter, maintenance doses should be given every 4 weeks. Recommended doses are: 500 mg for patients with body weight <60 kg; 750 mg for patients 60–100 kg; and 1 g for patients >100 kg. Abatacept is supplied lyophilized as single-use vials of 250 mg that must be reconstituted using the silicone-free syringes provided by the manufacturer.

INITIATING THERAPY

- All patients should be tested for reactivity to purified protein derivative. Patients with suspected latent tuberculosis should be treated prior to the institution of abatacept.
- Abatacept should not be administered concurrently with TNF inhibitors or anakinra due to an increase in the risk of serious infection.

SPECIAL PRECAUTIONS

- Patients should be monitored closely for infection during the transition from treatment with a TNF inhibitor to abatacept. The half-life of the discontinued TNF inhibitor should be considered before initiating abatacept.
- Abatacept should not be used in the setting of active infection, and considerable caution should be exercised before administering abatacept to patients with a history of recurrent, chronic, or latent infections.
- Abatacept can lead to exacerbations of chronic obstructive pulmonary disease and should be used cautiously in this setting.
- Live vaccinations should not be administered during, or within 3 months of discontinuing, therapy with abatacept.
- Abatacept is pregnancy category C.
- Mothers should not nurse their infants while taking abatacept.

COMPLICATIONS

- Infection. Most frequently reported include upper respiratory infections, sinusitis, bronchitis, and pneumonia.
- Malignancy. The risk is not known.
- Infusion-related events and hypersensitivity reactions.
- Chronic obstructive pulmonary disease exacerbations.

DISCONTINUING THERAPY

- Abatacept should be discontinued for the development of serious infection, malignancy, or hypersensitivity to the drug.

KEY POINTS

- Abatacept has demonstrated efficacy for rheumatoid arthritis that is refractory to therapy with DMARDs and/or TNF inhibitors.
- Infections were the most common adverse events in clinical trials of abatacept.
- Abatacept should not be used in combination with TNF inhibitors or with anakinra.

■ CYCLOPHOSPHAMIDE (CYC; CYTOXAN)

John H. Stone, MD, MPH

MECHANISM OF ACTION

- Alkylates various cellular constituents, leading to DNA cross-linking and disruption of transcription and translation.
- Depletes both B and T cells (with perhaps a greater effect on B cells), impacting both humoral and cellular immunity.
- Affects both proliferating and resting cells.

PHARMACOKINETICS

- Bioavailability: Oral CYC is rapidly absorbed and has a bioavailability of >75%.
- Metabolism: Metabolized in the liver to 4-hydroxycyclophosphamide and aldophosphoramide. Aldophosphoramide is then converted to phosphoramide mustard (the active metabolite) and the non-alkylating metabolite acrolein. (Of note, acrolein is

the metabolite that leads frequently to bladder toxicity through its exposure to the bladder wall). Phosphoramide mustard, which is highly protein-bound, is distributed to all tissues (including the central nervous system). This active metabolite of CYC is secreted in breast milk and assumed to cross the placenta.

- Half-life: 2–10 hours; 95% is excreted by the kidney.
- Elimination: Both active and inactive metabolites are excreted unchanged in the urine, with elimination complete by 48 hours.

USES IN RHEUMATIC DISEASE

CYC is a life-saving intervention in some patients with organ- or life-threatening rheumatic disease. Its therapeutic index is narrow, however, so the drug must be used with great caution and strict monitoring. Systemic vasculitis, SLE, and systemic sclerosis are the diseases in which CYC is used most commonly. With some exceptions, there are no unequivocal data favoring one schedule (daily or intermittent) or route of administration (oral or intravenous) over another in a particular disease.

Systemic Vasculitis

For most forms of systemic vasculitis, daily CYC is the preferred regimen of choice, principally because the limited data available to date in Wegener granulomatosis suggest that daily regimens are more likely to lead to sustained remissions (*Arthritis Rheum.* 1997;40:2099). However, intermittent CYC regimens (eg, every month) are probably equally effective in the induction of remission in systemic vasculitis (*Nephrol Dial Transplant.* 2001;16:2018). Full results of a European trial comparing daily CYC to intermittent CYC are pending. Other considerations in the choice of administration schedule and route are discussed in the dosing regimen section.

A. WEGENER GRANULOMATOSIS

In the 1970s, CYC converted severe Wegener granulomatosis from an invariably fatal condition to one that can be controlled in most cases, albeit with risk of substantial toxicity and a high likelihood (>50%) of eventual flares following remission. The usual starting dose in young patients with normal kidney function is 2 mg/kg/d. Dose adjustments for renal dysfunction and advanced age are important (see below).

B. MICROSCOPIC POLYANGIITIS

Because of the high frequency of major organ involvement in microscopic polyangiitis (alveolar hemorrhage, rapidly progressive glomerulonephritis, mononeuritis multiplex, and mesenteric vasculitis), CYC is usually indicated from the start of therapy.

C. CHURG-STRAUSS SYNDROME

Eosinophils are typically exquisitely sensitive to glucocorticoids. Nevertheless, at least 50% of patients with Churg-Strauss syndrome eventually require CYC as well. Patients with severe disease manifestations, such as vasculitic neuropathy, should be treated with CYC immediately.

D. IDIOPATHIC POLYARTERITIS NODOSA

Approximately half of all patients with polyarteritis nodosa not associated with hepatitis B may be treated with glucocorticoids alone. The other half usually require CYC. Patients with severe disease features should be treated with CYC immediately.

E. RHEUMATOID VASCULITIS

Patients with rheumatoid vasculitis who have scleritis, peripheral ulcerative keratitis, mononeuritis multiplex, significant cutaneous ulcerations, digital gangrene, evidence of mesenteric vasculitis, or other serious disease manifestations should be treated with CYC. Although CYC is effective in treating the synovitis of rheumatoid arthritis, the potential adverse-effect profile of this medication serves as a contraindication to its use in this disease except in the setting of vasculitis (or severe ocular manifestations, which often correlate with vasculitis).

F. BEHÇET DISEASE

Posterior uveitis (retinal vasculitis) and significant central nervous system disease are usually indications for CYC.

Systemic Lupus Erythematosus

In contrast to systemic vasculitis, evidence-based data favoring the use of intermittent CYC do exist for SLE (*N Engl J Med.* 1986;314:614; *Ann Intern Med.* 1996;125:549). CYC is particularly important in the treatment of proliferative glomerular lesions of SLE nephritis (eg, World Health Organization class 4 disease and diffuse proliferative glomerulonephritis). (Mycophenolate mofetil is now often used in favor of CYC for lupus nephritis, however; see the section on that agent.) The traditional National Institutes of Health (NIH) protocol for the treatment of lupus nephritis with intermittent CYC calls for 6 monthly pulses, followed by 18 months of "consolidation" therapy in which the patient receives intravenous CYC every 3 months (times 6), for a total duration of therapy of 24 months. Because of the potential hazards associated with this regimen, shorter courses of CYC are often used now, followed by mycophenolate mofetil.

Immunoablative cyclophosphamide therapy, an investigational use of this medication given with hematopoietic stem cell transplantation (*JAMA.* 2006; 295:559), is not discussed in this chapter.

Inflammatory Myopathy

CYC is rarely the initial treatment of choice for inflammatory myopathies but is sometimes required for patients whose disease is refractory to such second-line agents as azathioprine, methotrexate, and intravenous immune globulin.

Scleroderma

CYC is often used in the treatment of interstitial lung disease that occurs as a complication of diffuse scleroderma (*N Engl J Med.* 2006;354:2655).

DOSING REGIMEN

Under most circumstances, daily administration corresponds to oral use and intermittent therapy to intravenous administration. For patients who cannot take oral medications (eg. intubated patients), CYC may be administered in small daily intravenous doses equivalent to what would be given orally.

- Daily use: In the setting of normal renal function, the usual starting dose for CYC is 2 mg/kg/d. Adjustments for both renal dysfunction and advanced age are essential. Table 67–4 shows an algorithm for the adjustment of CYC dose according to creatinine clearance.
- Intermittent use: The NIH protocol for the use of pulse intravenous CYC is shown in Table 67–5. Patients with creatinine clearances >30 mL/min may receive 750 mg/m² body surface area, with subsequent upward adjustments of the monthly dose if tolerated to a maximum of 1000 mg/m² (see below). Patients with creatinine clearances <30 mL/min (including dialysis patients) should receive 500 mg/m² body surface area. Hemodialysis patients should undergo dialysis 12 hours after CYC (*Kidney Int.* 2002;61):1495).

Table 67–4. Algorithm for Adjusting CYC Dose Based on Creatinine Clearance

Creatinine Clearance[a] (mL/min)	CYC Dose (mg/kg/d)
>100	2.0
50–99	1.5
25–49	1.2
15–24	1.0
<15 or on dialysis	0.8

[a]Creatinine clearance calculated by the Cockroft equation: $CL_{cr} = [12Q - age]/\text{serum Cr in mg/dL}$ (*multiplied by a factor of 0.8 for women*).
CYC, cyclophosphamide.

Table 67–5. National Institutes of Health Pulse Intravenous CYC Protocol

Dosage
Creatinine clearance >30 mL/min: initially 750 mg/m² BSA. May increase to a maximum of 1000 mg/m² BSA if tolerated. Creatinine clearance <30 mL/min: initially 500 mg/m² BSA.

Monitoring of WBC count after CYC administration (between days 8 and 12)
If WBC nadir <1500/μL, reduce subsequent dose by 25%. If WBC nadir >4000/μL, increase subsequent doses to a maximum of 1000 mg/m² BSA.

Preparation and infusion
Mix in 150 mL normal saline or D_5W. Infuse over 60 minutes.

MESNA administration
Each MESNA dose is 20% of the CYC dose. Infuse MESNA immediately before CYC and every 3 hours thereafter, for a total of 4 doses[a].

Antiemetic regimen
Dexamethasone 10 mg orally 3–4 hours after CYC. Ondansetron 4–8 mg intravenously or orally starting 4 hours after CYC, then every 4 hours × 3. Granisetron 10 μg/kg intravenously 30 minutes before CYC.

Diuresis
In patients with normal cardiac function, hydration with $D_5$1/2NS at 150–200 mL/h for a total of 2–4 L. Bladder irrigation may be used if patient unable to tolerate intravenous fluids.

[a]This is sometimes decreased to a total of two doses.
WBC, white blood cell; CYC, cyclophosphamide; MESNA, 2-mercaptoethane sulfonate.

MONITORING THERAPY

In theory, with regard to infection, daily CYC should be safer than intermittent CYC because of the "titration" of the dose that is possible with careful monitoring of the white blood cell count. However, compared with intermittent CYC administered for the same length of time, daily CYC results in substantially more total CYC. In practice, infectious complications with daily CYC appear to be at least as common as with intermittent CYC. The reality of CYC is that *both* routes are potentially hazardous, and patients receiving the medication via either route must be monitored carefully.

Guidelines for using daily CYC safely are shown in Table 67–6. The most critical point in monitoring patients on CYC is checking a complete blood cell count not less often than every 2 weeks. Patients whose cell counts are borderline (eg, white blood cell counts in the

Table 67–6. Guidelines for the Safe Use of Daily CYC

Limit duration of CYC use (ideally 6–12 months or less, followed by a conversion—if appropriate—to a less toxic second-line agent).

Instruct patients to take CYC in the morning.

Instruct patients to drink eight 8-oz glasses of water daily.

Adjust dose to maintain the total white blood cell count greater than 3500/μL.

Decrease the dose in the setting of renal dysfunction (including the elderly, whose glomerular filtration rate is lower than that of younger patients).

Check complete blood cell counts (with differential) and serum creatinine levels every 2 weeks (more frequently for those with borderline counts). Urinalyses should be performed monthly.

Monthly urinalyses. Patients should notify their physicians immediately if dysuria develops (unfortunately, not all cases of CYC-induced bladder injury are symptomatic).

Long-term surveillance for CYC-induced bladder injury.

Always use *Pneumocystis jiroveci* prophylaxis.

CYC, cyclophosphamide.

range of 4000/μL) may need to have labs checked more frequently. Even if patients appear to tolerate daily CYC well for several months, there is usually a gradual decline in the white blood cell count that eventually requires dose adjustments.

For patients receiving intermittent CYC, white blood cell counts are checked about 10 days after the pulse of treatment. If the white blood cell count is $<1.5 \times 10^6$/L, the next dose should be decreased by 25%. If the white blood cell count nadir is $>4.0 \times 10^6$/L, the next dose may be increased (but should not exceed 1000 mg/m^2).

SPECIAL PRECAUTIONS

- Pregnancy and breastfeeding are strictly contraindicated.
- Daily CYC should be administered in the morning, to reduce the likelihood of adverse bladder effects. The risk of bladder toxicity is heightened if acrolein is permitted to reside in the bladder overnight. Induction of a brisk diuresis helps avoid CYC-induced cystitis.
- Patients taking CYC daily should drink eight 8-oz glasses of water a day. Those receiving intermittent CYC should receive pre- and post-CYC intravenous hydration (see Table 67–5).
- 2-Mercaptoethane sulfonate should be administered to patients receiving intermittent CYC (see Table 67–5).
- Prophylaxis against *Pneumocystis jiroveci* pneumonia is important for all patients taking CYC daily. Single-

strength trimethoprim-sulfamethoxazole (1 tablet daily), dapsone (100 mg/d), atovaquone (750 mg bid), and other strategies may be appropriate. The consensus about the need for such prophylaxis among patients with SLE who are receiving intermittent CYC is not as strong, but such infections occur occasionally in SLE patients treated in this fashion as well. Because allergies to trimethoprim-sulfamethoxazole are more common in SLE, alternatives to this medication may be prudent (dapsone is often preferred).

- Some data suggest that the subcutaneous administration of gonadotropin-releasing hormone agonists (eg, lupron) 10–14 days before the administration of intermittent CYC may be useful in preserving the ovulatory status of young women (*Arthritis Rheum.* 2006; 54:1608).

COMPLICATIONS

In the longitudinal study from the NIH involving 158 patients with Wegener granulomatosis, 42% of those treated with daily CYC (for a mean period of 2 years) suffered permanent treatment-related morbidity (*Ann Intern Med.* 1992;116:488). The common complications of CYC include the following:

- Bone marrow suppression: Neutropenia is the most common adverse effect of CYC on the bone marrow, followed by thrombocytopenia and anemia.
- Infection: Opportunistic infection is believed to correlate with the degree and duration of neutropenia.
- Gastrointestinal effects (eg, anorexia, nausea, and vomiting): The gastrointestinal side effects of CYC are more common with intermittent dosing but can usually be controlled adequately with the aggressive use of antiemetics.
- CYC-induced cystitis: Can occur as early as within several weeks of CYC use. Many patients (but not all) complain of severe dysuria. The development of CYC-induced cystitis is an indication for the immediate cessation of this drug and is a strong relative contraindication to future use of CYC in any form.
- Malignancy: A long-term risk, correlated with the overall quantity of CYC exposure. Hematopoietic malignancies (eg, leukemia and lymphoma) and bladder cancers are the most common types of CYC-associated cancers. Some evidence suggests that the combination of CYC and tumor necrosis factor inhibitors should be used cautiously, because of heightened concern about the risk of solid malignancies with this combination (*Arthritis Rheum.* 2006;54:1608).
- Infertility: 57% of women of child-bearing age became infertile on the NIH regimen of CYC administration.

Males are also at risk for infertility, although the risk has not been quantified precisely. Among women, age and duration of CYC use are strong predictors of the development of anovulation/early menopause, with an 18-year-old woman being substantially less likely than a 36-year-old woman to suffer this complication.

- Hepatitis: A reversible form of hepatocellular injury with cholestasis occurs in a minority of patients with CYC.
- Pneumonitis: Interstitial pulmonary inflammation and fibrosis are rare complications of CYC.
- Hypersensitivity reactions occur rarely in CYC, but are reported to occur. These are associated with fever, "drug rash," myalgias, liver function test abnormalities, gastrointestinal symptoms, and hypotension, and may sometimes be confused with the underlying disease.

DISCONTINUING THERAPY

For most patients, CYC should not be viewed as a long-term medication for the maintenance of remission. The aim of therapy should be to discontinue CYC in favor of a less toxic therapy after 3–6 months of treatment. The exception to this is SLE nephritis, in which longer courses (up to 2 years according to the NIH protocol) are sometimes prescribed. Tolerance of the long-term treatment regimens is poor, even in SLE. When it is time to discontinue CYC, no tapering is required.

LONG-TERM CONCERNS

- Malignancy: Daily CYC use is associated with a 33-fold increase in the risk of bladder cancer (*Ann Intern Med.* 1996;124:477). Moreover, cases of bladder cancer may occur a decade or more after discontinuation of the medication. Thus, continued surveillance of the urine is essential. Urine cytologies are not sensitive for cancer. The best method of screening is with annual or semiannual urinalyses screening for nonglomerular hematuria. Periodic cystoscopy for patients with known CYC-induced bladder injury is prudent, albeit the link between clinically-evident drug-induced cystitis and subsequent bladder cancer is not proven. The long-term risk of other forms of cancer is also increased among patients treated with CYC.

KEY POINTS

- CYC remains an essential medication in the treatment of many severe forms of rheumatic disease.
- Because of its multiple potential short- and long-term side effects, patients on CYC must be monitored closely and the medication should be discontinued in favor of a less toxic agent as soon as possible.

■ CHLORAMBUCIL (CHL; LEUKERAN)

John H. Stone, MD, MPH

Because of its narrow therapeutic window, the short-term risk of significant bone marrow dysfunction, and the long-term risk of lymphoproliferative disease, CHL is now employed in the treatment of rheumatic disease only in patients who cannot take cyclophosphamide (CYC). The usual reason for CHL use is the development of CYC-induced cystitis. Because of its uncommon use in rheumatic diseases, most of the literature on this agent and rheumatic illnesses is several decades old.

MECHANISM OF ACTION

- An alkylating agent. Cross-links DNA, leading to the disruption of transcription and translation.

PHARMACOKINETICS

- Bioavailability: Rapidly absorbed orally, with a bioavailability of >80%. Peak plasma concentrations occur 30–70 minutes after ingestion.
- Metabolism: Converted to phenylacetic acid mustard and other metabolites.
- Half-life: 1.5–1.7 hours.
- Clearance: The active metabolite phenylacetic acid mustard is excreted nearly entirely by the kidney.

USES IN RHEUMATIC DISEASE

CHL is used occasionally in systemic vasculitis (Wegener granulomatosis, polyarteritis nodosa, and Behçet disease), SLE, and (very rarely now) refractory rheumatoid arthritis. CHL is generally a default treatment in rheumatic disease, used only in patients who cannot take cyclophosphamide.

DOSING REGIMEN

- The usual starting dose is between 0.1 and 0.2 mg/kg/d (ie, in the range of 6–10 mg/d).

INITIATING THERAPY

- Patients who get as far down in the treatment algorithm to warrant consideration for CHL therapy have usually been treated with ample quantities of other immunosuppressive agents before that time. Consequently, they may be more susceptible to CHL-associated bone marrow toxicity, and additional caution is advised.

MONITORING THERAPY

Complete blood cell counts should be obtained on a weekly basis for patients taking CHL. Bone marrow aplasia may develop very rapidly in these patients, justifying this frequent interval of monitoring. Thrombocytopenia may be a particular problem with CHL.

SPECIAL PRECAUTIONS

Pregnancy and breast-feeding are strictly forbidden in patients taking CHL.

COMPLICATIONS

Most of the potential adverse effects of CHL are very similar to those observed in cyclophosphamide. The major exception is that CHL, unlike cyclophosphamide, does not have a propensity to induce bladder injury.

- Bone marrow suppression: May occur more suddenly in comparison to cyclophosphamide.
- Infection: *Pneumocystis jiroveci* prophylaxis and vigilance for other possible opportunistic infections is essential.
- Gastrointestinal effects (eg, anorexia, nausea, and vomiting).
- Infertility.
- Malignancy: The risk of malignancy, particularly of acute myelocytic leukemia, is even higher than with cyclophosphamide.

DISCONTINUING THERAPY

CHL should be prescribed for as short a time as possible. Once it has achieved its intended effect of controlling a refractory disease manifestation, it should be replaced by another safer medication designed to maintain disease control.

LONG-TERM CONCERNS

- Malignancy: The long-term concerns about the induction of bone marrow malignancies are greater with CHL than with cyclophosphamide.

KEY POINTS

- The principal role currently for CHL in the treatment of rheumatic disease is as a fallback position for patients who cannot take cyclophosphamide.

- CHL is effective in many rheumatic conditions, but its substantial toxicity profile greatly limits its use.

■ AZATHIOPRINE (AZA; IMURAN)

Philip Seo, MD, MHS, & John H. Stone, MD, MPH

MECHANISM OF ACTION

- Inhibits purine synthesis through its metabolite, 6-mercaptopurine.
- Inhibits the proliferation of B and T lymphocytes.
- Reduces antibody production.
- Decreases interleukin-2 secretion.

PHARMACOKINETICS

- Bioavailability: 60% (oral).
- Metabolism: Metabolized by glutathione in red blood cells to 6-mercaptopurine.
- Half-life: 3 hours.
- Clearance: Inactivated in the liver, gastrointestinal tract, and red blood cells by several enzymes, including xanthine oxidase and thiopurine methyltransferase (TPMT). The metabolites are excreted in the urine.

USES IN RHEUMATIC DISEASE

AZA is commonly used as a second-line agent in rheumatic disease, particularly in glucocorticoid- or cyclophosphamide-sparing roles, and is only rarely used as a first-line agent.

Lupus Nephritis

The efficacy of AZA for the maintenance of remission in lupus nephritis was shown in a prospective study in which 20 patients with membranous lupus nephritis were treated with prednisolone and oral cyclophosphamide for 6 months, followed by 6 months of prednisolone and AZA (*Lupus.* 1999;8:545). At the end of 12 months, 85% of patients were in complete or partial remission.

This regimen may be efficacious for other forms of lupus nephritis as well. In a retrospective study of 55 patients with diffuse proliferative glomerulonephritis, 89% of patients treated with the sequential use of cyclophosphamide and AZA were in complete or partial remission at the end of 12 months. Sixty-three percent remained in remission after 5 years (*Arthritis Rheum.* 2002;46:1003).

Cyclophosphamide-containing regimens were shown to be slightly superior to a regimen that used AZA in a longitudinal study from the National Institutes of Health (*N Engl J Med* 2003; 349:36).

Systemic Lupus Erythematosus

Although AZA is used as a glucocorticoid-sparing agent for the treatment of other manifestations of SLE (including arthritis, serositis, anemia, and neuropsychiatric lupus), it has not been studied rigorously for these indications.

Inflammatory Myopathy

AZA ranks with methotrexate as the glucocorticoid-sparing agent of choice in inflammatory myopathy. In one randomized controlled trial, treatment of polymyositis with AZA and glucocorticoids led to better long-term function than treatment with glucocorticoids alone (*Arthritis Rheum.* 1981;24:45).

Rheumatoid Arthritis

AZA is more effective than placebo for the treatment of rheumatoid arthritis; because of its associated toxicity and the availability of alternatives, however, it is not used for this indication.

Scleroderma

Anecdotal reports suggest that AZA may slow the progression of the cutaneous and pulmonary manifestations of scleroderma, but its role in the treatment of this disease, if any, remains unclear.

ANCA-Associated Vasculitis

The efficacy of AZA for the maintenance of remission in patients with ANCA-associated vasculitis was examined in a prospective, randomized controlled trial involving patients with Wegener granulomatosis and microscopic polyangiitis. Patients were treated with oral cyclophosphamide and prednisolone for 3 months (after which more than 90% were in remission). They were then randomized to continued therapy with cyclophosphamide or with AZA, and their prednisolone dose was tapered to 5 mg/d for the remainder of the trial. After 18 months of follow-up, there was no difference in the rate of relapse (*N Engl J Med.* 2003;349:36).

Behçet Disease & Other Vasculitides

The addition of AZA to glucocorticoid treatment in patients with Behçet disease was shown to preserve vision better than glucocorticoids alone in a double-blind, placebo-controlled trial (*Arthritis Rheum.* 1997;40:769).

In other forms of vasculitis (eg, polyarteritis nodosa) AZA is commonly used as a second-line agent to maintain disease remissions and diminish patients' requirements for glucocorticoids.

Spondyloarthropathies

With the emergence of methotrexate, and more recently biologic agents for the treatment of inflammatory arthritis, the role of AZA in the spondyloarthropathies is quite limited.

DOSING REGIMEN

- 1–2.5 mg/kg daily.

INITIATING THERAPY

- Test TPMT enzyme activity before starting AZA therapy (see section on special precautions, below). This can be accomplished directly, by measuring erythrocyte TPMT activity, or indirectly, by screening for common TPMT allelic variants. Both genotypic and phenotypic tests are now commercially available.
- Even in patients with normal TPMT enzyme activity, it is prudent to begin AZA at low doses (eg, 50 mg/d orally for several days) to monitor for violent gastrointestinal intolerance.
- If the patient is not TPMT-deficient and tolerates the low dose without gastrointestinal upset, AZA may be increased quickly to the target dose.
- Patients who have partial TPMT deficiency may be treated with AZA, but the therapy must be initiated at low doses (50 mg/d) and increased only with careful monitoring of blood counts (ie, weekly complete blood counts until a safe dose is established).
- Patients who have complete TPMT deficiency should not be treated with AZA.

MONITORING THERAPY

Complete blood cell counts and liver function tests should be performed every 2 weeks until a stable dose is achieved, then every 4–6 weeks thereafter.

SPECIAL PRECAUTIONS

- Complete TPMT deficiency is an absolute contraindication to the use of AZA, because such patients cannot metabolize the drug. Approximately 1 individual in 300 is homozygous for mutant TPMT alleles. However, 11% of the general population are heterozygous (ie, have one functional TPMT allele), placing them at increased risk for many of the toxicities commonly associated with AZA (eg, bone marrow suppression, hepatotoxicity, and gastrointestinal intolerance). For such patients, lower doses and great caution are required (*Ann Intern Med.* 1998;129:716). When possible, patients who are heterozygous for the TPMT mutation should be treated with alternative agents.

- Sulfasalazine may inhibit TPMT, and should be used cautiously in patients receiving AZA. The use of other agents that contain sulfa moieties, such as trimethoprim-sulfamethoxazole, is not contraindicated.
- AZA is not teratogenic, and when necessary, can be used in pregnant women. Its use during pregnancy has, however, been associated with premature births and low birth weight.
- Allopurinol, an inhibitor of xanthine oxidase, slows the elimination of AZA and can lead to life-threatening myelosuppression. As a rule, these two drugs should not be used in the same patient.
- In renal failure (ie, a creatinine clearance of less than 10 mL/min), the dosage of AZA should be decreased by 50%.

COMPLICATIONS

- Bone marrow suppression is dose-dependent. AZA frequently causes leukopenia, or less commonly, thrombocytopenia, both of which generally resolve with dose reduction. In SLE, distinguishing cytopenias related to the disease from those induced by therapy can be challenging. A short course of glucocorticoids (eg, 20 mg/d) may help resolve the issue.
- Gastrointestinal effects (eg, anorexia, nausea, and vomiting) are common and may be ameliorated by splitting the dose, reducing the dose, or taking the medication with meals. For many patients with gastrointestinal intolerance to AZA, however, alternative therapies must be found.
- Hepatitis and pancreatitis may occur with AZA use. Both of these side effects are reversible following cessation of the drug. Cholestasis may require dose reduction.
- Hypersensitivity reactions (which are associated with fever, rash, myalgias, liver function test abnormalities, gastrointestinal symptoms, and hypotension) are occasionally seen during the first few weeks of therapy, and may be mistaken for a flare of the underlying rheumatic illness (*J Nephrol.* 2003;16:272).

DISCONTINUING THERAPY

AZA should be discontinued in patients in whom severe leukopenia, thrombocytopenia, or gastrointestinal intolerance develops.

LONG-TERM CONCERNS

- The association between AZA use and the development of nondermatologic cancers is controversial. Renal transplant recipients treated with AZA seem to have an increased risk of malignancy (including non-Hodgkin lymphoma, Kaposi sarcoma, and skin carcinoma), but an increased risk of cancer has not been reported in patients receiving AZA for rheumatoid arthritis or inflammatory bowel disease (*Aliment Pharmacol Ther.* 2002;16:1225).
- AZA is now known to sensitize DNA to ultraviolet A radiation, increasing patient risk of skin cancer (*Science.* 2005;309:1871).
- AZA is known to decrease spermatogenesis and sperm viability in rats. Its effect on male fertility in humans is not known.
- Patients treated with AZA may experience more frequent bacterial and viral infections.

KEY POINTS

- AZA is useful in the treatment of lupus nephritis and vasculitis, particularly following cyclophosphamide as a remission maintenance agent.
- It is also useful as an adjunctive medication in the long-term therapy of polymyositis.
- AZA has an increasingly limited role in the treatment of spondyloarthropathies.
- Because of the availability of better medications, AZA is not used in the treatment of rheumatoid arthritis.
- Genotyping for TPMT (or an equivalent functional assay) should be performed before the initiation of AZA.

■ MYCOPHENOLATE MOFETIL (MMF; CELLCEPT)

Philip Seo, MD, MHS, & John H. Stone, MD, MPH

MECHANISM OF ACTION

- Lymphocytes are dependent on the de novo synthesis pathway of purine nucleotides, which is catalyzed by inosine monophosphate dehydrogenase.
- MMF reversibly inhibits the type II isoform of inosine monophosphate dehydrogenase, which is preferentially expressed by activated lymphocytes.
- Inhibits the proliferation of B and T lymphocytes.
- Decreases antibody production.

PHARMACOKINETICS

- Bioavailability: 94% (oral).
- Metabolism: Hydrolyzed to mycophenolic acid in the gastrointestinal tract almost immediately after absorption.
- Half-life: 11.6 hours.
- Clearance: Mycophenolic acid is conjugated in the liver to a glucuronide, an inactive metabolite that is excreted in the urine and feces.

USES IN RHEUMATIC DISEASE

Lupus Nephritis

A 12-month course of MMF and prednisolone proved effective in achieving remission in patients with diffuse proliferative lupus nephritis in a randomized controlled trial (*N Engl J Med.* 2005;353:2219). MMF has been used successfully to treat other forms of lupus nephritis as well.

Systemic Lupus Erythematosus

Treatment with MMF reduced disease activity (and significantly decreased oral glucocorticoid dose) in a prospective study of patients with manifestations of SLE refractory to other immunosuppressive agents (including cyclophosphamide, azathioprine, and methotrexate) (*Rheumatology.* 2002;41:876).

Inflammatory Myopathy

There are three case reports of patients with polymyositis or dermatomyositis successfully treated with MMF (*Neurology.* 2001;56:94; *Dermatology.* 2001;202:341; *Muscle Nerve.* 2002;25:286). In a case series of four patients, MMF was effective in controlling the cutaneous manifestations of dermatomyositis (*J Rheumatol.* 2000;27:1542).

Vasculitis

MMF was used to maintain remission in nine patients with Wegener granulomatosis and two patients with microscopic polyangiitis in an unrandomized, open-label study (*J Am Soc Nephrol.* 1999;10:1965). In another study, MMF was noted to be well-tolerated as a remission maintenance agent in Wegener granulomatosis, but disease flares were common (*Arthritis Rheum.* 2004;51:278). Another case series described three patients with refractory Takayasu arteritis who responded well to treatment with MMF (*Ann Intern Med.* 1999;130:422).

OTHER USES

MMF is being studied for the treatment of the cutaneous manifestations of scleroderma. There is some limited evidence that MMF may be efficacious for the treatment of rheumatoid arthritis, although it is not used for this indication.

DOSING REGIMEN

- 1.5–3.0 g/d in divided doses.

INITIATING THERAPY

- Start with lower doses at first (eg, 500 mg orally at bedtime for several days), which may promote tolerance to the gastrointestinal side effects, then rapidly increase to the target dosage.
- Most patients will tolerate MMF if taken twice daily. Some patients experience fewer gastrointestinal side effects if the total daily dose is split among three or four smaller doses.

MONITORING THERAPY

- Complete blood cell counts should be performed after the first 2 weeks of therapy, then once a month for the first year of therapy.

SPECIAL PRECAUTIONS

- MMF may be teratogenic. Women should have a pregnancy test before starting therapy and use contraception during therapy.
- Aluminum and magnesium hydroxide antacids and iron supplements decrease absorption of MMF.
- The maximum dose of MMF in patients with chronic renal failure (glomerular filtration rate <25 mL/min) should not exceed 2 g/d. Dose adjustment for hepatic insufficiency is not necessary.
- Attenuated vaccines should be avoided during therapy. Killed vaccines (including influenza and pneumococcal vaccines) are not contraindicated.

COMPLICATIONS

- Patients may develop leukopenia, which usually responds to dose reductions.
- Gastrointestinal effects (such as anorexia, nausea, vomiting, and diarrhea) are not uncommon, and may improve if the total daily dose is taken as three or four smaller doses, distributed throughout the day. A reduction in the total dose may be required. Enteric-coated mycophenolic acid (Myfortic) may provide an alternative for patients who develop intractable gastrointestinal intolerance.

- In four randomized, controlled trials of MMF in renal allograft transplant recipients, none of the patients treated with MMF developed *Pneumocystis jiroveci* infection (*Clin Infect Dis.* 2002;35:53). When used in conjunction with high doses of glucocorticoids, however, the use of *P jiroveci* prophylaxis is prudent.

DISCONTINUING THERAPY

- Contraception should be continued for 6 weeks after MMF has been stopped.

LONG-TERM CONCERNS

- In the transplant literature, immunosuppression with MMF has been associated with an increased incidence of opportunistic infections (especially cytomegalovirus) and lymphoproliferative disease.
- The long-term risk to patients with rheumatic illnesses treated with MMF is less clear.

KEY POINTS

- MMF is effective in the treatment of diffuse proliferative lupus nephritis and may allow patients to avoid cyclophosphamide altogether for this indication.
- There are some data supporting the use of MMF in the treatment of other manifestations of SLE as well.
- Although used for a wide variety of indications, there are few data supporting the use of MMF in the treatment of inflammatory myopathies, vasculitis, or scleroderma. MMF is not used in the treatment of rheumatoid arthritis.

■ RITUXIMAB (RITUXAN)

John H. Stone, MD, MPH

STRUCTURE

- Rituximab is a genetically-engineered chimeric murine/human monoclonal antibody directed against CD20, an antigen found on the surface of normal and malignant B lymphocytes. The antibody is an IgG1 kappa immunoglobulin containing murine light- and heavy-chain variable region sequences and human constant region sequences.

MECHANISM OF ACTION

- Rituximab binds specifically to the CD20 antigen, a hydrophobic transmembrane protein located on pre-B and mature B lymphocytes. Among other potential

functions, CD20 regulates early steps in the activation process for cell cycle initiation and differentiation. The Fab domain of the molecule binds to the CD20 antigen. The molecule's Fc domain recruits immune mediators that lead to B-cell lysis. Potential mechanisms include complement-dependent cytotoxicity, antibody-dependent cell mediated cytotoxicity, and apoptosis induction.

PHARMACOKINETICS

- Bioavailability: Rituximab is administered via intravenous infusion at intervals of approximately 1 week.
- Average half-life: The mean serum half-life is approximately 76 hours after the first infusion and 206 hours after the fourth. Rituximab is still detectable in patient sera 3–6 months after the completion of treatment.
- Rituximab results in depletion of circulating and tissue-based B cells (albeit the extent of tissue B-cell depletion in humans is not defined precisely and is likely incomplete). In RA, patients demonstrate complete peripheral B-cell depletion within 2 weeks of the first rituximab dose. Most patients maintain peripheral B-cell depletion for at least 6 months and typically longer. A small proportion of RA patients (4%) have peripheral B-cell depletion that lasts more than 3 years.
- Reductions in immunoglobulin levels: Mean immunoglobulin levels remain normal in most patients. Small proportions of patients experience decreased immunoglobulin levels compared to normal: IgM (7% of patients); IgG (2%); IgA (1%). The clinical consequences of this are not clear.

USES IN RHEUMATIC DISEASE

Rheumatoid Arthritis

The Food and Drug Administration has approved rituximab for the treatment of RA patients who have had inadequate responses to at least one tumor necrosis factor inhibitor. Rituximab is approved for use with methotrexate in the treatment of RA. In patients with active RA despite methotrexate, two 1000-mg infusions of rituximab 1 week apart provided significant improvement in symptoms at both 24 and 48 weeks (*N Engl J Med.* 2004;350:2572).

Systemic Lupus Erythematosus

In an open-label longitudinal analysis of 24 patients with SLE who had failed conventional therapy, rituximab (accompanied by intravenous cyclophosphamide and methylprednisolone) was associated with improvements in the British Isles Lupus Assessment Group score and certain laboratory parameters of disease (*Rheumatology (Oxford)*. 2005;44:1542). Additional data related to the use of rituximab in SLE come from small case series and case reports. Randomized trials of rituximab in SLE are ongoing presently. Some evidence suggests that compared with RA patients, those with SLE are less likely to have complete B-cell depletion and more likely to develop human anti-chimeric antibodies (HACA).

ANCA-Associated Vasculitis

Rituximab has been studied in several case series (including *Arthritis Rheum.* 2005;52:1) and one phase I trial (*Am J Respir Crit Care Med.* 2006;173:180). In these studies, patients have been treated concomitantly with 1-g pulses of methylprednisolone. Tolerance of rituximab has been good in these two studies. All patients have achieved swift B-cell depletion and entered at least temporary remissions, able to discontinue prednisone by 6 months. Disease flares have recurred in some cases following the return of B cells and ANCA. Some patients have been retreated with rituximab, with apparently good results. The combination of rituximab plus glucocorticoids is now being compared against cyclophosphamide and glucocorticoids in a randomized, double-blind, double-placebo trial of remission induction.

DOSING

- In non-Hodgkin's lymphoma, the standard dose of rituximab is 375 mg/m^2, administered in four weekly intravenous doses. This dose is also the dose under study in ANCA-associated vasculitis. For other rheumatic diseases, however, a different regimen has been employed. In RA, the dosing regimen approved by the FDA is 1000 mg intravenously times two (doses separated by 1 week).

INITIATING THERAPY

- Patients' immunizations should be complete before the administration of rituximab. The impact of B-cell depletion on immunization status is an area of ongoing study. No live vaccines should be administered within 4 weeks prior to the infusion of rituximab.
- Reactivation of certain viruses (eg, hepatitis B, cytomegalovirus, varicella-zoster, and herpes simplex) has been reported in patients with lymphoma receiving rituximab. It is recommended that the patient's hepatitis B and C status be checked before administering rituximab.
- In RA, rituximab is administered with a "mini-pulse" of methylprednisolone (100 mg) within 24 hours of the rituximab infusion. This glucocorticoid infusion is believed to help avoid infusion reactions that are commonly associated with rituximab. In ANCA-associated vasculitis, higher doses of glucocorticoids

have been employed: between 1 and 3 days of methylprednisolone (1 g/d) prior to rituximab, followed by daily prednisone tapered over approximately 6 months. Various glucocorticoid regimens have been employed in SLE.
- No published data are available currently about the combined use of rituximab and other biologic agents in rheumatic disease.

SPECIAL PRECAUTIONS

- Patients should be monitored closely for infection while on rituximab, particularly in view of the fact that such patients typically have been treated with other immunosuppressive agents at other points in their course.
- Rituximab should not be used in the setting of active infection, and considerable caution should be exercised before administering rituximab to patients with a history of recurrent, chronic, or latent infections.
- Rituximab is pregnancy category C.
- Mothers should not nurse their infants while taking rituximab.

COMPLICATIONS

The rituxmab label currently contains three WARNINGS:

1. Fatal infusion reactions within 24 hours. These infusion reactions followed complexes of signs and complications, including hypoxia, pulmonary infiltrates, acute respiratory distress syndrome, myocardial infarction, ventricular fibrillation, and cardiogenic shock. Eighty percent of such infusion reactions have occurred in association with the first infusion, with time to onset between 30 minutes and 2 hours.

    Severe infusion reactions of this nature are very rare. Far more common than severe infusion reactions are the much milder hypersensitivity reactions, accompanied by hypotension, a "scratchy" sensation in the throat, and bronchospasm may require temporary interruption of the infusion and continuation at a slower rate. Mild infusion reactions are often avoided or attenuated through the use of glucocorticoids (100–1000 mg), acetaminophen (650 mg), diphenhydramine (50 mg), and intravenous hydration prior to rituximab infusion.

2. Tumor lysis syndrome leading to acute renal failure. This has only been reported in non-Hodgkin's lymphoma patients treated with rituximab.

3. Severe mucocutaneous reactions. Fatal reactions have been reported, including Stevens-Johnson syndrome.

- Reactivation of hepatitis B with fulminant hepatitis, hepatic failure, and death has been reported in patients with hematologic malignancies treated with rituximab. Hepatitis B carrier status is not a contraindication to rituximab use, but patients with hepatitis B should be monitored closely for signs of active hepatitis B infection.
- Infections. Rituximab should be employed with caution in individuals who have histories of deep infections.
- HACA formation. Approximately 5% of RA patients treated with rituximab develop HACA, usually by week 24 following treatment initiation. Limited data are available on the safety or efficacy of rituximab retreatment in patients who develop HACA.

DISCONTINUING THERAPY

- Rituximab should be discontinued for the development of a severe infusion reaction or severe infection.

KEY POINTS

- Rituximab is approved for use in RA patients whose treatment responses to TNF inhibitors have been suboptimal. Studies of the use of this agent in other rheumatic diseases are ongoing.
- The medication should be administered in a controlled setting because of the risk of infusion reactions (severe ones are rare) and hypersensitivity reactions (common, but usually mild).
- The side-effect profile of this agent is generally favorable.

ALLOPURINOL

David B. Hellmann, MD

MECHANISM OF ACTION

- Blocks the production of uric acid by inhibiting the enzyme xanthine oxidase, which catalyzes the conversion of hypoxanthine to xanthine and of xanthine to uric acid. Thus, allopurinol reduces the level of uric acid in serum and urine.

PHARMACOKINETICS

- Bioavailability: High (80–90%) for oral allopurinol.
- Serum uric acid levels begin to fall slowly 24–48 hours after starting allopurinol.
- Metabolism: Metabolized to oxypurinol.
- Half-life: 1–3 hours for allopurinol and 18–30 hours for oxypurinol.
- Clearance: Allopurinol and metabolites are cleared by the kidney.

USES IN RHEUMATIC DISEASES

Gout

Allopurinol can help prevent recurrent attacks of gout by reducing serum uric acid levels (*N Engl J Med.* 1996;334:445). Since allopurinol has no anti-inflammatory effects, it has no role in the treatment of acute gouty arthritis. Allopurinol is indicated for treating patients who have the following: (1) recurrent gout attacks not prevented by or amenable to treatment with uricosuric agents, (2) tophi, or (3) renal uric acid stones. Because of its possible serious side effects, allopurinol is not indicated in the treatment of asymptomatic hyperuricemia.

DOSING

- Because abrupt changes in serum urate levels can provoke gout, allopurinol is usually initiated at 100 mg orally each day, and increased by 100 mg weekly until the serum uric acid level falls below 6 mg/dL or until the maximum recommended daily dose (800 mg) is reached.
- Colchicine (0.6 mg/d orally) is often administered during the first 6 months of allopurinol treatment to reduce the chance of provoking a gout flare when serum urate levels fall.
- After months or years of treatment, a smaller dose of allopurinol may be required to achieve the target serum uric acid level.
- The usual maintenance dose of allopurinol in most patients with normal renal function is 300 mg/d administered as a single daily dose.
- In the absence of side effects, allopurinol should be continued indefinitely. Intermittent use of allopurinol is a major cause of treatment failure.
- Doses greater than 300 mg should be given in divided doses.
- Because allopurinol is chiefly renally excreted, the dose must be reduced for renal insufficiency. Recommended maintenance doses of allopurinol are 200 mg/d for a creatinine clearance of 10–20 mL/min, and no more than 100 mg/d for a creatinine clearance less than 10 mL/min. Indeed, some clinicians recommend reducing allopurinol to 100 mg every 3 days when the creatinine clearance is 0 mL/min.

INITIATING THERAPY

- CBC with platelets, serum electrolytes, and creatinine; LFTs; and serum uric acid should be performed.

MONITORING THERAPY

- CBC counts, LFTs, and renal function tests should be monitored periodically, especially during the first few months of treatment.
- Serum uric acid level should be checked periodically during the first months of therapy to determine the dose of allopurinol needed to reduce the serum uric acid to less than 6.0 mg/dL.

SPECIAL PRECAUTIONS

General

- Allopurinol is contraindicated in persons who have had a previous severe hypersensitivity reaction.
- Hypersensitivity to allopurinol can cause life-threatening or fatal cutaneous reactions (including toxic epidermal necrolysis, vasculitis with desquamatous and exfoliative dermatitis accompanied by multiorgan failure). Allopurinol hypersensitivity may also cause severe hepatic reactions including elevations of LFTs accompanied by fever, eosinophilia, and rash. Allopurinol should be stopped immediately if a hypersensitivity reaction is suspected.

Drug Interactions

- The simultaneous use of allopurinol and azathioprine or mercaptopurine should be avoided or approached with great caution. Allopurinol inhibits the catabolism of azathioprine and mercaptopurine by xanthine oxidase and thereby increases their effect on bone marrow suppression. If concomitant use of allopurinol and azathioprine cannot be avoided, then the usual azathioprine dose should be reduced by 75% and the patient's CBC count should be monitored carefully.
- By an unknown mechanism, allopurinol can increase the risk of cytopenia from cyclophosphamide.
- Concomitant use of allopurinol and ampicillin or amoxicillin increases the risk of developing rash.
- Allopurinol increases the half-life of dicumarol.
- Concomitant use of diuretics and allopurinol may increase the risk of allopurinol toxicity.

COMPLICATIONS

- Approximately 2% of patients experience minor reactions to allopurinol (*N Engl J Med*. 2003;349:1647).

More severe hypersensitivity reactions chiefly affecting skin and liver occur rarely but can be life-threatening (see above).
- The most common complication of allopurinol is a maculopapular rash. Nausea, vomiting, diarrhea, or other gastrointestinal effects develop more infrequently in the absence of hypersensitivity reactions. Hematologic effects are rare except in patients taking myelosuppressive drugs (see above).
- Management of all hypersensitivity reactions includes immediately stopping allopurinol. The drug cannot be restarted in patients who have had severe hypersensitivity reactions. About half the patients with mild hypersensitivity reactions can be desensitized to allopurinol. The desensitization protocol involves reintroducing minute doses of allopurinol orally and increasing the dose gradually while monitoring the patient closely (*N Engl J Med*. 2003;349:1647). Febuxostat, a novel xanthine oxidase inhibitor that has not yet received FDA approval, could be used in patients who cannot tolerate allopurinol (*N Engl J Med*. 2005;353:2450).

KEY POINTS

- Allopurinol is effective in preventing reoccurrence of gout by inhibiting the production of uric acid.
- Because of (rare) fatal hypersensitivity reactions, allopurinol should be used cautiously in patients with gout and should not be used to treat asymptomatic hyperuricemia.

▪ COLCHICINE

David B. Hellmann, MD

MECHANISM OF ACTION

- Colchicine inhibits phagocytosis of urate crystals by neutrophils by impairing microtubule function.
- Colchicine has other broader anti-inflammatory effects: The drug impairs neutrophil metabolism, chemotaxis, and motility, and inhibits the release of chemotactic factor.
- In addition, colchicine interferes with the secretion of serum amyloid A protein, which is found in amyloid deposits in patients with familial Mediterranean fever.
- Toxic effects of colchicine may be related to its ability to inhibit cell division by interfering with the mitotic spindle.

PHARMACOKINETICS

- Orally administered colchicine is absorbed from the gastrointestinal system, partially metabolized by the liver, secreted in bile, and then partially reabsorbed. This enterohepatic circulation of colchicine helps account for the frequent gastrointestinal toxicity of orally administered colchicine.
- Colchicine is concentrated in leukocytes, where the half-life of the drug is 60 hours.
- Colchicine is eliminated chiefly in feces and to a lesser degree in urine.

USES IN RHEUMATIC DISEASES

Colchicine is approved by the Food and Drug Administration for the treatment of gout. However, it is not approved for familial Mediterranean fever, sarcoidosis arthropathy, pseudogout, Behçet disease, or other uses in rheumatic diseases.

Gout

Colchicine has two uses in gout. First, colchicine in high doses (see below) is an effective treatment for acute gouty arthritis. Second, colchicine in lower doses (see below) is frequently used as prophylaxis against recurrent attacks of gout (*N Engl J Med*. 1996;334:445).

Familial Mediterranean Fever

Colchicine helps prevent recurrent attacks of familial Mediterranean fever. Daily colchicine therapy also reduces the risk of systemic amyloidosis, a common complication of untreated familial Mediterranean fever (*N Engl J Med*. 2001;345:1748).

Sarcoidosis Arthropathy

Acute arthritis from sarcoidosis may respond to colchicine (*N Engl J Med*. 1960;263:778; *Arch Intern Med*. 1963;112:924).

Pseudogout

Colchicine is inconsistently effective in treating pseudogout.

Behçet Disease

In doses of 0.5–1.5 mg/d orally, colchicine has been effective as first-line therapy for the following manifestations of Behçet disease: oral ulcers, genital ulcers, and pseudofolliculitis (*N Engl J Med*. 1999;341:1284).

Other Uses in Rheumatic Diseases

Colchicine has been used to treat cutaneous manifestations of scleroderma, primary biliary cirrhosis, Sweet syndrome, and palmar fibromatosis.

DOSING

For prophylaxis against gout:

- Given as 0.6 mg orally once per day.
- Some patients may require 1.2–1.8 mg/d in divided doses to prevent recurrent gouty arthritis.
- The daily dose should not exceed 0.6 mg for those with renal insufficiency.

For treatment of acute gout:

- Usually given orally as 1 mg initially, followed by 0.5–0.6 mg orally every 1–2 hours until the patient improves or until abdominal discomfort or diarrhea develops or a total dose of 8 mg has been administered.
- Can be administered intravenously if oral dosing is not possible, but intravenous administration requires special precautions (see below).
- The usual initial intravenous dose is 2 mg diluted in 20–50 mL of normal saline and administered over 20 minutes through a well-functioning catheter (to avoid extravasation). Subsequent doses of 0.5–0.6 mg every 6 hours may be administered until the patient improves or until a cumulative dose of 4 mg is reached.
- Because of the risk of toxicity, intravenous colchicine should be avoided in a patient taking oral colchicine.
- Colchicine should never be administered subcutaneously or intramuscularly because doing so causes severe local irritation.

MONITORING THERAPY

- Serum creatinine and liver function tests should be checked before starting colchicine.

SPECIAL PRECAUTIONS

- Colchicine is contraindicated in patients with serious gastrointestinal, cardiac, or renal disease.
- Colchicine is contraindicated in patients with both renal and liver disease or failure.
- Colchicine is contraindicated in patients with blood dyscrasia or with a history of hypersensitivity reactions to the drug.
- Intravenous colchicine should be avoided or used with extreme caution because it can result in fatal bone marrow and multiorgan failure, especially when the

recommended doses are exceeded or when the patient has renal and/or liver insufficiency.

- Oral daily colchicine should not exceed 0.6 mg in patients who are over the age of 60 and/or have an elevated serum creatinine. Colchicine-induced neuromyopathy occurs most frequently in patients with renal insufficiency. Oral colchicine should generally be avoided in patients requiring hemodialysis.
- Fertile women should avoid colchicine unless they are using effective contraception. Colchicine is teratogenic in animals and may be unsafe during pregnancy for humans.

COMPLICATIONS

- Oral colchicine most commonly causes abdominal discomfort, nausea, and diarrhea. If these side effects develop, the drug should be stopped; once the gastrointestinal symptoms have resolved, the drug can be cautiously restarted at a lower dose. Gastrointestinal manifestations do not usually develop after the recommended dose of intravenous colchicine.
- Neuromyopathy may complicate long-term daily colchicine use. The clinical presentation resembles polymyositis with proximal muscle weakness and creatinine kinase (CK) enzyme elevations. Neuromyopathy requires stopping colchicine.
- Intravenous colchicine, especially at higher-than-recommended doses, can cause pancytopenia.

KEY POINTS

- Low-dose, daily colchicine effectively reduces recurrent episodes of gout.
- The high risks of intravenous colchicine limit its usefulness.

■ ANTI–TUMOR NECROSIS FACTOR AGENTS

Jonathan Graf, MD

FDA APPROVED MEDICATIONS

- Etanercept (Enbrel)
- Infliximab (Remicade)
- Adalimumab (Humira)

STRUCTURE

- Etanercept is a recombinant, dimeric fusion protein consisting of the soluble human p75 TNF receptor coupled to the Fc fragment of human IgG1 lacking the C_H1 domain.
- Infliximab is a "humanized" monoclonal antibody in which the antigen-binding regions of a mouse anti-TNF monoclonal antibody have been placed in the framework of a human IgG1 kappa antibody.
- Adalimumab is a recombinant, fully human monoclonal IgG1 kappa antibody.

MECHANISM OF ACTION

- TNF-α and TNF-β are cytokines that regulate a wide array of biological functions necessary for normal inflammatory and immune responses.
- TNF-α, through its binding to membrane-bound TNF receptors, mediates many of the proinflammatory processes implicated in inflammatory arthritis.
- Etanercept binds soluble TNF-α and TNF-β and prevents their association with cell-surface receptors.
- Both infliximab and adalimumab bind soluble as well as membrane-bound TNF-α and block cell signaling through TNF receptor pathways.

PHARMACOKINETICS

- Bioavailability: Etanercept (subcutaneous) 60%, adalimumab (subcutaneous) 64%. Infliximab is administered intravenously.
- Average half-life: Etanercept 4.25 days; infliximab 8–12 days; adalimumab 14 days.
- Clearance: The exact mechanisms of clearance for etanercept, infliximab, and adalimumab have not been definitively determined, although the reticuloendothelial system may play a role. No formal studies have been done to determine the effects of hepatic or renal impairment on clearance.

USES IN RHEUMATIC DISEASE
Rheumatoid Arthritis

Etanercept has been studied in diverse populations of adult patients with active RA, including patients with active RA despite previous therapy with at least one DMARD (*N Engl J Med.* 1997;337:141; *Ann Intern Med.* 1999;130:478) and DMARD-naïve patients with early RA (*N Engl J Med.* 2000;343:1586). Etanercept is superior to placebo as either monotherapy or add-on therapy with methotrexate (*N Engl J Med.* 1999;340:253) in relieving many of the signs and symptoms associated with RA.

In patients with active RA despite treatment with methotrexate, infliximab is superior to placebo in reducing the signs and symptoms of disease when given in concert with methotrexate (*N Engl J Med.* 2000;343:1594).

Adalimumab has been studied as monotherapy and in combination with methotrexate (*Arthritis Rheum.* 2003;48:35) and other DMARDS. It has also been studied in patients who have failed at least one previous DMARD, remained on stable doses of current DMARD therapy, or are DMARD-naíve. In all populations, adalimumab is superior to placebo in controlling the signs and symptoms of RA.

Etanercept (*Arthritis Rheum.* 2002;46:1443), infliximab (*N Engl J Med.* 2000;343:1594), and adalimumab (*Ann Rheum Dis.* 2002;61:311) have been shown to slow or inhibit the radiographic progression of joint destruction in rheumatoid arthritis.

Psoriatic Arthritis

All three of these anti-TNF agents are approved by the FDA for the treatment of psoriatic arthritis. Each has demonstrated efficacy as monotherapy in randomized, placebo-controlled studies (*Lancet.* 2000;356: 385; *Arthritis Rheum.* 2005;52:3279; *Arthritis Rheum.* 2005;52:1227; *Ann Rheum Dis.* 2005;64:1150).

Ankylosing Spondylitis

Etanercept and infliximab are both approved for managing the signs and symptoms of ankylosing spondylitis based on several published studies (*Arthritis Rheum.* 2005;52:582; *Ann Rheum Dis.* 2005;64:1557; *N Engl J Med.* 2002;346:1349; *Lancet.* 2002;359:1187).

Other Spondyloarthropathies

Small, open label studies suggest that etanercept and infliximab have efficacy in the treatment of undifferentiated spondyloarthropathy and reactive arthritis (*Arthritis Rheum.* 2005;53:613; *J Rheumatol.* 2002;29:118) and the axial and peripheral arthritis associated with inflammatory bowel disease (*Lancet.* 2000;356:1821). However, none of the anti-TNF agents have been rigorously studied in prospective, double-blinded placebo controlled studies for these diseases.

Juvenile Idiopathic Arthritis

Etanercept is the only anti-TNF agent to be approved by the FDA for the treatment of juvenile idiopathic arthritis. It has been rigorously studied in both short- and long-term clinical trials and has been found to be efficacious when used as monotherapy or as an addition to treatment with methotrexate (*N Engl J Med.* 2000;342:763).

Adult Still Disease

A small open-label study suggests that etanercept may reduce the signs and symptoms of adult Still disease (*Arthritis Rheum.* 2002;46:1171).

Wegener Granulomatosis

A large randomized study of etanercept added to standard therapy for Wegener granulomatosis (*N Engl J Med.* 2005;352:351) demonstrated no additional efficacy in maintaining remission.

DOSING

- Etanercept: Given either as a single, 50-mg injection once weekly or as a 25-mg subcutaneous injection twice weekly. Must be refrigerated and reconstituted in sterile solution before being administered.
- Infliximab: Infusion is given in a doctor's office or infusion center and takes approximately 2–3 hours to complete. Administered as an intravenous infusion beginning with a loading dose of 3 mg/kg at 0, 2, and 6 weeks. Dosing is usually maintained at 3 mg/kg every 8 weeks. Flexibility in dosing allows for the dose to be increased up to 10 mg/kg and/or the interval decreased to as little as every 4 weeks, depending on response to therapy.
- Adalimumab: Given as a single, 40-mg subcutaneous injection once every other week. Medication comes preloaded in a syringe, does not need to be reconstituted, and should be refrigerated before use. Dosing flexibility allows the medication to be given as often as 40 mg every week as clinical conditions warrant.

INITIATING THERAPY

- The risk of reactivation of latent tuberculosis should be assessed and should include, at a minimum, a baseline purified protein derivative prior to initiation of therapy. Many physicians obtain a chest radiograph as well.
- The risk of latent histoplasmosis and coccidioidomycosis infection should be considered in patients from endemic regions.
- No baseline or routine laboratory testing is officially recommended.
- Age-appropriate cancer screening, while not officially recommended, may be of benefit prior to initiating therapy.
- Patients are recommended not to receive live vaccinations after initiating or continuing therapy.
- Patients should be monitored for injection site or infusion reactions while receiving therapy.
- Anti-TNF agents should not be used in patients with a history of multiple sclerosis of any other demyelinating disease.

SPECIAL PRECAUTIONS

- TNF antagonists should not be used in patients with a history of latent tuberculosis unless they have completed an adequate course of prophylactic therapy.

- The TNF antagonists are contraindicated in patients with active acute or chronic infections.
- Patients receiving infliximab should have baseline screening for infection, including temperature and symptom assessment, prior to each infusion.
- Patients should be instructed to contact their physician if any symptoms of acute infection develop.
- The anti-TNF agents should not be used in patients with active or suspected malignancies.
- Hypersensitivity to an anti-TNF agent is a contraindication to its use.
- Patients with previous allergies to mouse-derived products should not receive infliximab.
- All anti-TNF agents are pregnancy category B.
- The use of anti-TNF agents in the setting of hepatic disease or renal failure has not been studied.
- Infliximab is specifically contraindicated in patients with moderate or severe congestive heart failure; extreme caution should be exercised for the other anti-TNF agents in this setting.

COMPLICATIONS

- Post-marketing surveillance of these agents has reported hospitalizations and deaths from serious infections, although randomized trials have not demonstrated an increased frequency of serious infections
- Blockade of TNF poses a theoretical risk of increased malignancy. There are post-marketing reports of lymphomas developing in patients treated with either etanercept or infliximab, but it remains to be determined if there is an actual increase in the incidence of malignancy.
- Etanercept and adalimumab are associated with a high degree of mild to moderate injection site reactions, including erythema, pruritus, pain, and/or swelling, reactions which are commonly self-limiting, early in the course of therapy.
- Infliximab is associated with a significant incidence of infusion reactions within 1–2 hours after receiving the therapy, including fever, chills, urticaria, and cardiopulmonary symptoms.
- Infliximab has been linked to a serum-sickness type of syndrome.
- The use of the anti-TNF agents, especially infliximab, can lead to the development of antibodies to the agent. Whether these antibodies influence efficacy or adverse reactions is uncertain.
- Anti-TNF agents can induce antinuclear antibodies and other autoantibodies, and rarely, a lupuslike syndrome.
- Use of anti-TNF agents may worsen symptoms of congestive heart failure.
- Rarely, a demyelinating syndrome has been observed in patients using anti-TNF agents.

- Cytopenias and aplastic anemia have been reported in sporadic cases of patients on anti-TNF agents.

DISCONTINUATING THERAPY

- TNF antagonists should be discontinued if active infection, malignancy, or a serious adverse event develops.
- Because of their relatively long half-lives, the immunosuppressive effects of infliximab and adalimumab should be considered when evaluating and treating those patients who have recently discontinued use of the drugs.

SUMMARY

- The TNF antagonists are effective in reducing the signs and symptoms and inhibiting structural joint damage of patients with moderate or severe rheumatoid arthritis. They are of proven efficacy in controlling the signs and symptoms of ankylosing spondylitis and psoriatic arthritis.
- Lack of long-term safety data, need for parenteral administration, and high cost should be considered when tailoring this therapy to specific patients.

■ BISPHOSPHONATES: ETIDRONATE (DIDRONEL), PAMIDRONATE (AREDIA), ALENDRONATE (FOSAMAX), RISEDRONATE (ACTONEL), IBANDRONATE (BONIVA), & ZOLEDRONIC ACID (ZOMETA)

Dolores Shoback, MD

MECHANISM OF ACTION

- Bind to bone matrix at sites of active resorption and act as antiresorptive or anticatabolic agents.
- Inhibit bone resorption by two mechanisms: (1) all bisphosphonates enhance osteoclast apoptosis; and (2) aminobisphosphonates (eg, pamidronate, alendronate, risedronate, ibandronate, and zoledronic acid) interfere with osteoclast function by blocking the mevalonate pathway and the geranylgeranylation of low-molecular-weight guanyl nucleotide (GTP) binding proteins (GTPases). These proteins are involved in the formation of the ruffled border of the osteoclast—a

cellular structure that enables the osteoclast to adhere tightly to bone matrix and allow resorption.

- Adhere avidly to bone and remain there for days, months, and even years. In vivo this translates into a long half-life for biologic action.

PHARMACOKINETICS

- Bioavailability: Poorly absorbed from the gastrointestinal tract—less than 1% of the administered dose even on an empty stomach (www.pdr.net; *Arch Intern Med.* 2001;161:353).
- Metabolism: Not substantially metabolized in vivo.
- Half-life: Depends on duration of therapy, specific compound, total amount administered, and rate of bone remodeling.
- Clearance: Renally cleared without significant in vivo metabolism.

USES IN RHEUMATIC DISEASES

Postmenopausal Osteoporosis

The efficacy of the oral bisphosphonates alendronate (10 mg/d) and risedronate (5 mg/d) in treating postmenopausal osteoporosis and preventing vertebral and hip fractures has been confirmed in several randomized, double-blind, placebo-controlled trials (*N Engl J Med.* 1995;333:1437; *Lancet.* 1996;348:1535; *JAMA.* 1999;282:1344; *N Engl J Med.* 2001;344:333). Alendronate (5 mg/d) has also been approved for the prevention of postmenopausal bone loss (*N Engl J Med.* 1998;338:485; *Ann Intern Med.* 1998;128:253).

Alendronate and risedronate reduce the incidence of new vertebral fractures by 40–50%. Risedronate is effective against vertebral fractures over 5 years of study (*Bone.* 2003;32:120). Hip fractures are reduced by approximately 50% for alendronate, compared with placebo. Risedronate significantly reduces hip fractures in postmenopausal women aged 70–79 in whom osteoporosis was diagnosed by low bone mineral density measurements. Women aged 80 years or older, enrolled on the basis of clinical risk factors for fracture (eg, poor eyesight, history of smoking, and fall-related injury) did not experience a decrease in hip fracture risk after 3 years of risedronate therapy. Weekly therapy with alendronate (70 mg/wk) is comparable to daily dosing (10 mg/d) as assessed by biochemical markers of bone turnover and bone mineral density at the lumbar spine and hip (*Aging.* 2000;12:1).

The newest bisphosphonate approved in the U.S. for the treatment and prevention of osteoporosis, ibandronate, has been tested in several dosing schedules. Ibandronate is approved to treat postmenopausal osteoporosis in dosages of 150 mg/mo or 2 mg intravenously every 3 months. In randomized controlled trials of women with osteoporosis, ibandronate (2.5 mg/d) for 3 years was shown to reduce the risk of new vertebral fractures by 62% versus placebo (*J Bone Miner Res.* 2004;19:1241). Nonvertebral fractures were not significantly reduced. In a 1-year, non-inferiority trial in osteoporotic women, several doses of ibandronate were compared, and 2.5 mg daily and 150 mg monthly were found to have comparable effects on bone mineral density and biochemical markers of bone turnover (*J Bone Miner Res.* 2005;20:1315). Studies with intravenous dosing (1 versus 2 mg every 3 months) showed greater effects on bone mineral density and biochemical markers at the 2-mg dose, which is the approved dose (*Bone.* 2004;34:881). No increased renal toxicity was seen with this regimen.

Currently, the three oral bisphosphonates offer considerable flexibility in oral dosing (daily, weekly, or monthly), and ibandronate has the option of quarterly intravenous dosing.

Glucocorticoid-Induced Osteoporosis

Alendronate and risedronate have been approved in the U.S. for the treatment and prevention of glucocorticoid-induced bone loss in men and women. The double-blind, placebo-controlled, multicenter trials with these agents included patients with a variety of rheumatologic, gastrointestinal, pulmonary, and dermatologic conditions. Patients were receiving either initial glucocorticoid therapy (*N Engl J Med.* 1998;339:292; *Arthritis Rheum.* 1999;42:2309) or chronic maintenance therapy with glucocorticoids (*N Engl J Med.* 1998;339:292; *J Bone Miner Res.* 2000;15:1006). The dose of glucocorticoid administered to patients enrolled in these trials was 7.5 mg of prednisone equivalents per day or more. Therapy with bisphosphonate or placebo was for 12 months, and in one case was followed by a 12-month, open-label extension (*Arthritis Rheum.* 2001;44:202). Primary outcomes were changes in lumbar spine bone mineral density. Secondary outcomes were changes in proximal femur bone mineral density, vertebral fractures, and changes in biochemical markers of bone turnover. Therapy with either bisphosphonate significantly increased bone mineral density at the lumbar spine and femoral neck compared with placebo-treated persons. Although the incidence overall of vertebral fractures was low in these trials, there were fewer patients with vertebral fractures (0.7%) who had been treated with alendronate at any dose (5 or 10 mg/d for 24 months or 2.5 mg/d for 12 months followed by 10 mg/d for 12 months) compared with those patients treated with placebo for 24 months (6.8%) (*Arthritis Rheum.* 2001;44:202). Similarly, patients treated with risedronate (5 mg/d for 12 months) experienced a statistically significant reduction in new vertebral fractures of 70% compared with placebo-treated patients (*Calcif Tissue Int.* 2000;67:277).

Osteoporosis in Men

Alendronate (10 mg/d) has been approved for the treatment of low bone mass in men. This drug increases bone mineral density at the spine, femoral neck, and total body, decreasing the vertebral fracture incidence (*N Engl J Med.* 2000;343:604; *J Clin Endocrinol Metab.* 2001;86:5252; *Rheum Int.* 2004;24:110). Studies have confirmed the efficacy of risedronate (5 mg/d) in men with osteoporosis treated for 1 year (compared to controls treated with calcium and vitamin D supplements) (*Rheum Int.* 2005;7:1). Risedronate significantly increased bone mineral density after 1 year of therapy and produced a significant decrease (60%) in new vertebral fractures compared to the control groups. Risedronate is not specifically approved by FDA for the therapy of osteoporosis in men.

Paget Disease of Bone

Both oral alendronate and risedronate are approved for the treatment of this disease (*J Bone Miner Res.* 2001;16:1379). Risedronate improves both the elevated alkaline phosphatase and the pain due to Paget disease after 3 months of therapy (30 mg/d) (*Bone.* 1998;22:51; *J Clin Endocrinol Metab.* 1998;83:1906). In one series, risedronate was also shown to enhance radiologic healing of pagetic lesions (*Bone.* 2000;26:263). In a randomized, double-blind trial comparing risedronate (30 mg/d for 2 months) to etidronate (400 mg/d for 6 months), a higher percentage of patients normalized their alkaline phosphatase values on risedronate (73%) versus etidronate (15%). The maintenance of a normal alkaline phosphatase at 6 months after therapy was more common in patients treated with risedronate (77%) versus etidronate (15%). Patients on risedronate were also noted to have greater reduction in skeletal pain. Alendronate has also been successfully used to treat Paget disease. In a randomized, double-blind trial comparing alendronate (40 mg/d for 6 months) with placebo, there was a mean decline in alkaline phosphatase levels of 73%, which was markedly greater than placebo-treated patients who experienced no significant change in this parameter (*Am J Med.* 1996;171:341). In this same study, approximately 50% of patients showed a normalization of alkaline phosphatase levels and a radiologically documented improvement in their bone lesions. In a double-blind, randomized trial comparing alendronate (40 mg/d) with etidronate (400 mg/d) for 6 months, alendronate was shown to be superior. Alkaline phosphatase activity decreased to a greater extent (by 79% with alendronate compared with 44% with etidronate) (*J Clin Endocrinol Metab.* 1996;81:961). In addition, alendronate was able to normalize alkaline phosphatase activity in 63% of patients, which was significantly greater than the efficacy of etidronate—only 17% of patients normalized this parameter with 6 months of therapy.

OTHER USES

Bisphosphonates have been successfully used in the prevention of skeletal complications (bone pain, pathologic fractures, spinal cord compression, and hypercalcemia) in patients with solid tumors and multiple myeloma (pamidronate: *J Clin Oncol.* 1998;16:593; zoledronic acid: *Cancer.* 2001;91:1191; *Cancer Pract.* 2002;10:219). Although skeletal-related complications are reduced with this therapy in multiple myeloma, no survival advantage over placebo has been observed (*J Clin Oncol.* 2002;20:719).

Intravenous bisphosphonates are the treatment of choice for hypercalcemia of malignancy (pamidronate: *Am J Med.* 1993;95:297; zoledronic acid: *J Clin Oncol.* 2001;19:558).

DOSING REGIMEN

- Alendronate: 70 mg orally once weekly for osteoporosis (*J Bone Miner Res.* 2002;17:1998). Weekly alendronate (35 mg/wk) has also been approved for the prevention of postmenopausal bone loss (*J Bone Miner Res.* 2002;17:1998).
- Risedronate: 35 mg orally once weekly for osteoporosis (*Calcif Tissue Int.* 2002;71:103).
- Ibandronate: 150 mg orally once monthly (*J Bone Miner Res.* 2005;20:1315) or 2 mg intravenously every 3 months (*Bone.* 2004;34:881) for osteoporosis.
- Oral bisphosphonates are best absorbed on an empty stomach, 30–60 minutes before breakfast, with 8 oz of water and while remaining upright.

INITIATING THERAPY

- Weekly oral alendronate, risedronate, or ibandronate are used with adequate daily calcium and vitamin D supplementation to treat osteoporosis. Therapy can be initiated on the basis of bone mineral density measurements or the history of fragility fractures in a patient at high risk for bone loss.

MONITORING THERAPY

- The efficacy of bisphosphonate therapy to increase bone mineral density can be monitored on an annual or semiannual basis in patients with osteoporosis.
- A reduction in bone resorption can also be assessed by measuring biochemical markers of bone turnover (eg, urinary excretion of or serum levels of N-telopeptide, osteocalcin, or bone-specific alkaline phosphatase).

Urinary measurements of bone markers are particularly subject to variation.

- In treating Paget disease of bone, regular monitoring of alkaline phosphatase is advised along with periodic skeletal radiologic evaluation to assess the response to therapy.

SPECIAL PRECAUTIONS

- Because bisphosphonates have a long half-life in bone and significantly reduce skeletal remodeling, their use is strongly discouraged in growing children (except in very unusual circumstances) and in women of childbearing age.
- Bisphosphonates should be used with great care, if at all, in patients with renal insufficiency.

COMPLICATIONS

- Daily, long-term alendronate and risedronate therapy for glucocorticoid-induced or postmenopausal osteoporosis may cause gastrointestinal irritation, especially abdominal pain, and less commonly, esophagitis, ulceration, and bleeding (*N Engl J Med.* 1996;335:1016). Weekly administration of both alendronate and risedronate or monthly therapy with ibandronate has obviated most concerns regarding gastrointestinal adverse events. Additional minor adverse events have included headache, nausea, and body pain, which have generally been mild.
- Patients receiving intensive, higher-dose daily oral bisphosphonates (alendronate and risedronate) for Paget disease of bone should be closely monitored for upper gastrointestinal adverse events.
- Acute phase reactions, characterized by joint pains, myalgias, and fever within 24–48 hours of the infusion, can develop in patients receiving intravenous aminobisphosphonates (pamidronate, ibandronate, and zoledronic acid). Such reactions occur in <10% of patients receiving these therapies and are self-limited.
- Patients with mild renal insufficiency (serum creatinine <2.5 mg/dL) do not need doses of bisphosphonate adjusted for renal function. Long-term oral bisphosphonates are not recommended in patients with serum creatinine >2.5 mg/dL.
- Alendronate, risedronate, and ibandronate are not recommended for use in patients with renal insufficiency (creatinine clearances <30 or 35 mL/min) (www.pdr.net).
- Intravenous zoledronic acid (4 mg infused over 15 minutes) has the potential for inducing renal failure, and patients with significant renal insufficiency (serum creatinine ≥3.0 mg/dL) should not receive this medica-

tion. Renal function should be assessed before each dose of intravenous bisphosphonate.
- Preexisting renal dysfunction, multiple cycles of zoledronic acid, and concurrent use of other nephrotoxic agents enhance the risk of further renal functional deterioration with intravenous bisphosphonates. In cases in whom baseline creatinine clearance is between 30 and 60 mL/min, the recommended dose of zoledronic acid should be decreased accordingly (www.pdr.net).
- Vitamin D deficiency should be excluded prior to the administration of intravenous bisphosphonates in particular since symptomatic hypocalcemia has been reported in such individuals after these agents.
- Although oral bisphosphonates are not contraindicated for use with nonsteroidal anti-inflammatory agents, the potential for increased upper gastrointestinal adverse effects with such a combination suggests that careful clinical monitoring is indicated.
- Second- and third-generation bisphosphonates (alendronate, risedronate, and ibandronate) used in established treatment regimens for osteoporosis have not been associated with the development of osteomalacia by bone biopsy studies. Older first-generation bisphosphonates (eg, etidronate), when used in high doses for conditions like Paget disease, must be used with care. There is the potential for the accumulation of such agents in bone over time with the subsequent induction of a mineralization defect, low bone turnover, and frank osteomalacia (*J Clin Endocrinol Metab.* 1996;81:961).

LONG-TERM CONCERNS

- It is unclear how long women with ongoing postmenopausal bone loss or men with idiopathic or hypogonadism-induced osteoporosis should be treated. Therapy for years with oral alendronate, risedronate, or ibandronate leads to a large skeletal reservoir of these drugs that may have long-term effects—yet unknown—on the repair of microdamage to the skeleton. Thus far, excessive clinical fracture risk with 10 or 7 years of therapy with alendronate or risedronate, respectively, has not been observed (*J Clin Endocrinol Metab.* 2000;85:3109; *Calcif Tiss Int.* 2003;72:402; *Calcif Tiss Int.* 2004;75:469; *N Engl J Med.* 2004;350:1189).
- An uncommon but worrisome complication of therapy with intravenous (zoledronic acid and pamidronate) and oral (alendronate) therapy is osteonecrosis of the jaw. In a series of 119 patients with this complication, there were 48, 32, 36, and 3 cases in patients who had taken zoledronic acid, pamidronate, pamidronate followed by zoledronic acid, and alendronate, respectively

(*J Oral Maxillofac Surg.* 2005;63:1567). In this series, 97.5% of patients had an underlying malignancy. Other comorbid conditions that predispose to this disabling complication are ongoing dental procedures (eg, tooth extraction), preexisting dental conditions, and other therapies such as chemotherapy, radiation, and glucocorticoids. Patients who will be starting long-term therapy with potent intravenous bisphosphonates should be counseled regarding this potential complication and treated for any active dental or periodontal problem prior to bisphosphonate therapy. Invasive dental procedures should be avoided while on intravenous bisphosphonate treatment if possible.

KEY POINTS

- Bisphosphonates are the most bone-selective agents currently available for the treatment of a variety of metabolic bone diseases including osteoporosis, Paget disease, and the skeletal complications of malignancy. They demonstrate excellent therapeutic efficacy and can be used in both oral and intravenous formulations depending on the disease state.

■ PARATHYROID HORMONE (1–34): TERIPARATIDE (FORTEO)

Dolores Shoback, MD

MECHANISM OF ACTION

- Relatively low doses activate parathyroid hormone receptors in bone to produce anabolic effects that stimulate new bone formation as opposed to the catabolic effects of parathyroid hormone on bone to increase resorption

PHARMACOKINETICS

- Bioavailabililty: Administered in daily subcutaneous injections and rapidly absorbed with a peak in serum levels within 30 minutes of injection with ~95% bioavailability of the administered dose. By 3 hours after injection, serum levels of peptide are undetectable.
- Metabolism and clearance: No studies have been done with teriparatide, but PTH (1–84) is metabolized by hepatic and extrahepatic mechanisms and then renally cleared.
- Half-life: After subcutaneous injection ~1 hour

USES IN RHEUMATIC DISEASES

Postmenopausal Osteoporosis

The anabolic PTH-derived peptide teriparatide is administered as a subcutaneous injection of 20 μg daily. In a large randomized, controlled trial in women with osteoporosis, this dose substantially increased lumbar spine (9.7%) and femoral neck (2.8%) bone mineral density after 19 months of therapy (*N Engl J Med.* 2001;344:1434). New vertebral fractures were reduced by 65%, while nonvertebral fractures were decreased 53%. Teriparatide is indicated for severe osteoporosis with or without fractures and is approved for a maximum of 24 months of use.

Osteoporosis in Men

Teriparatide is approved for the treatment of male osteoporosis. This agent increases bone mineral density at the spine (5.9%) and femoral neck (1.5%) after 10 months of therapy, compared to placebo (*J Bone Miner Res.* 2003;18:9).

DOSING REGIMEN

- Teriparatide: 20 μg subcutaneously each day for a maximum of 2 years

INITIATING THERAPY

- Teriparatide is indicated for treating men and women with osteoporosis at high risk for fracture. This includes patients with a history of prior fractures or with multiple risk factors or who have failed other therapies.
- In men or women with severe osteoporosis, teriparatide can be started instead of bisphosphonate therapy and is then followed with chronic antiresorptive therapy with a bisphosphonate.

SPECIAL PRECAUTIONS

- Because preclinical testing in rats showed an induction of osteosarcoma with high daily doses of teriparatide, the agent carries an FDA black box warning. It is contraindicated in several groups of patients including: children with open epiphyses, patients with bone metastases, patients with Paget disease of bone, individuals with prior skeletal radiation, and subjects with unexplained elevation of the alkaline phosphatase level.

COMPLICATIONS

- Teriparatide at the recommended dose is unlikely to cause persistent hypercalcemia. Approximately 11% of women and 6% of men on teriparatide had at least one serum calcium value over 10.6 mg/dL (*N Engl J Med.* 2001;344:1434) but this was self-limited. Persistent elevations in serum calcium in teriparatide-treated patients generally can be managed with a dose reduction in calcium and/or vitamin D. No increased risk of renal stones or hypercalciuria (urinary calcium >300 mg/d) was seen. Minor adverse effects included headache, nausea, and leg cramps.

KEY POINTS

- Teriparatide is the only approved anabolic therapy for osteoporosis and induces the largest changes in bone mineral density among the approved therapies for this disease.

Index

Note: Page numbers followed by a *t* indicate tables; numbers followed by an *f* indicate figures.